Biobehavioral Approaches to Pain

T0178381

Rhonda J. Moore
Editor

Biobehavioral Approaches to Pain

Foreword by Judith A. Paice

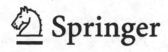

Editor
Rhonda J. Moore
Bethesda, MD
USA
moorer2001uk@yahoo.co.uk

ISBN: 978-1-4419-2684-5   e-ISBN: 978-0-387-78323-9
DOI 10.1007/978-0-387-78323-9

springer.com

It has been said that a person reaches in three directions: Inward, to oneself, up to G-d, and out to others. The miracle of life is that in truly reaching in any one direction, one embraces all three. (Rebbe Nachman of Breslov)

This book is dedicated first and foremost to G-d, the most high for his love, guidance, and many blessings. It is also dedicated to the memory of my father, friend and colleague R. Calvin Wilson (11/26/1926–06/10/ 2006). He was a man that had a profound and positive impact on my life, my thinking, and on my desire to embrace this miracle called life.

I will love and miss you always. Know you are never forgotten, and may you rest in peace.

Preface

Who except the Gods can live time through forever without any pain.

Aeschylus (BC 525–456)

Hunger, love, pain, fear are some of the inner forces which rule the individual's instinct for self-preservation.

Albert Einstein (1879–1955)

Two thousand years ago St. Paul called his painful affliction "the thorn in the flesh" and a "messenger from Satan" which only God could remove. St. Augustine echoed this sentiment stating, "the greatest evil is physical pain." The concept of pain as punishment for one's sins lasted for centuries and evolved into a "warning" of impending doom. Historically, attempts at defining and quantifying pain have been akin to trying to control and corral a herd of feral housecats.

The current definition of pain by the International Association for the Study of Pain (IASP) as, "an unpleasant sensory and emotional experience associated with actual or potential tissue damage, or described in terms of such damage" is certainly inadequate. Advances in neuroscientific and biobehavioral aspects of pain, as demonstrated in this volume, promise to help clarify the multifaceted phenomenon of pain as more than simply an unpleasant sensory assault. This will afford a more comprehensive definition.

We now know that the velocity of neuronal transmission leading to the perception of nociceptive stimuli through supraspinal brain centers may be inconstant. Variations in nerve conductivity, that was once thought to be relatively fixed, along with synaptic neurochemical alterations may lead to a delayed or altered recognition of pain. Responses to painful stimuli, at times reflexive though primarily subjective, are the most difficult to predict and especially to measure. Emblematic of this is The Facial Action Coding System (FACS), based on pain reactions such as grimacing, nasolabial fold deepening, and brow furrowing.. FACS is one of several schemes attempting to measure degrees of pain. Psychometric and psychosocial evaluations are also used, with varying degrees of success, in identifying the ramifications of an individual's unique responses to pain.

Because of the Gestalt of cultural, behavioral, emotional, and spiritual components in painful ideation, the best portrayals of pain, for millennia, have been through poetry, philosophy, art, and music. Individual examination of each of the integral entities within neuroscience, though exciting and promising, cannot alone explain the wondrous complexity and plasticity of the human nervous system and man's "experience" with pain.

The microanatomy of pain mechanisms, once thought to be fully elucidated, is in a constant state of flux. The immune–glial cell contribution to neuropathic pain is one of a constellation of continually evolving discoveries in neuroscience. Gene research and therapies have opened a vast frontier for understanding how the nervous system works. Consider the discovery of the gene responsible for the neurochemical defect in patients with Congenital Insensitivity to Pain. Advances in PET and SPECT scanning, fMRI, Electroencephalography, Deep Brain Stimulation, and MR spectroscopy, along with technical advances in neurochemistry and molecular neurobiology, should expand our ability to correlate biobehavioral aspects of pain to the hard neurosciences exponentially.

In this volume, Dr Rhonda Moore has established a holistic template for understanding the complex nature of pain. The neuroanatomy and neurophysiology of nociceptive reception and perception are fundamental and evolving. Along with this, crucial biobehavioral elements responsible for an individual's response to pain must be integrated in any reasonable definition. These include, but are not limited to, gender, cultural, emotional, genetic, societal and spiritual factors. To honestly evaluate an individual's painful experience, inclusive of neuroscience, one must consider it a "perfect storm" of all that is implicit in understanding human behavior. In the selection of the contributors' and subject matter for this book, Dr. Moore has accomplished this. This multidimensional approach in defining pain in all of its ramifications will have a profound impact in clinical medicine and beyond.

Houston, TX   Richard M. Hirshberg

Forward

Pain finds its way everywhere, into my vision, my feelings,
my sense of judgment; it's an infiltration...
Alphonse Daudet, *In the Land of Pain*, 1840–1897

Pain is all encompassing. To the person suffering from it, pain infiltrates all aspects of the individual's life. Pain is indiscriminate; it affects everyone at some time during their life, regardless of age, gender, race, or geography. For those unfortunate individuals who experience chronic, persistent pain, their lives are forever changed.

There is much that we can do to address the needs of those in pain. To do so effectively, scientists, clinicians, and policy experts must be informed regarding a wide range of topics. In the past decades, this has become incredibly overwhelming. The scope of our knowledge base in pain has exploded, ranging from understanding the basic mechanisms of pain at a molecular level to discerning the larger role of biological, environmental, emotional and psychosocial processes that affect the individual, and beyond, to realizing the societal implications of pain and its treatment. Because the scope is so broad, multidisciplinary perspectives are critical. This is true in the treatment of pain, as well as in our understanding of this complex phenomenon.

This comprehensive text addresses the rapidly expanding scope of the field of pain by providing a forum for experts from many disciplines to share their wisdom on a variety of topics. From addressing the larger impact of pain, to describing specific syndromes and special populations, this text takes a multidisciplinary and biobehavioral approach throughout each chapter. The authors are internationally recognized experts representing an authoritative and global viewpoint. Furthermore, the authors embody many specialties, from the basic sciences to psychology, medicine, philosophy, ethics and public policy, providing the reader a deeper understanding of the many facets of pain.

Biobehavioral Approaches to Pain has been expertly edited by Rhonda J. Moore, PhD, who as a medical anthropologist, is uniquely qualified to explore this topic from a universal perspective. Specialists in pain will find this rich perspective refreshing. Those new to the field will discover an extraordinary synopsis of the complexity of this fascinating syndrome. Ultimately, the field will benefit from this text as scientists, policy analysts, and clinicians use this information to further enrich our understanding as we explore new mechanisms and treatments. Finally, patients will benefit as this new information is translated into safe and effective therapies provided by multidisciplinary teams of informed clinicians.

Chicago, IL   Judith A. Paice

Acknowledgements

> If you concentrate on finding whatever is good in every situation, you will discover that your life will suddenly be filled with gratitude, a feeling that nurtures the soul.
> ~ Rabbi Harold Kushner ~

> "No duty is more urgent than that of returning thanks."
> ~ Unknown ~

The beginning and completion of an edited volume is never an individual endeavor. Others always assist along the way. At this time I thank those individuals who were supportive of this edited volume. I begin by thanking my collaborators for their enthusiasm, commitment and support of this project. I could not have completed this volume without your fine insight and the wisdom of your words. I thank Bill Tucker, Khristine Queja, James Russo of the New York editorial offices of the Springer Publishing house and Sharmila Krishnamurthy (Project Manager at Integra India) on their assistance with the publication of this edited volume. Their encouragement, kindness, support and patience made this dream a reality.

I am also indebted to the encouraging words and the kindness of my colleagues, friends and family. I thank Kirt Vener, PhD, Ken Bielat, PhD, Bob Kruth, Clara Murphy, and C. Michael Kerwin, PhD, MPH, Rosalind Naimke, BS and Ricardo Rawle, BS (all of the Special Review and Logistics Branch at the National Cancer Institute in Rockville, MD) for their support of this intellectual endeavor.

I trained as a cultural and medical anthropologist and the works of David Spiegel, MD (Stanford Medical School), Robert Dantzer (PhD) (University of Illinois), Steve Coles, PhD (UCLA), Linda R. Watkins, PhD (University of Colorado), Elaine Scarry, PhD (Harvard University), Howard Spiro, MD (Yale School of Medicine), Polly Matzinger, PhD (National Institute of Allergy and Infectious Diseases (NIAID), NIH), Viktor Emil Frankl, M.D., Ph.D. (Professor of Neurology and Psychiatry at the University of Vienna, Austria, Deceased), Arthur Frank (University of Calgary), Arthur Kleinman, MD (Harvard Medical School) and David Morris, PhD (University of Virginia) have all served as inspiration for my ideas and musings on this subject matter even as I take full responsibility for what has been written. I thank Steve Coles, PhD (UCLA) for hiskind words, and support of my ideas. It has meant so much more than I can say. I also thank Richard Hirshberg, MD (Houston, TX), who is always unfailing in his sincerity, support, friendship, kindness, generosity and inspiring conversations. I thank Judy Paice, PhD (Northwestern) for her keen intellect and enthusiasm. I thank John Adler, MD (Stanford Medical School) for his great sense of humor, great conversations and intellectual encouragement. I thank my mum, Juanita Moore, and all my friends, including SKYY, Dorota Doherty, PhD (Perth, Australia), Gloria Valentine (The Hoover Institution at Stanford University), Ralph Zinner, MD (The University of Texas MD Anderson Cancer Center, Houston, TX), Jean Wong, RN (Bethesda, MD), Ines Ruiz, MBA, Wilfredo Bermudez, RN, Dianne M. Gray, (Office of Acquisitions, Prevention, Control and Population Sciences Branch, National Cancer Institute, NIH) and my very best friend in the whole world, Lee O. Carter, Jr., MS (Houston, Texas). I am a better person because of you all, and I thank each of you for your friendship, kindness, and care all these years.

Rockville, MD   Rhonda J. Moore

Contents

Contributors

Elie D. Al-Chaer, MS, PhD, JD is Associate Professor of Pediatrics, Medicine, Neurobiology and Developmental Sciences at the University of Arkansas for Medical Sciences. His research explores the neural mechanisms associated with pain symptoms refractory to conventional treatments. In particular, his work focuses on defining the neurogenic components of functional gastrointestinal disorders, and exploring the interactive dynamics of gender, stress and sensorimotor pathways, and their roles in pain processing.

Fabrizio Benedetti, MD is Professor of Physiology and Neuroscience at the University of Turin Medical School and at the National Institute of Neuroscience in Italy. His current scientific interests are the placebo effect across diseases, pain in dementia, and intraoperative neurophysiology for mapping the human brain.

Giovanni Cucchiaro, MD is Assistant Professor in the Department of Anesthesiology and Critical Care Medicine, at The Children's Hospital in Philadelphia and University of Pennsylvania Medical School. His research interests include chronic pain management in children, regional anesthesia and research on central pathways of pain transmission.

Barry Eliot Cole, M.D., MPA is Executive Director, American Society of Pain Educators, a non-profit professional organization dedicated to training healthcare professionals to become Credentialed Pain Educators (CPEs). His research interests include chronic pain management and pain education.

Doris K. Cope, MD is Board Certified in both Anesthesiology and Pain Medicine. She has served as a Board Examiner in both fields. She is Professor and Vice Chair for Pain Medicine, Department of Anesthesiology, and Director of the UPMC Pain Medicine Division at the University of Pittsburgh School of Medicine. A noted authority on the history of anesthesiology, Dr. Cope is also interested in chronic pain management including the uses of gene therapies for the treatment of chronic pain conditions.

Pieter U. Dijkstra PT, MT, PhD Clinical Epidemiologist is an Associate Professor and a researcher with the Center for Rehabilitation, the Northern

Center for Health Care Research, and the Department of Oral and Maxillofacial Surgery at the University Medical Center Groningen, University of Groningen, in the Netherlands. His research interests include rehabilitation medicine and pain research.

Aram Dobalian, PhD, MPH, JD is Assistant Professor in the Department of Health Services at the UCLA School of Public Health and a Research Health Scientist with the HSR&D Center of Excellence for the Study of Healthcare Provider Behavior at the VA Greater Los Angeles Healthcare System. His research interests include health services research in the context of chronic illness, bioterrorism, hurricanes, and other natural and human-caused disasters.

Sydney M. Dy, MD, MSc is an Assistant Professor at the Health Services Research Center, Department of Health Policy and Management, Johns Hopkins Bloomberg School of Public Health; and in the Departments of Medicine and Oncology, Johns Hopkins School of Medicine. Her research interests include improving quality, use of technology, and access to care for patients facing serious and terminal illnesses; quality of health care; and inner-city health care.

Jan H.B. Geertzen, MD, PhD is a Physiatrist and Professor in Rehabilitation Medicine at the Center for Rehabilitation and the Graduate School for Health Research, University Medical Centre Groningen, University of Groningen, in the Netherlands. His research interests include amputation and prosthetics, and specific pain syndromes such as phantom pain and Complex Regional Pain Syndromes.

James Hallenbeck, MD is Assistant Professor of Medicine at the Stanford University Medical School. His clinical research interests include hospice and palliative care with emphases on physician education, cultural aspects of end-of-life care, and healthcare system issues.

Howard A. Heit, MD, FACP, FASAM is board certified in internal medicine and gastroenterology. He is also certified in addiction medicine and as a medical review officer (MRO) by the American Society of Addiction Medicine. Dr. Heit was the recipient of the 2007 Marie Nyswander Award from the International Association for Pain and Chemical Dependency. Dr. Heit's publications are on the interface of pain and addiction, patient-centered urine drug testing and federal regulations for prescribing controlled substances.

Richard Hirshberg, MD (retired) was Chief of Neurosurgery at the St. Joseph's Hospital in Houston, TX. He also completed groundbreaking clinical work that led to the identification of a pathway in the posterior funiculus in the dorsal column that signals visceral pain.

Francis J. Keefe, PhD is Professor of Psychiatry and Behavioral Sciences and Director of the Pain Prevention and Treatment Research Program at Duke

University. His major research centers on how individuals copes with disease-related pain. He has published over 200 papers on this topic, is the Psychology Section Editor for the journal, *Pain*, and serves on scientific advisory panels dealing with chronic pain. His current research include the effects of mammography pain on sustained mammography adherence in breast cancer survivors, teaching couples how to better communicate about pain, and partner-assisted pain coping skills training for patients having advanced cancer.

Ed Keogh, PhD is Senior Lecturer in the Department of Psychology and Centre for Pain Research, both at the University of Bath in the United Kingdom. His main research interest is in sex differences in pain, with a focus on mechanisms that might help explain why such differences exist. Other interests include the role of psychological factors in pain, such as emotions, cognition and coping, as well as a general interest in cognitive-behavioral approaches to pain management.

William R. Lariviere, PhD Dr. Lariviere received his training in the laboratories of Ronald Melzack and Jeffrey Mogil, currently at McGill University in Montréal, Québec, Canada. His postdoctoral work, funded provincially (FCAR fellowship of Québec) and nationally (NSERC of Canada), investigates the fundamental genetic relationships among animal models of pain and hypersensitivity widely used in basic pain research, how they relate to each other and to clinical pain states. He has spoken at several national and international meetings and continues to contribute significantly with publications in leading journals in the field. Is Assistant Professor of Anesthesiology at the University of Pittsburgh School of Medicine. His research interests include the genetics of variability in pain and analgesia, stress and pain interactions, and the use of gene therapies for the treatment of chronic pain.

Arthur G. Lipman, PharmD, FASHP is University Professor, Department of Pharmacotherapy, College of Pharmacy; Adjunct Professor Anesthesiology, School of Medicine; and Director of Clinical Pharmacology, Pain Management Center, University Health Care at the University of Utah Health Sciences Center. He is editor of the Journal of Pain & Palliative Care Pharmacotherapy and an editor in the Pain Palliative and Supportive Care Collaborative Review Group of the international Cochrane Collaboration on Evidence-based Medicine. His research focuses on pain and palliative care pharmacotherapy.

Alexander J. MacGregor, MD is Professor of Medicine at the University of Norwich (UK), and an honorary consultant to the Twin & Genetic Epidemiology Unit, St Thomas' Campus, King's College London. St Thomas' has the UK's largest database of twins, and is the most detailed cohort of adult twins in the world with hundreds of measurements for each twin. Twin studies offer features that uniquely enhance our ability to localize genes and understand their function. His research explores the heritability of pain in humans.

Patrick Mansky, MD is Director of the Integrative Medicine Consult Service and Clinical Investigator in the Oncology Program of the National Center for Complementary and Alternative Medicine (NCCAM) at the National Institutes of Health (NIH). He is trained in medical and pediatric oncology. His research interests include the role of complementary and alternative medicine for the management of cancer and cancer related symptoms.

Dagfin Matre, PhD is a research scientist in the Department of Occupational Musculoskeletal Disorders, National Institute of Occupational Health in Oslo, Norway. His research interests include pain modulation, chronic pain development and the use of imaging technologies to better understand pain.

Bill McCarberg, MD practices family medicine at Kaiser Permanente in San Diego and is an assistant clinical professor (voluntary) for the University of California, San Diego. He is also president of the Western Pain Society, and has served on the board of directors of the American Pain Society from 2000 to 2003, and chairs several committees for various pain-related organizations, including the American Academy of Pain Medicine, the American Pain Society, and the National Institutes of Health. His research interests include chronic pain management and pain in the older person.

Lance M. McCracken, PhD is Consultant Clinical Psychologist and Clinical Lead of the Pain Management Unit, Royal National Hospital for Rheumatic Diseases at the University of Bath in the United Kingdom. His research interests include behavioral, cognitive, and social influences on disability and suffering, psychological treatment methods and mechanisms, and medication use.

Shana McDaniel, MD is a practicing anesthesiologist in San Diego, California. She received her medical education at the University of Vermont College of Medicine. She completed an anesthesiology residency and palliative medicine fellowship at the Stanford School of Medicine in Palo Alto, California.

Rhonda J. Moore, PhD is at the National Cancer Institute at the National Institutes of Health in Rockville, MD. Trained as a medical anthropologist, her research interests include clinical pain management, pharmacology, clinical trials and cancer related pain and suffering.

Judith Paice, PhD is Professor of Research in the Division of Hematology/Oncology at the Northwestern University Medical School. Her clinical work is in the management of cancer-related pain. Her current research is on the study of chemotherapy-induced peripheral neuropathy associated with paclitaxel.

Antonella Pollo, MD is Assistant Professor in the Department of Neuroscience, University of Turin Medical School and the National Institute of Neuroscience, Turin, Italy. Her current scientific interests are the placebo and nocebo effect across diseases and physiological conditions and pain in dementia.

Laura Porter, PhD is Assistant Professor of Psychiatry and Behavioral Sciences at Duke University. She is also a licensed psychologist whose research focuses on interventions to help patients and their family members adjust to the symptoms and psychological demands associated with cancer and other chronic illnesses.

Caroline M. Reavley, MBBS, FRCA is a consultant in Anaesthesia at Norfolk and Norwich University Hospitals NHS Foundation Trust. Her interests include Cardiothoracics, Pain Research and Anaesthesia.

Ben A. Rich, JD, PhD is Professor and School of Medicine Alumni Association Endowed Chair of Bioethics at the UC Davis School of Medicine. He also currently holds joint academic appointments in the Departments of Internal Medicine and Anesthesiology and Pain Medicine. His research interests include informed consent, advance directives, pain management, and end-of-life care.

Rebecca L. Robinson, MS is a health outcomes researcher with the Eli Lilly and Company. Her interests include pharmacoeconomics studies of pain related syndromes and pain management.

Tamara J. Somers, PhD is a postdoctoral fellow at Duke University in the Psychiatry and Behavioral Sciences Department. Trained as a clinical psychologist, her research interests focus on promoting health behaviors to increase quality of life in individuals with disease or at risk of disease development.

Howard M. Spiro, MD is currently Professor Emeritus of Medicine at Yale University School of Medicine and is the former head of the Gastroenterology section and Program for Humanities in Medicine at Yale. He is also author of Clinical Gastroenterology McGraw-Hill Health Professions Division (June 1, 1995), Empathy and the Practice of Medicine (Yale University Press, 1993), The Power of Hope (Yale University Press, 2004), The Optimist: Meditations on Medicine (Science and Medicine, 2004), Doctors, Patients and Placebos (Yale University Press, 1988), Facing Death: Where Culture, Religion, and Medicine Meet (Yale University Press, 1988), and The Yale Guide to Careers in Medicine and the Health Professions: Pathways to Medicine in the 21st Century (The Institution for Social and Policy St) (Yale University Press, 2003). His research interests include clinical medicine, placebo and nocebo research, clinician-patient communication, and the role of narrative and medicine.

Jamie M. Stagl, BA obtained her underqraduate degree in psychology at American University. Since June 2007, she has been working as a fellow in the NIH Postbaccalaureate Intramural Research Training Award (IRTA) program in NCCAM's Oncology Program in the Division of Intramural

Research in clinical research data management. Her research areas of interest include mind-body approaches in Psychooncology.

Michele Sterling, PhD MPhty Bphty is Associate Director, Centre for National Research on Disability and Rehabilitation Medicine (CONROD) and Director of the Rehabilitation (Medical and Allied Health) Research Program (CONRD) at the University of Queensland in Australia. She is also a Senior Lecturer in the Division of Physiotherapy, School of Health and Rehabilitation Sciences. Her research interests include the physical and psychological factors underlying whiplash associated disorders; the prediction of outcome following whiplash injury, improving the timing and nature of interventions for whiplash and neck pain and the clinical translation of research findings to clinical practice.

Catherine M. Stoney, PhD is at the National Center for Complementary and Alternative Medicine at the National Institutes of Health (NCCAM-NIH). Her research interests include affective disorders, mind-body medicine, clinical and neurobiological aspects of the placebo effect, and clinical trial design and methodology.

Jennie C. I. Tsao, PhD is Associate Professor in the UCLA Pediatric Pain Program, Department of Pediatrics, at the David Geffen School of Medicine at UCLA. Her research interests center on the relationships among pain, anxiety, drug use and health outcomes, including pain-related functioning and utilization of conventional and alternative medical care.

Tuan Diep Tran, MD, PhD is an Assistant Professor with University of Medicine and Pharmacy at the Ho Chi Minh City in Vietnam. His research interests include pain management and the uses of imaging techniques such as magnetoencephalography and functional MRI for the measurement of acute and chronic pain.

Thomas R. Vetter, MD, MPH is Director of Pain Treatment and Associate Professor of Anesthesiology at the University Of Alabama School Of Medicine. He is also Associate Professor of Health Policy and Organization at the University of Alabama at Birmingham School of Public Health. His research interests include patient-reported outcomes, in particular health-related quality of life, and the application of economic evaluation methods in the adult and pediatric acute and chronic pain management arenas. He also has an interest in healthcare disparities with regards to access to chronic pain treatment.

Kevin K. Vowles, PhD is a Clinical Psychologist in the Pain Management Unit, Royal National Hospital for Rheumatic Diseases at the University of Bath in the United Kingdom. His research interests include behavioral, cognitive, and social influences on disability and suffering, and psychological approaches to treating pain.

Lonnie K. Zeltzer, MD is Professor of Pediatrics, Anesthesiology, Psychiatry and Biobehavioral Sciences and Director, UCLA Pediatric Pain Program at the UCLA Mattel Children's Hospital. Her research interests include biopsychosocial models of pain, the experience of chronic pain in pediatric populations, laboratory models of acute pain in children, and complementary/alternative (CAM) approaches to pain management.

Dawn Wallerstedt, MSN, CRNP is a Research Nurse Practitioner at NIH NCAAM. Since 2002, she has been working with Dr. Patrick Mansky, conducting clinical Research Studies using CAM Modalities in people with cancer and cancer Survivors. Her research areas of interest include botanical medicine and mind-body approaches, particularly in the medical applications of hypnotherapy.

Introduction

"Being ill like this combines shock – this time I will die – with a pain and agony that are unfamiliar, that wrench me out of myself. "
From Harold Brodkey's This Wild Darkness: The Story of my Death. Owl Books, 1997

"Nothing begins, and nothing ends, That is not paid with moan. For we are born in other's pain, And perish in our own."
From Daisy by Frances Thompson (1859–1907)

"Everyone who is born holds dual citizenship, in the kingdom of the well and in the kingdom of the sick. Although we all prefer to use only the good passport, sooner or later each of us is obliged, at least for a spell, to identify ourselves as citizens of that other place."
From Susan Sontag's Illness as Metaphor. Farrar Straus and Giroux, 1988

Pain has long been regarded as an unpleasant sensory consequence of neuronal activity in specific nociceptive pathways that is triggered by noxious stimuli, inflammation, or damage to the nervous system activity.[1–9] Yet classic models of disease and pain mechanisms do not adequately explain the commonly observed discrepancies between the extent of the pathology and levels of reported pain. They also fail to adequately describe the impact of these factors on the experience of illness and subsequent disability.[3–7] For instance, pain is not only a sensory event. It is also a significant cause of suffering and even existential questioning, as pain is also subjective, thus treatment for many chronic pain syndromes is an inexact science.[8–9]

Recent studies over the past decade have begun to explore a biobehavioral approach, one that considers the interactive role of biological, environmental, cultural, emotional and psychosocial processes that affect the development and course of illness and disease.[6–7] Illness here is defined as the subjective experience of a disease or disorder. In contrast, disease is defined as an objective biological event involving the disruption of specific body structures, or organ systems.[6,10–14] Similarly, pain is a subjective experience that results from the transduction, transmission or modulation of sensory information. This physiologic input is filtered via the individual's socio-cultural framework, learning and experience, genetic, history, affective or emotional states, as well as, past and current psychological status.

Given these findings, it is increasingly clear that pain is a biobehavioral experience. Pain is multi-factorial and multidimensional, encompassing socio-cultural, psychologic, spiritual (existential), emotional and physiologic components. Long term chronic pain also sets the stage for the emergence of a complex set of physiologic, mental, emotional, and psychosocial changes that are an integral part of the chronic pain problem and add greatly to the burden of the patient who is in pain. Chronic pain is also associated with an increased incidence in psychiatric disorders, emotional and existential suffering. Yet, despite recent advances in the assessment and management of chronic pain, many chronic pain patients still suffer unnecessarily due to inadequate evaluation, assessment, monitoring and treatment.[9] The intactness of the self, the individual's sense of coherence and integrity, comes not only from intactness of the body mind but from the perceived wholeness of the web of relationships with self and others.[15] This perception and experience of intactness is compromised by chronic pain. Thus the challenge lies in understanding how these biologic, environmental, cultural existential, emotional and psychosocial processes influence and interact with one another to influence the development and maintenance of chronic pain states.[6,16–18]

The broad aim of this edited volume is to take a multidisciplinary as well as a biobehavioral approach to understanding the effective management, evaluation and treatment of pain. This book is organized as a set of chapters. The collaborators for this project are from diverse clinical settings, including the United States, Brazil, the Netherlands, Denmark, Italy, Vietnam, the United Kingdom, and Africa. And also includes a number of international experts in the topics of their chapters. The chapter included in this book spans research and expertise from the fields of genetics, biology, psychology, anthropology neuroanatomy, neurology, oncology, clinical medicine, substance abuse and pharmacology, pharmacoeconomics, gerontology, pediatrics, health services research, health disparities, pain imaging, transportation and rehabilitation, narrative approaches, palliative care, as well as insights from philosophy, ethics and public policy.[6]

The following topics covered in this edited volume are briefly summarized as follows:

Acute Versus Chronic Pain: What Are the Differences?

Distinctions between acute and chronic pain are commonly made. Whether this type of distinction between categories of pain conditions based on chronicity is entirely useful is perhaps a matter for further consideration. In this chapter titled, "The Experience of Pain and Suffering from Acute and Chronic Pain" by

Lance McCracken and Kevin Vowles (The University of Bath, UK) provides a reviews the clinical, biologic and psychological distinctions and similarities between acute and chronic pain, examines the transition between the two, and considers the usefulness of these categories.

The Neuroanatomy of Pain and Pain Pathways

The chapter titled "The Neuroanatomy of Pain and Pain Pathways" by Elie Al-Chaer, PhD, JD (University of Arkansas, USA) highlights recent advances in our knowledge of the pain system including our understanding of nociceptors, the processing of nociceptive information in the spinal cord, brainstem, thalamus, and cerebral cortex and of descending pathways that modulate nociceptive activity.

The Genetic Epidemiology of Pain

One of the more fundamental questions concerning pain in populations is the extent to which its occurrence is determined by constitutional factors as opposed to potentially modifiable factors in the environment to which an individual is exposed throughout life. In the chapter titled "The Genetic Epidemiology of Pain" by Alex MacGregor and Caroline Reavley (University of East Anglia, Norwich, UK) explores this important question and how it can be addressed through studies of the genetic epidemiology of pain.[19]

Pain and the Placebo Effect

Insight regarding the neurobiological basis of the top-down modulation of pain represents a challenge in pain research and many efforts are currently devoted to the development of models illustrating its "modus operandi". One such model is offered by placebo analgesia, i.e. the lessening of pain experienced in response to a therapeutic act devoid of intrinsic analgesic activity. The chapter titled "Pain and the Placebo Effect" by Antonella Pollo and Fabrizio Benedetti (University of Turin, Italy) will provide the reader with an understanding of how the pain experience can be directly and indirectly impacted by placebo and nocebo effects. These include placebo treatment, either in the form of a drug or a physical manipulation, extending the concept of placebo and nocebo to include all aspects of the context surrounding the care of the patient.

The Narrative Approach to Pain

Understanding the meaning of pain in the clinical context generally begins with the patient self-report, or narrative. However, the pain of chronic illness can contribute to a breakdown in the taken-for-granted experience of reality as shared.[4] Narrative accounts can also be viewed as interpretive edifices designed to rationalize and come to terms with the disruption in the ordinary flow of life caused by pain and chronic and severe illness.[20-21] It also provides tellers with an opportunity to impose order on otherwise disconnected events, and to create continuity between past, present, and imagined worlds.[21] In the chapter titled, "The Narrative Approach to Pain", Howard Spiro (The Yale University of Medicine) describes the Narrative Approach to Pain. In oncologic practice, narrative calls the physician back to the story the patient tells, shoves attention from the cancer/tumor back to the patient, moves the physician focus from the statistics of the controlled clinical trial to the pains of the subjects/patients, from considering only their survival to enhancing their comfort and their way of life and sometimes, death.

Psychosocial and Partner-Assisted Biopsychosocial Interventions for Disease-Related Pain

Pain is a biopsychosocial experience. In the chapter titled "Understanding and Enhancing Patient and Partner Adjustment to Disease-Related Pain: A Biopsychosocial Perspective", Frank Keefe, Tamara Somers and Laura Porter (Duke University/ Duke University Cancer Center) discuss those factors that influence patient and partner adjustment to disease-related pain within a biopsychosocial framework and provide an overview of biopsychosocial approaches involving partners in pain management. The chapter is divided into three sections. In the first section, they present a biopsychosocial model that can be used to understand how patients and their partners adjust to disease-related pain. In the second section, they describe factors that influence patient and partner adjustment to both arthritis pain and cancer pain and how these factors are influenced by patient and partner pain management interventions. Finally, they highlight important future directions for clinical and research efforts in this area.

Sex Differences in Pain Perception

The findings on gender highlight the importance of taking into account disparities between males and females in their experience of pain. In "Sex Differences in Pain", Ed. Keogh (The University of Bath, UK) provides a review of the current evidence for the variability in human pain experiences, as ascribed to the sex of the individual, as well as considering some of the reason why such differences exist. As will become apparent, not only are there important biological differences that help to explain why men and women may differ, but there are a range of psychological and socio-cultural factors that need to be considered when attempting to account for sex-specific variations in pain and analgesia.

Children and Pain

One of the primary duties of medicine is to reduce pain and suffering. This aim has often been a poorly fulfilled duty especially in the pediatric patient. Indeed, the tendency toward under medication for pain is even more pronounced in children than in adults. In "Pain in Children", Giovanni Cucchiaro (Children's Hospital of Philadelphia [CHOP]) discusses the biobehavioral assessment, management and treatment of pain in children. First, he defines the neurobiology and behavioral of pain in children. Then he proceeds to describe the epidemiology of acute and chronic pain in several clinical pain populations including headache, central regional pain syndrome (CPRS), and abdominal pain. He then evaluates the different factors that directly impact acute and chronic pain management in these previously mentioned populations. Finally, he describes evidence based best practices for the effective assessment, management and treatment of pain in children, as well as, future directions for the field.

Pain in the Elderly

In "Pain in the Older Person", Bill McCarberg and Barry Cole (Kaiser Permanente, CA, and American Society of Pain Educators, Montclair, NJ) explore the topic of pain in the older person. First they describe the neurophysiology of aging in the older person. Then they proceed to discuss the following: the measurement of pain in the cognitively intact and non-intact patients; psychosocial and behavioral issues associated with pain in this clinical population, the treatment of pain in the older person based upon diagnostic and physiology, complementary and alternative methods for pain; and pain at the end of life. Finally, they conclude this discussion of pain in the older person, and make some suggestions in terms of where the field might go from this point forward.

Healthcare Economic Evaluation of Chronic Pain: Measuring the Economic, Social and Personal Impact of Chronic Pain and its Management

Chronic pain is one of the most costly, disabling, and burdensome conditions afflicting patients and our society at large. The aim of "Healthcare Economic Evaluation of Chronic Pain: Measuring the Economic, Social and Personal Impact of Chronic Pain and its Management" by Rebecca Robinson and Thomas Vetter (Eli Lilly and Company and the University of Alabama School of Medicine) is to provide an overview of the social and personal costs of chronic pain and the role of healthcare economic evaluation methods within the context of chronic pain management, using a standardized and scientific approach. The types of healthcare economic evaluations, the categories of cost incorporated in healthcare economic evaluations, the possible perspectives of a healthcare economic evaluation, and a framework for assessing healthcare economic evaluations will first be discussed. The application of such evaluation methods will then be described for two very common, specific chronic pain conditions, namely, chronic low back pain and fibromyalgia.

Lastly, the implications and challenges related to the clinical application of healthcare economic evaluations of chronic pain treatment will be described.

Chemotherapy Induced Peripheral Neuropathies (CIPNs): A Biobehavioral Approach

Pain is the most common symptom that brings patients to a clinician's office, yet it remains one of the least understood. Chemotherapy-induced peripheral neuropathies are damage to the peripheral nervous system, the system that transmits information between the central nervous system (e.g. the brain and spinal cord) and the rest of the body, caused by some chemotherapy agents. In this chapter, Rhonda Moore (National Cancer Institute, NIH) offers a biobehavioral approach to understanding Chemotherapy Induced Peripheral Neuropathies (CIPNs). CIPNs are defined. This is followed by a description of the epidemiology, behavioral symptoms, barriers and risk factors associated with the development of CIPN. She suggests that injury to peripheral nerves after chemotherapeutic treatments initiates immune to brain communication, which further modulates the biological mechanisms through which life experiences and behavior potentially reinforce and likely perpetuate the experience of chronic long-term neuropathic pain.

Pain and the Use of Health Services among Persons Living with HIV

"Pain and Use of Health Services Among Persons Living with HIV" by Aram Dobalian, Jennie C.I. Tsao, and Lonnie K. Zeltzer (The University of California Los Angeles) summarize the role of pain in HIV and begin with a synopsis of epidemiologic studies on the prevalence of pain symptoms with a focus on chronic pain. This is followed by a synthesis of the existing evidence-base on pain and the use of health services using Andersen's Behavioral Model of Health Services Use and includes discussions of both conventional health services and complementary and alternative medicine (CAM) approaches where such studies exist. They then address the role of comorbid psychological disorders and substance abuse in the use of health services among persons experiencing pain. Finally, the chapter describes gaps in existing knowledge regarding the role of pain in the use of health services among persons living with HIV. Future directions in this field are also described.

Pain Measurement

Chronic pain is under evaluated, under assessed and under treated. In "Pain Measurement", Sydney Morss Dy, The Johns Hopkins School of Medicine/ The Johns Hopkins School of Public Health (JHUPH) builds on evidence-based systematic reviews and expert panels aiming to standardize and improve the quality of care. Dr. Dy describes tools and interventions aimed at more general populations and for vulnerable populations, where appropriate.

Finally, where applicable, she also describes differences among populations and how pain management interacts with other physical, psychiatric symptoms and psychosocial issues. Future directions are also proposed.

Phantom Pain

Phantom Pain, a neuropathic pain syndrome, which results from functional changes in the peripheral and central pain pathways is challenging to treat.[22] Despite the various explanations, the underlying mechanisms and the etiology of phantom pain are still not completely understood.[22–24] In "Phantom Pain", Jan Geertzen and Pieter Dijkstra (Department of Rehabilitation, University Hospital Groningen, Netherland), take a biobehavioral approach to the study of Phantom Limb Pain which highlights the way biological, neurological, psychosocial and environmental factors all play a significant role in the experience of phantom limb pain and phantom limb sensations.

Pain: Substance Abuse Issues in the Treatment of Pain

Pain patients in recovery from the disease of addiction faces multiple barriers to appropriate pharmacologic pain management. These barriers may be insurmountable if the addictive disease is both active and dominant. The healthcare professional must know and understand federal regulations for prescribing a controlled substance to a pain patient with or without a history of addiction. In "Pain: Substance Abuse Issues in the Treatment of Pain", Howard Heit and Arthur Lipman describe substance abuse issues in the treatment of pain patients. This chapter will also provide healthcare providers with the information they need to treat pain patients who also have a history of addiction.

Uses of Complementary and Alternative Medicine for Pain

Individuals who are living with chronic and debilitating conditions, particularly those that are resistant to conventional treatments, are increasingly turning toward Complementary and Alternative Medicine (CAM) modalities for symptomatic relief. In this chapter, Catherine Stoney and Patrick Mansky (The National Center for Complementary and Alternative Medicine (NCCAM), The National Institutes of Health, Bethesda, MD) discuss those CAM modalities for which the most investigations have been employed, including massage, acupuncture, Reiki, hypnosis, Yoga, and Tai Chi. Future directions for this field are also discussed.

Imaging Modalities for Pain

Information transfer in the brain takes place by electrical conduction along axons and chemical interaction between neurons. Functional brain imaging is a general term for techniques measuring correlates of neuronal activity. The techniques used most often are functional magnetic resonance imaging (fMRI), positron emission tomography (PET), single photon emission computed tomography (SPECT), electroencephalography (EEG), magnetoencephalography (MEG) and MR spectroscopy.[25] Although there are a variety of important imaging techniques; in "Imaging Modalities for Pain", Dagfin Matre (University of Oslo, Norway) and Tuan Diep Tran (University of Medicine and Pharmacology, Ho Chi Mihn City, Vietnam) discuss MEG, fMRI, and PET which are three of the main functional imaging methods used to study pain.

Pain, Transportation Issues and Whiplash: A Biobehavioral Approach

The development of pain following a motor vehicle crash (MVC) is a relatively common occurrence. In "Pain, Transportation Issues and Whiplash", Michele Sterling (the University of Queensland, Australia) takes a biobehavioral approach to discuss whiplash associated disorders (WAD), a condition that is more readily accepted to arise as a consequence of motor vehicle trauma. The symptoms, possible injury mechanisms and manifestations, both physical and psychological of the condition are outlined. There are overlapping features between WAD and conditions with more widespread pain and these are described. Finally evidence based best practices for the assessment and management of whiplash will be discussed, and future therapeutic strategies are explored.

Gene Therapies for Chronic Pain

Gene therapy shows great potential to assist numerous patients with inadequate relief of inflammatory or neuropathic pain, or intractable pain associated with advanced cancer. In "Gene Therapy for Chronic Pain", Lariviere and Cope (University of Pittsburgh, USA) provide a brief overview of the methods of gene therapy and of preclinical findings in animal models of prolonged inflammatory, neuropathic and cancer pain. Future directions for this field are also discussed.

Palliative Care and Pain Management in the United States

Palliative care focuses on the whole person: body, mind, and spirit. In "Palliative Care and Pain Management in the United States", Hallenbeck and McDaniel (Stanford University Medical School/Veteran's Administration, Palo Alto, CA) discuss the cultural evolution of the modern palliative care movement. Then they provide a more detailed discussion of the relationship between palliative care and pain management and contrast the clinical worlds of "palliative care" and "pain management" as practiced in the United States. Finally, they review the impact palliative care has had on evidence based practice.

Pain in Society: Ethical Perspectives and Public Policy Concerns

In "Pain in Society: Ethical Issues and Public Policy Concerns", Ben Rich (University of California Davis) provides an overview of the ambivalence that Western society has demonstrated toward those who suffer pain and how those who are in a position to provide relief should respond to it. Despite an incredible amount and diversity of activity in recent years, this ambivalence persists and manifests itself in law and public policy that prompts many health care professionals to decry that they are truly between the proverbial "rock and hard place" when it comes to caring for patients who report and seek prompt and effective relief from pain. This chapter provides insight into the ethics of pain in society and public policy concerns.

In sum, Chronic pain remains a global public health care problem. Indeed, pain remains the most common symptom that brings patients to a doctor's office, yet it remains one of the least understood. While this edited volume is clearly not wholly representative of every chronic pain condition or issue; it can and should be read as an attempt to try and understand some of the challenges underlying how certain biologic, environmental, existential, emotional and psychosocial processes interact to influence the development and maintenance of long term chronic pain.

The Experience of Pain and Suffering from Acute and Chronic Pain

Lance M. McCracken and Kevin E. Vowles

Introduction

Pain can create huge problems, whether this pain is transient "everyday pain," acute post surgical pain, recurrent disease-related pain, or long-standing persistent pain. These problems include disturbed daily functioning, emotional suffering, poor general health, high healthcare use, and high healthcare costs, among others (e.g., Breivik, Collett, Ventafridda, Cohen, & Gallacher, 2006). However, while pain is ubiquitous in human experience, these consequences do not occur in all cases. For researchers and healthcare providers to better understand and manage pain, it is important to accurately discriminate differing pain experiences, identify their initiating causes, and identify the influences that both maintain the pain itself and determine impacts of pain on the daily lives of pain sufferers.

Surely, it is important to pursue a deeper understanding of the *processes* by which pain, suffering, and disability develop and persist, and the means to effectively address these in treatment. Distinctions between acute and chronic pain are commonly made. Whether this type of distinction, based on the chronicity of the pain conditions, is entirely useful is perhaps a matter for further consideration. This chapter will review distinctions and similarities between the experiences of acute and chronic pain, examine the transition between the two, and consider the usefulness of these categories.

Acute Pain

Acute pain is pain of a transient or short-lived nature, from seconds to weeks in duration. Acute pain is a particularly frequent experience, both in the form of fleeting pain that may have little impact, and short term pain associated with significant distress and interference with activities. Point prevalence for acute

L.M. McCracken (✉)
Pain Management Unit, Royal National Hospital for Rheumatic Disease, Bath BA1
1RL, UK
e-mail: Lance.McCracken@rnhrd.nhs.uk

R.J. Moore (ed.), *Biobehavioral Approaches to Pain*,
DOI 10.1007/978-0-387-78323-9_1, © Springer Science+Business Media, LLC 2009

pain, based on a large survey in Finland, for example, is 15% for women and 12% for men (Sasstamoinen, Leino-Rjas, Laaksonen, & Lahelma, 2005). Data from the UK suggest that in older samples these prevalence rates are likely to be several times higher. Here 71% of survey respondents age 50 and older report pain for one day or longer in the past four weeks (Thomas, Peat, Harris, Wilkie, & Croft, 2004). Episodic non-specific low back pain in adults is very common (Deyo, Rainville, & Kent, 1992; McCormick, 1995), with one estimate suggesting that up to 44% of individuals are affected by at least transient back pain in any given year (Picavet & Schouten, 2003).

Most episodes of acute pain resolve quickly with the passage of time and do not require any medical treatment. This includes, for example, most episodes of acute back pain that occur without any associated longer-term difficulties in emotional or physical functioning (Pengel, Herbert, Maher, & Refshauge, 2003; Thomas et al., 1999). A number of studies suggest that up to 90% of individuals seeking treatment for low back pain report being pain free within approximately four weeks of pain onset (e.g., Coste, Delecoeuillerie, Cohen de Lara, Le Parc, & Paolaggi, 1994; Deyo & Tsui-Wu, 1987). When pain remains for more than three months, but less than one year, recovery rates are reduced, but still average approximately 60% across studies (Grotle, Brox, Glomstrød, Lønn, & Vøllestad, 2007; Jones et al., 2006; Poiraudeau et al., 2006; Schiøttz-Christensen et al., 1999). Nonetheless, in spite of the generally positive prognosis, one episode of low back pain increases the risk of future episodes (Von Korff, Deyo, Cherkin, & Barlow, 1993), and once low back pain has been present, it may only partially remit, or can reoccur (Elliott, Smith, Hannaford, Smith, & Chambers, 2002; Gureje, Simon, & Von Korff, 2001).

In the relative minority of cases where treatment is sought, medications such as non-steroidal anti-inflammatories (NSAIDs) can be helpful, but certainly do not provide complete relief for all (Van Tulder, Koes, & Bouter, 1997). In fact, purely medical approaches, and a biomedical model generally, do not appear wholly adequate for understanding or managing the experience of acute pain much of the time. For example, a long history of pain studies repeatedly shows inconsistent relations between tissue damage, diagnostic test results, measures of physiological mechanisms presumed to underlie pain, and the actual reports of pain and functioning (e.g., Grotle, Vøllestad, Veierød, & Brox, 2004; Kroenke & Mangelsdorff, 1989). Even the experience of tightly controlled, standardized, pain stimuli is often associated with wide variations in pain ratings across different individuals and even in the same individual across time (Bonica, 1990).

The experience and outcome of acute pain are associated with a number of psychological factors. For example, pre-procedure anxiety, distress or expectations reliably predict pain reports in response to medical or dental procedures, a phenomenon documented across multiple procedures and across the lifespan (Bernard & Cohen, 2006; Lang, Sorrell, Rodgers, & Lebeck, 2006; Litt, 1996; McNeil, Sorrell, & Vowles, 2006). Similarly, variables such as pain expectations and fear-avoidance beliefs predict general disability in acute back pain (Grotle et al., 2004) and work-related disability in a sample of patients with mixed acute pain conditions (Ciccone & Just, 2001), in each case at levels that appears similar to samples of patients with chronic pain. Further, psychosocial factors, and not physical or physiological factors, are almost invariably among the strongest predictors of longer term prognoses following acute pain (Grotle et al., 2007; Linton, 2000; Pincus, Burton, Vogel, & Field, 2002). Therefore, it appears important to consider psychosocial processes to adequately explain how acute pain has its influence on the behavior of the pain sufferer, particularly when the experience is associated with significant levels of distress and disability.

Chronic Pain

Chronic pain is longstanding pain, most commonly defined as lasting more than 3 months. It appears that most people with chronic pain *in the community* have pain of low intensity and/or low disability (e.g., Elliott et al., 2002), although a large minority do suffer with significant psychological problems, perhaps 35% (Von Korff et al., 2005). In contrast, a greater number of those with chronic pain seen *in primary or specialty care* settings have both significant psychological impacts and impaired daily activities (e.g., Blyth, March, Brnabic, & Cousins, 2004; Gureje et al., 2001). As many as 54% of those who seek treatment for chronic pain suffer with significant depression (Banks & Kerns, 1996), 17–29% with anxiety disorders, and 15–28% with a substance use disorder (Dersh, Polatin, & Gatchel, 2002). Other significant problems include anger (Lombardo, Tan, Jensen, & Anderson, 2005), cognitive issues such as reduced concentration and memory (Sjøgren, Christrup, Peterson, & Hojsted, 2005), sexual dysfunction (Kwan, Roberts, & Swalm, 2005), and sleep disturbance (Smith, Perlis, Smith, Giles, & Carmody, 2000).

As with acute pain, biomedical models of chronic pain and the treatments they yield, including pharmacological, interventional, and surgical, are not entirely adequate, particularly in the long term. For example, according to existing quantitative reviews and meta-analyses, only one in every three to four people treated with anticonvulsant medications for neuropathic pain achieves a 50% reduction in pain that would not have been achieved with a placebo, while minor adverse reactions occur in up to one of every four people treated (Wiffen et al., 2005). Opioids are only marginally more effective for short term pain relief than non-opioid medication or placebo. Moreover, their longer term efficacy remains unclear (Martell et al., 2007). Epidural steroid injections for low back pain demonstrate no beneficial impacts on function, future needs for surgery, or long term pain relief, and achieve only minimal reductions in pain over the short term (i.e., mean reduction of 15%; Armon et al., 2007). Furthermore, studies of more invasive interventions (i.e., surgery, spinal cord stimulators, and implantable drug delivery systems) only rarely include measures of functioning (Turk & Swanson, 2007), and when they do, functional improvements are achieved in only a minority of cases, ranging from 22.8 to 37.5% of patients treated (e.g., Fritzell et al., 2001; Kumar, Nath, & Wyatt, 1991; Paice, Penn, & Shott, 1996). See also Turk and Swanson (2007) for a recent review of the efficacy and cost-effectiveness of treatments for chronic pain.

The basis for the unimpressive results of medically focused interventions may lie in the fact that they do not adequately address the biopsychosocial processes that play a crucial in the suffering and disability of chronic pain. Psychological models that specify the processes by which chronic pain leads to disability and suffering have varied over the years. They have, however, tended to evolve in directions that include both more specific and more integrative processes. Unidimensional models of personality factors, traditional operant behavioral, or exclusively cognitive factors, have given way to, as we say, integrative behavioral, cognitive, and social models such as the fear-avoidance model (Vlaeyen & Linton, 2000), a socially sensitive model of catastrophizing (e.g., Sullivan et al., 2001; Buenaver, Edwards, & Haythornthwaite, 2007), and to fully functional and contextual models to better understand chronic pain (e.g., McCracken, 2005).

One well-known specific process of suffering in the current literature is catastrophizing. The data regarding catastrophizing and chronic pain show that this cognitive process of helplessness, magnification, and rumination is associated with pain severity, depression, disability, and employment status. Remarkably, these results appear generalizable across a variety of pain groups including those with musculoskeletal pain (Severeijns, van den Hout, Vlaeyen, & Picavet, 2002; Sullivan, Stanish, Waite, Sullivan, & Tripp, 1998), neuropathic pain (Sullivan, Lynch, & Clarke, 2005), temperomandibular disorder (Turner, Mancl, & Aaron, 2004), and spinal cord injury pain (Turner, Jensen, Warns, & Cardenas, 2002). Yet, the precise mechanism by which catastrophizing exerts its impact on emotional, physical, and social functioning, is less clear. We would argue, however, that these processes, which are sometimes considered a reflection of communal coping or schema activation (Sullivan et al., 2001), may be alter-natively considered a result of cognitive fusion, loss of contact with the present moment, and experiential avoidance (see Hayes, Luoma, Bond, Masuda, & Lillis, 2006).

The data from a pain-specific "fear-avoidance" model are similarly strong and persuasive. When persons with chronic pain experience fear or anxiety, and act to avoid their pain, they suffer more emotional impact overall and they function relatively poorly. This is a reliable finding in low back pain (Crombez, Vlaeyen, Heuts, & Lysens, 1999), general musculoskeletal pain (McCracken, Spertus, Janeck, Sinclair, and Wetzel, 1999), rheumatoid arthritis (Strahl, Kleinknecht, & Dinnel, 2000), and osteoarthritis (Heuts et al., 2004). Other studies have shown that reduction in fear and avoidance is a critically important process in successful multidisciplinary treatment for chronic pain (e.g., McCracken, Gross, & Eccleston, 2002), and that exposure-based treatments specifically designed to address fear and avoidance appear effective for chronic low back pain (Vlaeyen, de Jong, Geilen, Heuts, & van Breukelen, 2002), and for

complex regional pain syndrome (de Jong et al., 2005). The proposed processes behind the fear and avoidance model are a blend of respondent and
operant processes in tandem with processes of physical deconditioning or
"disuse," hypervigilance, and possibly muscular reactivity (Vlaeyen & Linton,
2000). These various processes are not yet well integrated into a coherent
psychological model, are not yet supported by empirical evidence in all cases,
and the specific nature of the cognitive processes within the fear-avoidance
model seems especially unclear (i.e., how do thoughts translate into emotional
responses or determine actions?). It appears likely that further development of
this model would yield significant dividends for treatment development.

The Transition from Recent Onset Pain to Long-Term Distress and Disability

As noted, psychosocial factors seem to be among the strongest available
predictors of short or long term functioning in relation to pain conditions,
while biomedical, physiological, or mechanical factors have not been as consistently predictive. Furthermore, historical factors, such as history of trauma
or abuse, appear to be only marginal predictors of eventual development of a
long-term pain problem (Linton, 2000; Young Casey, Greenberg, Nicassio,
Harpin, & Hubbard, in press).

In a quantitative review of 37 prospective studies of risk factors relating to
back and neck pain, Linton (2000) reported that the vast majority of studies
found that levels of stress, mood difficulties, and anxiety during the acute stages
of pain were reliably predictive of continuing pain-related difficulties over the
longer term. In particular, greater levels of avoidance behavior and beliefs,
passivity, distress, and anxiety were the strongest and most consistent predictors
of poorer long term prognosis (Linton, 2000). This general conclusion is consistent with more recent studies as well (e.g., Grotle et al., 2007; Jones et al., 2006).

Pain-related fear appears to have a strong relation with longer term prognosis, consistent with the well-established links between these types of fears,
distress, and disability in chronic pain (see Leeuw et al., 2007 for a review).
While at least one study has found that the relations among pain-related fear,
distress, and disability are not as strong in acute pain as in chronic pain (Sieben,
Portegijs, Vlaeyen, & Knottnerus, 2005), other data show that they are similar
(Grotle et al., 2004), and available evidence suggests that this relation is nonetheless important. For example, Fritz, George, and Delitto (2001) found that
pain-related fear specific to work predicted disability four weeks later and
Sieben, Vlaeyen, Tuerlinckx and Portegijs (2002) showed that duration and
severity of such fear increased the risk of persistent disability. Interestingly, such
fear also appears to predict the inception of back pain or future difficulties in pain
free individuals (Linton, Buer, Vlaeyen, & Hellsing, 2000; Buer & Linton, 2002).
In an interesting twist in research methods, it has been found that primary care

physicians who report elevated levels of pain-related fear themselves are less likely to follow established treatment guidelines for low back pain (Poiraudeau et al., 2006), which can be another contributory factor to patient suffering.

Two recent studies have tested a classification system to prospectively identify those at risk of long term disabling low back pain among persons seeking care for low back pain.. Both studies were performed in primary care settings; one study was based in the United States (Von Korff & Miglioretti, 2006) and the other in the United Kingdom (Dunn, Croft, Main, & Von Korff, 2008). Each attempted to predict the presence of low back pain one year later. Predictive elements were a mixture of pain specific variables, including pain severity, duration, and number of sites, as well as measures of pain-related interference and symptoms of depression. Both studies were able to correctly identify approximately 90% of those who were deemed most at risk of having back pain one year later (i.e., "probable" risk), and approximately 50% of those deemed at a lower risk level (i.e., "possible" risk). The authors of both studies conclude that defining acute, subacute, or chronic pain based solely on duration is not likely to be helpful. Rather, they recommend that any risk assessment should include an assessment of additional elements as well, including pain-related interference and emotional functioning.

In summary, the literature on the transition from acute to chronic pain as a whole suggests that the issue cannot be simply reduced to one of duration, rather, there is a need to look for processes that influence how one reacts to, or how behavior is influenced by, the experience of acute pain. The most predictive elements appear to be based around pain-related fear, general levels of distress and passivity, and the interference that pain creates in day-to-day functioning.

Preventing the Development of Chronic Pain Following Episodes of Acute Pain

Consistent with studies of the transition from acute to chronic pain, prevention efforts have explored the key role of psychosocial factors following acute pain episodes. Invasive interventions and medicines, while potentially helpful for shorter-term symptom reduction, may be considerably less useful in preventing the occurrence of longer-term difficulties (Fordyce, 1995; McCracken & Turk, 2002; Nelemans, deBie, deVet, & Sturman, 2001). Prescribed exercise regimens also appear effective only over the shorter term, whereas longer-term efficacy appears negligible in comparison to sham interventions (Pengel et al., 2007). It seems that the most useful medical approaches include methods to insure patients spend as little time as possible inactive, such as no more than two days in bed, and then continue with normal activities in order to speed recovery (Deyo, Diehl, & Rosenthal, 1986; Deyo et al., 1992; Hagen, Hilde, Jamtvedt, & Winnem, 2004; McCormick, 1995).

With regard to prevention of disability, education alone and other minimal interventions appear insufficient for many patients. A study by Jellema and colleagues (2005a) indicated that a primary care based treatment for acute low back pain consisting of approximately 20 minutes of education and limited goal setting did not reliably decrease future disability or work absence. Following a secondary analysis, these authors concluded that the treatment was particularly ineffective when the relevant psychosocial factors were not correctly identified, or when interventions failed to have a noticeable impact on these factors (Jellema et al., 2005b). The findings of this randomized controlled trial are consistent with other analyses that have failed to find a significant preventative effect of education or information alone (e.g., booklets; Burton, Waddell, Tillotson, & Summerton, 1999; Cherkin, Deyo, Street, Hunt, & Barlow, 1996; Frost, Haahr, & Andersen, 2007; Roberts et al., 2002).

Effective treatments, therefore, will almost certainly include more than education alone, will focus beyond medical or biological factors alone, and will explicitly target the resumption of "normal" everyday activities. For instance, treatments incorporating methods from cognitive-behavioral therapy (CBT) have been tested as preventative interventions, as a focus on daily functioning and on the psychosocial processes that underpin it is an integral part of many applications of CBT. Such treatments generally involve some education, but more importantly, also include exposure-based methods and skills training. CBT methods directly address emotional functioning, which, as noted, is so often a core part of the experience of persistent pain. Published trials of CBT for acute pain, again primarily low back pain, demonstrate reductions in sick leave, health care use, and disability (Von Korff et al., 1998; Linton & Andersson, 2000; Moore, von Korff, Cherkin, Saunders, & Lorig, 2000, Damush et al., 2003). CBT even appears useful in those reporting acute pain that is not associated with significant distress or disability. Linton and colleagues, for example, found that reductions in disability were approximately threefold in non-clinical patients and ninefold in patients presenting for treatment who viewed themselves as "at risk" for long-term disability in comparison to individuals assigned to control conditions receiving education only (Linton & Andersson, 2000; Linton & Ryberg, 2001). Dahl and colleagues report a similar finding in a group of nurses at risk for prolonged disability (Dahl & Nilsson, 2001) and among public service employees at risk of long-term disability due to pain or stress (Dahl, Wilson, & Nilsson, 2004).

Common and Distinct Elements of Suffering in Acute and Chronic Pain

...people in pain often report suffering from pain when they feel out of control, when the pain is overwhelming, when the source of pain is unknown, when the meaning of pain is dire, or when the pain is without end (Cassell, 2004, p. 35).

With this statement Eric Cassell provides a descriptive analysis of pain-related suffering that is distinctly concordant with the best current technical analyses. Both those with short term pain and long term pain suffer when they are not able to do what their normal lives ask them to do, or when this capacity appears threatened. Again, uncertainty is a direct recipe for anxiety, worry, or fear. When pain is either known to mean, or merely thought to mean, a loss of what is valued, suffering occurs as well. And, finally, those with *chronic* pain merely have one more realistic reason for distress, but even those who simply think and *believe* that their pain will be unending essentially suffer from unending pain, because believing this is true makes the person feel that it is true.

Statistically speaking, most people with short term pain will continue to function fairly well or fully recover functioning, even if many will have a recurrence of symptoms (e.g., Cassidy, Cote, Carroll, & Kristman, 2005; Von Korff et al., 1993). Once pain is persistent and to some degree disabling, on the other hand, half or more of patients do not recover from their symptoms or disability (e.g., Carey, Garrett, & Jackman, 2000; Elliott et al., 2002; Gureje et al., 2001; Vingard et al., 2002). Patients with short term pain likely have had short term pain before and have experienced that they recovered, which may lead them to feel, and act, as if this will occur. They may even notice a process of change in how they feel as time passes following the onset of their pain, while long term pain patients do not experience this and may even perceive an increase in pain over time. Human behavior being what it is, however, those in acute pain may suffer as if it will not end, and those with chronic pain may take actions each day *as if* their pain will end, despite all evidence to the contrary. In some cases these actions and the moments of "hope" that are associated with them are transient experiences that eventually, sometimes recurrently, give way to the reality of treatment failures and the direct experience of unending pain. Both people with short term and long term pain can get caught up in their own thinking and distress such that they lose contact with the reality of their circumstances, take actions that both defy this reality, and, in one way or another, fail to achieve their goals.

Logic says that the passage of time means positive learning and adjustment, as a result of trial and error, if nothing else, but this is not always the case. Likewise, it is in some ways reasonable to assume that the longer pain continues, the worse the consequences and the greater the problems for the pain sufferer. Interestingly, it is not clear that data bear out either of these scenarios. For example, in data from patients seeking treatment for pain, we rarely, if ever, find correlations between the chronicity of pain and measures of pain severity, anxiety, depression, disability, or healthcare use, either in secondary care (e.g., McCracken & Eccleston, 2005) or tertiary care (e.g., McCracken, Vowles, & Eccleston, 2004) settings. In fact, subgroups of patients empirically classified in terms of pain intensity, disability, and psychosocial variables are found not to differ on duration of pain (e.g., Denison, Asenlof, Sanborgh, & Lindberg, 2007), suggesting that this may not be a clinically relevant variable at least in the ranges of subacute and chronic pain. It has been suggested that, "it may be more meaningful to distinguish characteristic levels of pain intensity, pain-related disability, and pain persistence than to classify patients as acute or chronic." (Von Korff et al., 1993, p. 855). We might suggest that it is more meaningful to understand the current processes of suffering and disability and the factors that will lead related behavior patterns to persist, or to change.

While it appears true that both those with short term and long term pain will have occasions of suffering, and behaving as if their pain is either temporary or unending, there are other real differences between these groups. Patients with chronic pain will have a longer history of failures to control their pain or to otherwise find relief. They also will have a history of accumulated social contacts that either increasingly recognize their pain and disability behavior as aspects of "who they are," or who, alternatively, present a consistently disbelieving or sceptical attitude about their pain and behavior that persists without anything apparently being "wrong." Ironically, both, collusion with the disabled role or frank disbelief in the legitimacy of the problem, can perpetuate a behavior pattern of chronic pain, the former by reinforcing a stable "sense of self" concordant with chronic pain and disability (Crombez, Morley, McCracken, Sensky, & Pincus, 2003,) and the latter by setting up a pattern of resistance to "being wrong" (McCracken, 2005). Pain for a short time after an injury is "normal" and meets accepting and supportive social responses accordingly, however, chronic pain does not appear normal, particularly due to the unclear association with a diagnosable underlying cause, and inconsistent behavior patterns in different situations, and thus, can meet punishing responses and can be alienating for the chronic pain sufferer.

There is at least one set of physical factors that have been long thought to be an etiologically pertinent difference between acute and chronic pain, that is patterns of low activity, or disuse, and concomitant physical deconditioning (e.g., Bortz, 1984). These factors in tandem have been regarded as significant perpetuating factors in models of chronic pain-related disability due to the passage of time. Interestingly, reviews of the literature regarding disuse, deconditioning, and chronic low back pain conclude that, "the presence of deconditioning and disuse in chronic low back pain as factors contributing to chronicity in chronic pain is not confirmed by the literature presented in this review." (Verbunt et al., 2003, p. 19), and, "the most notable finding of this review is the lack of any strong evidence supporting the existence of physical deconditioning symptoms regarding cardiovascular capacity and paraspinal muscles in chronic low back pain patients." (Smeets et al., 2006, p. 689). So, at least based on these expert reviews on chronic low back pain, deconditioning appears not to be present in chronic pain and, therefore, cannot be a distinguishing factor between short term and long term pain.

Developing Approaches to Pain and Suffering

It is an interesting time of new developments in the psychology of pain and suffering. In psychology more broadly there is an increasing growth of what are referred to as "third wave" therapies (Hayes, 2004). Within pain management approaches, this refers to developments that follow the first wave, or operant approaches, and second wave, or first generation cognitive-behavioral approaches. These developments are fully integrative with previous approaches in that they are environmental, behavioral, and fully cognitive in focus. However, they differ in some important ways as well, such as in their explicit functional and contextual focus on acceptance, mindfulness, and values (McCracken, 2005). Data from more than 25 studies in this area support a particular model of human behavior and suffering, a process-oriented model proposing that suffering results from unsuccessful attempts to control unwanted psychological experiences, loss of contact with the present situation, failures of behavior to be guided by important purposes, and general entanglement in restrictive verbal-cognitive influences on behavior patterns (Hayes, Luoma, Bond, Masuda, & Ellis, 2006). Data from early treatment trials support the effectiveness of this approach to chronic pain (e.g., Dahl et al., 2004; Vowles & McCracken, in press). Wider success from the same treatment model outside of chronic pain, for depression, diabetes self-management, psychosis, and work stress, for example, and suggests that it may be generally applicable, including for less complex and shorter term pain (see Hayes et al., 2006 for a review). Future work in this area would benefit from a continued focus on the processes in successful treatment for pain and on comparisons of these treatment approaches with alternate approaches, including biomedical or other psychological methods.

Summary

The experience of pain, regardless of whether it is classified as acute or chronic, is a common and essentially unavoidable part of the human experience. As such it will continue to create significant short and long term difficulties in a substantial proportion of the population. If healthcare providers are to be ideally positioned to address these difficulties, then they will want to understand the key influences on the experience of pain, particularly those that are therapeutically manipulable.

Over time, many of the variables that were once identified as relevant contributors to pain, pain-related suffering, and disability, have failed to demonstrate sufficient utility. These variables include pain location, results from certain diagnostic tests, certain clinical test results, personality classifications, and certain aspects of psychological history. Even pain duration, the very basis for the distinction between "acute" and "chronic" pain, within many ranges, fails to suggest clear clinical action or to discriminate those who will do well from those who will suffer long term interference with daily functioning. Instead, a remarkably consistent group of predictors of current and future functioning include contemporaneous behavior patterns and the cognitive and emotional influences on those behavioural behavior patterns. These include variables such as catastrophizing, fear and avoidance, and the processes that produce both these responses and their effects.

Treatments for acute and chronic pain that are based on a general cognitive-behavioral model appear effective for acute pain, for the prevention of chronic pain, and for the rehabilitation of chronic pain. As the frameworks we apply to the problem of pain gradually shift and change, we may increasingly understand such issues as duration of pain in new ways, and we may, as a result, gain an increasingly practical focus on the problem that yields a more precise analyses and more effective treatments.

References

Armon, C., Argoff, C.E., Samuels, J., Bacleonja, M.M. (2007). Therapeutics and Technology Assessment Subcommittee of the American Academy of Neurology. *Neurology, 68,* 1526–1632.

Banks, S. M., & Kerns, R. D. (1996). Explaining high rates of depression in chronic pain: A diathesis-stress framework. *Psychological Bulletin, 119,* 95–110.

Bernard, R. S., & Cohen, L. L. (2006). Parent anxiety and infant pain during pediatric immunizations. *Journal of Clinical Psychology in Medical Settings, 13,* 282–287.

Blyth, F. M., March L. M., Brnabic, A. J. M., & Cousins, M. J. (2004). Chronic pain and frequent use of health care. *Pain, 111,* 51–58.

Bonica, J. J. (1990). History of pain concepts and theories. In J. J. Bonica (Ed.), *The management of pain* (pp. 2–17). Philadelphia: Lea & Fibiger.

Bortz, W. M. (1984). The disuse syndrome. *Western Journal of Medicine, 141,* 691–694.

Breivik, H., Collett, B., Ventafridda, V., Cohen R., & Gallacher, D. (2006). Survey of chronic pain in Europe: Prevalence, impact on daily life, and treatment. *European Journal of Pain, 10,* 287–333.

Buenaver, L. F., Edwards, R. R., & Haythornthwaite, J. A. (2007). Pain-related catastrophizing and perceived social responses: Inter-relationships in the context of chronic pain. *Pain, 127,* 234–242.

Buer, N., & Linton, S. J. (2002). Fear-avoidance beliefs and catastrophizing: Occurrence and risk factor in back pain and ADL in the general population. *Pain, 99,* 485–491.

Burton, A. K., Waddell, G., Tillotson, K. M., & Summerton, N. (1999). Information and advice to patients with back pain can have a positive effect: A randomized controlled trial of a novel educational booklet in primary care. *Spine,* 24:2484–2491.

Carey, T. S., Garrett, J. M., & Jackman, A. M. (2000). Beyond good prognosis: Examination of an inception cohort of patients with chronic low back pain. *Spine, 25,* 115–120.

Cassell, E. J. (2004). The nature of suffering and the goals of medicine (2nd ed.). New York: Oxford University Press.

Cassidy, J. D., Cote. P., Carroll, L. J., & Kristman, V. (2005). Incidence and course of low back pain episodes in the general population. *Spine, 30,* 2817–2823.

Cherkin, D. C., Deyo R. A., Street, J. H., Hunt, M., & Barlow, W. (1996). Pitfalls of patient education: Limited success of a program for back pain in primary care. *Spine,* 21, 345–355.

Ciccone, D. S., & Just N. (2001). Pain expectancy and work disability in patients with acute and chronic pain: A test of the fear avoidance hypothesis. *The Journal of Pain, 2,* 181–194.

Coste, J., Delecoeuillerie, G., Cohen de Lara, A., Le Parc, J. M., & Paolaggi, J. B. (1994). Clincial course and prognostic factors in acute low back pain: An inception cohort study in primary care practice. *British Medical Journal, 308,* 577–580.

Crombez, G., Morley, S., McCracken, L. M., Sensky, T., & Pincus, T. (2003). Self, identity and acceptance in chronic pain. In J. O. Dostrovsky, D. B. Carr, & M. Koltzenburg (Eds.), *Proceedings on the 10th World Congress on Pain* (pp. 651–659). Seattle: IASP Press.

Crombez, G., Vlaeyen, J. W. S., Heuts, P. H. T. G., & Lysens, R. (1999). Pain-related fear is more disabling then the pain itself: Evidence on the role of pain-related fear in chronic back pain disability. *Pain, 80*, 329–339.

Dahl, J. C., & Nilsson, A. (2001). Evaluation of a randomized preventive behavioural medicine work site intervention for public health workers at risk for developing chronic pain. *European Journal of Pain, 5*, 421–432.

Dahl, J. C., Wilson, K. G., & Nilsson, A. (2004). Acceptance and commitment therapy and the treatment of persons at risk for long-term disability resulting from stress and pain symptoms: A preliminary randomized trial. *Behavior Therapy, 35*, 785–801.

Damush, T. M., Weinberger, M., Perkins, S. M., Rao, J. K., Tierney, W. M., Qi, R., et al. (2003). The long-term effects of a self-management program for inner-city primary care patients with acute low back pain. *Archives of Internal Medicine, 163*, 2632–2638.

de Jong, J. R., Vlaeyen, W. S. J., Onghena, P., Cuypers, C., den Hollander, M., & Ruijgrok, J. (2005). Reduction of pain-related fear in complex regional pain syndrome type I: The application of graded exposure in vivo. *Pain, 116*, 264–275.

Denison, E., Asenlof, P., Sanborgh, M., & Lindberg, P. (2007). Musculoskeletal pain in primary care health care: Subgroups based on pain intensity, disability, self-efficacy, and fear-avoidance variables. *The Journal of Pain, 8*, 67–74.

Dersh, J., Polatin, P. B., & Gatchel, R. J. (2002). Chronic pain and psychopathology: Research findings and theoretical considerations. *Psychosomatic Medicine, 64*, 773–786.

Deyo, R. A., Diehl, A. K., & Rosenthal, M. (1986). How many days of bed rest for acute low back pain? A randomised clinical trial. *New England Journal of Medicine, 315*, 1064–1070.

Deyo, R. A., Rainville, J., & Kent, D. L. (1992). What can the history and physical examination tell us about low back pain? *Journal of the American Medical Association, 268*, 760–765.

Deyo, R. A., & Tsui-Wu, Y. J. (1987). Descriptive epidemiology of low-back pain and its related medical care in the United States. *Spine, 12*, 264–268.

Dunn, K. M., Croft, P. R., Main, C. J., & Von Korff, M. (2008). A prognostic approach to defining chronic pain: Replication in a UK primary care low back pain population. *Pain, 135*, 48–54.

Elliott, A. M., Smith, B. H., Hannaford, P. C., Smith, W. C., & Chambers, W. A. (2002). The course of chronic pain in the community: Results of a 4-year follow-up study. *Pain, 99*, 299–307.

Fordyce, W. E. (Ed). (1995). *Back pain in the workplace: Management of disability in non-specific conditions*. Seattle: IASP Press.

Fritz, J. M., George, S. Z., & Delitto, A. (2001). The role of fear-avoidance beliefs in acute low back pain: Relationships with current and future disability and work status. *Pain, 94*, 7–15.

Fritzell, P., Olle, H., Wessberg, P., & Nordwall, A., Swedish Lumbar Spine Study Group. (2001). Lumbar fusion versus nonsurgical treatment for chronic low back pain: A multi-center randomized controlled trial from the Swedish lumbar spine study group. *Spine, 26*, 2521–2534.

Frost, P., Haahr, J., & Andersen, J. H. (2007). Reduction of pain-related disability in working populations: A randomized intervention study of the effects of an educational booklet addressing psychosocial risk factors and screening workplaces for physical health hazards. *Spine, 32*, 1949–1954.

Grotle, M., Brox, J. I., Glomstrød, B., Lønn, J. H., & Vøllestad, N. K. (2007). Prognostic factors in first-time care seekers due to acute low back pain. *European Journal of Pain, 11*, 290–298.

Grotle, M., Vøllestad, N. K., Veierød, M. B., & Brox, J. I. (2004). Fear-avoidance beliefs and distress in relation to disability in acute and chronic low back pain. *Pain, 112*, 343–352.

Gureje, O., Simon, G. E., & Von Korff, M. (2001). A cross-national study of the course of persistent pain in primary care. *Pain, 92,* 195–200.

Hagen, K. B., Hilde, G., Jamtvedt, G., & Winnem, M. (2004). Bed rest for acute low-back pain and sciatica. *Cochrane Database of Systematic Reviews, 4,* Art. No.: CD001254. DOI:10.1002/14651858.CD001254.pub2.

Hayes, S. C. (2004). Acceptance and commitment therapy, relational frame theory, and the third wave of behavior therapy. *Behavior Therapy, 35,* 639–665.

Hayes, S. C., Luoma, J. B., Bond, F. W., Masuda, A., & Lillis, J. (2006). Acceptance and Commitment Therapy: Model, processes and outcomes. *Behaviour Research and Therapy, 44,* 1–25.

Heuts, P. H. T. G., Vlaeyen, J. W. S., Roelofs, J., de Bie, R. A., Aretz, K., van Weel, C., et al. (2004). Pain-related fear and daily functioning in patients with osteoarthritis. *Pain, 110,* 228–235.

Jellema, P., van der Windt, D. A. W. M., van der Horst, H. E., Blankenstein, A. H., Bouter, L. M., & Stalman, W. A. B. (2005a). Why is a treatment aimed at psychosocial factors not effective in patients with (sub)acute low back pain? *Pain, 118,* 350–359.

Jellema, P., van der Windt, D. A. W. M., van der horst, H. E., Twisk, J. W. R., Stalman, W. A. B., & Bouter, L. M. (2005b). Should treatment of (sub)acute low back pain be aimed at psychosocial prognostic factors? Cluster randomized clinical trial in general practice. *British Medical Journal, 331,* 84–90.

Jones, G. T., Johnson, R. E., Wiles, N. J., Chaddock, C., Potter, R. G., Roberts, C., et al. (2006). Predicting persistent disabling low back pain in general practice: A prospective cohort study. *British Journal of General Practice, 56,* 334–341.

Kroenke, K., & Mangelsdorff, A. D. (1989). Common symptoms in ambulatory care: Incidence, evaluation, therapy, and outcome. *The American Journal of Medicine, 86,* 262–266.

Kwan, K. S. H., Roberts, L. J., & Swalm, D. M. (2005). Sexual dysfunction and chronic pain: The role of psychological variables and impact on quality of life. *European Journal of Pain, 9,* 643–52.

Kumar, K., Nath, R., & Wyatt, G. M. (1991). Treatment of chronic pain by epidural spinal cord stimulation: A 10-year experience. *Journal of Neurosurgery, 75,* 402–407.

Lang, A. J., Sorrell, J. T., Rodgers, C. S., & Lebeck, M. M. (2006). Anxiety sensitivity as a predictor of labor pain. *European Journal of Pain, 10, 263–270.*

Leeuw, M., Goossens, M. E. J. B., Linton, S. J., Crombez, G., Boersma, K., & Vlaeyen, J. W. S. (2007). The fear-avoidance model of musculoskeletal pain: Current state of scientific evidence. *Journal of Behavioral Medicine, 30,* 77–94.

Linton, S. J. (2000). A review of psychological risk factors in back and neck pain. *Spine, 25,* 1148–1156.

Linton, S. J., & Andersson, T. (2000). Can chronic disability be prevented? A randomized trial of a cognitive-behavior intervention and two forms of information for patients with spinal pain. *Spine, 25,* 2825–2831.

Linton, S. J., Buer, N., Vlaeyen, J. W. S., & Hellsing, A. -L. (2000). Are fear-avoidance beliefs related to a new episode of back pain? A prospective study. *Psychological Health, 14,* 1051–1059.

Linton, S. J., & Ryeberg, M. (2001). A cognitive-behavioral group intervention as prevention for persistent neck and back pain in a non-patient population: A randomized controlled trial. *Pain, 90,* 83–90.

Litt, M. D. (1996). A model of pain and anxiety associated with acute stressors: Distress in dental procedures. *Behaviour Research and Therapy, 34,* 459–476.

Lombardo, E. R., Tan, G., Jensen, M. P., & Anderson, K. O. (2005). Anger management style and associations with self-efficacy and pain in male veterans. *The Journal of Pain, 6,* 765–70.

Martell, B. A., O'Connor, P. G., Kerns, R. D., Becker, W. C., Morales, K. H., Kosten, T. R., et al. (2007). Systematic review: Opioid treatment for chronic back pain: Prevalence, efficacy, and association with addiction. *Annals of Internal Medicine, 146,* 116–127.

McCormick, A. (1995). *Morbidity statistics from general practice: Fourth national study 1991–1992. A study carried out by the Royal College of General Practitioners, the Office of Population Censuses and Surveys, and the Department of Health*. London: HMSO.

McCracken, L. M. (2005). Contextual cognitive-behavioral therapy for chronic pain. Seattle, WA: IASP Press.

McCracken, L. M., & Eccleston, C. (2005). A prospective study of acceptance of pain and patient functioning with chronic pain. *Pain, 118*, 164–169.

McCracken, L. M., Gross, R. T., & Eccleston, C. (2002). Multimethod assessment of treatment process in chronic low back pain: Comparison of reported pain-related anxiety with directly measured physical capacity. *Behaviour Research and Therapy, 40*, 585–594.

McCracken, L. M., Spertus, I. L., Janeck, A. S., Sinclair, D., & Wetzel, F. T. (1999). Behavioral dimensions of adjustment in persons with chronic pain: Pain-related anxiety and acceptance. *Pain, 80*, 283–289.

McCracken, L. M., & Turk, D. C. (2002). Behavioral and cognitive behavioral treatment for chronic pain: Outcomes, predictors of outcomes, and treatment process. *Spine, 27*, 2564–2573.

McCracken, L. M., Vowles, K. E., & Eccleston, C. (2004). Acceptance of chronic pain: Component analysis and a revised assessment method. *Pain, 107*, 159–166.

McNeil, D. W., Sorrell, J. T., & Vowles, K. E. (2006). Emotional and environmental determinants of dental pain. In D. I. Mostofsky, A. Forgione, & D. Giddon (Eds.), *Behavioral dentistry* (pp. 79–99). Ames, Iowa: Blackwell Publishing.

Moore, J. E., von Korff, M., Cherkin, D., Saunders, K., & Lorig, K. (2000). A randomized trial of a cognitive-behavioural program for enhancing back pain self care in a primary care setting. *Pain, 88*,145–153.

Nelemans, P. J., de Bie, R. A., de Vet, H. C. W., & Sturman, F. (2001). Injection therapy for subacute and chronic benign low back pain. *Spine, 26*, 501–515.

Paice, J. A., Penn, R. D., & Shott, S. (1996). Intraspinal morpine for chronic pain: A retrospective, multicenter study. *Journal of Pain and Symptom Management, 11*, 71–80.

Pengel, L. H. M., Herbert, R. D., Maher, C. G., & Refshauge, K. M. (2003). Acute low back pain: Systematic review of its prognosis. *British Medical Journal, 327*, 323–328.

Pengel, L. H. M., Refshaug, K. M., Maher, C. G., Nicholas, M. K., Herbert, R. D., & McNair, P. (2007). Physiotherapist-directed exercise, advice, or both for subacute low back pain. *Annals of Internal Medicine, 146*, 787–796.

Picavet, H. S. J., & Schouten, J. S. A. G. (2003). Musculoskeletal pain in the Netherlands: Prevalences, consequences and risk groups, the DMC(3)-study. *Pain, 102*, 167–178.

Pincus, T., Burton, A. K., Vogel, S., & Field, A. P. (2002). A systematic review of psychological factors as predictors of chronicity/disability in prospective cohorts of low back pain. *Spine, 27*, E109–120.

Poiraudeau, S., Rannou, F., Le Henanff, A., Coudeyre, E., Rozenberg, S., Huas, D., et al. (2006). Outcome of subacute low back pain: Influence of patients' and rheumatologists' characteristics. *Rheumatology, 45*, 718–723.

Roberts, L., Little, P., Chapman, J., Cantrell, T., Pickering, R., & Langridge, J. (2002). The back home trial: General practitioner-supported leaflets may change back pain behaviour. *Spine, 27*, 1821–1828.

Sasstamoinen, P., Leino-Arjas, P., Laaksonen, M., & Lahelma, E. (2005). Socio-economic differences in the prevalence of acute, chronic, and disabling chronic pain among ageing employees. *Pain, 114*, 364–371.

Schiøttz-Christensen, B., Nielsen, G. L., Hansen, V. K., Schødt, T., Sørensen, H. T., & Olesen, F. (1999). Long-term prognosis of acute low back pain in patients seen in general practice: A 1-year prospective follow-up study. *Family Practice, 16*, 223–232.

Severeijns, R., van den Hout, M. A., Vlaeyen, J. W. S., & Picavet, H. S. J. (2002). Pain catastrophizing and general health status in a large Dutch community sample. *Pain, 99*, 367–376.

Sieben, J. M., Portegijs, P. J. M., Vlaeyen, J. W. S., & Knottnerus, J. A. (2005). Pain-related fear at the start of a new low back pain episode. *European Journal of Pain, 9*, 635–641.

Sieben, J. M., Vlaeyen, J. W. S., Tuerlinckx, S., & Portegijs, P. J. (2002). Pain-related fear in acute low back pain: The first two weeks of a new episode. *European Journal of Pain, 6*, 229–237.

Sjøgren, P., Christrup, L. L., Peterson, M., & Højsted, J. (2005). Neuropsychological assessment of chronic non-malignant pain patients treated in a multidisciplinary pain centre. *European Journal of Pain, 9*, 453–62.

Smeets, R. J. E. M., Wade, D., Hidding, A., Van Leeuwen, P. J. C. M., Vlaeyen J. W. S., & Knottnerus, J. A. (2006). The association of physical deconditioning and chronic low back pain: A hypothesis-oriented systematic review. *Disability and Rehabilitation, 28*, 673–693.

Smith, M. T., Perlis, M. L., Smith, M. S., Giles, D. E., & Carmody, T. P. (2000). Sleep quality and presleep arousal in chronic pain. *Journal of Behavioral Medicine, 23*, 1–13.

Strahl, C., Kleinknecht, R. A., & Dinnel, D. L. (2000). The role of pain anxiety, coping, and pain self-efficacy in rheumatoid arthritis patient functioning. *Behaviour Research and Therapy, 38*, 863–873.

Sullivan, M. J. L., Lynch, M. E., & Clark, A. J. (2005). Dimensions of catastrophic thinking associated with pain experience and disability in patients with neuropathic pain conditions. *Pain, 113*, 310–315.

Sullivan, M. L. J., Stanish, W., Waite, H., Sullivan, M., & Tripp, D. A. (1998). Catastrophzing, pain, and disability in patients with soft tissue injuries. *Pain, 77*, 253–260.

Sullivan, M. J. L., Thorn, B., Haythorthwaite, J. A., Keefe, F., Martin, M., Bradley, L. A., et al. (2001). Theoretical perspectives on the relation between catastrophizing and pain. *The Clinical Journal of Pain, 17*, 52–64.

Thomas, E., Peat, G., Harris, L., Wilkie, R., & Croft, P. R. (2004). The prevalence of pain and pain interference in a general population of older adults: Cross-sectional findings from the North Staffordshire Osteoarthritis Project (NorStOP). *Pain, 110*, 361–368.

Thomas, E., Silman, A. J., Croft, P. J., Papageorgiou, A. C., Jayson, M. I., & Macfarlane, G. J. (1999). Predicting who develops chronic low back pain in primary care: A prospective study. *British Medical Journal, 318*, 1662–1667.

Turk, D. C., & Swanson, K. (2007). Efficacy and cost-effectiveness treatment for chronic pain: An analysis and evidence-based synthesis. In M. Schatman & A. Campbell (Eds.) *Chronic pain management: Guidelines for multidisciplinary program development* (pp. 15–38). New York, Informa.

Turner, J. A., Jensen, M. P., Warms, C. A., & Cardenas, D. D. (2002). Catastrophizing is associated with pain intensity, psychological distress, and pain-related disability among individuals with chronic pain after spinal cord injury. *Pain, 98*, 127–134.

Turner, J. A., Mancl, L., & Aaron, L. A. (2004). Pain-related catastrophzing: A daily process study. *Pain, 110*, 103–111.

Van Tulder, M. W., Koes, B. W., & Bouter, L. M. (1997). Conservative treatment of acute and chronic nonspecific low back pain: A systematic review of randomized controlled trials of the most common interventions. *Spine, 22*, 2128–2156.

Verbunt, J. A., Seelen, H. A., Vlaeyen, J. W. S., van de Heijden, G. J., Heuts, P. H., Pons, K., et al. (2003). Disuse and deconditioning in chronic low back pain: Concepts and hypotheses on contributing mechanisms. *European Journal of Pain, 7*, 9–21.

Vingard, E., Mortimer, M., Wiktorin C., Pernold, G., Fredriksson, K., Nemeth G., et al. (2002). Seeking care for low back pain in the general population. *Spine, 27*, 2159–2165.

Vlaeyen, J, W. S., de Jong, J., Geilen, M., Heuts, P. H. T. G., & van Breukelen, G. (2002). The treatment of fear of movement/(re)injury in chronic low back pain: Further evidence on the effectiveness of exposure in vivo. *The Clinical Journal of Pain, 18*, 251–261.

Vlaeyen, J. W. S., & Linton, S. J. (2000). Fear-avoidance and its consequences in chronic musculoskeletal pain: A state of the art. *Pain, 85*, 317–332.

16   L.M. McCracken and K.E. Vowles

Von Korff, M., Crane, P., Lane, M., Miglioretti, D. L., Simon, G., Saunders, K., et al. (2005). Chronic spinal pain and physical-mental comorbidity in the United States: Results from the national comorbidity survey replication. *Pain, 113*, 331–339.

Von Korff, M., Deyo, R. A., Cherkin D., & Barlow, W. (1993). Back pain in primary care: Outcomes at 1 year. *Spine, 18*, 855–862.

Von Korff, M., & Miglioretti, D. L. (2006). A prospective approach to defining chronic pain. In H. Flor, E. Kalso, & J. O. Dostrovsky (Eds.), *Proceedings of the 11th world congress on pain* (pp. 761–769). Seattle: IASP Press.

Von Korff, M., Moore, J. E., Lorig, K., Cherkin, D. C., Saunders, K., Gonzalez, V. M., et al. (1998). A randomized trial of a lay person-led self-management group intervention for back pain patients in primary care. *Spine, 23*, 2608–2615.

Vowles, K. E., & McCracken, L. M. (2008). Acceptance and values-based action in contextual cognitive behavioral therapy for chronic pain: A study of effectiveness and treatment process. *Journal of Consulting and Clinical Psychology, 76*, 397–407.

Wiffen, P., Collins, S., McQuary, H., Carroll, D., Jadad, A., & Moore, A. (2005). Anticonvulsant drugs for acute and chronic pain. *Cochrane Database Systematic Reviews,* Issue 3, Article Number: CD001133.

Young Casey, C., Greenberg, M. A., Nicassio, P. M., Harpin, R. E., & Hubbard, D. (2008). Transition from acute to chronic pain and disability: A model including cognitive, affective, and trauma factors. *Pain, 134*, 69–79.

The Neuroanatomy of Pain and Pain Pathways

Elie D. Al-Chaer

Introduction

Our fascination with pain mechanisms possibly dates back to our awareness of our existence. Yet our study of pain pathways only gained focus with the reflex theory advanced by René Descartes in 1664 (Descartes, 1664) and was rejuvenated time and again by a number of subsequent theories, such as the specificity theory (Schiff, 1858) and the sensory interaction theory (Noordenbos, 1959). On the other hand, pattern and neuromatrix theories have discounted the specific function assigned to anatomic components of the nervous system (e.g. Berkley & Hubscher, 1995a; Melzack, 1999; Nafe, 1934), particularly when it comes to pain processing; but they have been faced with challenges of their own, not the least of which is translating their theoretical framework into clinical applications. This chapter highlights recent advances in our knowledge of the pain system including our understanding of nociceptors, of the processing of nociceptive information in the spinal cord, brainstem, thalamus, and cerebral cortex and of descending pathways that modulate nociceptive activity. Some of this information might potentially lead to improvements in patient care.

Peripheral Pathways

Peripheral sensory nerves are composed of the axons of somatic and visceral sensory neurons and the connective tissue sheaths that enfold them (epineurium, perineurium, and endoneurioum; Ross, Romrell, & Kaye, 1995). These axons may be myelinated or unmyelinated. The large myelinated sensory axons belong to the Aβ class and are predominantly somatic, whereas the small myelinated axons belong to the Aδ group and along with the unmyelinated

E.D. Al-Chaer (✉)
Pediatrics, Internal Medicine, Neurobiology and Developmental Sciences, College of Medicine, University of Arkansas for Medical Sciences, Biomedical Research Center, Bldg. II, Suite 406-2, 4301 West Markham, Slot 842, Little Rock, AR 72205, USA
e-mail: ealchaer@uams.edu

R.J. Moore (ed.), *Biobehavioral Approaches to Pain*,
DOI 10.1007/978-0-387-78323-9_2, © Springer Science+Business Media, LLC 2009

fibers (often referred to as C fibers), they innervate both somatic and visceral tissues (Al-Chaer & Willis, 2007). As a general rule, only small myelinated and umyelinated fibers are involved in pain processing; however, in some cases of peripheral neuropathy, large myelinated fibers have also been implicated (e.g. see Kajander & Bennett, 1992).

Nociceptors

Nociceptors are defined as sensory receptors activated by stimuli that threaten to damage or actually damage a tissue (Sherrington, 1906). They have been described in most of the structures of the body that give rise to pain sensation, including the skin, muscle, joints, and viscera (Willis & Coggeshall, 2004). Some nociceptors are unresponsive to mechanical stimuli unless they are sensitized by tissue injury or inflammation. These are referred to as "silent nociceptors" (Häbler, Jänig, & Koltzenburg, 1990; Lynn & Carpenter, 1982; Schaible & Schmidt, 1983) and have been described in joint, cutaneous and visceral nerves. Human studies involving microneurography and microstimulation in peripheral nerves have demonstrated that activation of nociceptors results in pain (Ochoa & Torebjörk, 1989). The quality of the pain sensation depends on the tissue innervated; e.g., stimulation of cutaneous Aδ nociceptors leads to pricking pain (Konietzny, Perl, Trevino, Light, & Hensel, 1981), whereas stimulation of cutaneous C nociceptors results in burning or dull pain (Ochoa & Torebjörk, 1989). However, it is important to keep in mind that pain does not always result from activation of nociceptors. Examples include cases of central pain following damage to the central nervous system (Boivie, Leijon, & Johansson, 1989), functional pain residual to neonatal injury (Al-Chaer, Kawasaki, & Pasricha, 2000) or activation of motivational-affective circuits that can also mimic pain states, particularly in patients with anxiety, neurotic depression, or hysteria (Chaturvedi, 1987; Merskey, 1989).

Peripheral Sensitization and Primary Hypersensitivity

Sensitization of nociceptors is commonly defined as an increase in the firing rate and a reduction in threshold of the nociceptor. In silent nociceptors, sensitization causes an "awakening" by effecting the development of spontaneous discharges and causing the receptors to become more sensitive to peripheral stimulation (Schaible & Schmidt, 1985, 1988). Sensitization depends on the activation of second-messenger systems by the action of inflammatory mediators released in the damaged tissue, such as bradykinin, prostaglandins, serotonin, and histamine (Birrell, McQueen, Iggo, & Grubb., 1993; Davis, Meyer, & Campbell, 1993; Dray, Bettaney, Forster, & Perkins, 1988; Schepelmann, Messlinger, Schraible, & Schmidt, 1992). A hallmark of the sensitization of peripheral nociceptors is sensory hypersensitivity classified as primary hyper-algesia or allodynia.

Hyperalgesia is defined as an increase in the painfulness of a noxious stimu-lus and a reduced threshold for pain (LaMotte, Thalhammer, & Robinson, 1983; Meyer & Campbell, 1981; see Bonica, 2001). Primary hyperalgesia is felt at the site of injury and is believed to be a consequence of the sensitization of nociceptors during the process of inflammation (LaMotte, Thalhammer, Torebjörk, & Robinson, 1982; LaMotte et al., 1983; Meyer & Campbell, 1981). Allodynia is a related phenomenon in which non-noxious stimuli pro-duce painful responses. One of the most common examples of allodynia is pain produced by lightly touching burned skin.

Primary Afferents: Somatic and Visceral

The nociceptors described above run in peripheral nerves as they extend towards the skin surface or other target organs in the periphery (muscles or viscera). They represent peripheral processes of dorsal root ganglion (DRG) cells, or in the case of the head and neck, trigeminal ganglion cells. These cells are organized as groups of neurons in the peripheral nervous system and form two longitudinal chains along either side of the spinal cord (see Willis & Coggeshall, 2004).

Whereas somatic afferents innervate peripheral tissues following a dermato-mal distribution, afferents innervating visceral organs are broadly subdivided into splanchnic and pelvic afferents that follow the path of sympathetic and parasympathetic efferents that project to the gut wall (see Al-Chaer & Traub, 2002). Somatic afferents that innervate the striated musculature of the pelvic floor project to the sacral spinal cord via the pudendal nerve (Grundy et al., 2006). Visceral afferents have multiple receptive fields extending over a rela-tively wide area. Those in the serosa and mesenteric attachments respond to distortion of the viscera during distension and contraction. Other endings detect changes in the submucosal chemical milieu following injury, ischemia or infection and may play a role in generating hypersensitivity. Intramural spinal afferent fibers have collateral branches that innervate blood vessels and enteric ganglia. These contain and release neurotransmitters during local axon reflexes that influence blood flow, motility and secretory reflexes in the gastro-intestinal tract (Maggi & Meli, 1988; for a review of the neurochemistry of visceral afferents, see Al-Chaer & Traub, 2002). Spinal afferents on route to the spinal cord also give off collaterals that innervate prevertebral sympathetic ganglia neurons. The same sensory information is thereby transmitted to infor-mation processing circuits in the spinal cord, enteric nervous system (ENS) and prevertebral ganglia. The main transmitters are calcitonin gene-related peptide (CGRP) and substance P, and both peptides are implicated in the induction of neurogenic inflammation. (Grundy et al. 2006)

Chemical Mediators

The activity of nociceptors can be affected by adequate stimuli, such as strong mechanical, thermal, or chemical stimuli (see Willis, 1985; Willis & Coggeshall, 2004), and also by chemical actions on surface membrane receptors of their axons. A battery of chemical mediators, including biogenic amines (such as glutamate, [gamma]-aminobutyric acid (GABA), histamine, serotonin, norepinephrine) (Dray, Urban, & Dickenson, 1994; McRoberts et al., 2001), opiates (Joshi, Su, Porreca, & Gebhart, 2000; Su, Sengupta, & Gebhart, 1997), purines, prostanoids, proteases cytokines, and other peptides (such as bradykinin, substance P, and CGRP) act in a promiscuous manner on a range of receptors expressed upon any one sensory ending (Kirkup, Brunsden, & Grundy, 2001).

Three distinct processes are involved in the actions of these substances on afferent nerves. First, by direct activation of receptors coupled to the opening of ion channels present on nerve terminals, the terminals are depolarized and firing of impulses is initiated. Second, by sensitization that develops in the absence of direct stimulation and results in hyperexcitability to both chemical and mechanical modalities. e.g., opiate receptors are ineffective in modulating the normal activity of joint nociceptors, but they were shown to become effective after the development of inflammation (Stein, 1994). Sensitization may also involve post-receptor signal transduction that includes G-protein coupled alterations in second messenger systems which in turn lead to phosphorylation of membrane receptors and ion channels that control excitability of the afferent endings. Third, by genetic changes in the phenotype of mediators, channels and receptors expressed by the afferent nerve, for example after peripheral nerve injury, many afferent fibers express newly formed adrenoreceptors (Bossut & Perl, 1995; Campbell, Meyer, & Raja, 1992; Sato & Perl, 1991; Xie, Yoon, Yom, & Chung, 1995); a change in the ligand-binding characteristics or coupling efficiency of these newly expressed receptors could alter the sensitivity of the afferent terminals. Neurotrophins, in particular nerve growth factor and glial-derived neurotropic factor, influence different populations of visceral afferents and play an important role in adaptive responses to nerve injury and inflammation (McMahon, 2004; Bielefeldt, Lamb, & Gebhart, 2006).

Central Pathways

Peripheral sensory information carried by primary afferents converges onto the CNS via the dorsal roots. The first synapse in the transmission of noxious information from the periphery to the brain is in the superficial dorsal horn of the spinal cord, which is comprised of lamina I and II (the marginal zone and substantia gelatinosa, respectively) (Sorkin & Carlton, 1997) . Lamina I of the spinal cord plays a key role in the modulation of pain transmission; its neurons have distinct response properties compared to neurons deeper in the dorsal horn (e.g. lamina V). The majority of these lamina I neurons are nociceptive-specific in their responses, a smaller number are polymodal nociceptive with an additional response to noxious cold, and a very few neurons are wide dynamic range (WDR). In lamina V the large majority are WDR so that information transmitted from dorsal horn neurons is almost entirely nociceptive in lamina I but spans the innocuous through the noxious range in lamina V. Lamina I neurons exhibit higher thresholds for excitation and generally have smaller mechanical and heat-evoked responses and receptive fields when compared to deeper dorsal horn neurons. By contrast to lamina II, which is comprised mainly of small intrinsic neurons terminating locally (Woolf & Fitzgerald, 1983), lamina I neurons typically have long axons thus allowing projection to higher CNS centers (Todd, 2002). The predominant ascending output from lamina I neurons appears to be the spino-parabrachial pathway in the rat (Hylden, Anton, & Nahin, 1989; Light, Sedivec, Casale, & Jones, 1993; Todd, 2002); however, a small proportion of lamina I neurons appears to project contralaterally via the lateral spinothalamic tract (STT), a key pathway for pain, itch and temperature (Craig & Dostrovsky, 2001; Marshall, Shehab, Spike, & Todd, 1996; Wall, Bery, & Saade, 1988). Neurons in the deep dorsal horn (lamina V–VI), however, have predominant projections in the STT. In recent years, lamina X neurons located around the central canal, have been shown to respond to somatic and visceral stimulation in the innocuous and noxious ranges (Al-Chaer, Lawand, Westlund, & Willis, 1996b). Despite their morphological diversity, some of these neurons have long axons projecting in the dorsal column to the caudal medulla, specifically to the dorsal column nuclei.

Pathways in the Ventral (Anterior) Quadrant

The Spinothalamic Tract

The spinothalamic tract (STT) is a major ascending pathway in primates and humans. It is classically associated with pain and temperature sensations and generally believed to mediate the sensations of pain, cold, warmth, and touch (Gybels & Sweet, 1989; Willis, 1985; Willis & Coggeshall, 2004). This belief is based largely on the results of anterolateral cordotomies performed to relieve pain (Foerster & Gagel, 1932; Spiller & Martin, 1912; White & Sweet, 1969) or deficits due to selective damage to the spinal cord by disease or trauma (Gowers, 1878; Head & Thompson, 1906; Noordenbos & Wall, 1976; Spiller, 1905). It is further reinforced by results of experimental studies of primates in which behavioral responses to noxious stimuli measured before and after spinal lesions were consistent with the clinical evidence (Vierck & Luck, 1979; Vierck, Greenspan, & Ritz, 1990; Yoss, 1953).

The STT arises largely from neurons in the dorsal horn of the spinal cord and projects to various areas in the thalamus (see Willis & Coggeshall, 2004). The locations of the cells of origin of the STT have been mapped in the rat, cat and monkey using retrograde tracing (Apkarian & Hodge, 1989a, 1989b; Carstens & Trevino, 1978; Craig, Linington, & Kniffki, 1989; Giesler, Menétrey, & Basbaum, 1979; Kevetter & Willis, 1982; Willis, Kenshalo, & Leonard, 1979) and antidromic activation methods (Albe-Fesssard, Levante, & Lamour, 1974a, 1974b; Giesler, Menétrey, Guilbaud, & Besson, 1976; Trevino, Maunz, Bryan, & Willis, 1972; Trevino, Coulter, & Willis, 1973). In monkeys, a large fraction of STT cells is located in the lumbar and sacral enlargements, and these cells are concentrated in the marginal zone and neck of the dorsal horn in laminae I and IV–VI (Apkarian & Hodge, 1989a; Willis et al., 1979). However, some spinothalamic cells are located in other laminae, including lamina X, which is around the central canal, and in the ventral horn. Tracing studies demonstrate that the STT distributes projections to several thalamic nuclei and that each have different anatomical and functional associations and, conversely, that the STT originates in several different cell groups that each have different anatomical and functional characteristics (Albe-Fessard, Berkley, Kruger, Ralston, & Willis, 1985; Apkarian & Hodge, 1989a, 1989b, 1989c; Boivie, 1979; Burton & Craig, 1983; Craig et al., 1989; Le Gros Clark, 1936; Mantyh, 1983; Mehler, Feferman, & Nauta, 1960; Willis et al., 1979). Comparison of the populations of STT cells projecting to the lateral thalamus, including the ventral posterior lateral nucleus, and those projecting to the medial thalamus, including the central lateral nucleus, show clear differences between the two (Craig & Zhang, 2006; Willis et al., 1979). Laterally projecting STT neurons are more likely to be situated in laminae I and V, whereas medially projecting cells are more likely to be situated in the deep dorsal horn and in the ventral horn. Most of the cells project to the contralateral thalamus, although a small fraction project ipsilaterally.

In general, the axons of STT neurons decussate through the ventral white commissure at a very short distance from the cell body (Willis et al., 1979). They initially enter the ventral funiculus and then shift into the lateral funiculus as they ascend. Axons from STT cells of lamina I ascend more dorsally in the lateral funiculus than do the axons of STT cells in deeper layers of the dorsal horn (Apkarian & Hodge, 1989b). Clinical evidence from anterolateral cordotomies indicates that spinothalamic axons in the anterolateral quadrant of the spinal cord are arranged somatotopically. At cervical levels, spinothalamic axons representing the lower extremity and caudal body are placed more laterally and those representing the upper extremity and rostral body more anteromedially (Hyndman & Van Epps, 1939; Walker, 1940). Recordings from spinothalamic axons in monkeys are consistent with this scheme (Applebaum, Beall, Foreman, & Willis, 1975).

In primates, STT axon terminals exist in the following nuclei: the caudal and oral parts of the ventral posterior lateral nucleus (VPLc and VPLo) (Olszewski, 1952), the ventral posterior inferior nucleus (VPI), the medial part of the posterior complex (POm), the central lateral (CL) nucleus, the ventral medial nucleus, and other intralaminar and medial thalamic nuclei (Apkarian &

Hodge, 1989c; Apkarian & Shi, 1994; Berkley, 1980; Boivie, 1979; Craig, Bushnell, Zhang, & Blomqvist, 1994; Gingold, Greenspan, & Apkarian, 1991; Kerr, 1975; Mantyh, 1983; Mehler et al., 1960; Mehler, 1962).

Primate STT cells that project to the lateral thalamus generally have receptive fields on a restricted area of the contralateral skin (Willis, Trevino, Coulter, & Maunz, 1974). Cells that project to the region of the CL nucleus in the medial thalamus may also collateralize to the lateral thalamus; these cells have response properties identical to those of STT cells that project just to the lateral thalamus (Giesler, Yezierski, Gerhart, & Willis, 1981), except for their larger receptive fields. Most of the neurons show their best responses when the skin is stimulated mechanically at a noxious intensity. However, many STT cells also respond to innocuous mechanical stimuli or noxious heating of the skin (Chung, Kenshalo, Gerhart, & Willis, 1979; Craig et al., 1994; Ferrington, Sorkin, & Willis, 1987; Kenshalo, Leonard, Chung, & Willis, 1979; Price & Mayer, 1975; Price, Hayes, Ruda, & Dubner, 1978; Surmeier, Honda, & Willis, 1986a, 1986b; Willis et al., 1974). Some spinothalamic neurons respond to stimulation of receptors in muscle (Foreman, Schmidt, & Willis, 1979), joints (Dougherty, Sluka, Sorkin, Westlund, & Willis, 1992), or viscera (Al-Chaer, Feng, & Willis, 1999; Ammons, 1989a, 1989b; Blair, Wenster, & Foreman, 1982; Blair, Ammons, & Foreman, 1984; Milne, Foreman, Giesler, & Willis, 1981).

These observations clearly suggest that the STT comprises several distinct components that each convey ascending activity selectively associated with different spinal functions (Craig & Zhang, 2006; Craig et al., 1989; Klop, Mouton, Kuipers, & Holstege, 2005; Stepniewska, Sakai, Qi, & Kaas, 2003; Truitt, Shipley, Veening, & Coolen, 2003;). Whether these distinct components imply segregated functions vis-à-vis the processing of pain information within the STT remains uncertain.

Several other pathways accompany the spinothalamic tract in the white matter of the ventrolateral quadrant of the spinal cord. These include the spinomesencephlic tract, the spinoreticular tracts, and several spino-limbic tracts. For a detailed review of these pathways, see Willis and Coggeshall (2004) and Willis and Westlund (1997).

Pathways in the Dorsal (Posterior) Quadrant

A number of pathways believed to be involved in pain processing originate in the dorsal horn and have axons that project in the dorsolateral and dorsal white matter of the spinal cord; these include the spinocervical pathway and the postsynaptic dorsal column.

Spinocervical Pathway

The spinocervical pathway originates from neurons in the spinal cord dorsal horn and relays in the lateral cervical nucleus in segments C1 and C2 (reviewed in Willis, 1985; Willis & Coggeshall, 2004). The axons of neurons of the lateral cervical nucleus decussate and then ascend with the medial lemniscus to the thalamus (Ha, 1971). A lateral cervical nucleus has been identified in several species, including rat, cat, and monkey (see Mizuno, Nakano, Imaizumi, & Okamoto, 1967). A comparable nucleus has been observed in at least some human spinal cords (Truex, Taylor, Smythe, & Gildenberg, 1965).

In cats, the cells of origin are situated mostly in lamina IV, although some are situated in adjacent laminae of the dorsal horn and in deeper layers (Brown, Fyffe, Noble, Rose, & Snow, 1980; Craig, 1978). The axons of spinocervical tract neurons ascend in the dorsal part of the lateral funiculus to the upper cervical level (Nijensohn & Kerr, 1975) and terminate in the lateral cervical nucleus. Cervicothalamic neurons project to the contralateral VPL nucleus and the medial part of the posterior complex (Berkley, 1980; Boivie, 1980; Smith & Apkarian, 1991). Many of the cells also give off collaterals to the midbrain (Willis & Coggeshall, 2004). Some spinocervical tract cells respond to noxious stimuli, both in cats (Brown & Franz, 1969; Cervero, Iggo, & Molony, 1977) and in monkeys (Bryan, Coulter, & Willis, 1974; Downie, Ferrington, Sorkin, & Willis, 1988); therefore, the spinocervical is considered a potential pathway through which nociceptive signals can reach the lateral thalamus.

The Dorsal Column

The dorsal funiculus, also referred to as the dorsal column (DC) in animals or the posterior column in man, contains collateral branches of primary afferent fibers that ascend from the dorsal root entry level all the way to the medulla (Willis & Coggeshall, 2004). In addition, it contains the ascending axons of tract cells of the dorsal horn (Angaut-Petit, 1975a, 1975b; Petit, 1972; Rustioni, 1973; Uddenburg, 1966, 1968). These tract cells form the postsynaptic dorsal column pathway (PSDC), which along with primary afferent axons, travel in the dorsal column and synapse in the dorsal column nuclei. The dorsal funiculus is subdivided into two components known as the fasciculus gracilis, containing the ascending afferents from levels caudal to the mid-thoracic region, and the fasciculus cuneatus, containing the ascending afferents that originate from mid-thoracic to upper cervical levels. The gracilis and cuneatus fasciculi terminate at the level of the lower medulla in the nucleus gracilis and the nucleus cuneatus respectively, collectively known as the dorsal column nuclei.

Classical teaching holds that the DC subserves graphesthesia, two-point discrimination, and kinesthesia. This concept was adopted at the turn of the 20th century (Brown-Sequard, 1868; Head & Thompson, 1906; Stanley, 1840; see also Davidoff, 1989) and was based on the pathologic alterations observed in certain disease states associated with DC lesions and on the skimpy knowledge of spinal tracts available at that time. On the other hand, the evidence for the importance of the DC pathway in the transmission of visceral nociceptive information is compelling. It rests on studies which highlight the great effectiveness of limited midline myelotomy in reducing intractable pelvic cancer pain in humans (Gildenberg & Hirshberg, 1984; Hirshberg, Al-Chaer, Lawand, Westlund, & Willis, 1996; Hitchcock, 1970, 1974; Schwarcz, 1976, 1978) and on a number of ground-breaking experimental observations (Al-Chaer, Lawand, Westlund, & Willis, 1996a, 1996b; Al-Chaer, Feng, & Willis, 1998a, 1998b; Al-Chaer et al., 1999; see also Willis, Al-Chaer, Quast, & Westlund, 1999).

In an early report on visceral nociceptive fibers in the DC, awake human subjects experienced unbearable, excruciating pain when the DC or medial aspect of the nucleus gracilis was probed mechanically (Foerster & Gagel, 1932). The pain was referred to the sacral region and perineum. Subsequent studies observed that the sensation of visceral distension was retained following extensive anterolateral cordotomy (White, 1943) and that the sensation of duodenal distension was unaffected by a differential spinal block which abolished the sensation of cutaneous pinprick (Sarnoff, Arrowood, & Chapman, 1948) suggesting that these sensations were mediated by a posterior column pathway.

More direct clinical evidence comes from successful neurosurgical procedures aimed at treating intractable visceral pain. These procedures have often accidentally severed DC axons in and around the midline. Commissural myelotomy was introduced as a technique to produce bilateral analgesia by interrupting the decussating axons of the spinothalamic and spinoreticular tracts by means of a longitudinal midline incision extending over several segments (Armour, 1927). The rostro-caudal extent of commissural myelotomy was later reduced to a localized lesion made stereotaxically by inserting a metal electrode into the midline at the C1 level with the patient awake (Hitchcock, 1970, 1974; Schwarcz, 1976, 1978). The clinical result was an unexpectedly widespread distribution of pain relief, similar to that found with open commissural myelotomy, despite the small extent of the lesion and its location well rostral to the decussation of most of the STT. Similar successes were reported later using limited midline myelotomy to treat pelvic visceral cancer pain (Gildenberg & Hirshberg, 1984). This result compelled a major revision in thinking regarding pain pathways in the spinal cord (Gybels & Sweet, 1989). Hirshberg et al. reported eight clinical cases where pelvic visceral cancer pain was successfully treated using a limited posterior midline myelotomy (1996). The lesion was placed in the midline at the T10 level of the spinal cord and extended a few mm rostrocaudally. Following surgery the pelvic pain was found to be markedly reduced or eliminated without any demonstrable postoperative neurological deficit. The extent of the lesion in one of the patients was examined histologically postmortem and was found to interrupt axons of the posterior columns at and adjacent to the midline and anteriorly to the level of the posterior gray commissure. More recent studies have lent further support for the concept that neurosurgical interruption of a midline posterior column pathway provides significant pain relief without causing adverse neurological sequelae in cancer patients with visceral pain refractory to other therapies (Kim & Kwon, 2000; Nauta, Hewitt, Westlund, & Willis, 1997; Nauta et al., 2000).

Early experimental evidence that described the DC as the pathway of splanchnic afferents was obtained in rabbits, cats and dogs (Amassian, 1951) and led to the conclusion that the sense of visceral distension may be dependent on the integrity of this afferent projection system. Responses to splanchnic nerve stimulation, were recorded "in logical time relationships", in the ipsilateral fasciculus gracilis of the spinal cord, the ipsilateral nucleus gracilis, the region of decussation of the medial lemniscus, the medial lemniscus at various levels in the medulla, pons and caudal thalamus and in the ventral posterior lateral (VPL) nucleus of the thalamus, suggesting a continuous pathway for splanchnic input that "parallels that for proprioception from the limbs and trunk" (Aidar, Geohegan, & Ungewitter, 1952). Nociceptive activity, including responses to uterine and vaginal distension, has also been demonstrated in neurons of the DC nuclei (Angaut-Petit, 1975a, 1975b; Berkley & Hubscher, 1995a, 1995b; Cliffer, Hasegawa, & Willis, 1992; Ferrington, Downie, & Willis, 1988). These nociceptive responses could be triggered by unmyelinated primary afferent fibers that have been shown to ascend in the dorsal column directly to the DC nuclei (Conti, De Biasi, Giuffrida, & Rustioni, 1990; Patterson, Coggeshall, Lee, & Chung, 1990; Patterson, Head, McNeill, Chung, & Coggeshall, 1989). Alternatively, they could be mediated through the postsynaptic dorsal column pathway (Bennett, Seltzer, Lu, Nishikawa, & Dubner, 1983; Bennett, Nishikawa, Hoffert, & Dubner, 1984; Noble & Riddell, 1988; Uddenburg, 1968). More recent studies in primates and rodents have shown that a lesion of the DC can dramatically reduce the responses of neurons in the VPL nucleus of the thalamus (Al-Chaer et al., 1996a, 1988; Al-Chaer, Feng, & Willis, 1998a; Ness, 2000) and in the DC nuclei (Al-Chaer et al., 1996b, 1999; Berkley & Hubscher, 1995a) to mechanical distension of normal and acutely inflamed colons. These studies have identified the DC as being more important in visceral nociceptive transmission than the spinothalamic and spinoreticular tracts. In rats and monkeys, colorectal distension stimulates the firing of viscerosensitive VPL thalamic neurons. After a DC lesion at T10 level, the responses are reduced despite ongoing stimulation. A similar lesion of the STT at T10 does not achieve the same effect (Al-Chaer et al., 1996a, 1998a). The DC also has a role in signaling epigastric nociception (Feng et al., 1998; see Willis et al., 1999).

The correspondence between these functional studies in experimental animals and the findings from human neurosurgical studies is consistent with accumulating evidence that strongly supports the concept that the DC projection system is critical for visceral pain sensation.

Postsynaptic Dorsal Column Pathway

The postsynaptic dorsal column (PSDC) pathway arises from cells distributed medial to laterally in lamina III in the dorsal horn, as well as from a few cells just lateral to lamina X (Bennett et al., 1983; Giesler, Nahin, & Madsen, 1984; Rustioni, 1973, 1974; Rustioni et al., 1979). The trajectories of postsynaptic dorsal

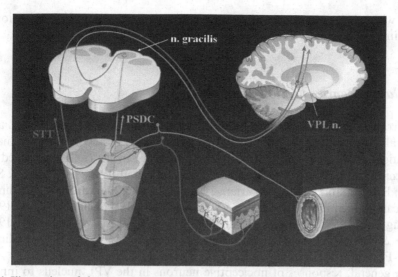

Fig. 1 Illustration of the postsynaptic dorsal column (PSDC) and the spinothalamic tract (STT) as they arise in the dorsal horn of the spinal cord and ascend towards the brainstem and eventually the thalamus. The PSDC pathway synapses on neurons in the dorsal column nuclei (DCN; the nucleus gracilis is labeled); axons of DCN neurons subsequently cross the midline and ascend in the medial lemniscus to converge onto thalamic neurons. The axons of STT neurons cross the midline at the dorsal horn level and ascend to the VPL nucleus of the thalamus in the anterolateral quadrant of the cord. Peripheral input is shown from the colon mainly onto the PSDC pathway and from the skin mainly onto the STT to illustrate the relative importance of these pathways in the nociception arising from these tissues respectively

column fibers are somatotopically organized in the dorsal column (Cliffer & Giesler, 1989; Hirshberg et al., 1996; Wang, Willis, & Westlund, 1999).

Although the PSDC pathway may not have a role in cutaneous pain (Al-Chaer et al., 1996b, 1999; Giesler & Cliffer, 1985), the postsynaptic dorsal column cells in rats and monkeys were shown to respond to both mechanical and chemical irritation of viscera (Al-Chaer et al., 1996b, 1999). They receive inputs from the colon, the ureter, the pancreas and epigastric structures (see Willis et al., 1999). Presumably, the visceral information is relayed together with cutaneous epicritic information in the medial lemniscus to the thalamus (Willis & Westlund, 1997). An illustration of the STT and the PSDC trajectories in the spinal cord to the thalamus can be seen in Fig. 1.

Representation of Nociceptive Sensation in the Brain

In contrast to most other sensory modalities, the neuroanatomical substrates in the brain for pain sensation in general and visceral pain in particular, have only recently begun to be elucidated. Major advances in this field have come through functional anatomical and physiological studies in non-human primates and rats, which have identified substrates that underlie findings from functional imaging and microelectrode studies in humans.

Thalamic Representation of Pain

Electrophysiological recordings made of nociceptive responses in the VPL and ventral posteromedial (VPM) nuclei of the thalamus in rats and monkeys by many investigators showed that neurons in these thalamic nuclei can be activated by nociceptive stimulation of the periphery (Al-Chaer et al. 1996a; Apkarian & Shi, 1994; Brüggemann, Shi, & Apkarian, 1994; Bushnell & Duncan, 1987; Bushnell, Duncan, & Tremblay, 1993; Casey & Morrow, 1983, 1987; Chandler et al., 1992; Chung et al., 1986; Duncan, Bushnell, Oliveras, Bastrash, & Tremblay, 1993; Gaze & Gordon, 1954; Kenshalo, Giesler, Leonard, & Willis, 1980; Pollin & Albe-Fessard, 1979; Yokota, Nishikawa, & Koyama, 1988).

In general, responses of nociceptive neurons in the VPL nucleus to innocuous cutaneous mechanical stimuli are weak, in contrast to their responses to noxious mechanical stimuli (Casey & Morrow, 1983, 1987; Chung et al., 1986; Kenshalo et al., 1980). The location of the neurons in the VPL nucleus is somatotopic but their receptive fields are relatively small and situated on the contralateral side. Almost all of the VPL neurons tested were shown by antidromic activation to project to the SI cortex (Kenshalo et al., 1980). Surprisingly, most neurons (85%) in the VPL nucleus respond to both cutaneous and visceral stimuli (Al-Chaer et al., 1996a, 1998b; Brüggemann et al., 1994; Chandler et al., 1992). Although the cutaneous input is somatotopic, the visceral input is not viscerotopic (Brüggemann et al., 1994).

Investigations of visceral inputs into the thalamus were made using electrical stimulation of visceral nerves (Aidar et al., 1952; Dell & Olson, 1951; McLeod, 1958; Patton & Amassian, 1951), or natural stimulation of visceral organs (Chandler et al., 1992; Davis & Dostrovsky, 1988; Emmers, 1966; Rogers, Novin, & Butcher, 1979). In monkeys, the medial thalamus receives viscerosomatic input via thoracic STT neurons (Ammons, Girardot, & Foreman, 1985), whereas neurons in the lateral thalamus are activated by input through the STT and the DC (Al-Chaer et al., 1998a). Lateral thalamic neurons can also be excited by colorectal distension or urinary bladder distension and by convergent input elicited by noxious stimulation of somatic receptive fields in proximal lower body regions (Chandler et al., 1992). In fact, the majority of lateral thalamic somatosensory neurons in squirrel monkeys receive somatovisceral and viscero-visceral inputs from naturally-stimulated visceral organs (Brüggemann et al., 1994). In the rat, neurons in and near the thalamic ventrobasal complex respond to stimulation of different visceral organs, including the uterus, the cervix, the vagina and the colon (Al-Chaer et al., 1996a, Berkley, Guilbaud, Benoist, & Gaultron, 1993). Colorectal distension or colon inflammation excites neurons in the ventral posterolateral nucleus of thalamus (Al-Chaer et al., 1996a; Berkley et al., 1993; Brüggemann et al., 1994) and in the medial thalamus at the level of the nucleus submedius (Kawakita, Sumiya, Murase, & Okada, 1997).

Microstimulation in the region of the thalamic principal sensory nucleus (the ventrocaudal nucleus) – a nucleus that corresponds to the ventral posterior nucleus in the cat and the monkey (Hirai & Jones, 1989; Jones, 1985) – can evoke a sensation of angina in humans (Lenz et al., 1994) and trigger in some cases pain "memories" (Davis, Tasker, Kiss, Hutchison, & Dostrovsky, 1995). Electrical stimulation of the thalamic ventrobasal complex in animals inhibits viscerosensory processing in normal rats but facilitates visceral hypersensitivity in rats with neonatal colon pain (Saab, Park, & Al-Chaer, 2004). These observations coupled with an extensive repertoire of experimental data suggest that the thalamus, particularly the posterolateral nucleus, is involved in the processing of visceral information, including both noxious and innocuous visceral inputs.

Nociceptive neurons also exist in the VPI and POm nuclei (Casey & Morrow, 1987; Apkarian & Shi, 1994; Pollin & Albe-Fessard, 1979). The cutaneous receptive fields of neurons in the VPI nucleus are somatotopically organized but tend to be larger than those of the VPL nociceptive neurons and presumably project to the SII cortex (Friedman, Murray, O'Neill, & Mishkin, 1986). The cells studied in the monkey POm nucleus had small, contralateral nociceptive receptive fields. The POm nucleus projects to the retroinsular cortex in monkeys (Burton & Jones, 1976).

Cortical Pain Processing

Anatomical, physiological, and lesion data implicate multiple cortical regions in the complex experience of pain (Head & Holmes, 1911; Kenshalo, Chudler, Anton, & Dubner, 1988; White & Sweet, 1969). These regions include primary and secondary somatosensory cortices, anterior cingulate cortex, insular cortex, and regions of the frontal cortex. Nevertheless, the role of different cortical areas in pain processing remains controversial. Studies of cortical lesions and cortical stimulation in humans did not uncover a clear role of various cortical areas in the pain experience and more recent human brain-imaging studies are not always consistent in revealing pain-related activation of somatosensory areas (see Bushnell et al., 1999). Despite this controversy, the application of functional magnetic resonance imaging (fMRI) and positron emission tomography (PET) has identified a network of brain areas that process painful sensation from a number of somatic regions including chronic pain states (see Apkarian, Bushnell, Treede, & Zubieta, 2005; Matre and Tuan, this volume; Peyron et al., 2000; Veldhuijzen et al., 2007) and from a number of visceral organs such as the esophagus (Aziz et al., 1997), stomach (Ladabaum et al., 2001) and the anorectum (Hobday et al., 2001). Results of these studies show activation of the primary somatosensory cortex (S1) by a range of noxious stimuli. These studies also confirm the somatotopic organization of S1 pain responses, thus supporting the role of S1 in pain localization. Other imaging data that implicate S1 in the sensory aspect of pain perception note that S1 activation is modulated by cognitive manipulations that alter perceived pain intensity but not by manipulations that alter unpleasantness, independent of pain intensity (Baliki et al., 2006).

Visceral sensation, on the other hand, is primarily represented in the secondary somatosensory cortex (S2). Unlike somatic sensation, which has a strong homuncular representation in S1, visceral representations in the primary somatosensory cortex are vague and diffuse (Aziz et al., 1997). This might account for visceral sensation being poorly localized in comparison with somatic sensation. Nevertheless, visceral sensation is represented in paralimbic and limbic structures (e.g., anterior insular cortex, amygdala, anterior and posterior cingulate cortex), and prefrontal and orbitofrontal cortices (Mertz et al., 2000; Silverman et al., 1997), areas that purportedly process the affective and cognitive components of visceral sensation (Derbyshire, 2003).

Differential cortical activation is also seen when comparing sensation from the visceral and somatic regions of the gastrointestinal tract, for example, sensations from the esophagus versus the anterior chest wall (Strigo, Duncan, Boivin, & Bushnell, 2003) or the rectum versus the anal canal (Hobday et al., 2001). Brain processing for esophageal and anterior chest wall sensations occur in a common brain network consisting of secondary somatosensory and parietal cortices, thalamus, basal ganglia and cerebellum (Strigo et al., 2003). Yet, differential processing of sensory information from these two areas occurred within the insular, primary sensory, motor, anterior cingulate and prefrontal cortices. These findings are consistent with other studies which highlight similarities in the visceral and somatic pain experience and might also explain the individual's ability to distinguish between the two modalities and generate differential emotional, autonomic and motor responses when each modality is individually stimulated.

Descending Modulatory Pathways

In addition to the afferent pathways that process nociceptive signals at different levels of the neuraxis, pain processing involves a number of modulatory controls that exist throughout the nervous system and function to enhance or dampen the intensity of the original signal or to modify its quality. At the level of the spinal cord, input from non-nociceptive and nociceptive afferent pathways can interact to modulate transmission of nociceptive information to higher brain centers. In addition, the brain contains modulatory systems that affect the conscious perception of sensory stimuli. Spinal nociceptive transmission is subject to descending modulatory influences from supraspinal structures e.g., periaqueductal gray, nucleus raphe magnus, locus ceruleus, nuclei reticularis gigantocellularis, and the ventrobasal complex of the thalamus (see Besson & Chaouch, 1987; Hodge, Apkarian, & Stevens, 1986]; Light, 1992; Peng, Lin, & Willis, 1996b; Willis, 1982). Descending modulation can be inhibitory, facilitatory or both depending on the context of the stimulus or the intensity of the descending signal (Saab et al., 2004; Zhuo & Gebhart, 2002). The descending influence from the ventromedial medulla is mediated mainly by pathways traveling in the dorsolateral spinal cord (Zhuo & Gebhart, 2002) and can be inhibitory or facilitatory based on stimulus intensity. In contrast, descending control from the thalamus is context-specific in that it may facilitate or inhibit spinal nociceptive processing depending upon the presence or absence of central sensitization (Saab et al., 2004). For instance, serotonergic (Peng, Lin, & Willis, 1995), noradrenergic (Peng, Lin, & Willis, 1996a; Proudfit, 1992), and to a lesser extent dopaminergic projections are major components of descending modulatory pathways (Dahlström & Fuxe, 1964, 1965), in addition to a major role played by opiates and enkephalins (Duggan & North, 1984; Duggan, Hall, & Headley, 1977).

Gender Differences in Pain Processing

Gender differences are a hallmark of pain perception particularly visceral pain; however, little is known about the biological causes of these differences (Fillingim, 2000; Keogh, this volume). Recent studies have shown that estrogen receptors located on nociceptive neurons in the spinal cord play an important role in the sexually-differentiated responses of these neurons to nociceptive visceral stimuli (Al-Chaer, unpublished observations). Similarly gender differences have been reported in the cortical representation of pain. Activation in the sensory-motor and parieto-occipital areas is common in both males and females following rectal distension; however, greater activation in the anterior cingulate/prefrontal cortices have been found in women (Kern et al., 2001). These actual gender differences in the processing of sensory input substantiate reports that perceptual responses are exaggerated in female patients with chronic pain.

Conclusion

It is important to keep in mind that these pathways, while seemingly anatomically segregated and traditionally perceived as conveying specific perceptions of pain, are in fact functionally dynamic, interactive polymodal channels for visceral, cutaneous, muscular and proprioceptive sensations, in addition to possible motor, autonomic and not as yet defined functions. As such, the STT as well as the DC can be regarded as interactive polymodal channels for visceral, somatic and autonomic events with sorted priorities for the sake of immediate, reliable and simple readings of acute and transient but complex situations. These breakthroughs in defining pain mechanisms and pathways have advanced the field of pain research and management particularly in the areas of drug development. However, despite these extraordinarily impressive scientific advances in our understanding of the mechanisms of pain and describing some of its pathways, the field is beset by similarly and equally impressive stalemates and retreats in the actual management and cure of pain. After all, knowledge about pain and its mechanisms is only useful to the extent it helps the sufferer.

For pain relief, we naturally use anything that works; historically we used trephination, opiates and willow bark. Today, regardless of their site of action, we continue to use some of the same techniques that worked albeit in different pharmaceutical formulae and more controlled environments... but the nervous system seems to be extremely resistant to switching off pain!

Future Directions

Basic translational research in the immediate and extended future can be expected to maintain ongoing progress in each of the following areas:

1. Continued mechanistic focus on the basic science of pain that includes the molecular basis for peripheral sensitization of sensory receptors by inflammatory mediators, selectivity of central pain-related transmission pathways, and higher-order central processing of nociceptive information from the periphery.
2. Integration of imaging technology and classic neurophysiologic and neuropharmacologic approaches for improved understanding of the neurobiology of pain.
3. Expanded investigation of the psychoneuroendocrine pathways, which are not only responsible for alteration of function during psychogenic stress and the exacerbation of chronic pain states, but which also may be partly responsible for gender differences in pain.
4. Enhanced focus on the identification of drug targets on neuronal elements of the nervous system and on nonneuronal cell types, such as glia, which release substances that alter the activity of neurons (Saab, Wang, Gu, Garner, & Al-Chaer, 2007).

Acknowledgments The author would like to thank Ms. Kirsten Garner for assistance with editing the manuscript. This work was supported by NIH Grant RR020146.

References

Aidar, O., Geohegan, W. A., & Ungewitter, L. H. (1952). Splanchnic afferent pathways in the central nervous system. *Journal of Neurophysiology*, *15*, 131–138.
Al-Chaer, E. D., & Traub, R. J. (2002). Biological basis of visceral pain: Recent developments. *Pain*, *96*(3), 221–225.

Al-Chaer, E. D., & Willis, W. D. (2007). Neuroanatomy of visceral pain: Pathways and processes. In P. J. Pasricha, W. D. Willis, & G. F. Gebhart (Eds.), *Chronic abdominal and visceral pain: Theory and practice* (pp. 33–44). New York: Informa Health Care, Inc.

Al-Chaer, E. D., Lawand, N. B., Westlund, K. N., & Willis, W. D. (1996a). Visceral nociceptive input into the ventral posterolateral nucleus of the thalamus: A new function for the dorsal column pathway. *Journal of Neurophysiology, 76,* 2661–2674.

Al-Chaer, E. D., Lawand, N. B., Westlund, K. N., & Willis, W. D. (1996b). Pelvic visceral input into the nucleus gracilis is largely mediated by the postsynaptic dorsal column pathway. *Journal of Neurophysiology, 76,* 2675–2690.

Al-Chaer, E. D., Feng, Y., & Willis, W. D. (1998a). A role for the dorsal column in nociceptive visceral input into the thalamus of primates. *Journal of Neurophysiology, 79,* 3143–3150.

Al-Chaer, E. D., Feng, Y., & Willis, W. D. (1998b). Visceral pain: A disturbance in the sensorimotor continuum? *Pain Forum, 7*(3), 117–125.

Al-Chaer, E. D., Feng, Y., & Willis, W. D. (1999). A comparative study of viscerosomatic input onto postsynaptic dorsal column and spinothalamic tract neurons in the primate. *Journal of Neurophysiology, 82*(4), 1876–1882.

Al-Chaer, E. D., Kawasaki, M., & Pasricha, P. J. (2000). A new model of chronic visceral hypersensitivity in adult rats induced by colon irritation during postnatal development. *Gastroenterology, 119*(5), 1276–1285.

Albe-Fesssard, D., Levante, A., & Lamour, Y. (1974a). Origin of spinothalamic and spinoreticular pathways in cats and monkeys. *Advances in Neurology, 4,* 157–166.

Albe-Fesssard, D., Levante, A., & Lamour, Y. (1974b). Origin of spino-thalamic tract in monkeys. *Brain Research, 65,* 503–509.

Albe-Fessard, D., Berkley, K. J., Kruger, L., Ralston, H. J. III, & Willis, W. D., Jr (1985). Diencephalic mechanisms of pain sensation. *Brain Research Reviews, 9,* 217–296.

Amassian, V. E. (1951). Fiber groups and spinal pathways of cortically represented visceral afferents. *Journal of Neurophysiology, 14,* 445–460.

Ammons, W. S. (1989a). Primate spinothalamic cell responses to ureteral occlusion. *Brain Research, 496,* 124–30.

Ammons, W. S. (1989b). Electrophysiological characteristics of primate spinothalamic neurons with renal and somatic inputs. *Journal of Neurophysiology, 60,* 1121–30.

Ammons, W. S., Girardot, M. N., & Foreman, R. D. (1985). T2–T5 spinothalamic neurons projecting to medial thalamus with viscerosomatic input. *Journal of Neurophysiology, 54,* 73–89.

Angaut-Petit, D. (1975a). The dorsal column system: I. Existence of long ascending postsynaptic fibres in the cat's fasciculus gracilis. *Experimental Brain Research, 22,* 457–470.

Angaut-Petit, D. (1975b). The dorsal column system: II. Functional properties and bulbar relay of the postsynaptic fibres of the cat's fasciculus gracilis. *Experimental Brain Research, 22,* 471–493.

Apkarian, A. V., & Hodge, C. J. J. (1989a). The primate spinothalamic pathways: I. A quantitative study of the cells of origin of the spinothalamic pathway. *Journal of Comparative Neurology, 288,* 447–473.

Apkarian, A. V., & Hodge, C. J. J. (1989b). The primate spinothalamic pathways: II. The cells of origin of the dorsolateral and ventral spinothalamic pathways. *Journal of Comparative Neurology, 288,* 474–492.

Apkarian, A. V., & Hodge, C. J. J. (1989c). Primate spinothalamic pathways: III. Thalamic terminations of the dorsolateral and ventral spinothalamic pathways. *Journal of Comparative Neurology, 288,* 493–511.

Apkarian, A. V., & Shi, T. (1994). Squirrel monkey lateral thalamus. I. Somatic nociresponsive neurons and their relation to spinothalamic terminals. *Journal of Neuroscience, 14,* 6779–95.

Apkarian, A. V., Bushnell, M. C., Treede, R. D., & Zubieta, J. K. (2005). Human brain mechanisms of pain perception and regulation in health and disease. *European Journal of Pain, 9*(4), 463–484.

Applebaum, A. E., Beall, J. E., Foreman, R. D., & Willis, W. D. (1975). Organization and receptive fields of primate spinothalamic tract neurons. *Journal of Neurophysiology, 38,* 572–86.

Armour, D. (1927). On the surgery of the spinal cord and its membranes. *Lancet, 2,* 691–697.

Aziz, Q., Andersson, J. L., Valind, S., Sundin, A., Hamdy, S., Jones, A. K., et al. (1997). Identification of human brain loci processing esophageal sensation using positron emission tomography. *Gastroenterology, 113,* 50–9.

Baliki, M. N., Chialvo, D. R., Geha, P. Y., Levy, R. M., Harden, R. N., Parrish, T. B., et al. (2006). Chronic pain and the emotional brain: Specific brain activity associated with spontaneous fluctuations of intensity of chronic back pain. *Journal of Neuroscience, 26*(47), 12165–12173.

Bennett, G. J., Seltzer, Z., Lu, G. W., Nishikawa, N., & Dubner, R. (1983). The cells of origin of the dorsal column postsynaptic projection in the lumbosacral enlargements of cats and monkeys. *Somatosensory Research, 1,* 131–49.

Bennett, G. J., Nishikawa, N., Lu, G. W., Hoffert, M. J., & Dubner, R. (1984). The morphology of dorsal column postsynaptic (DCPS) spino-medullary neurons in the cat. *Journal of Comparative Neurology, 224,* 568–78.

Berkley, K. J. (1980). Spatial relationships between the terminations of somatic sensory and motor pathways in the rostral brainstem of cats and monkeys. I. Ascending somatic sensory inputs to lateral diencephalon. *Journal of Comparative Neurology, 193,* 283–317.

Berkley, K. J., & Hubscher, C. H. (1995a). Are there separate central nervous system pathways for touch and pain? *Nature Medicine, 1*(8), 766–773.

Berkley, K. J., & Hubscher, C. H. (1995b). Visceral and somatic sensory tracks through the neuraxis and their relation to pain: Lessons from the rat female reproductive system. In: G. F. Gebhart (Ed.), *Visceral Pain* (pp. 195–216). Seattle: IASP Press.

Berkley, K. J., Guilbaud, G., Benoist, J., & Gautron, M. (1993). Responses of neurons in and near the thalamic ventrobasal complex of the rat to stimulation of uterus, cervix, vagina, colon, and skin. *Journal of Neurophysiology, 69,* 557–568.

Besson, J. M., & Chaouch, A. (1987). Peripheral and spinal mechanisms of nociception. *Physiological Reviews, 67,* 67–186.

Bielefeldt, K., Lamb, K., & Gebhart, G.F. (2006). Convergence of sensory pathways in the development of somatic and visceral hypersensitivity. *American Journal of Physiology. Gastrointestinal and Liver Physiology, 291*(4), G658–G665.

Birrell, G. J., McQueen, D. S., Iggo, A., & Grubb, B. D. (1993). Prostanoid-induced potentiation of the excitatory and sensitizing effects of bradykinin on articular mechanonociceptors in the rat ankle joint. *Neuroscience, 54,* 537–44.

Blair, R. W., Wenster, R. N., & Foreman, R. D. (1982). Responses of thoracic spinothalamic neurons to intracardiac injection of bradykinin in the monkey. *Circulation Research, 51,* 83–94.

Blair, R. W., Ammons, W. S., & Foreman, R. D. (1984). Responses of thoracic spinothalamic and spinoreticular cells to coronary artery occlusion. *Journal of Neurophysiology, 51,* 636–48.

Boivie, J. (1979). An anatomical reinvestigation of the termination of the spinothalamic tract in the monkey. *Journal of Comparative Neurology, 186,* 343–370.

Boivie, J. (1980). Thalamic projections from lateral cervical nucleus in monkey. A degeneration study. *Brain Research, 198*(1), 13–26.

Boivie, J., Leijon, G., & Johansson, I. (1989). Central post-stroke pain—a study of the mechanisms through analyses of the sensory abnormalities. *Pain, 37,* 173–85.

Bonica, J. J. (2001). *Bonica's management of pain* (3rd ed.) J. D. Loeser (Ed.). Philadelphia, PA: Lippincott Williams and Wilkins.

Bossut, D. F., & Perl, E. R. (1995). Effects of nerve injury on sympathetic excitation of A[delta] mechanical nociceptors. *Journal of Neurophysiology, 73,* 1721–23.

Brown, A. G., & Franz, D. N. (1969). Responses of spinocervical tract neurones to natural stimulation of identified cutaneous receptors. *Experimental Brain Research, 7*, 231–49.

Brown, A. G., Fyffe, R. E. W., Noble, R., Rose, P. K., & Snow, P. J. (1980). The density, distribution and topographical organization of spinocervical tract neurones in the cat. *Journal of Physiology, 300*, 409–28.

Brown-Sequard, E. (1868). Lectures on the physiology and pathology of the central nervous system and on the treatment of organic nervous affections. *Lancet, 2*, 593–823.

Brüggemann, J., Shi, T., & Apkarian, A. V. (1994). Squirrel monkey lateral thalamus. II. Viscerosomatic convergent representation of urinary bladder, colon, and esophagus. *Journal of Neuroscience, 14*, 6796–814.

Bryan, R. N., Coulter, J. D., & Willis, W. D. (1974). Cells of origin of the spinocervical tract in the monkey. *Experimental Neurology, 42*, 574–86.

Burton, H., & Craig, A. D. (1983). Spinothalamic projections in cat, raccoon and monkey: A study based on anterograde transport of horseradish peroxidase. In: G. Macchi, A. Rustioni & R. Spreafico (Eds.), *Somatosensory integration in the thalamus* (pp. 17–41). New York: Elsevier.

Burton, H., & Jones, E. G. (1976). The posterior thalamic region and its cortical projection in New World and Old World monkeys. *Journal of Comparative Neurology, 168*, 249–302.

Bushnell, M. C., & Duncan, G. H. (1987). Mechanical response properties of ventroposterior medial thalamic neurons in the alert monkey. *Experimental Brain Research, 67*, 603–14.

Bushnell, M. C., Duncan, G. H., & Tremblay, N. (1993). Thalamic VPM nucleus in the behaving monkey. I. Multimodal and discriminative properties of thermosensitive neurons. *Journal of Neurophysiology, 69*, 739–752.

Bushnell, M. C., Duncan, G. H., Hofbauer, R. K., Ha, B., Chen, J. I., & Carrier, B. (1999). Pain perception: Is there a role for primary somatosensory cortex? *Proceedings of the National Academy of Science of the USA, 96*(14), 7705–7709.

Campbell, J. N., Meyer, R. A., & Raja, S. N. (1992). Is nociceptor activation by alpha-1 adrenoreceptors the culprit in sympathetically maintained pain? *American Pain Society Journal, 1*, 3–11.

Carstens, E., & Trevino, D. L. (1978). Laminar origins of spinothalamic projections in the cat as determined by the retrograde transport of horseradish peroxidase. *Journal of Comparative Neurology, 182*, 151–166.

Casey, K. L., & Morrow, T. J. (1983). Ventral posterior thalamic neurons differentially responsive to noxious stimulation of the awake monkey. *Science, 221*, 675–7.

Casey, K. L., & Morrow, T. J. (1987). Nociceptive neurons in the ventral posterior thalamus of the awake squirrel monkey: Observations on identification, modulation, and drug effects. In: J. M. Besson, G. Guilbaud, & M Peschanski (Eds.), *Thalamus and pain* (pp. 211–226). Amsterdam: Exerpta Medica.

Cervero, F., Iggo, A., & Molony, V. (1977). Responses of spinocervical tract neurones to noxious stimulation of the skin. *Journal of Physiology, 267*, 537–58.

Chandler, M. J., Hobbs, S. F., Qing-Gong, F., Kenshalo, D. R., Blair, R. W., & Foreman, R. D. (1992). Responses of neurons in ventroposterolateral nucleus of primate thalamus to urinary bladder distension. *Brain Research, 571*, 26–34.

Chaturvedi, SK. (1987). Prevalence of chronic pain in psychiatric patients. *Pain, 29*, 231–237.

Chung, J. M., Kenshalo, D. R., Gerhart, K. D., & Willis, W. D. (1979). Excitation of primate spinothalamic neurons by cutaneous C-fiber volleys. *Journal of Neurophysiology, 42*, 1354–69.

Chung, J. M., Surmeier, D. J., Lee, K. H., Sorkin, L. S., Honda, C. N., Tsong, Y., et al. (1986). Classification of primate spinothalamic and somatosensory thalamic neurons based on cluster analysis. *Journal of Neurophysiology, 56*, 308–27.

Cliffer, K. D., & Giesler, G. J., Jr. (1989). Postsynaptic dorsal column pathway of the rat. III. Distribution of ascending afferent fibers. *Journal of Neuroscience, 9*, 3146–68.

Cliffer, K. D., Hasegawa, T., & Willis, W. D. (1992). Responses of neurons in the gracile nucleus of cats to innocuous and noxious stimuli: Basic characterization and antidromic activation from the thalamus. *Journal of Neurophysiology, 68*, 818–832.

Conti, F., De Biasi, S., Giuffrida, R., & Rustioni, R. (1990). Substance P-containing projections in the dorsal columns of rats and cats. *Neuroscience, 34*, 607–21.

Craig, A. D. (1978). Spinal and medullary input to the lateral cervical nucleus. *Journal of Comparative Neurology, 181*, 729–44.

Craig, A., & Dostrovsky, J. (2001). Differential projections of thermoreceptive and nociceptive lamina I trigeminothalamic and spinothalamic neurons in the cat. *Journal of Neurophysiology, 86*, 856–870.

Craig, A. D., & Zhang, E. T. (2006). Retrograde analyses of spinothalamic projections in the macaque monkey: Input to posterolateral thalamus. *Journal of Comparative Neurology, 499* (6), 953–964.

Craig, A. D., Linington, A. J., & Kniffki, K. D. (1989). Cells of origin of spinothalamic projections to medial and/or lateral thalamus in the cat. *Journal of Comparative Neurology, 289*, 568–585.

Craig, A. D., Bushnell, M. C., Zhang, E. T., & Blomqvist, A. (1994). A thalamic nucleus specific for pain and temperature sensation. *Nature, 372*, 770–3.

Dahlström, A., & Fuxe, K. (1964). Evidence for the existence of monoamine-containing neurons in the central nervous system. I. Demonstration of monoamines in the cell bodies of brain stem neurones. *Acta Physiologica Scandinavica, 62*(suppl 232), 1–55.

Dahlström, A., & Fuxe, K. (1965). Evidence for the existence of monoamine neurons in the central nervous system. II. Experimentally induced changes in the intraneuronal amine levels of bulbospinal neurons systems. *Acta Physiologica Scandinavica, 64*(suppl 247), 1–36.

Davidoff, R. A. (1989). The dorsal columns. *Neurology, 39*, 1377–1385.

Davis, K. D., & Dostrovsky, J. O. (1988). Properties of feline thalamic neurons activated by stimulation of the middle meningeal artery and sagittal sinus. *Brain Research, 454*, 89–100.

Davis, K. D., Meyer, R. A., & Campbell, J. N. (1993). Chemosensitivity and sensitization of nociceptive afferents that innervate the hairy skin of monkey. *Journal of Neurophysiology, 69*, 1071–81.

Davis, K. D., Tasker, R. R., Kiss, Z. H. T., Hutchison, W. D., & Dostrovsky, J. O. (1995). Visceral pain evoked by thalamic microstimulation in humans. *NeuroReport, 6*, 369–374.

Dell, P., & Olson, R. (1951). Projections thalamiques, corticales et cerebelleuses des afferences viscerales vagales. *Comptes rendus des séances de la Société de biologie et de ses filiales, 145*, 1084–1088.

Derbyshire, S. W. (2003). A systematic review of neuroimaging data during visceral stimulation. *American Journal of Gastroenterology, 98*, 12–20.

Descartes, R. (1664). *L'Homme.* Paris: e. Angot.

Dougherty, P. M., Sluka, K. A., Sorkin, L. S., Westlund, K. N., & Willis, W. D. (1992). Neural changes in acute arthritis in monkeys. I. Parallel enhancement of responses of spinothalamic tract neurons to mechanical stimulation and excitatory amino acids. *Brain Reearchs Reviews, 17*, 1–13.

Downie, J. W., Ferrington, D. G., Sorkin, L. S., & Willis, W. D. (1988). The primate spinocervicothalamic pathway: Responses of cells of the lateral cervical nucleus and spinocervical tract to innocuous and noxious stimuli. *Journal of Neurophysiology, 59*, 861–85.

Dray, A., Bettaney, J., Forster, P., & Perkins, M. N. (1988). Bradykinin-induced stimulation of afferent fibres is mediated through protein kinase C. *Neuroscience Letters, 91*, 301–7.

Dray, A., Urban, L., & Dickenson, A. (1994). Pharmacology of chronic pain. *Trends in Pharmacological Sciences, 15*(6), 190–197.

Duggan, A. W., & North, R. A. (1984). Electrophysiology of opioids. *Pharmacological Reviews, 35*, 219–81.

Duggan, A. W., Hall, J. G., & Headley, P. M. (1977). Enkephalins and dorsal horn neurones of the cat: Effects on responses to noxious and innocuous skin stimuli. *British Journal of Pharmacology*, *61*, 399–408.

Duncan, G. H., Bushnell, M. C., Oliveras, J. L., Bastrash, N., & Tremblay, N. (1993). Thalamic VPM nucleus in the behaving monkey. III. Effects of reversible inactivation by lidocaine on thermal and mechanical discrimination. *Journal of Neurophysiology*, *70*, 2086–96.

Emmers, R. (1966). Seperate relays of tactile, pressure, thermal, and gustatory modalities in the cat thalamus. *Proceedings of the Society for Experimental Biology and Medicine*, *121*, 527–531.

Feng, Y., Cui, M., Al-Chaer, E. D., & Willis, W. D. (1998). Epigastric antinociception by cervical dorsal column lesions in rats. *Anesthesiology*, *89*(2), 411–420.

Ferrington, D. G., Sorkin, L. S., & Willis, W. D. (1987). Responses of spinothalamic tract cells in the superficial dorsal horn of the primate lumbar spinal cord. *Journal of Physiology*, *388*, 681–703.

Ferrington, D. G., Downie, J. W., & Willis, W. D. (1988). Primate nucleus gracilis neurons: Responses to innocuous and noxious stimuli. *Journal of Neurophysiology*, *59*, 886–907.

Fillingim R. B. (Ed.) (2000). *Sex, gender, and pain*. Progress in Pain Research and Management, volume 17. Seattle: IASP Press.

Foerster, O., & Gagel, O. (1932). Die Vorderseitenstrangdurchschneidung beim Menschen. Eine klinisch-patho-physiologisch-anatomische Studie. *Zeitschrift für die Gesamte Neurologie und Psychiatrie*, *138*, 1–92.

Foreman, R. D., Schmidt, R. F., & Willis, W. D. (1979). Effects of mechanical and chemical stimulation of fine muscle afferents upon primate spinothalamic tract cells. *Journal of Physiology*, *286*, 215–31.

Friedman, D. R., Murray, E. A., O'Neill, J. B., & Mishkin, M. (1986). Cortical connections of the somatosensory fields of the lateral sulcus of macaques: Evidence for a corticolimbic pathway for touch. *Journal of Comparative Neurology*, *252*, 323–47.

Gaze, R. M., & Gordon, G. (1954). The representation of cutaneous sense in the thalamus of the cat and monkey. *Journal of Experimental Physiology*, *39*, 279–304.

Giesler, G. J., Jr, & Cliffer, K. D. (1985). Postsynaptic dorsal column pathway of the rat. II. Evidence against an important role in nociception. *Brain Research*, *326*(2), 347–356.

Giesler, G. J. J., Menétrey, D., Guilbaud, G., & Besson, J. (1976). Lumbar cord neurons at the origin of the spinothalamic tract in the rat. *Brain Research*, *118*, 320–324.

Giesler, G. J. J., Menétrey, D., & Basbaum, A. I. (1979). Differential origins of spinothalamic tract projections to medial and lateral thalamus in the rat. *Journal of Comparative Neurology*, *184*, 107–126.

Giesler, G. J., Yezierski, R. P., Gerhart, K. D., & Willis, W. D. (1981). Spinothalamic tract neurons that project to medial and/or lateral thalamic nuclei: Evidence for a physiologically novel population of spinal cord neurons. *Journal of Neurophysiology*, *46*, 1285–308.

Giesler, G. J., Nahin, R. L., & Madsen, A. M. (1984). Postsynaptic dorsal column pathway of the rat. I. Anatomical studies. *Journal of Neurophysiology*, *51*, 260–75.

Gildenberg, P. L., & Hirshberg, R. M. (1984). Limited myelotomy for the treatment of intractable cancer pain. *Journal of Neurology, Neurosurgery & Psychiatry*, *47*, 94–96.

Gingold, S. I., Greenspan, J. D., & Apkarian, A. V. (1991). Anatomic evidence of nociceptive inputs to primary somatosensory cortex: Relationship between spinothalamic terminals and thalamocortical cells in squirrel monkeys. *Journal of Comparative Neurology*, *308*, 467–90.

Gowers, W. R. (1878). A case of unilateral gunshot injury to the spinal cord. *Transactions of the Clinical Society of London*, *11*, 24–32.

Grundy, D., Al-Chaer, E. D., Aziz, Q., Collins, S. M., Ke, M., Tache, Y., et al. (2006). Fundamentals of neurogastroenterology: Basic science. *Gastroenterology*, *130*(5), 1391–1411.

Gybels, J. M., & Sweet, W. H. (Eds.) (1989). Neurosurgical treatment of persistent pain. Basel: Karger.

Ha, H. (1971). Cervicothalamic tract in the Rhesus monkey. *Experimental Neurology, 33,* 205–12.

Häbler, H. J., Jänig, W., & Koltzenburg, M. (1990). Activation of unmyelinated afferent fibres by mechanical stimuli and inflammation of the urinary bladder in the cat. *Journal of Physiology, 425,* 545–562.

Head, H., & Holmes, G. (1911). Sensory disturbances from cerebral lesions. *Brain, 34,* 102–254.

Head, H., & Thompson, T. (1906). The grouping of afferent impulses within the spinal cord. *Brain, 29,* 537–741.

Hirai, T., & Jones, E. G. (1989). A new parcellation of the human thalamus on the basis of histochemical staining. *Brain Research Reviews, 14,* 1–34.

Hirshberg, R. M., Al-Chaer, E. D., Lawand, N. B., Westlund, K. N., & Willis, W. D. (1996). Is there a pathway in the posterior funiculus that signals visceral pain? *Pain, 67,* 291–305.

Hitchcock, E. R. (1970). Stereotactic cervical myelotomy. *Journal of Neurology, Neurosurgery & Psychiatry, 33,* 224–230.

Hitchcock, E. R. (1974). Stereotactic myelotomy. *Proceedings of the Royal Society of Medicine, 67,* 771–772.

Hobday, D. I., Aziz, Q., Thacker, N., Hollander, I., Jackson, A., & Thompson, D. G. (2001). A study of the cortical processing of ano-rectal sensation using functional MRI. *Brain, 124,* 361–8.

Hodge, C. J., Apkarian, A. V., & Stevens, R. T. (1896). Inhibition of dorsal-horn cell responses by stimulation of the Kölliker-Fuse nucleus. *Journal of Neurosurgery, 65,* 825–33.

Hylden, J. L., Anton, F., & Nahin, R. L. (1989). Spinal lamina I projection neurons in the rat: Collateral innervation of parabrachial area and thalamus. *Neuroscience, 28,* 27–37.

Hyndman, O. R., & Van Epps, C. (1939). Possibility of differential section of the spinothalamic tract. *Archives of Surgery, 38,* 1036–53.

Jones, E. G. (1985). *The Thalamus.* New York: Plenum.

Joshi, S. K., Su, X., Porreca, F., & Gebhart, G. F. (2000). Kappa-Opioid receptor agonists modulate visceral nociception at a novel, peripheral site of action. *Journal of Neuroscience, 20,* 5874–5879.

Kajander, K. C., & Bennett, G. J. (1992). Onset of a painful peripheral neuropathy in rat: A partial and differential deafferentation and spontaneous discharge in A beta and A delta primary afferent neurons. *Journal of Neurophysiology, 68*(3), 734–744.

Kawakita, K., Sumiya, E., Murase, K., & Okada, K. (1997). Response characteristics of nucleus submedius neurons to colo-rectal distension in the rat. *Neuroscience Research, 28*(1), 59–66.

Kenshalo, D. R., Leonard, R. B., Chung, J. M., & Willis, W. D. (1979). Responses of primate spinothalamic neurons to graded and to repeated noxious heat stimuli. *Journal of Neurophysiology, 42,* 1370–89.

Kenshalo, D. R., Giesler, G. J., Leonard, R. B., & Willis, W. D. (1980). Responses of neurons in primate ventral posterior lateral nucleus to noxious stimuli. *Journal of Neurophysiology, 43,* 1594–614.

Kenshalo, D. R., Chudler, E. H., Anton, F., & Dubner, R. (1988). SI cortical nociceptive neurons participate in the encoding process by which monkeys perceive the intensity of noxious thermal stimulation. *Brain Research, 454,* 378–382.

Kern, M. K., Jaradeh, S., Arndorfer, R. C., Jesmanowicz, A., Hyde, J., & Shaker, R. (2001). Gender differences in cortical representation of rectal distension in healthy humans. *American Journal of Physiology – Gastrointestinal and Liver Physiology, 281,* G1512–23.

Kerr, F. W. L. (1975). The ventral spinothalamic tract and other ascending systems of the ventral funiculus of the spinal cord. *Journal of Comparative Neurology, 159,* 335–56.

Kevetter, G. A., & Willis, W. D. (1982). Spinothalamic cells in the rat lumbar cord with collaterals to the medullary reticular formation. *Brain Research, 238*, 181–185.

Kim, Y. S., & Kwon, S. J. (2000). High thoracic midline dorsal column myelotomy for severe visceral pain due to advanced stomach cancer. *Neurosurgery, 46*(1), 85–92.

Kirkup, A. J., Brunsden, A. M., & Grundy, D. (2001). Receptors and transmission in the brain-gut axis: Potential for novel therapies. I. Receptors on visceral afferents. *American Journal of Physiology – Gastrointestinal and Liver Physiology, 280*, G787–G794.

Klop, E. M., Mouton, L. J., Kuipers, R., & Holstege, G. (2005). Neurons in the lateral sacral cord of the cat project to periaqueductal grey, but not to thalamus. European Journal of Neuroscience, 21, 2159–2166.

Konietzny ,F., Perl, E. R., Trevino, D., Light, A., & Hensel, H. (1981). Sensory experiences in man evoked by intraneural electrical stimulation of intact cutaneous afferent fibers. *Experimental Brain Research, 42*, 219–22.

Ladabaum, U., Minoshima, S., Hasler, W. L., Cross, D. Chey, W. D., & Owyang, C. (2001). Gastric distention correlates with activation of multiple cortical and subcortical regions. *Gastroenterology, 120*, 369–76.

LaMotte, R. H., Thalhammer, J. G., Torebjörk, H. E., & Robinson, C. J. (1982). Peripheral neural mechanisms of cutaneous hyperalgesia following mild injury by heat. *Journal of Neuroscience, 2*, 765–81.

LaMotte, R. H., Thalhammer, J. G., & Robinson, C. J. (1983). Peripheral neural correlates of magnitude of cutaneous pain and hyperalgesia: A comparison of neural events in monkey with sensory judgments in human. *Journal of Neurophysiology, 50*, 1–26.

Le Gros Clark, W. E. (1936). The termination of ascending tracts in the thalamus of the macaque monkey. *Journal of Anatomy, 71*, 7–40.

Lenz, F. A., Gracely, R. H., Hope, E. J., Baker, F. H., Rowland, L. H., Dougherty, P. M., et al. (1994). The sensation of angina can be evoked by stimulation of the human thalamus. *Pain, 59*, 119–125.

Light, A. R. (1992). *The initial processing of pain and its descending control: Spinal and trigeminal systems*. Basel: Karger.

Light, A., Sedivec, M., Casale, E., & Jones, S. (1993). Physiological and morphological characteristics of spinal neurones projecting to the parabrachial region of the cat. *Somatosensory and Motor Research, 10*, 309–325.

Lynn, B., & Carpenter, S. E. (1982). Primary afferent units from the hairy skin of the rat hind limb. *Brain Research, 238*(1), 29–43.

Maggi, C. A., & Meli, A. (1988). The sensory-efferent function of capsaicin-sensitive sensory neurons. General Pharmacology, *19*, 1–43.

Mantyh, P. W. (1983). The spinothalamic tract in the primate: A re-examination using wheatgerm agglutinin conjugated to horseradish peroxidase. *Neuroscience, 9*, 847–862.

Marshall, G. E., Shehab, S. A., Spike, R. C., & Todd, A. J. (1996). Neurokinin-1 receptors on lumbar spinothalamic neurons in the rat. *Neuroscience, 72*, 255–263.

McLeod, J. G. (1958). The representation of the splanchnic afferent pathways in the thalamus of the cat. *Journal of Physiology, 94*, 439–452.

McMahon, S. B. (2004). Sensitisation of gastrointestinal tract afferents. *Gut, 53*, ii13–ii15.

McRoberts, J. A., et al. (2001). Role of peripheral N-methyl-D-aspartate (NMDA) receptors in visceral nociception in rats. *Gastroenterology, 120*, 1737–1748.

Mehler, W. R. (1962). The anatomy of the so-called "pain tract" in man: An analysis of the course and distribution of the ascending fibers of the fasciculus anterolateralis. In: J. D. French, & R. W. Porter (Eds.), *Basic research in paraplegia* (pp. 26–55). Springfield: Charles C Thomas.

Mehler, W. R., Feferman, M. E., & Nauta, W. J. H. (1960). Ascending axon degeneration following anterolateral cordotomy. An experimental study in the monkey. *Brain, 83*, 718–750.

Melzack, R. (1999). From the gate to the neuromatrix. *Pain* 6, S121–S126.
Merskey, H. (1989). Pain and psychological medicine. In: P. D. Wall & R. Melzack (Eds.), *Textbook of pain*, 2nd ed. (pp. 656–66). Edinburgh: Churchill-Livingstone.
Mertz, H., Morgan, V., Tanner, G., Pickens, D., Price, R., Shyr, Y., et al. (2000). Regional cerebral activation in irritable bowel syndrome and control subjects with painful and nonpainful rectal distention. *Gastroenterology*, *18*, 842–8.
Meyer, R. A., & Campbell, J. N. (1981). Myelinated nociceptive afferents account for the hyperalgesia that follows a burn to the hand. *Science*, *213*, 1527–9.
Milne, R. J., Foreman, R. D., Giesler, G. J., & Willis, W. D. (1981). Convergence of cutaneous and pelvic visceral nociceptive inputs onto primate spinothalamic neurons. *Pain*, *11*, 163–83.
Mizuno, N., Nakano, K., Imaizumi, M., & Okamoto, M. (1967). The lateral cervical nucleus of the Japanese monkey (Macaca fuscata). *Journal of Comparative Neurology*, *129*, 375–84.
Nafe, J. P. (1934). The pressure, pain and temperature senses. In: C. A. Murchison (Ed.), *Handbook of general experimental psychology*. Worcester, MA: Clark University Press.
Nauta, H. J., Hewitt, E., Westlund, K. N., & Willis, W. D. (1997). Surgical interruption of a midline dorsal column visceral pain pathway. Case report and review of the literature. *Journal of Neurosurgery*, *86* (3), 538–542.
Nauta, H. J., Soukup, V. M., Fabian, R. H., Lin, J. T., Grady, J. J., Williams, C. G., et al. (2000). Punctate midline myelotomy for the relief of visceral cancer pain. *Journal of Neurosurgery*, *92* (2 Suppl), 125–130.
Ness, T. J. (2000). Evidence for ascending visceral nociceptive information in the dorsal midline and lateral spinal cord. *Pain*, *87*(1), 83–88.
Nijensohn, D. E., & Kerr, F. W. L. (1975). The ascending projections of the dorsolateral funiculus of the spinal cord in the primate. *Journal of Comparative Neurology*, *161*, 459–70.
Noble, R., & Riddell, J,S. (1988). Cutaneous excitatory and inhibitory input to neurones of the postsynaptic dorsal column system in the cat. *Journal of Physiology*, *396*, 497–513.
Noordenbos W. (1959). *Pain*. Amsterdam: Elsevier.
Noordenbos, W., & Wall, P. D. (1976). Diverse sensory functions with an almost totally divided spinal cord. A case of spinal cord transection with preservation of part of one anterolateral quadrant. *Pain*, *2*, 185–95.
Ochoa, J., & Torebjörk, E. (1989). Sensations evoked by intraneural microstimulation of C nociceptor fibres in human skin nerves. *Journal of Physiology*, *415*, 583–599.
Olszewski, J. (1952). *The thalamus of Macaca mulatta*. New York: Karger.
Patterson, J. T., Head, P. A., McNeill, D. L., Chung, K., & Coggeshall, R. E. (1989). Ascending unmyelinated primary afferent fibers in the dorsal funiculus. *Journal of Comparative Neurology*, *290*, 384–90.
Patterson, J. T., Coggeshall, R. E., Lee, W. T., & Chung, K. (1990). Long ascending unmyelinated primary afferent axons in the rat dorsal column: Immunohistochemical localizations. *Neuroscience Letters*, *108*, 6–10.
Patton, H. D., & Amassian, V. E. (1951). Thalamic relay of splanchnic afferent fibers. *American Journal of Physiology*, *167*, 815–816.
Peng, Y. B., Lin, Q., & Willis, W. D. (1995). The role of 5HT3 receptors in periaqueductal gray-induced inhibition of nociceptive dorsal horn neurons in rats. *Journal of Pharmacology and Experimental Therapeutics*, *276*, 116–24.
Peng, Y. B., Lin, Q., & Willis, W. D. (1996a). Involvement of[alpha]2-adrenoreceptors in the periaqueductal gray-induced inhibition of dorsal horn cell activity in rats. *Journal of Pharmacology and Experimental Therapeutics*, *278*(1), 125–35.
Peng, Y. B., Lin, Q., & Willis, W. D. (1996b). Effects of GABA and glycine receptor antagonists on the activity and PAG-induced inhibition of rat dorsal horn neurons. *Brain Research*, *736*(1–2), 189–201.
Petit, D. (1972). Postsynaptic fibres in the dorsal columns and their relay in the nucleus gracilis. *Brain Research*, *48*, 380–384.

Peyron, R., et al. (2000). Parietal and cingulate processes in central pain. A combined positron emission tomography (PET) and functional magnetic resonance imaging (fMRI) study of an unusual case. *Pain, 84*(1), 77–87.

Pollin, B., & Albe-Fessard, D. (1979). Organization of somatic thalamus in monkeys with and without section of dorsal spinal tracts. *Brain Research, 173*, 431–49.

Price, D. D., & Mayer, D. J. (1975). Neurophysiological characterization of the anterolateral quadrant neurons subserving pain in *M. mulatta. Pain, 1*, 59–72.

Price, D. D., Hayes, R. L., Ruda, M. A., & Dubner, R. (1978). Spatial and temporal transformations of input to spinothalamic tract neurons and their relation to somatic sensation. *Journal of Neurophysiology, 41*, 933–47.

Proudfit, H. K. (1992). The behavioral pharmacology of the noradrenergic descending system. In: J. -M. Besson & G. Guilbaud (Eds.), *Towards the use of noradrenergic agonists for the treatment of pain* (pp. 119–36). New York: Elsevier.

Rogers, R. C., Novin, D., & Butcher, L. L. (1979). Hepatic sodium and osmoreceptors activate neurons in the ventrobasal thalamus. *Brain Research, 168*, 398–403.

Ross, M. H., Romrell, L. J., & Kaye, G. I. (1995). *Histology; A text and Atlas* (3rd ed.). Baltimore: Williams & Wilkins.

Rustioni, A. (1973). Non-primary afferents to the nucleus gracilis from the lumbar cord of the cat. *Brain Research, 51*, 81–95.

Rustioni, A. (1974). Non-primary afferents to the cuneate nucleus in the brachial dorsal funiculus of the cat. *Brain Research, 75*, 247–59.

Rustioni, A., Hayes, N. L., & O'Neill, S. (1979). Dorsal column nuclei and ascending spinal afferents in macaques. *Brain, 102*, 95–125.

Saab, C. Y., Park, Y. C., & Al-Chaer, E. D. (2004). Thalamic modulation of visceral nociceptive processing in adult rats with neonatal colon irritation. *Brain Research, 1008*(2), 186–192.

Saab, C. Y., Wang, J., Gu C., Garner K. N., & Al-Chaer E. D. (2007). Microglia: A newly discovered role in visceral hypersensitivity? *Neuron Glia Biology* doi:10.1017/S1740925X07000439

Sarnoff, S. J., Arrowood, J. G., & Chapman, W. P. (1948). Differential spinal block. IV. The investigation of intestinal dyskinesia, colonic atony, and visceral afferent fibers. *Surgery, Gynecology & Obstetrics, 86*, 571–581.

Sato, J., & Perl, E. R. (1991). Adrenergic excitation of cutaneous pain receptors induced by peripheral nerve injury. *Science, 251*, 1608–10.

Schaible, H. G., & Schmidt, R. F. (1983). Activation of groups III and IV sensory units in medial articular nerve by local mechanical stimulation of knee joint. *Journal of Neurophysiology, 49*, 35–44, 1983.

Schaible, H. G., & Schmidt, R. F. (1985). Effects of an experimental arthritis on the sensory properties of fine articular afferent units. *Journal of Neurophysiology, 54*, 1109–22.

Schaible, H. G., & Schmidt, R. F. (1988). Time course of mechanosensitivity changes in articular afferents during a developing experimental arthritis. *Journal of Neurophysiology, 60*, 2180–95.

Schepelmann, K., Messlinger, K., Schaible, H. G., & Schmidt, R. F. (1992). Inflammatory mediators and nociception in the joint: Excitation and sensitization of slowly conducting afferent fibers of cat's knee by prostaglandin I2. *Neuroscience, 50*, 237–47.

Schiff, J. M. (1858). *Lehrbuch der physiologie des menschen I: Muskel and nervenphysiologie* (pp. 234: 253–255). Lahr: M Schauenburg.

Schwarcz, J. R. (1976). Stereotactic extralemniscal myelotomy. *Journal of Neurology, Neurosurgery and Psychiatry, 39*, 53–57.

Schwarcz, J. R. (1978). Spinal cord stereotactic techniques, trigeminal nucleotomy and extralemniscal myelotomy. *Applied Neurophysiology, 41*, 99–112.

Sherrington, C. S. (1906). *The integrative action of the nervous system* (2nd ed., 1947). New Haven: Yale University Press.

Silverman, D. H., Munakata, J. A., Ennes, H., Mandelkern, M. A., Hoh, C. K., & Mayer, E. A. (1997). Regional cerebral activity in normal and pathological perception of visceral pain. *Gastroenterology, 112*, 64–72.

Smith, M. V., & Apkarian, A. V. (1991). Thalamically projecting cells of the lateral cervical nucleus in monkey. *Brain Research, 555*, 10–8.

Sorkin, L., & Carlton, S. (1997). Spinal anatomy and pharmacology of afferent processing. In T. Yaksh, C. Lynch, W. Zapol, M. Maze, J. Biebuyck & L. Saidman (Eds.), *Anesthesia. Biologic Foundations* (pp. 577–610). Philadelphia: Lippincott-Raven.

Spiller, W. G. (1905). The occasional clinical resemblance between caries of the vertebrae and lumbothoracic syringomyelia, and the location within the spinal cord of the fibres for the sensations of pain and temperature. *University of Pennsylvania Medical Bulletin, 18*, 147–54.

Spiller, W. G., & Martin, E. (1912). The treatment of persistent pain of organic origin in the lower part of the body by division of the anterolateral column of the spinal cord. *Journal of the American Medical Association, 58*, 1489–90.

Stanley, E. (1840). A case of disease of the posterior columns of the spinal cord. *Medico-chirurgical Transactions, 23*, 80–84.

Stein, C. (1994). Peripheral opioid analgesia: Mechanisms and therapeutic applications. In: J. M. Besson, G. Guilbaud & H. Ollat H (Eds.), *Peripheral neurons in nociception: Physio-pharmacological aspects* (pp. 157–65). Paris: John Libbey Eurotext.

Stepniewska, I., Sakai, S.T,, Qi, H. X., & Kaas, J. H. (2003). Somatosensory input to the ventrolateral thalamic region in the macaque monkey: Potential substrate for parkinsonian tremor. *Journal of Comparative Neurology, 455*, 378–395.

Strigo, I. A., Duncan, G. H., Boivin, M., & Bushnell, M. C. (2003). Differentiation of visceral and cutaneous pain in the human brain. *Journal of Neurophysiology, 89*, 3294–303.

Su, X., Sengupta, J. N., & Gebhart, G. F. (1997). Effects of kappa opioid receptor-selective agonists on responses of pelvic nerve afferents to noxious colorectal distension. *Journal of Neurophysiology, 78*, 1003–1012.

Surmeier, D. J., Honda, C. N., & Willis, W. D. (1986a). Responses of primate spinothalamic neurons to noxious thermal stimulation of glabrous and hairy skin. *Journal of Neurophysiology, 56*, 328–50.

Surmeier, D. J., Honda, C. N., & Willis, W. D. (1986b). Temporal features of the responses of primate spinothalamic neurons to noxious thermal stimulation of hairy and glabrous skin. *Journal of Neurophysiology, 56*, 351–68.

Todd, A. (2002). Anatomy of primary afferents and projection neurones in the rat spinal dorsal horn with particular emphasis on substance P and the neurokinin 1 receptor. *Experimental Physiology, 87*, 245–249.

Trevino, D. L., Maunz, R. A., Bryan, R. N., & Willis, W. D. (1972). Location of cells of origin of the spinothalamic tract in the lumbar enlargement of cat. *Experimental Neurology, 34*, 64–77.

Trevino, D. L., Coulter, J. D., & Willis, W. D. (1973). Locations of cells of origin of spinothalamic tract in lumbar enlargement of the monkey. *Journal of Neurophysiology, 36*, 750–761.

Truex, R. C., Taylor, M. J., Smythe, M. Q., & Gildenberg, P. L. (1965). The lateral cervical nucleus of cat, dog and man. *Journal of Comparative Neurology, 139*, 93–104.

Truitt, W. A., Shipley, M. T., Veening, J. G., & Coolen, L. M. (2003). Activation of a subset of lumbar spinothalamic neurons after copulatory behavior in male but not female rats. *Journal of Neuroscience, 23*, 325–331.

Uddenburg, N. (1966). Studies on modality segragation and second-order neurons in the dorsal funiculus. *Experientia, 15*, 441–442.

Uddenburg, N. (1968). Functional organization of long, second-order afferents in the dorsal funiculus. *Experimental Brain Research, 4*(4), 377–382.

Veldhuijzen, D. S., et al. (2007). Imaging central pain syndromes. Current Pain & Headache Reports, *11*(3), 183–189.

Vierck, C. J., & Luck, M. M. (1979). Loss and recovery of reactivity to noxious stimuli in monkeys with primary spinothalamic cordotomies, followed by secondary and tertiary lesions of other cord sectors. *Brain, 102*, 233–48.

Vierck, C. J., Greenspan, J. D., & Ritz, L. A. (1990). Long-term changes in purposive and reflexive responses to nociceptive stimulation following anterolateral chordotomy. Journal of Neuroscience, *10*, 2077–95.

Walker, A. E. (1940). The spinothalamic tract in man. *Archives of Neurology and Psychiatry, 43*, 284–98.

Wall, P., Bery, J., & Saade, N. (1988). Effects of lesions to rat spinal cord lamina I cell projection pathways on reactions to acute and chronic noxious stimuli. *Pain, 35*, 327–339.

Wang, C. C., Willis, W. D., & Westlund, K. N. (1999). Ascending projections from the area around the spinal cord central canal: A Phaseolus vulgaris leucoagglutinin study in rats. *Journal of Comparative Neurology, 415*(3), 341–367.

White, J. C. (1943). Sensory innervation of the viscera: Studies on visceral afferent neurones in man based on neurosurgical procedures for the relief of intractable pain. *Research Publications Association for Research in Nervous and Mental Disease, 23*, 373–390.

White, J. C., & Sweet, W. H. (1969). *Pain and the neurosurgeon.* Springfield: Charles C Thomas.

Willis, W. D. (1982). Control of nociceptive transmission in the spinal cord. In: D. Ottoson (Ed.), *Progress in sensory physiology 3.* Berlin: Springer-Verlag.

Willis, W. D. (1985). *The pain system.* Basel: Karger.

Willis, W. D., & Coggeshall, R. E. (2004). *Sensory mechanisms of the spinal cord*, 3rd ed. New York: Plenum Press.

Willis, W. D., & Westlund, K. N. (1997). Neuroanatomy of the pain system and of the pathways that modulate pain. Journal of Clinical Neurophysiology, *14*(1), 2–31.

Willis, W. D., Trevino, D. L., Coulter, J. D., & Maunz, R. A. (1974). Responses of primate spinothalamic tract neurons to natural stimulation of hindlimb. *Journal of Neurophysiology, 37*, 358–72.

Willis, W. D., Kenshalo, D. R. J., & Leonard, R. B. (1979). The cells of origin of the primate spinothalamic tract. *Journal of Comparative Neurology, 188*, 543–574.

Willis, W. D., Al-Chaer, E. D., Quast, M. J., & Westlund, K. N. (1999). A visceral pain pathway in the dorsal column of the spinal cord. *Proceedings of the National Academy of Sciences (USA), 96*(14), 7675–7679.

Woolf, C., & Fitzgerald, M. (1983). The properties of neurons recorded in the superficial dorsal horn of the rat spinal cord. *Journal of Comparative Neurology, 221*, 313–328.

Xie, J., Yoon, Y. W., Yom, S. S., & Chung, J. M. (1995). Norepinephrine rekindles mechanical allodynia in sympathectomized neuropathic rat. *Analgesia, 1*, 107–13.

Yoss, R. E. (1953). Studies of the spinal cord. Part 3. Pathways for deep pain within the spinal cord and brain. *Neurology, 3*, 163–75.

Yokota, T., Nishikawa, Y., & Koyama, N. (1988). Distribution of trigeminal nociceptive neurons in nucleus ventralis posteromedialis of primates. In: R. Dubner, G. F. Gebhart, M. R. Bond (Eds.), *Pain research and clinical management*, vol. 3 (pp. 555–9). Amsterdam: Elsevier.

Zhuo, M., & Gebhart, G. F. (2002). Facilitation and attenuation of a visceral nociceptive reflex from the rostroventral medulla in the rat. *Gastroenterology, 122*, 1007–1019.

The Genetic Epidemiology of Pain

Alex J. MacGregor and Caroline M. Reavley

Chronic pain is common among populations worldwide and presents a significant burden both to individuals and to society through its negative impact on daily activities, social and working lives (Moulin et al. 2002; Cosby et al. 2005; Breivik et al. 2006; Chung & Wong 2007). One of the most fundamental questions concerning pain in populations is the extent to which its occurrence is determined by constitutional factors as opposed to potentially modifiable factors in the environment to which an individual is exposed throughout life. This can be addressed through studies of genetic epidemiology and is the focus of this chapter.

Evidence for a genetic contribution to pain is well established through animal studies, but the genetic contribution to pain in humans is only now starting to be fully recognised. The inherently subjective nature of pain and ethical considerations surrounding studies of pain are important limiting factors. In this chapter we review the epidemiological evidence that assesses the influence of genetic and environmental factors on the variation in clinical pain in human populations. We also examine how the increasingly widespread data on the contribution of individual genes fits within this framework. Finally, we propose some future directions for this field.

Genetic Influences on Pain at the Population Level: The Evidence

The multidimensional nature of pain and the consequent difficulties in definition, assessment and measurement make it a singularly difficult subject for genetic studies. The concept of pain encompasses a set of biological entities that range from the pathophysiological basis of pain perception itself to pain in its wider psychological and social context. Given this broad, heterogeneous and inherently complex remit, it is manifestly too ambitious at the outset to expect

A.J. MacGregor (✉)
Twin Research and Genetic Epidemiology Unit, Kings College, London, UK;
University of East Anglia, Norwich UK
e-mail: alex.macgregor@kcl.ac.uk A.Macgregor@uea.ac.uk

R.J. Moore (ed.), *Biobehavioral Approaches to Pain*,
DOI 10.1007/978-0-387-78323-9_3, © Springer Science+Business Media, LLC 2009

to be able to produce a simple satisfactory model that explains the contribution of genetic factors to all aspects of human pain experience. Nevertheless by focusing attention on specific aspects of pain, for example by examining responses to painful stimuli, the clinical pain experienced in disease along with psychological aspects that might explain and modify pain behaviours, it is possible to begin to piece together a picture of the genetic contribution to pain incrementally.

Evidence that points to a genetic influence on pain related traits at the population level can come from several sources. Ethnic and gender differences in pain reporting are indicative, as is clustering of pain related traits in families. The obvious difficulty in interpreting this information is in disentangling genetic effects from those of the shared cultural and family environment.

Studies of monozygotic (MZ) and dizygotic (DZ) twins provide a well established approach to separating the genetic factors from those in the shared family and cultural environment. MZ twins are genetically identical while DZ twins share on average only half their genetic material. If it is assumed that both types of twin share their family environment to the same extent, a greater similarity among traits in MZ when compared with DZ twin pairs can be attributed directly to genetic factors.

Quantitative analysis of data that compare correlations in traits among MZ and DZ twins allows phenotypic variation (P) measured in the population to be divided into a genetic component (G) and into environmental components that are common to the family environment of the twins (C) and unique to each twin (E). The proportion of population variation that can be attributed to genetic variation (the ratio G/P) is termed heritability. Data on heritability of traits related to pain is becoming increasingly widely available.

Classical evidence supporting a genetic influence on pain from twin studies provides justification for subsequent more focused genetic enquiry into the action of individual genes. This is an area that is advancing rapidly. The increasing availability of genotyping technology has led to a profusion of information available from association studies of individual genes that relate to pain phenotypes. This information is adding an important extra dimension to the task of unravelling the genetic basis of human pain perception.

Cultural, Social and Gender Influences on Pain

An influence of the social, cultural and gender factors in determining differences in pain reporting between individuals has been suggested in the scientific literature for over five decades. In their 1990 review, Zatzick and Dimsdale (1990) identified 13 studies that had examined differences in laboratory-induced pain using a variety of models among a number of different ethnic groups. Overall, pain tolerance varied widely: the greatest variation was seen in the affective rather than neurosensory aspects of pain. However, individuals' attitudes to pain showed no consistent pattern among the ethnic groups studied and there was also no consistent discernable difference between ethnic groups in their ability to discriminate painful stimuli.

More recently, the topic has been reviewed by Fillingim (2004) who has conducted an updated review that included several studies that had used more sophisticated methods of psychophysical pain assessment. Among these, the strongest comparative data examine the differences in pain responses between African Americans and Whites where some consistent differences appear to have emerged. In several reports, African Americans demonstrated a lower tolerance when compared with Whites for specific painful stimuli including heat pain, ischemic pain and cold pressor pain (Campbell et al. 2005; Rahim-Williams et al. 2007). African Americans also demonstrated higher ratings for pain unpleasantness and intensity, and were shown to use passive pain coping strategies more commonly than Whites. These reports concur with a range of studies of clinical pain in which African Americans have been recorded as reporting greater levels of pain than Whites for a range of conditions including migraine (Stewart et al. 1996), postoperative pain (Faucett et al. 1994), myofascial pain (Nelson et al. 1996) and chronic noncancer pain (Green et al. 2003). Taken together they provide evidence to suggest that ethnicity can have a direct influence on aspects of pain sensitivity and reporting.

Gender differences in pain responses have also been the focus of much interest (See also Keogh this volume). A number of studies have shown men to exhibit greater stoicism and a lesser willingness to report pain than women (Zatzick & Dimsdale 1990; Robinson et al. 2001). Ovarian hormones have been shown to influence pain sensitivity (Riley III et al. 1999). There are several studies indicating that men exhibit more robust responses to experimentally induced pain (Berkley 1997; Wiesenfeld-Hallin 2005). In one study based on positron emission tomography (PET), women were shown to be more likely than men to perceive a thermal stimulus as painful (Paulson et al. 1998). The most striking difference between the two sexes was in the degree of activation of the prefrontal cortex, a possible reflection of different affective responses. Sex differences have also been seen in analgesic responsiveness (Fillingim & Gear 2004). κ opioid receptor antagonists have been shown to be less effective as analgesics in men than in women in dental postoperative pain (Gear et al. 1996). PET scanning studies have indicated gender differences in activation in the μ opioid system after exposure to equivalent levels of pain (Zubieta et al. 2002).

Despite an increasing awareness of ethnic and gender variation in the response to pain; considerable caution needs to be exercised in interpreting the results of studies of this type that purport to show differences between ethnic and gender groups. Experimental studies of pain sensitivity are frequently based on small sample sizes. The choice and selection of subjects can have an important bearing on results of the assessments. The results are also known to be exquisitely situation dependent: the gender of the operator, the precise language used in delivering the test and in reporting results all have been demonstrated to exert subtle influences that render the observations of differences in pain reporting between ethnic and gender groups particularly prone to misinterpretation (Zatzick & Dimsdale 1990).

It is also clearly incorrect to directly infer that differences in pain responses and pain reporting between ethnic and gender reflect the action of genetic factors since cultural and social influences on pain reporting are profound and undisputed. Nevertheless, the existence of variation in ethnic and gender groups means that it is justifiable to consider genetic factors as one of the possible contributing causes and to focus interest on study designs that can distinguish between genetic and environmental effects with greater precision.

Twin and Family Studies

Family studies have provided much evidence to support a dominating influence of the shared family environment on attitudes to pain and on pain behaviour. Examples include two studies published by Turkat showing that family pain models can exert an influence on pain behaviour in both healthy and diseased individuals (Turkat & Guise 1983; Turkat & Noskin 1983). Studies of college students have shown similar results (Lester et al. 1994). Poor models of pain tolerance in family members predict an earlier onset and greater severity of post-operative pain following thoracotomy (Bachiocco et al. 1993). Similarities have been observed in the way in which children and their mothers describe pain (Campbell 1975). In the experimental setting, pain tolerance to finger pressure is influenced by a subject's prior exposure to other individuals with either a high or low tolerance to painful stimulation. Other factors shown to influence pain reporting include family size and socio-economic status, the position in the sibship, the quality of relationships with parents including early experiences of abuse, and early loss of family members (Payne & Norfleet 1986).

These studies have provided additional insight into the strength of environmental influences determining the familial clustering of pain and generally support the view that early family environment shapes future pain behaviour by vicarious learning through exposure to pain and suffering in a family member (Turk et al. 1987). However, as with studies of ethnicity and gender, these data also provide justification to look more closely at the potential contribution of genetic factors.

Genetic Influences on Diseases Characterised by Pain

Several clinical disease states are characterised by pain and many of these have been the subject of classical twin studies seeking to determine the relative influences of genetic and environmental factors (Table 1). The majority have shown a significant heritable component, although the degree of genetic

Table 1 Heritability of diseases in which pain is a significant component

	Heritability	Reference
Chronic widespread pain	48–54%	Kato et al. (2006)
Low back pain	52–68%	MacGregor et al. (2004)
Neck pain	35–58%	MacGregor et al. (2004)
Shoulder and elbow pain	50%	Hakim et al. (2003)
Temporomandibular pain	Nil	Michalowicz et al. (2000)
Migraine	34–58%	Mulder et al. (2003)
Tension headache	44–48%	Russell et al. (2007)
Gastro-oesophageal reflux pain	43%	Mohammed et al. (2003)
Functional bowel disorder	57%	Morris-Yates et al. (1998)
Chronic pelvic pain	41%	Zondervan et al. (2005)
Menstrual pain	55%	Treloar et al. (1998)

contribution varies considerably and for certain painful diseases, for example temporomandibular joint disease, a heritable component appears to be absent.

Twin data are frequently criticised for tending to overstate heritability because of their reliance on the assumption that the degree of environmental sharing in MZ and DZ twins is similar. However, the majority of studies reporting genetic influences in painful diseases were conducted in representative adult population samples among twins living apart. The level of genetic contribution is unlikely to be solely explained by any differences in the MZ and DZ shared environment (Khoury et al. 1988). These findings provide robust and persuasive evidence that genetic factors have a dominating influence on the variation in clinical pain.

What is uncertain in evidence of this type is how the genetic influences are mediated. In a number of these diseases (lower back and neck pain are two examples) the degree of pain reported is not tightly coupled to the degree of observed physical damage favouring the hypothesis that genetic factors directly influence pain pathways in these conditions. However, it is difficult to exclude the possibility that the chief genetic influence might be mediated through determining disease susceptibility or severity. This issue would be better addressed directly by studying clinical pain in response to a standardised stimulus, for example a surgical injury, delivered in a uniform setting. This is a situation that rarely arises in observational studies and is more readily obtained through laboratory based studies of experimental pain.

Genetic Influences on Experimental Pain

Among rodents, nociceptive and analgesic sensitivity show strain-specific variation that equates to heritability estimates of individual traits that range from of 28 to 76% (Mogil 1999). Data on the heritability of responses to painful stimuli in man have been much more limited and it is only relatively recently that a fuller picture of the heritability of experimental pain has begun to emerge through classical twin studies (Table 2).

Table 2 Heritability of responses to experimental pain in man

	Heritability
UK Twin Registry Study, 1997 (MacGregor et al. 1997)	
Pressure pain threshold	10%
UK Twin Registry Study, 2007 (Norbury et al. 2007)	
Heat pain threshold	53%
Acid iontophoresis	31%
ATP iontophoresis	11%
Pain during burn induction	34%
Skin flare	Nil
Pinprick hyperalgesia	55%
Thermal hyperalgesia	Nil
Brush evoked allodynia	25%
Danish Twin Registry Study, 2007 (Nielsen et al. 2008)	
Heat pain	26%
Cold pressor pain	60%

The first study of this type was conducted by ourselves in 1997 among 269 MZ and 340 DZ female-female adult twin volunteers from the UK twin registry (MacGregor et al. 1997). The study assessed pressure pain thresholds using a variable pain dolorimeter with measurements taken at the forehead. All twins were healthy with no intercurrent illness or chronic pain.

The responses among twin pairs were highly correlated, with an intraclass correlation coefficient in MZ twins of 0.57 and in DZ twins of 0.51. Neither estimate was substantially altered after adjusting for a range of potential confounding variables including age, current tobacco and alcohol use, current analgesic use, psychological status assessed by the general health questionnaire, and social class. The pattern of correlations confirmed that there was familial clustering of this trait, but suggested that the primary influence was from the shared environment of the twins. The excess margin of correlation in MZ over DZ twins was only slight and indicated that genetic factors contributed at most 10% to the variation that was observed.

The results were consistent with the data that suggest the importance of the shared environmental and family pain models in shaping pain responses. However, extrapolating from the results of a single pain modality to pain responsiveness in general presents difficulties, especially given the wide variation in genetic contribution to individual nociceptive responses seen in animal models (Mogil 1999). Further, there was concern in this particular study that the twin pairs were assessed together, which might have tended to inflate the influence of the shared environment and underestimate a potential genetic effect.

We have since extended this work to consider a wider range of painful stimuli in a rigorously controlled experimental setting in which individual twins were blinded to their co-twin's responses (Norbury et al. 2007). The set of stimuli were chosen to reflect both acute and chronic pain. Baseline heat pain threshold was measured at the forearm using a 32 mm probe heated from 32°C at a rate of 0.5°C /second until the subject first perceived a change from a feeling of heat to a feeling of pain. Visual analogue scale (VAS) ratings of pain induced during the iontophoresis of adenosine triphosphate (ATP) and hydrochloric acid were also assessed. The twins were exposed to a 45°C thermal burn. Pain during the induction of the burn was measured by VAS. In the 15 min following the burn, measurements were also made of the area of skin flare, the area of post-burn allodynia to brush stroke (brush-evoked allodynia), and the area of hyperalgesia assessed by application of a von Frey filament (punctate hyper-algesia) and by repeat measurement of the heat pain threshold at the burn site (thermal hyperalgesia). The study was conducted in 51 MZ and 47 DZ female-female twins. As in the earlier study, all were healthy and on no analgesic medication.

The heritabilities of the responses assessed in the study are shown in Table 2. The majority of responses showed a genetic contribution, although this varied widely among the variables and no heritable contribution was found for post burn hyperalgesia or for skin flare area. The data did not support an important influence from the shared environment for all variables in which a heritable component was detected.

Similar findings have also been reported recently by Nielsen et al. (2008) in a study in which cold-pressor pain and contact heat pain were assessed in 53 MZ and 39 DZ twin pairs from the Norwegian twin registry. Their protocol assessed supramaximal pain sensitivity with heat pain measured using a thermode start-ing at 43°C increasing by 1°C increments until the VAS exceeded 50%. Cold pressor pain was assessed by immersion in cold water (0–2.5°C for 60s). From their results, they estimated that 60% of the variance in cold-pressor pain and 26% of the variance in heat pain was genetically mediated.

The variation in heritability estimates among measures of pain responsive-ness in these studies accords with observations made in rodents that suggest that genetic mediation of nociceptive sensitivity is specific to the noxious stimulus (Mogil 1999). Animal studies have also shown clustering in pain responses defined by stimulus modality (Mogil et al. 1999). In the UK data, modest phenotypic correlation was seen for certain variables, including heat pain threshold, pain during burn induction, ATP and acid iontophoresis. This raises the possibility that heritability of nociception might be explained by a limited set of common genetic factors.

The relevance of these findings to clinical pain can be questioned. Although experimental pain is both distant to and distinct from pain experienced in disease, certain experimental measurements can be directly related to clinical pain. In patients undergoing surgery for example, pre-operative pain ratings assessed following a thermal burn protocol similar to that used in the UK twins are strongly correlated with postoperative pain (Werner et al. 2004). Preopera-tive pressure pain assessment has also been shown to predict postoperative pain and analgesic consumption in women undergoing surgery (Hsu et al. 2005). Thus it is conceivable that the genetic signals detected in these twins and those seen in clinical pain states may well relate to similar underlying mechanisms.

Genetic Influences on Affective, Cognitive and Behavioural Aspects of Pain

The experience of pain is bound tightly to that of emotion as well as to an individual's understanding of the nature and significance of the painful stimulus and to their behavioural response to it (Gatchel et al. 2007). The relationship of pain to anxiety and depression has received considerable attention. Around 50% of patients with fibromyalgia acknowledge that they are anxious (Wolfe et al. 1990); depression is equally common among those with chronic pain (Dersh et al. 2006). Levels of anxiety influence both experimental pain reporting and clinical pain. In surgical patients, anxiety influences the degree of post-operative pain and the length of surgical stay (de Groot et al. 1997). The role of cognition and beliefs about pain is also supported by a number of empirical observations. Fear and anticipation of pain have an impact of pain tolerance and level of function (Vlaeyen & Linton 2000). This can in turn be reflected in maladaptive avoidance pain behaviours and pain avoidance strategies. Anger and frustration are also critical components of the pain experience. Anger is frequently reported among those with chronic pain and has been related to the intensity and unpleasantness of pain (Wade et al. 1990).

In many respects, affect and behaviour are an integral part of an individual's experience of pain that cannot be considered in isolation. However, from an epidemiological perspective it is valid to question whether personality and behavioural traits might predispose to the onset or modify the expression of pain. Some of the strongest data on risk factors for the development of chronic pain come from studies of musculoskeletal pain. Magni et al. (1994) assessed 2,324 participants in the US National Health and Nutrition Survey both for the presence of musculoskeletal pain and the presence of depression over a period of 10 years. Depressive symptoms at year 1 significantly predicted the development of chronic musculoskeletal pain at year 8 with an odds ratio of 2.14 for the depressed subjects compared with the non-depressed subjects. A systematic review of data from 18 prospective cohort studies of low back pain has emphasised the importance of psychological factors in the development of chronic symptoms (Pincus et al. 2002). The review showed strong evidence to support increased risk of persisting pain and disability among subjects with pre-existing psychological distress or depressive mood, and among those reporting multiple physical symptoms. High scores on tests designed to detect somatisation and maladaptive illness behaviours have been recently identified as being the most important predictor of the development of chronic widespread pain in a community-based cohort (Gupta et al. 2007).

Many of the affective and behavioural traits that are related to the onset and persistence and response to pain are now recognised to have a genetic basis. Twin studies of anxiety and depression show heritabilities of 30–40% (Leonardo & Hen 2006). Psychological distress as assessed by the general health questionnaire has been shown to have a heritability of 35% (Rijsdijk et al. 2003). Coping strategies relevant to pain have also been the subject of twin studies conducted in a number of groups, with one study suggesting that a range of coping styles shared a common genetic component (Kendler et al. 1991; Busjahn et al. 1999). Self reported fear and fear conditioning have been shown to a have heritable basis (Hettema et al. 2008). Anger expression has been estimated to have a heritability of 30% (Wang et al. 2005). Most of these measures were assessed in healthy subjects and were not evaluated with direct reference to clinical or experimental pain experienced by the study subjects. However, they provide strong evidence that many of the psychological factors that are themselves related to pain have a genetic basis and it is likely that this list will be extended in future studies targeting pain psychology in twins.

The extension of twin and family study methodology to the emotions and behavioural responses in the context of clinical and experimental pain is likely to further resolve the genetic basis of pain reporting. The use of scanning techniques including positron emission tomography and functional magnetic resonance imaging may also have an important contribution in quantitative assessment (Gatchel et al. 2007; Matre & Tran this volume). However, for the present, the observations that affective and behavioural aspects of pain are likely themselves to have significant and distinguishable genetic determinants has important implications. Studies investigating the genetic basis of pain in clinical disease states and in experimental settings need to account for affective and behavioural aspects of the pain phenotype if the precise effects of individual genes are to be clearly distinguished. The presence of genetic determinants underlying these phenotypes may limit the effectiveness of pain management strategies targeted at modifying affective and pain behaviour and may indicate a need to develop approaches that are targeted to genetically susceptible individuals.

Genetic Association Studies in Pain

The breadth of the potential mechanisms for genetic action in pain together with the increasing availability of genotype data provides enormous scope for identifying the specific action of individual genes. The search has to an extent been spurred on by the success of genetic studies in rodents that have pinpointed the action of several genes involved in nociceptive sensitivity in a number of well defined experimental settings (Mogil & Max 2006).

Examples of reported associations between individual genes and pain related phenotypes are shown in Table 3 which considers associations in the

Table 3 Examples of genes implicated in pain in man through genetic association studies

Protein	Gene	Trait/Stimulus	Reference
Painful clinical traits			
Catechol-O-methyl transferase	COMT	Fibromyalgia	Gursoy et al. (2003)
		Temporomandibular joint pain	Diatchenko et al. (2005)
Collagen 9	COL9A3	Sciatica	Paassilta et al. (2001)
GTP cyclohydrolase	GHC1	Pain following surgical discectomy	Tegeder et al. (2006)
Hypocretin receptor	HCRTR2	Migraine	Schurks et al. (2007)
Major histocompatability complex	HLA-DR	Complex regional pain	van de Beek et al. (2003)
	HLA-A and B	Postherpetic neuralgia	Sato et al. (2002)
Monoamine oxidise A	MAOA	Fibromyalgia	Gursoy et al. (2007)
Serotonin receptor	5HTA	Fibromyalgia	Bondy et al. (1999)
Serotonin transporter	5-HTT	Fibromyalgia	Offenbaecher et al. (1999)
Experimental pain responses			
δ opioid receptor	OPRD1	49 degree thermal stimulus	Kim et al. (2004)
Catechol-O-methyl transferase	COMT	Thermal pain	Diatchenko et al. (2006)
		Heat and cold sensation	Kim et al. (2006)
		Hypertonic saline infusion	Zubieta et al. (2003)
Fatty acid amide hydrolase	FFAH	Heat and cold sensation	Kim et al. (2006)
GTP cyclohydrolase	GHC1	Heat, ischaemic and pressure pain sensitivity	Tegeder et al. (2006)
Melanocortin 1 receptor	MC1R	Tolerance to electrical pulse stimulation	Mogil et al. (2005)
		Thermal and ischaemic pain	Mogil et al. (2003)
Sparteine/debrisoquine oxygenase	CYP2D6	Cold pressor test	Sindrup et al. (1993)
Transient receptor potential	TRPA1	Heat and cold sensation	Kim et al. (2006)
Vallinoid receptor subtype 1	TPRV1	Cold withdrawal	Kim et al. (2006)
Psychological and behavioural traits associated with pain			
Catechol- O-methyl transferase	COMT	Anxiety	Olsson et al. (2007)
		Pain catastrophising	George et al. (2007)

Table 3 (continued)

Protein	Gene	Trait/Stimulus	Reference
Corticotrophin releasing hormone receptor	CRH-R1	Depression	Liu et al. (2006)
Monoamine oxidase-A	MAOA-	Depression	Brummett et al. (2007)
Serotonin receptor	5-HT1A	Depression	Albert & Lemonde (2004)
Serotonin transporter	5-HTT	Depression	Caspi et al. (2003)
		Coping strategies	Wilhelm et al. (2007)
Serotonin transporter regulator	5-HTTLPR	Trait anxiety	Melke et al. (2001)
		Fear processing	Brocke et al. (2006)
Tryptophan hydroxylase	THP2	Depression	Zill et al. (2004)
Monoamine oxidase-A	MAOA	Anger expression	Yang et al. (2007)

framework of clinical pain, experimental pain, and psychological, cognitive and behavioural phenotypes that have been related to pain. As in the foregoing discussion of heritability, interpreting whether these genes relate to clinical disease, pain pathways or ancillary phenotypes that modify pain experience presents an obvious challenge. In sciatica, for example the association with collagen genes is most likely to reflect the disease process of disc degeneration rather than the pain that is related to it (Paassilta et al. 2001). It is also necessary to be cautious in interpreting the results of individual association studies in isolation because of the well established risk of type I error and publication bias (Cardon & Bell 2001). Few of the reported findings have been replicated (Hirschhorn et al. 2002). However, a number of genetic associations have emerged through these studies that provide a plausible explanation of how genetic variation might have a direct influence in established pain mechanisms.

Catecholamine-O-methyltransferase (COMT) is an enzyme with a range of biological features that include the regulation of catecholamine and enkephalin levels (Mannisto & Kaakkola 1999). A functional polymorphism of the COMT gene that reduces the enzyme's thermostability has been reported to influence pain processing. Zubieta et al. (Zubieta et al. 2003) performed PET scanning in 29 healthy volunteers who were subjected to intensity controlled sustained pain induced by the infusion of small amounts of hypertonic saline into the masseter muscle. Control subjects were injected with isotonic saline. Polymorphic variation in COMT accounted for downstream alteration in the functional responses of μ opioid neurotransmitters by inducing differences in μ opioid activation in a number of regions of the brain including the thalamus and amygdala. Polymorphic variation also influenced the clinical report of pain in study subjects. The volume of iso-tonic saline needed to reach a similar level of pain intensity was related to the COMT activity of their genotype.

Variations of the COMT gene have been linked with differing levels of pain sensitivity and variable propensity for developing temporo-mandibular joint disorder pain (Diatchenko et al. 2005). Interestingly the gene has also been associated with a number of clinical pain phenotypes including fibromyalgia (Gursoy et al. 2003), and with anxiety and depression (Stein et al. 2005; Massat et al. 2005). A recent study by George et al. (2007) showed an interaction between COMT genotype and catastrophising to predict postoperative pain following shoulder surgery.

Other genes that have been identified in pain processing include the vanilloid receptor subtype 1 gene (TRPV1) and the δ opioid receptor subtype 1 gene (OPRD1) which have been associated with hand withdrawal latency to submersion in cold water and to pain ratings to varying cutaneous thermal stimuli. (Kim et al. 2004; Kim et al. 2006). The TRPV1 $Val^{585}Val$ allele led to longer cold withdrawal times in female European Americans. A polymorph-ism in the OPRD1 gene appeared to be important for pain rating to a 49°C thermal stimulus.

GTP cyclohydrolase (GCH1) is the rate-limiting enzyme for tetrahydro-biopterin synthesis and is a key modulator of peripheral neuropathic and inflammatory pain. In an analysis of Caucasians participating in an observa-tional study of surgical discectomy, Tegeder et al. (2006) demonstrated that a haplotype of the GCH1 gene was associated with less pain persistence in the first postoperative year. Healthy individuals with the pain protective haplo-type showed reduced experimental pain sensitivity to thermal and ischaemic pain together with reduced levels of lymphocyte GHC1 upregulation.

Polymorphisms in CYP2D6 that encode sparteine/debrisoquine oxidase involved in activating codeine by o-demethylation to morphine have also been associated with a number of aspects of the pain response. Poor metabo-lisers show reduced efficacy for codeine with respect to both clinical and experimental pain (Sindrup et al. 1990; Poulsen et al. 1996) and also exhibit a decreased basal pain threshold and tolerance, which might reflect an impaired ability to synthesise endogenous morphine (Sindrup et al. 1993). These polymorphisms are common in the population and are found in ~10% of Caucasians, and in 2% of Asian and African Americans.

The melanocortin-1-gene has also been implicated in determining pain responsiveness (Mogil et al. 2005). Variant melanocortin receptors in women are associated with enhanced analgesia from the κ opioid agonist pentazocine after thermal and ischaemic pain testing (Mogil et al. 2003). This may provide one explanation for the differences that have been observed between men and women for κ opioid analgesia that has been reported in the setting of clinical pain.

The Multifactorial Model

The question of how genes that have been identified as determining the individual aspects of the pain phenotype might act together in combination to explain pain in an individual remains a considerable challenge. However, some early attempts have been made to address this issue through multivariate analyses conducted in twins. The approach involved studying the distribution of correlated traits simultaneously in MZ and DZ twin pairs and allows an assessment of the extent to which the phenotypic correlation can be explained by genetic and shared environmental factors that are shared between the traits themselves.

In our own data on back and neck pain reporting in twins we examined the extent to which the interrelationship with structural changes as assessed on magnetic resonance image (MRI) scanning and measures of psychological distress as assessed by the GHQ might be related (MacGregor et al. 2004). These variables were heritable in their own right and associated with the report of pain. For both MRI degeneration and GHQ, the relationship with pain reporting was mediated through shared genetic factors. However these accounted for only a small part of the heritability of pain reporting overall. Similar findings have recently been reported by Battié et al. (2007).

In the Swedish Twin Cohort, Kato (2007) has examined the relationship between chronic widespread pain (CWP) and a set of diseases that are more commonly reported in subjects with CWP (including irritable bowel syndrome, chronic fatigue, recurrent headache) together with measures of self reported anxiety and depression. In a multivariate analysis, two latent factors, both with a substantial heritable component could be identified as explaining the common occurrence of these traits. Both latent factors loaded on all traits; however the first loaded most heavily with depression and anxiety, the second most heavily on CWP and the diseases associated with it. The interpretation was that the genetic contribution to CWP could be best explained in terms of distinct genetically determined affective and physiological components. These findings are reminiscent of the affective and neurosensory explanations used to describe the patterns of familial clustering of pain in a range of settings discussed earlier.

These analyses confirm the view that the genetic contribution to pain is multifactorial in nature. However, they raise the possibility that some of the complexity of genetic studies of pain might be resolved by identifying clusters of phenotypes that share a common genetic basis.

Conclusions

Pain is a complex phenotype that presents many challenges to epidemiologists seeking to identify the causes of variation in populations. There is a clear role for the environment and the contribution of culture, social factors and learning to the development and expression of pain. However, data from a number of sources also support a genetic contribution not only to pain processing, but also to the expression of pain in disease, and to the psychological and behavioural aspects that may modify the expression of pain. The precise contribution of individual genes is becoming increasingly well characterised, with polymorphisms implicated in a few key physiological pain pathways. Evidence also supports the possibility that common genetic mechanisms underlie pain reporting across a range of clinical and experimental settings.

The technologies available for quantitative research into the determinants of pain have undergone a revolution in recent years. Knowledge of genomewide polymorphisms, together with the ability to identify the expression of genes in tissues and to detect physiological processes on dynamic images of the nervous system bring the capacity to develop biologically comprehensive models of pain. Global efforts to collect high quality clinical data among representative and informative populations including twins, and advances in design both in human and animal studies of experimental pain will allow these technologies to be exploited in full. These new approaches hold the promise of significant advances in explaining the basis of inter-individual differences in pain. It is hoped that this will lead to the development of new and better targeted therapies.

Acknowledgments Thanks to Tim Spector, Steve McMahon, Tim Norbury and the participants in the UK Twin Registry.

References

Albert, P. R. & Lemonde, S. 2004, "5-HT1A receptors, gene repression, and depression: guilt by association", *Neuroscientist.*, vol. 10, no. 6, pp. 575–593.

Bachiocco, V., Scesi, M., Morselli, A. M., & Carli, G. 1993, "Individual pain history and familial pain tolerance models: relationships to post-surgical pain", *Clin. J. Pain*, vol. 9, no. 4, pp. 266–271.

Battie, M. C., Videman, T., Levalahti, E., Gill, K., & Kaprio, J. 2007, "Heritability of low back pain and the role of disc degeneration", *Pain*, vol. 131, no. 3, pp. 272–280.

Berkley, K. J. 1997, "Sex differences in pain", *Behav. Brain Sci.*, vol. 20, no. 3, pp. 371–380.

Bondy, B., Spaeth, M., Offenbaecher, M., Glatzeder, K., Stratz, T., Schwarz, M., de Jonge, S., Kruger, M., Engel, R. R., Farber, L., Pongratz, D. E., & Ackenheil, M. 1999, "The T102C polymorphism of the 5-HT2A-receptor gene in fibromyalgia", *Neurobiol. Dis*, vol. 6, no. 5, pp. 433–439.

Breivik, H., Collett, B., Ventafridda, V., Cohen, R., & Gallacher, D. 2006, "Survey of chronic pain in Europe: prevalence, impact on daily life, and treatment", *Eur. J. Pain*, vol. 10, no. 4, pp. 287–333.

Brocke, B., Armbruster, D., Muller, J., Hensch, T., Jacob, C. P., Lesch, K. P., Kirschbaum, C., & Strobel, A. 2006, "Serotonin transporter gene variation impacts innate fear processing: Acoustic startle response and emotional startle", *Mol. Psychiatry*, vol. 11, no. 12, pp. 1106–1112.

Brummett, B. H., Krystal, A. D., Siegler, I. C., Kuhn, C., Surwit, R. S., Zuchner, S., Ashley-Koch, A., Barefoot, J. C., & Williams, R. B. 2007, "Associations of a regulatory polymorphism of monoamine oxidase-A gene promoter (MAOA-uVNTR) with symptoms of depression and sleep quality", *Psychosom. Med.*, vol. 69, no. 5, pp. 396–401.

Busjahn, A., Faulhaber, H. D., Freier, K., & Luft, F. C. 1999, "Genetic and environmental influences on coping styles: a twin study", *Psychosom. Med.*, vol. 61, no. 4, pp. 469–475.

Campbell, J. D. 1975, "Illness is a point of view: the deveopment of childrens's concepts of illness", *Chil Develop*, vol. 46, pp. 92–100.

Campbell, C. M., Edwards, R. R., & Fillingim, R. B. 2005, "Ethnic differences in responses to multiple experimental pain stimuli", *Pain*, vol. 113, no. 1–2, pp. 20–26.

Cardon, L. R. & Bell, J. I. 2001, "Association study designs for complex diseases", *Nat. Rev. Genet.*, vol. 2, no. 2, pp. 91–99.

Caspi, A., Sugden, K., Moffitt, T. E., Taylor, A., Craig, I. W., Harrington, H., McClay, J., Mill, J., Martin, J., Braithwaite, A., & Poulton, R. 2003, "Influence of life stress on depression: moderation by a polymorphism in the 5-HTT gene", *Science*, vol. 301, no. 5631, pp. 386–389.

Chung, J. W. & Wong, T. K. 2007, "Prevalence of pain in a community population", *Pain Med.*, vol. 8, no. 3, pp. 235–242.

Cosby, A. G., Hitt, H. C., Thornton-Neaves, T., McMillen, R. C., Koch, K., Sitzman, B. T., Pearson, E. J., & Parvin, T. S. 2005, "Profiles of pain in Mississippi: results from the Southern Pain Prevalence Study", *J. Miss. State Med. Assoc.*, vol. 46, no. 10, pp. 301–309.

de Groot, K. I., Boeke, S., van den Berge, H. J., Duivenvoorden, H. J., Bonke, B., & Passchier, J. 1997, "The influence of psychological variables on postoperative anxiety and physical complaints in patients undergoing lumbar surgery", *Pain*, vol. 69, no. 1–2, pp. 19–25.

Dersh, J., Gatchel, R. J., Mayer, T., Polatin, P., & Temple, O. R. 2006, "Prevalence of psychiatric disorders in patients with chronic disabling occupational spinal disorders", *Spine*, vol. 31, no. 10, pp. 1156–1162.

Diatchenko, L., Nackley, A. G., Slade, G. D., Bhalang, K., Belfer, I., Max, M. B., Goldman, D., & Maixner, W. 2006, "Catechol-O-methyltransferase gene polymorphisms are associated with multiple pain-evoking stimuli", *Pain*, vol. 125, no. 3, pp. 216–224.

Diatchenko, L., Slade, G. D., Nackley, A. G., Bhalang, K., Sigurdsson, A., Belfer, I., Goldman, D., Xu, K., Shabalina, S. A., Shagin, D., Max, M. B., Makarov, S. S., & Maixner, W. 2005, "Genetic basis for individual variations in pain perception and the development of a chronic pain condition", *Hum. Mol. Genet.*, vol. 14, no. 1, pp. 135–143.

Faucett, J., Gordon, N., & Levine, J. 1994, "Differences in postoperative pain severity among four ethnic groups", *J. Pain Symptom. Manage.*, vol. 9, no. 6, pp. 383–389.

Fillingim, R. B. 2004, "Social and Environmantal Influences on Pain: Implications for Pain Genetics," in *The Genetics of Pain*, J. S. Mogil, ed., IASP Press, Seattle, pp. 283–303.

Fillingim, R. B. & Gear, R. W. 2004, "Sex differences in opioid analgesia: clinical and experimental findings", *Eur. J. Pain*, vol. 8, no. 5, pp. 413–425.

Gatchel, R. J., Peng, Y. B., Peters, M. L., Fuchs, P. N., & Turk, D. C. 2007, "The biopsychosocial approach to chronic pain: scientific advances and future directions", *Psychol. Bull.*, vol. 133, no. 4, pp. 581–624.

Gear, R. W., Miaskowski, C., Gordon, N. C., Paul, S. M., Heller, P. H., & Levine, J. D. 1996, "Kappa-opioids produce significantly greater analgesia in women than in men", *Nat. Med.*, vol. 2, no. 11, pp. 1248–1250.

George, S. Z., Wallace, M. R., Wright, T. W., Moser, M. W., Greenfield, W. H., III, Sack, B. K., Herbstman, D. M., & Fillingim, R. B. 2007, "Evidence for a biopsychosocial influence on shoulder pain: Pain catastrophizing and catechol-O-methyltransferase (COMT) diplotype predict clinical pain ratings", *Pain*.

Green, C. R., Baker, T. A., Sato, Y., Washington, T. L., & Smith, E. M. 2003, "Race and chronic pain: A comparative study of young black and white Americans presenting for management", *J. Pain*, vol. 4, no. 4, pp. 176–183.

Gupta, A., Silman, A. J., Ray, D., Morriss, R., Dickens, C., Macfarlane, G. J., Chiu, Y. H., Nicholl, B., & McBeth, J. 2007, "The role of psychosocial factors in predicting the onset of chronic widespread pain: results from a prospective population-based study", *Rheumatology (Oxford)*, vol. 46, no. 4, pp. 666–671.

Gursoy, S., Erdal, E., Herken, H., Madenci, E., Alasehirli, B., & Erdal, N. 2003, "Significance of catechol-O-methyltransferase gene polymorphism in fibromyalgia syndrome", *Rheumatol. Int.*, vol. 23, no. 3, pp. 104–107.

Gursoy, S., Erdal, E., Sezgin, M., Barlas, I. O., Aydeniz, A., Alasehirli, B., & Sahin, G. 2007, "Which genotype of MAO gene that the patients have are likely to be most susceptible to the symptoms of fibromyalgia?", *Rheumatol. Int.*

Hakim, A. J., Cherkas, L. F., Spector, T. D., & MacGregor, A. J. 2003, "Genetic associations between frozen shoulder and tennis elbow: a female twin study", *Rheumatology (Oxford)*, vol. 42, no. 6, pp. 739–742.

Hettema, J. M., Annas, P., Neale, M. C., Fredrikson, M., & Kendler, K. S. 2008, "The Genetic Covariation Between Fear Conditioning and Self-Report Fears", *Biol. Psychiatry*, Mar 15, vol. 63, no. 6, pp. 587–93.

Hirschhorn, J. N., Lohmueller, K., Byrne, E., & Hirschhorn, K. 2002, "A comprehensive review of genetic association studies", *Genet. Med.*, vol. 4, no. 2, pp. 45–61.

Hsu, Y. W., Somma, J., Hung, Y. C., Tsai, P. S., Yang, C. H., & Chen, C. C. 2005, "Predicting postoperative pain by preoperative pressure pain assessment", *Anesthesiology*, vol. 103, no. 3, pp. 613–618.

Kato, K. 2007, *Genetic epidemiological studies of the functional somatic syndromes*, PhD, Karolinska Institutet.

Kato, K., Sullivan, P. F., Evengard, B., & Pedersen, N. L. 2006, "Importance of genetic influences on chronic widespread pain", *Arthritis Rheum*, vol. 54, no. 5, pp. 1682–1686.

Kendler, K. S., Kessler, R. C., Heath, A. C., Neale, M. C., & Eaves, L. J. 1991, "Coping: a genetic epidemiological investigation", *Psychol. Med.*, vol. 21, no. 2, pp. 337–346.

Khoury, M. J., Beaty, T. H., & Liang, K. Y. 1988, "Can familial aggregation of disease be explained by familial aggregation of environmental risk factors?", *Am J Epidemiol*, vol. 127, no. 3, pp. 674–83.

Kim, H., Mittal, D. P., Iadarola, M. J., & Dionne, R. A. 2006, "Genetic predictors for acute experimental cold and heat pain sensitivity in humans", *J. Med. Genet.*, vol. 43, no. 8, p. e40.

Kim, H., Neubert, J. K., San Miguel, A., Xu, K., Krishnaraju, R. K., Iadarola, M. J., Goldman, D., & Dionne, R. A. 2004, "Genetic influence on variability in human acute experimental pain sensitivity associated with gender, ethnicity and psychological temperament", *Pain*, vol. 109, no. 3, pp. 488–496.

Leonardo, E. D. & Hen, R. 2006, "Genetics of affective and anxiety disorders", *Annu. Rev. Psychol.*, vol. 57, pp. 117–137.

Lester, N., Lefebvre, J. C., & Keefe, F. J. 1994, "Pain in young adults: I. Relationship to gender and family pain history", *Clin. J. Pain*, vol. 10, no. 4, pp. 282–289.

Liu, Z., Zhu, F., Wang, G., Xiao, Z., Wang, H., Tang, J., Wang, X., Qiu, D., Liu, W., Cao, Z., & Li, W. 2006, "Association of corticotropin-releasing hormone receptor1 gene SNP and haplotype with major depression", *Neurosci. Lett.*, vol. 404, no. 3, pp. 358–362.

MacGregor, A. J., Andrew, T., Sambrook, P. N., & Spector, T. D. 2004, "Structural, psychological, and genetic influences on low back and neck pain: a study of adult female twins", *Arthritis Rheum*, vol. 51, no. 2, pp. 160–167.

MacGregor, A. J., Griffiths, G. O., Baker, J., & Spector, T. D. 1997, "Determinants of pressure pain threshold in adult twins: evidence that shared environmental influences predominate", *Pain*, vol. 73, no. 2, pp. 253–257.

Magni, G., Moreschi, C., Rigatti-Luchini, S., & Merskey, H. 1994, "Prospective study on the relationship between depressive symptoms and chronic musculoskeletal pain", *Pain*, vol. 56, no. 3, pp. 289–297.

Mannisto, P. T. & Kaakkola, S. 1999, "Catechol-O-methyltransferase (COMT): biochemistry, molecular biology, pharmacology, and clinical efficacy of the new selective COMT inhibitors", *Pharmacol. Rev.*, vol. 51, no. 4, pp. 593–628.

Massat, I., Souery, D., Del Favero, J., Nothen, M., Blackwood, D., Muir, W., Kaneva, R., Serretti, A., Lorenzi, C., Rietschel, M., Milanova, V., Papadimitriou, G. N., Dikeos, D.,

Van Broekhoven, C., & Mendlewicz, J. 2005, "Association between COMT (Val158Met) functional polymorphism and early onset in patients with major depressive disorder in a European multicenter genetic association study", *Mol. Psychiatry*, vol. 10, no. 6, pp. 598–605.

Melke, J., Landen, M., Baghei, F., Rosmond, R., Holm, G., Bjorntorp, P., Westberg, L., Hellstrand, M., & Eriksson, E. 2001, "Serotonin transporter gene polymorphisms are associated with anxiety-related personality traits in women", *Am. J. Med. Genet.*, vol. 105, no. 5, pp. 458–463.

Michalowicz, B. S., Pihlstrom, B. L., Hodges, J. S., & Bouchard, T. J., Jr. 2000, "No heritability of temporomandibular joint signs and symptoms", *J. Dent. Res.*, vol. 79, no. 8, pp. 1573–1578.

Mogil, J. S. 1999, "The genetic mediation of individual differences in sensitivity to pain and its inhibition", *Proc. Natl. Acad. Sci. U.S.A*, vol. 96, no. 14, pp. 7744–7751.

Mogil, J. S. & Max, M. B. 2006, "The genetics of pain," in *Wall and Melzack's Textbook of Pain*, Fifth edn, S. B. McMahon & M. Koltzenburg, eds., Elsevier, pp. 159–174.

Mogil, J. S., Ritchie, J., Smith, S. B., Strasburg, K., Kaplan, L., Wallace, M. R., Romberg, R. R., Bijl, H., Sarton, E. Y., Fillingim, R. B., & Dahan, A. 2005, "Melanocortin-1 receptor gene variants affect pain and mu-opioid analgesia in mice and humans", *J. Med. Genet.*, vol. 42, no. 7, pp. 583–587.

Mogil, J. S., Wilson, S. G., Bon, K., Lee, S. E., Chung, K., Raber, P., Pieper, J. O., Hain, H. S., Belknap, J. K., Hubert, L., Elmer, G. I., Chung, J. M., & Devor, M. 1999, "Heritability of nociception II. 'Types' of nociception revealed by genetic correlation analysis", *Pain*, vol. 80, no. 1–2, pp. 83–93.

Mogil, J. S., Wilson, S. G., Chesler, E. J., Rankin, A. L., Nemmani, K. V., Lariviere, W. R., Groce, M. K., Wallace, M. R., Kaplan, L., Staud, R., Ness, T. J., Glover, T. L., Stankova, M., Mayorov, A., Hruby, V. J., Grisel, J. E., & Fillingim, R. B. 2003, "The melanocortin-1 receptor gene mediates female-specific mechanisms of analgesia in mice and humans", *Proc. Natl. Acad. Sci. U.S.A*, vol. 100, no. 8, pp. 4867–4872.

Mohammed, I., Cherkas, L. F., Riley, S. A., Spector, T. D., & Trudgill, N. J. 2003, "Genetic influences in gastro-oesophageal reflux disease: a twin study", *Gut*, vol. 52, no. 8, pp. 1085–1089.

Morris-Yates, A., Talley, N. J., Boyce, P. M., Nandurkar, S., & Andrews, G. 1998, "Evidence of a genetic contribution to functional bowel disorder", *Am. J. Gastroenterol.*, vol. 93, no. 8, pp. 1311–1317.

Moulin, D. E., Clark, A. J., Speechley, M., & Morley-Forster, P. K. 2002, "Chronic pain in Canada–prevalence, treatment, impact and the role of opioid analgesia", *Pain Res. Manag.*, vol. 7, no. 4, pp. 179–184.

Mulder, E. J., Van Baal, C., Gaist, D., Kallela, M., Kaprio, J., Svensson, D. A., Nyholt, D. R., Martin, N. G., MacGregor, A. J., Cherkas, L. F., Boomsma, D. I., & Palotie, A. 2003, "Genetic and environmental influences on migraine: a twin study across six countries", *Twin. Res.*, vol. 6, no. 5, pp. 422–431.

Nelson, D. V., Novy, D. M., Averill, P. M., & Berry, L. A. 1996, "Ethnic comparability of the MMPI in pain patients", *J. Clin. Psychol.*, vol. 52, no. 5, pp. 485–497.

Nielsen, C. S., Stubhaug, A., Price, D. D., Vassend, O., Czajkowski, N., & Harris, J. R. 2008, "Individual differences in pain sensitivity: Genetic and environmental contributions", *Pain* May, vol. 136, no. 1–3, pp. 21–9.

Norbury, T. A., MacGregor, A. J., Urwin, J., Spector, T. D., & McMahon, S. B. 2007, "Heritability of responses to painful stimuli in women: a classical twin study", *Brain*, vol. 130, no. Pt 11, pp. 3041–3049.

Offenbaecher, M., Bondy, B., de Jonge, S., Glatzeder, K., Kruger, M., Schoeps, P., & Ackenheil, M. 1999, "Possible association of fibromyalgia with a polymorphism in the serotonin transporter gene regulatory region.", *Arthritis Rheum*, vol. 42, no. 11, pp. 2482–8.

Olsson, C. A., Byrnes, G. B., Anney, R. J., Collins, V., Hemphill, S. A., Williamson, R., & Patton, G. C. 2007, "COMT Val(158)Met and 5HTTLPR functional loci interact to predict persistence of anxiety across adolescence: results from the Victorian Adolescent Health Cohort Study", *Genes Brain Behav.*, vol. 6, no. 7, pp. 647–652.

Paassilta, P., Lohiniva, J., Goring, H. H., Perala, M., Raina, S. S., Karppinen, J., Hakala, M., Palm, T., Kroger, H., Kaitila, I., Vanharanta, H., Ott, J., & Ala-Kokko, L. 2001, "Identification of a novel common genetic risk factor for lumbar disk disease", *JAMA*, vol. 285, no. 14, pp. 1843–1849.

Paulson, P. E., Minoshima, S., Morrow, T. J., & Casey, K. L. 1998, "Gender differences in pain perception and patterns of cerebral activation during noxious heat stimulation in humans", *Pain*, vol. 76, no. 1–2, pp. 223–229.

Payne, B. & Norfleet, M. A. 1986, "Chronic pain and the family: a review", *Pain*, vol. 26, no. 1, pp. 1–22.

Pincus, T., Burton, A. K., Vogel, S., & Field, A. P. 2002, "A systematic review of psychological factors as predictors of chronicity/disability in prospective cohorts of low back pain", *Spine*, vol. 27, no. 5, p. E109–E120.

Poulsen, L., Brosen, K., Arendt-Nielsen, L., Gram, L. F., Elbaek, K., & Sindrup, S. H. 1996, "Codeine and morphine in extensive and poor metabolizers of sparteine: pharmacokinetics, analgesic effect and side effects", *Eur. J. Clin. Pharmacol.*, vol. 51, no. 3–4, pp. 289–295.

Rahim-Williams, F. B., Riley, J. L., III, Herrera, D., Campbell, C. M., Hastie, B. A., & Fillingim, R. B. 2007, "Ethnic identity predicts experimental pain sensitivity in African Americans and Hispanics", *Pain*, vol. 129, no. 1–2, pp. 177–184.

Rijsdijk, F. V., Snieder, H., Ormel, J., Sham, P., Goldberg, D. P., & Spector, T. D. 2003, "Genetic and environmental influences on psychological distress in the population: General Health Questionnaire analyses in UK twins", *Psychol. Med.*, vol. 33, no. 5, pp. 793–801.

Riley, J. L., III, Robinson, M. E., Wise, E. A., & Price, D. D. 1999, "A meta-analytic review of pain perception across the menstrual cycle", *Pain*, vol. 81, no. 3, pp. 225–235.

Robinson, M. E., Riley, J. L., III, Myers, C. D., Papas, R. K., Wise, E. A., Waxenberg, L. B., & Fillingim, R. B. 2001, "Gender role expectations of pain: relationship to sex differences in pain", *J. Pain*, vol. 2, no. 5, pp. 251–257.

Russell, M. B., Levi, N., & Kaprio, J. 2007, "Genetics of tension-type headache: A population based twin study", *Am. J. Med. Genet. B Neuropsychiatr. Genet*, Dec 5, vol. 144B, no. 8, pp. 982–6.

Sato, M., Ohashi, J., Tsuchiya, N., Kashiwase, K., Ishikawa, Y., Arita, H., Hanaoka, K., Tokunaga, K., & Yabe, T. 2002, "Association of HLA-A*3303-B*4403-DRB1*1302 haplotype, but not of TNFA promoter and NKp30 polymorphism, with postherpetic neuralgia (PHN) in the Japanese population", *Genes Immun.*, vol. 3, no. 8, pp. 477–481.

Schurks, M., Limmroth, V., Geissler, I., Tessmann, G., Savidou, I., Engelbergs, J., Kurth, T., Diener, H. C., & Rosskopf, D. 2007, "Association between migraine and the G1246A polymorphism in the hypocretin receptor 2 gene", *Headache*, vol. 47, no. 8, pp. 1195–1199.

Sindrup, S. H., Brosen, K., Bjerring, P., Arendt-Nielsen, L., Larsen, U., Angelo, H. R., & Gram, L. F. 1990, "Codeine increases pain thresholds to copper vapor laser stimuli in extensive but not poor metabolizers of sparteine", *Clin. Pharmacol. Ther.*, vol. 48, no. 6, pp. 686–693.

Sindrup, S. H., Poulsen, L., Brosen, K., Ardendt-Nielsen, L., & Gram, L. F. 1993, "Are poor metabolisers of sparteine/debrisoquine less pain tolerant than extensive metabolisers?", *Pain*, vol. 53, pp. 335–349.

Stein, M. B., Fallin, M. D., Schork, N. J., & Gelernter, J. 2005, "COMT polymorphisms and anxiety-related personality traits", *Neuropsychopharmacology*, vol. 30, no. 11, pp. 2092–2102.

Stewart, W. F., Lipton, R. B., & Liberman, J. 1996, "Variation in migraine prevalence by race", *Neurology*, vol. 47, no. 1, pp. 52–59.

Tegeder, I., Costigan, M., Griffin, R. S., Abele, A., Belfer, I., Schmidt, H., Ehnert, C., Nejim, J., Marian, C., Scholz, J., Wu, T., Allchorne, A., Diatchenko, L., Binshtok, A. M., Goldman, D., Adolph, J., Sama, S., Atlas, S. J., Carlezon, W. A., Parsegian, A., Lotsch, J., Fillingim, R. B., Maixner, W., Geisslinger, G., Max, M. B., & Woolf, C. J. 2006, "GTP cyclohydrolase and tetrahydrobiopterin regulate pain sensitivity and persistence", *Nat. Med.*, vol. 12, no. 11, pp. 1269–1277.

Treloar, S. A., Martin, N. G., & Heath, A. C. 1998, "Longitudinal genetic analysis of menstrual flow, pain, and limitation in a sample of Australian twins", *Behav. Genet.*, vol. 28, no. 2, pp. 107–116.

Turk, D. C., Flor, H., & Rudy, T. E. 1987, "Pain and families. I. Etiology, maintenance, and psychosocial impact", *Pain*, vol. 30, no. 1, pp. 3–27.

Turkat, I. D. & Guise, B. J. 1983, "The effects of vicarious experience and stimulus intensity on pain termination and work avoidance", *Behav. Res. Ther.*, vol. 21, no. 3, pp. 241–245.

Turkat, I. D. & Noskin, D. E. 1983, "Vicarious and operant experiences in the etiology of illness behavior: a replication with healthy individuals", *Behav. Res. Ther.*, vol. 21, no. 2, pp. 169–172.

van de Beek, W. J., Roep, B. O., van der Slik, A. R., Giphart, M. J., & van Hilten, B. J. 2003, "Susceptibility loci for complex regional pain syndrome", *Pain*, vol. 103, no. 1–2, pp. 93–97.

Vlaeyen, J. W. & Linton, S. J. 2000, "Fear-avoidance and its consequences in chronic musculoskeletal pain: a state of the art", *Pain*, vol. 85, no. 3, pp. 317–332.

Wade, J. B., Price, D. D., Hamer, R. M., Schwartz, S. M., & Hart, R. P. 1990, "An emotional component analysis of chronic pain", *Pain*, vol. 40, no. 3, pp. 303–310.

Wang, X., Trivedi, R., Treiber, F., & Snieder, H. 2005, "Genetic and environmental influences on anger expression, John Henryism, and stressful life events: the Georgia Cardiovascular Twin Study", *Psychosom. Med.*, vol. 67, no. 1, pp. 16–23.

Werner, M. U., Duun, P., & Kehlet, H. 2004, "Prediction of postoperative pain by pre-operative nociceptive responses to heat stimulation", *Anesthesiology*, vol. 100, no. 1, pp. 115–119.

Wiesenfeld-Hallin, Z. 2005, "Sex differences in pain perception", *Gend. Med.*, vol. 2, no. 3, pp. 137–145.

Wilhelm, K., Siegel, J. E., Finch, A. W., Hadzi-Pavlovic, D., Mitchell, P. B., Parker, G., & Schofield, P. R. 2007, "The long and the short of it: associations between 5-HTT genotypes and coping with stress", *Psychosom. Med.*, vol. 69, no. 7, pp. 614–620.

Wolfe, F., Smythe, H. A., Yunus, M. B., Bennett, R. M., Bombardier, C., Goldenberg, D. L., Tugwell, P., Campbell, S. M., Abeles, M., Clark, P., & . 1990, "The American College of Rheumatology 1990 Criteria for the Classification of Fibromyalgia. Report of the Multicenter Criteria Committee", *Arthritis Rheum*, vol. 33, no. 2, pp. 160–172.

Yang, J. W., Lee, S. H., Ryu, S. H., Lee, B. C., Kim, S. H., Joe, S. H., Jung, I. K., Choi, I. G., & Ham, B. J. 2007, "Association between Monoamine Oxidase A Polymorphisms and Anger-Related Personality Traits in Korean Women", *Neuropsychobiology*, vol. 56, no. 1, pp. 19–23.

Zatzick, D. F. & Dimsdale, J. E. 1990, "Cultural variations in response to painful stimuli", *Psychosom. Med.*, vol. 52, no. 5, pp. 544–557.

Zill, P., Baghai, T. C., Zwanzger, P., Schule, C., Eser, D., Rupprecht, R., Moller, H. J., Bondy, B., & Ackenheil, M. 2004, "SNP and haplotype analysis of a novel tryptophan hydroxylase isoform (TPH2) gene provide evidence for association with major depression", *Mol. Psychiatry*, vol. 9, no. 11, pp. 1030–1036.

Zondervan, K. T., Cardon, L. R., Kennedy, S. H., Martin, N. G., & Treloar, S. A. 2005, "Multivariate genetic analysis of chronic pelvic pain and associated phenotypes", *Behav. Genet.*, vol. 35, no. 2, pp. 177–188.

Zubieta, J. K., Heitzeg, M. M., Smith, Y. R., Bueller, J. A., Xu, K., Xu, Y., Koeppe, R. A.,
    Stohler, C. S., & Goldman, D. 2003, "COMT val158met genotype affects mu-opioid
    neurotransmitter responses to a pain stressor", *Science*, vol. 299, no. 5610, pp. 1240–1243.
Zubieta, J. K., Smith, Y. R., Bueller, J. A., Xu, Y., Kilbourn, M. R., Jewett, D. M., Meyer, C.
    R., Koeppe, R. A., & Stohler, C. S. 2002, "mu-opioid receptor-mediated antinociceptive
    responses differ in men and women", *J. Neurosci.*, vol. 22, no. 12, pp. 5100–5107.

Pain and the Placebo Effect

Antonella Pollo and Fabrizio Benedetti

Psychological Modulation of Pain

Since ancient times it has been recognized that many psychological factors can strongly influence and modulate the multidimensional experience of pain. Attending a distracting toy can make a distressed child stop crying, and expectation of pain relief can lessen the unpleasantness of stomach-aches. Attention, emotions, suggestions and expectations, anxiety, fear, mood are among the best known examples of factors that can shape the processing of nociceptive information as it travels from the spinal cord to higher centers in the brain.

The understanding of the neurobiological basis of this top-down modulation of pain represents a challenge in pain research and many efforts are currently devoted to the development of models illustrating its "modus operandi". One such model is offered by placebo analgesia, i.e. the lessening of pain experienced in response to a therapeutic act devoid of intrinsic analgesic activity. As it will be detailed in this chapter, placebo analgesia is mediated by expectation and/or conditioning, involving the modulation of neural activity in a number of centers of the so-called "pain matrix". But the comprehension of what goes on inside our nervous system when we trust the clinician handing us a sugar pill and boosting our expectation of pain relief goes beyond the boundaries of pain research, yielding precious information on the links between mental activity and body functions, and contributing to a unitary vision of psyche and soma.

The aim of this chapter is to provide the reader with an understanding of how the pain experience can be affected by a placebo treatment, either in the form of a drug or a physical manipulation, extending the concept of placebo to include all aspects of the context surrounding the care of the patient.

A. Pollo (✉)
Dipartimento di Neuroscienze, Università degli Studi di Torino, Corso Raffaello 30, I-10125 Torino, Italy
e-mail: antonella.pollo@unito.it

R.J. Moore (ed.), *Biobehavioral Approaches to Pain*,
DOI 10.1007/978-0-387-78323-9_4, © Springer Science+Business Media, LLC 2009

The Placebo Effect and Its Measurement

To evaluate the pharmacological action of a new drug in a clinical trial, it is crucial to compare the effect following its administration with that elicited in a control group receiving a sham treatment, similar in all respects to the treatment under investigation but lacking the drug active principle. This group is known as the placebo arm of the clinical trial and the overall effect observed in it is usually, although wrongly, considered as the placebo effect. The symptom amelioration in the placebo arm can in fact be due to a number of different factors, only one of which is the placebo effect. All these factors can be conveniently lumped together as nonspecific when the aim is to conduct a pharmacological analysis, but must be carefully dissected when investigating the placebo effect itself. The first and most important source of confusion is the natural history, that is, the time course of a symptom or disease, in the absence of any external intervention. For example, pain can undergo spontaneous fluctuations in time: a remission right after placebo administration could then be mistakenly interpreted as placebo analgesia, or cause an overestimation of the placebo effect, while the opposite can occur if a pain exacerbation sets in (Fields & Levine, 1984). Another aspect to be considered is a statistical phenomenon called regression to the mean, whereby patients in pain seeking medical advice are likely to obtain pain measurement scores which on a second evaluation are lower than they were at the first visit. In other words, chances are that they undergo the first test near the peak of a pain fluctuation, while the pain may have subsided at the time of the second visit, thus inducing a false impression of improvement (Davis, 2002). Other possible confounding problems are biases, errors in the detection of relief (judgment errors), or concurrent actions of simultaneously intervening agents, for instance the soothing action of the cold swab onto which a placebo painkiller has been sprayed. Thus, only carefully designed experimental studies targeting on the placebo can demonstrate the real psychobiological placebo response, that is, the effect remaining when all other possible sources of improvement have been ruled out. Conversely, the attempt to assess the extent of placebo effects from the analysis of clinical trials conducted for pharmacological reasons, even when they include a natural history group, can be misleading, thus conducting to erroneous conclusions (Hrobjartsson & Gotzsche, 2001; Vase, Riley, & Price, 2002; Wampold, Minami, Callen Tierney, Baskin, & Bhati, 2005; Thorn, 2007 and the commentaries therein).

When referring to the outcome of an inert treatment, the terms placebo effect and placebo response are often used as synonyms. To be strictly correct, however, the first refers to the effect observed in the control group of a clinical trial, thus including any cause of improvement other than the drug being tested, while the second defines the causal relationship between a placebo and its effect in a single individual, and is thus more aptly investigated when searching for the psychobiological process involved. Still, given the difficulties outlined above, which make it very hard to identify the placebo response as such in a single individual, it is usually in a group of subjects that the response is statistically evidenced.

From the Sugar Pill to Context Effects: Conditioning and Expectation

For a long time, the word placebo has been equated with "sugar pill". It was widespread practice to give a carbohydrate tablet as a means of detecting the mystifying patient (identified through the success of the sham therapy), or as a compassionate remedy to the terminally ill. However, the aim of "pleasing the patient", as the latin etymology *placēre* suggests, can clearly be achieved not only with drugs, but also with any medical treatment ranging from physical cures to psychotherapy. What matters is not the sugar, of course, but its symbolic significance, which can be attached to virtually anything (Brody, 2000). Moerman (2002) has proposed to substitute the term *placebo response* with *meaning response*, to underscore the importance of the patient's beliefs about the treatment and stress what is present (something inducing the expectation of a benefit) rather than what is absent (a chemical or manipulation of proven specific efficacy). The raised expectation then triggers an internal change which in turn determines a specific experience, e.g. a reduction of pain (Kirsch, 1985, 1990, 1999).

Thus, the concept of placebo must be extended to embrace all aspects of the therapeutic act. In this sense, we may affirm that the placebo effect is a context effect, produced by the global perception of the cure, i.e. the ensemble of all the features contributing to it, like the physician's words, the sight and smell of the environment, the memory of past experiences in similar situations (Di Blasi, Harkness, Ernst, Georgiou, & Kleijnen, 2001; Benedetti, 2002).

Manipulating the context can then result in the modulation of the placebo response. A large body of evidence points to the role of expectations in shaping the response to a sham treatment. For example, grading the degree of expectation produces graded responses: the same placebo cream applied onto three contiguous skin areas induces a progressively stronger analgesia, according to the strength of the accompanying words ("it is a powerful/weak analgesic cream") (Price et al., 1999). Moving from the experimental to the clinical setting, changing the symbolic meaning of a basal infusion in postoperative patients impacts on their analgesic request. In spite of all patients receiving a physiological solution, those who believed that they would receive an analgesic drug demanded significantly less painkillers than those who believed that they would receive no pain reliever at all. Interestingly, the belief certainty also mattered: a group of patients with uncertain expectations, warned that they could receive either a painkiller or a placebo in a double blind protocol, requested an intermediate dose of analgesics (Pollo et al., 2001). Non verbal clues are equally important. Deceiving clinicians as to the substance (placebo or drug) being administered to two groups of patients, when in fact both groups received a placebo, resulted in a bigger effect in the group believed by the clinicians to receive a drug (Gracely, Dubner, Deeter, & Wolskee, 1985). This suggests that in the interaction between a patient and his clinician also unintentionally conveyed impressions are important.

It has also been demonstrated that the influence of the context on the outcome of a therapy is mediated by a conditioning process. In this process, the repeated co-occurrence of an unconditioned response to an unconditioned stimulus (e.g. salivation after the sight of food) with a conditioned stimulus (e.g. a bell ringing) induces a conditioned response (i.e., salivation that is induced by bell ringing alone). Likewise, aspects of the clinical setting (e.g. taste, color, shape of a tablet, as well as white coats, or the peculiar hospital smell) can also act as conditioned stimuli, eliciting a therapeutic response in the absence of an active principle, just because they have been paired with it in the past (Wikramasekera, 1985; Siegel, 1985, 2002; Ader, 1997). In a series of studies, Voudouris and colleagues applied a protocol whereby conditioning was achieved by pairing a placebo analgesic cream with a painful stimulation, which was surreptitiously reduced with respect to a baseline condition to mislead the subject regarding the analgesic effect. In this way, a direct comparison could be made between a conditioned and an unconditioned group. Pain reduction following conditioning was invariably larger, indicating the effectiveness of conditioning in mediating a placebo response (Voudouris, Peck, & Coleman, 1985, 1989, 1990).

The two mechanisms of conditioning and expectation are not mutually exclusive. It has been argued that in the course of conditioning, by learning that the unconditioned stimulus (food or pain decrease) will follow the conditioned one (bell or pill), the subject does in fact learn what to expect (Montgomery & Kirsch, 1997; Reiss, 1980; Rescorla, 1988). Both mechanisms have been shown to be at work in the same experimental protocol, testing pain tolerance in arm ischemic pain (Amanzio & Benedetti, 1999). In a group of subjects a series of pain tolerance measurements were made in control conditions, after conditioning with a potent analgesic (morphine) and after a placebo. The increase in pain tolerance in this last trial reflects the simultaneous action of conditioning and expectation, because the subjects were instructed that they would receive the same potent analgesic drug as during the conditioning trials. If, on the other hand, the subjects were told that they would be given only an antibiotic to prevent infection, thus selectively eliminating the contribution of expectation, a placebo increase was still observed, although smaller. Similarly, a lower effect was also shown when the placebo was given without prior conditioning with morphine, just with the accompanying instruction inducing expectation of pain relief. Thus, it appears that the two mechanisms can be triggered independently and that their outcomes are additive.

A selective role for conditioning, without the contribution of anticipatory processes, can also be demonstrated for physiological functions controlled by the subconscious domain, like those involving the immune system or neuroendocrine secretions (Pacheco-López, Engler, Niemi, & Schedlowski, 2006). In mice, development of autoimmune disease was dramatically modified by classical conditioning of immunosuppression, pairing placebo saccharin with the immunosuppressant cyclophosphamide (Ader & Cohen, 1982). In multiple sclerosis patients, decrements in peripheral leukocyte counts induced by cyclophosphamide could be conditioned by pairing the drug with a strongly flavoured beverage (Giang et al., 1996). In healthy subjects, a similar conditioning with cyclosporine A produced immunosuppression after placebo, as assessed by depressed mRNA expression of IL-2 and interferon-gamma, and lymphocyte proliferation (Goebel et al., 2002).

In another experimental protocol, placebo modulation of growth hormone (GH) and cortisol secretion could be obtained after conditioning with sumatriptan (a selective $5-HT_{1B/1D}$ receptor agonist stimulating GH and inhibiting cortisol secretion). It was not possible to reverse this modulation by inducing the opposite expectation in the subjects. Also, suggestion alone, in the absence of conditioning, was unable to induce placebo hormonal modulation. However, when a similar expectation/conditioning competition protocol was applied to placebo analgesia, where cognitive conscious processes play an important role, it was indeed possible to reverse the effect achieved by conditioning by expectations of hyperalgesia (Benedetti et al., 2003; see also below, placebo and nocebo). Thus, it appears that in unconscious processes only conditioning is important in mediating the placebo response, with no effect of expectation, while in conscious processes both expectation and conditioning play a role, with conditioning possibly acting through a learning process inducing expectation.

The Neurobiology of the Placebo Effect

What exactly happens in the patient's brain experiencing pain relief after a trust-inspiring clinician assures him that the sham medicament he has just delivered will shortly take effect? The same thing that happened over and over many centuries back, when medicine was still in its infancy and shamans half-unknowingly exploited the powers of the human mind: endogenous opioids are released.

The involvement of endogenous opioids in placebo analgesia was first proposed by Levine, Gordon, and Fields (1978) by studying dental postoperative pain. In their patients, the opiate antagonist naloxone reduced the probability of a positive placebo response. Following that pioneering study, many accurate and carefully designed experiments confirmed the efficacy of naloxone in blocking placebo analgesia (Benedetti, 1996; Fields & Levine, 1984; Grevert, Albert, & Goldstein, 1983; Levine & Gordon, 1984). Gradually, many lines of evidence converged to corroborate a model whereby pain can be placebo-modulated through the secretion of endogenous opioids in the brain. In the cerebrospinal fluid of placebo-responders the peak concentration of β-endorphin was more than twice that of placebo non-responders (Lipman et al., 1990). The naloxone-sensitive effect showed a strict site specificity, being possible to reverse the placebo response of a cream applied on different body parts together with locally circumscribed instructions as to where the cream would produce analgesia (Benedetti, Arduino, & Amanzio, 1999a). Therefore, it seems that the endogenous opioid system is somatotopically organized. Opioids released by the central nervous system after a placebo procedure also showed the typical side-effects of exogenously administered narcotics. Measuring minute ventilation during and after conditioning with buprenorphine in thoracotomized patients resulted in depression of the respiratory centers with both the drug and the subsequently administered placebo, an effect which could be prevented by naloxone (Benedetti, Amanzio, Baldi, Casadio, & Maggi, 1999b). The β-adrenergic sympathetic system was also inhibited during placebo-induced expectation of analgesia, as shown by slowed heart rate and reduced β-adrenergic spectral component of heart rate variability, once again in a naloxone-sensitive way. It is not known however, whether the effect on the heart is mediated by the pain reduction or caused by a direct action of endogenous opioids (Pollo, Vighetti, Rainero, & Benedetti, 2003). Indirect evidence for a role of endogenous opioids is provided also by the involvement of the opioid antagonist cholecystokinin (CCK). The CCK antagonist proglumide potentiated the placebo analgesic response in a model of experimental ischemic pain, suggesting an inhibitory role for CCK in placebo analgesia (Benedetti, Amanzio, & Maggi, 1995). The overlapping distribution of opioid and CCK peptides and their receptors, and the proposed existence of regulatory loops between the two systems (Noble & Roques, 2003) suggest that placebo responses can be regulated by the opposing actions of promoting endogenous opioids, and inhibiting endogenous CCK peptides (see also below, placebo and nocebo).

Notwithstanding this compelling evidence, not all placebo responses seem to be opioid-dependent. In some situations, an effect can still occur after blockade of opioid mechanisms by naloxone (Gracely, Dubner, Wolskee, & Deeter, 1983; Vase, Robinson, Verne, & Price, 2005). In the study by Amanzio and Benedetti (1999) on experimental ischemic arm pain, a complete blockade could be observed when the placebo analgesic response was induced by means of cognitive expectation cues and conditioning with morphine, alone or in combination. In contrast, when the conditioning procedure was carried out with ketorolac, a non-opioid drug, the effect of naloxone was greatly diminished (but still present), if suggestions were associated, but totally abolished if conditioning was unaccompanied by expectation. These results point to the existence of specific non-opioid systems which can act independently. Almost nothing is known at present of these non-opioid mechanisms and additional research is needed to better clarify their action. The effects of conditioning and expectation are summarized in Fig. 1.

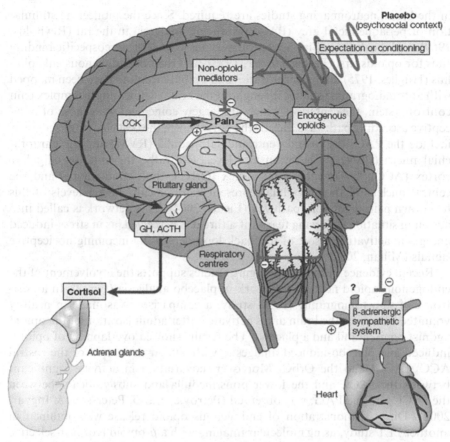

Fig. 1 Cascade of biochemical events after placebo administration. Placebo administration, along with verbal suggestions of analgesia (psychosocial context) might reduce pain through opioid and/or non-opioid mechanisms by expectation and/or conditioning mechanisms. The respiratory centers might also be inhibited by opioid mechanisms. The β-adrenergic sympathetic system of the heart is also inhibited during placebo analgesia, although the mechanism is not known (either reduction of the pain itself and/or the direct action of endogenous opioids). Cholecystokinin (CCK) counteracts the effects of the endogenous opioids, thereby antagonizing placebo analgesia. Placebos can also act on serotonin-dependent growth hormone (GH) and cortisol secretion, in both the pituitary and adrenal glands, thereby mimicking the effect of the analgesic drug sumatriptan. ACTH, adrenocorticotrophic hormone (From Colloca and Benedetti, 2005)

How the Brain Produces Placebo Analgesia – The Neuroimaging Studies

Neurochemical and pharmacological studies are providing satisfying, albeit still incomplete, answers to the question of *what* mediates placebo analgesia. In order to gain information about *where* and *when* placebo analgesia is generated in the brain, neuroimaging studies are required. Since the pioneering stimulation of periaqueductal grey (PAG) producing analgesia in the rat (Reynolds, 1969), and the discovery in the central nervous system of stereospecific binding sites for opioids first (Pert & Snyder, 1973), and then of endogenous enkephalins (Hughes, 1975), high concentrations of opioid receptors have been mapped with autoradiographic studies throughout the brain, delineating a complex pain control system, the centers of which are largely coincident with those of nociceptive ascending pathways. Beside the dorsal horn, the best characterized areas include the PAG, the rostral ventromedial medulla (RVM) and the parabrachial nuclei (PBN) at the brainstem level. Rostrally, the anterior cingulate cortex (ACC), the orbitofrontal cortex (OrbC), the hypothalamus and the central nucleus of the amygdala represent hierarchically higher levels of this top-down pain regulatory pathway (Fields, 2004). This network is called into action in situations inducing fear or if a threat is perceived, as in stress-induced analgesia, activating a sort of feedback loop depressing incoming nociceptive signals (Millan, 2002).

Recent evidence from neuroimaging studies supports the involvement of the endogenous opioid neuronal network in placebo analgesia (Fig. 2). In a positron emission tomography (PET) study, a comparison was made in healthy volunteers between the brain areas activated after administration of the opioid agonist remifentanil and a placebo. The results showed overlapping of opioid-induced and placebo-induced analgesia, with similar activation of the rostral ACC (rACC) and the OrbC. Moreover, covariation in activity, significant between the rACC and the lower pons/medulla and subsignificant between the rACC and the PAG, was observed (Petrovic, Kalso, Petersson, & Ingvar, 2002). Direct demonstration of endogenous opioid release was obtained in another PET study, using molecular imaging with a μ-opioid receptor-selective radiotracer, a sensitive technique showed to effectively reveal the activation of opioid neurotransmission as a reduction of the in vivo availability of μ-opioid receptors to bind the radiolabeled tracer (Bencherif, Fuchs, Sheth, Dannals, Campbell, & Frost, 2002). After placebo, decreased binding was observed in pregenual rACC, insula, nucleus accumbens and dorsolateral prefrontal cortex (DLPFC); in all areas except DLPFC, this decrease was correlated with placebo reduction of pain intensity reports (Zubieta et al., 2005). A connectivity analysis recently identified placebo dependent contributions of rACC activity with bilateral amygdalae and the PAG, confirming the cognitive role of rACC as a crucial control area for antinociception (Bingel, Lorenz, Schoell, Weiller, & Büchel, 2006).

Beside supporting the function of endogenous opioids, neuroimaging studies also provide interesting data to corroborate the role of expectation. In a functional magnetic resonance imaging (fMRI) study, not only did placebo administration induce a decrease in the activation of pain regions such as thalamus, ACC and insula (correlated with the decrease in pain intensity report), but also an increase in DLPFC activity in the anticipatory phase. The latter was negatively correlated with the signal reduction in thalamus, ACC and insula and

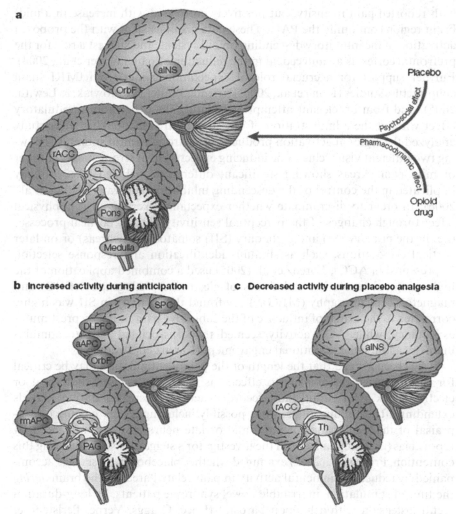

Fig. 2 Summary of brain imaging studies with the different brain regions that are involved in placebo analgesia. **a** | Brain regions activated by both the administration of a placebo and the administration of an opioid drug, which indicates that mental events (psychosocial effect) and painkillers (pharmacodynamic effect) might have similar effects on the brain (data from Petrovic et al., 2002). **b** | Detailed representation of the brain regions that are activated by the administration of a placebo. During the anticipatory phase, the activated regions are likely to represent the activation of a cognitive-evaluative network. **c** | During placebo analgesia, there is a decrease in the activity of different brain areas that are involved in pain processing, thus indicating an effect of the placebo on pain transmission (data from Wager et al., 2004). aAPC, anterior anterior prefrontal cortex; aINS, anterior insula; DLPFC, dorsolateral prefrontal cortex; OrbF, orbitofrontal cortex; PAG, periacqueductal grey; rACC, rostral anterior cingulate cortex; rmAPC, rostral medial anterior prefrontal cortex; SPC, superior parietal cortex; Th, thalamus (The entire figure is from Colloca and Benedetti, 2005)

with reported pain intensity, but positively correlated with increase in a mid-brain region containing the PAG. These data are consistent with the proposed activation of the inhibitory descending opioid system, and suggest a role for the prefrontal cortex as an antecedent in the reduction of pain (Wager et al., 2004). Further support for a crucial role of expectation comes from fMRI sham acupuncture studies (Kong et al., 2006; Pariente, White, Frackowiak, & Lewith, 2005), and from an elegant attempt at isolating the expectation modulatory effect without the administration of any dummy treatment. This latter study analyzed the regional activation produced by a strong painful stimulus following two different visual clues, one inducing expectation of strong pain, the other of mild pain. Areas showing significant differences included those already implicated in the control of the descending inhibitory pathway (Keltner et al., 2006). In order to discriminate whether expectancy exerts its psychophysical effect through changes of the perceptual sensitivity of early cortical processes (i.e. in the primary (SI) and secondary (SII) somatosensory areas) or on later cortical elaborations, such as stimulus identification and response selection (represented in ACC), Lorenz et al. (2005) used a combined application of the high temporal resolution techniques of electroencephalography (EEG) and magnetoencephalography (MEG). They found that activity in SII was highly correlated to the extent of influence of the subjective pain rating by prestimulus expectancy, while ACC activity seemed to be associated only to stimulus intensity and related attentional engagement (Lorenz et al., 2005).

It has been argued that the length of the painful stimulation may be critical for the measurement of placebo effects, as most studies used short heat or electric shock pain stimuli and recorded activity decreases during periods extending after stimulus offset, thus possibly including a later cognitive reappraisal of the significance of pain, and/or late neural activity influenced by report bias (i.e. compliance with the investigator's suggestions). Addressing this contention, Price et al. (2007) examined whether placebo analgesia was accompanied by reductions in neural activity in pain-related areas of the brain *during* the time of stimulation, in irritable bowel syndrome patients, by long-duration rectal distension with a balloon barostat (Price, Craggs, Verne, Perlstein, & Robinson, 2007). They found that placebo analgesia was accompanied by reductions in brain activity similar to those resulting from lowering the strength of stimulation (in the thalamus, somatosensory cortex, insula and ACC), and that these reductions occurred during the stimulus presentation itself, not just when subjects reported pain. Notably, this study was conducted on a clinically relevant model of placebo analgesia and showed large placebo effects, consistent with the described discrepancy in magnitude between placebo responses in the experimental and clinical settings (Charron, Rainville, & Marchand, 2006).

As pain is a psychologically constructed experience, including not only sensory, but also affective and cognitive evaluation of the potential for harm, it is important to discriminate whether a placebo diminishes the pain experience by acting on one, all or a combination of the pain components. Moreover, a placebo may act by afferent pain fiber inhibition, but its effect could also be mediated centrally, by changes in specific pain regions (Wager et al., 2004). The high individual variability of the neurochemical response to placebo administration observed by Zubieta et al. (2005) was addressed by the same authors in a subsequent paper, where they tested by multiple regression models the influence on the activation of endogenous opioid neurotransmission of both expectation and experience of pain (i.e. the level of pain inducing "need" or motivation for pain relief). Their results indicate that the internal emotional state, the pain affective characteristics and the subject's pain sensitivity are important determinants of the differences observed (Zubieta, Yau, Scott, & Stohler, 2006). Thus, it appears that many factors may interact in shaping the placebo response, not only directly, but also through the modulation of other possible aspects like anxiety, attention or habituation. Although evidence is building up that nociceptive processing on one side, and pain affect, evaluation and judgement on the other, both contribute to the overall experience of placebo analgesia (Wager, Matre, & Casey, 2006; Matre, Casey, & Knardahl, 2006; Kong et al., 2006), a thorough grasping of the intricate interactions among the players of the game still eludes us.

Placebo and Nocebo

When a placebo is given with the explicit intent of improving the patient symptoms, or when the context surrounding the therapy acts in the same way, with or without awareness of the actors involved, what follows is a positive result. But conditioning and expectation can also work in the opposite direction, tilting the balance toward the negative side. What ensues then is a worsening of the patient condition, called a nocebo effect, from the latin nocēre, to harm (Kissel & Barrucand, 1964; Hahn, 1985). For example, nocebo hyperalgesia can be obtained by giving an inert treatment accompanied by verbal suggestions of worsening and the direction of the response can be directly influenced by cognitive manipulation (Dworkin, Chen, LeResche, & Clark, 1983).

For ethical reasons, it is difficult to devise studies investigating the nocebo effect, especially in the clinical setting. Consequently, we know much less about it than we know about the placebo effect. However, recent experiments in healthy volunteers and animals are beginning to yield fruitful results (Benedetti, Amanzio, Vighetti, & Asteggiano, 2006; Benedetti, Lanotte, Lopiano, & Colloca, 2007). A nocebo pain response could be evoked in post-operative patients by inducing negative expectations, and the pain increase following a saline infusion could be prevented by the CCK antagonist proglumide, in a dose-dependent way. The blockade by proglumide is not mediated by endogenous opioids, as it is unaffected by naloxone (Benedetti, Amanzio, Casadio, Oliaro, & Maggi, 1997). In search of an alternative mechanism of action of the CCK system, attention has been focused on anxiety, known to be enhanced by CCK and attenuated by CCK antagonists in animal models (Lydiard, 1994) and to be associated with hyperalgesia (Hebb, Poulin, Roach, Zacharko, & Drolet, 2005; Andre et al., 2005). In fact, the expectation of pain increase is a highly anxiogenic process, likely to be interfered with by drugs with anxiolytic activity, dampening CCK-boosted pain perception. Supporting this hypothesis, in a study on healthy volunteers employing the protocol of experimental ischemic arm pain, Benedetti et al. (2006) showed that nocebo hyperalgesia is accompanied by increased levels of adrenocorticotropic hormone (ACTH) and cortisol, which indicates hyperactivity of the hypothalamic-pituitary-adrenal (HPA) axis, consistent with a stress response. Following administration of a benzodiazepine anxiolytic drug (diazepam), both HPA hyperactivity and nocebo hyperalgesia were blocked, suggesting a key role for anxiety in both effects. However, when proglumide was given together with nocebo suggestions only hyperalgesia was completely prevented, with no effect on HPA axis. This suggests that CCK acts specifically on nocebo/anxiety-induced hyperalgesia, rather than on the more general process of nocebo-induced anxiety. In other words, nocebo suggestions induce anxiety, which in turn separately induces both HPA and pain enhancement. While diazepam acts on anxiety, thus blocking both effects, proglumide acts only on the pain pathway, downstream of the nocebo-induced anxiety.

Thus, placebo analgesia and nocebo hyperalgesia appear to be the two sides of the same coin, with opposing pain modulation mediated by the antagonist action of the opioid and CCK systems. Different context factors can act favourably or unfavourably on pain perception, pulling the rope in opposite directions, with the resulting balance depending on the prevailing influence. An example of contrasting influence is shown in the study by Benedetti et al. (2003), where the analgesic response, induced by pharmacological pre-conditioning with ketorolac together with placebo suggestions, could be turned into a hyperalgesic one just by reversing the verbal instructions.

As for placebo analgesia, brain imaging techniques have also helped shed light on the circuitry underlying nocebo hyperalgesia. In the case of nocebo, however, most studies have so far centered on negative expectations, without the concrete administration of any inert substance or sham physical manipulation. Strictly speaking, the effects described should then be defined as "nocebo-related" effects. Drawing on the notion that perceived unpleasantness of innocuous stimuli can be amplified by negative expectation, as shown by increased fMRI responses in ACC and insula (Sawamoto et al., 2000), which are regions whose activation can also be demonstrated during pain anticipation (Koyama, Tanaka, & Mikami, 1998; Porro et al., 2002; Porro, Cettolo, Francescato, & Baraldi, 2003), a number of recent studies have provided insight as to how pain experience can be enhanced by negative expectation. By combining psychophysical and fMRI techniques, a strict correlation was shown between the magnitude of expected pain and the level of activation of pain areas such as thalamus, insula, PFC and ACC (Koyama, McHaffie, Laurienti, & Coghill, 2005). By using MEG and EEG, it was demonstrated that SII-localized pain-evoked potentials were increased, in parallel with pain reporting, by cues announcing strong pain. This suggests a modulation of sensory gain of nociceptive stimuli (Lorenz et al., 2005). The effect of high or low expectancy was directly compared in a fMRI study where two different visual clues were employed to condition the subject to expect a high or low noxious thermal stimulus. When the high expectancy red light was then paired with the high painful stimulus, activation in the ipsilateral caudal anterior cingulate cortex, the head of the caudate, cerebellum, and the contralateral nucleus cuneiformis was significantly higher than when the same stimulus was paired with the low expectancy blue light (Keltner et al., 2006). Some of the brain areas involved overlap with those implicated in descending modulatory processes, suggesting that nocebo-related effect might be mediated by descending facilitatory pathways, from cortical regions activated by expectancy to brainstem nuclei where nociceptive ascending projections converge. Further data are needed to confirm this hypothesis, as imaging studies including administration of a nocebo are still missing.

Clinical Implications of Placebo Analgesia

As an example of how complex endogenous phenomena blend perception, affect and motivation into the construct of pain, placebo analgesia is of great interest to scientists enquiring the forming of human experience and the neurophysiological basis of mind-body interaction. But its clinical implications are of at least equal significance and patients may greatly benefit from the application of research findings, on placebo in general and on placebo analgesia in particular.

The Role of Expectation on the Outcome of a Clinical Trial: The "Principle of Uncertainty"

We have learned that expectation can powerfully influence the perception of pain. This posits a general caveat on the results of all clinical trials. The placebo control group should by definition serve the purpose of ruling out all factors other than the principle under investigation. But expectation of improvement is not usually among the controlled variables. A study on acupuncture has showed that results could be drastically reversed by redistributing the subjects according to what they believed was their group of assignment. In other words, no differences were found with the standard grouping, but the subjects expecting real acupuncture reported significant less pain than those believing to be in the sham group, regardless of the real assignment (Bausell, Lao, Bergman, Lee, & Berman, 2005). Similar results were obtained in another study, extended to a 6-month follow-up in a large sample (Linde et al., 2007). Any drug has the potential of interacting with patient expectations, thus the ascription of its effect to the pharmacodynamic or the psychosocial component can be difficult, if not impossible. If the very act of administering a therapeutic agent can induce in the patient's brain the activation of nonspecific pathways which have nothing to do with the specific action of the drug, then the clinician faces the same dilemma confronted by the physicist trying to locate an electron in the atom's orbit, but displacing it by the very act of measurement (Heisenberg uncertainty principle; Colloca & Benedetti, 2005). A possible solution is offered by a different design of clinical trials, comparing the effects of a drug administered openly and in a hidden way, i.e. without the patient's knowledge, thus shutting down the expectation mechanism. In fact, when the context around the therapy was eliminated, the placebo component of the drug's action was abolished, resulting in significantly lower analgesic efficacy (Amanzio, Pollo, Maggi, & Benedetti, 2001). Notably, in this way it is possible to analyze the placebo effect without actually giving a placebo, thus circumventing potential ethical limitations to the use of placebos in clinical practice (Colloca, Lopiano, Lanotte, & Benedetti, 2004).

The Placebo Therapeutic Potential

An obvious clinical exploitation of the placebo effect is offered by its therapeutic potential. If the psychosocial (context) component of a therapy needs to be eliminated in order to isolate pharmacological effects tested in clinical trials, it should on the contrary be enhanced as much as possible in routine clinical practice, to maximize the benefit of the therapeutic act. In fact, this is just what medicine took advantage of in its pre-scientific era.

The above mentioned greater effect of analgesics in the open respect to the hidden administration (Amanzio et al., 2001) was paralleled by a specular finding whereby the relapse of pain was faster and of larger intensity after open, rather than hidden, interruption of morphine analgesic therapy (Benedetti et al., 2003). Thus, a double target may be achieved, maximizing therapy outcome on one side and minimizing drug intake, along with side effects and tolerance, on the other.

The optimization of the psychosocial context can be achieved in countless ways, ranging from changing the symbolic meaning of the cure (as in the study by Pollo et al., 2001) to the improvement of therapist-patient interaction, whereby correct attitudes and appropriate words can positively impact on the patient's expectation and belief brain circuitry (Benedetti, 2002). Finding the time to promote trust and establish personal relationships is of special importance in our epoch of overcrowded hospitals and hastened clinical agendas. Concurrently, we must also be aware of the harm that can be done by the opposite approach, whereby negligence and distrust can act as nocebos, lessening the effectiveness of therapeutic agents.

Patients Without Expectations

A final word of caution must be spent concerning the approach to cognitively impaired patients. Pain treatment in the elderly poses special problems due to chronic pain, frail metabolism and concurrent illnesses, but particularly hampering is the inability to communicate and purposefully interact with the caregiver (see also McCarberg, this volume). In light of the role played by the context, it is reasonable to wonder whether in these patients a painkiller has the same effect as in a cognitively intact person. Following this reasoning, Benedetti et al. (2006) applied the open-hidden paradigm to Alzheimer's disease (AD) patients and found that the effect provoked by the psychosocial context in the open condition was completely lost, with comparable analgesia produced by lidocaine on venipuncture pain in the open and in the hidden condition. Moreover, a correlation was found between disruption of placebo effect, cognitive scores and disconnection of frontal lobes from the rest of the brain (Benedetti et al., 2006). Thus, analgesic, and possibly also other therapies, in AD and other neurodegenerative conditions might have to be revised, to make up for the loss of placebo-related mechanisms and contribute to the best possible quality of life in these patient populations.

Conclusions

Placebo analgesia should not be considered as the product of a deceptive therapy given to please the patient. Rather, it is a physiologically sound phenomenon, rooted in brain circuitry and biochemistry, the mechanisms of which we are finally beginning to unravel. They are providing us with a vision of mind-body interactions, enabling us to believe that we can influence our well being, if not by sheer willpower, at least by employing means known to act on our central nervous system. Placebo effects are not limited to analgesia, as described in this chapter, but extend to many conditions other than pain, with depression, neuroendocrine functions and motor performance being the most actively investigated. There seem to exist specific neural mechanisms responsible in each instance, suggesting that expectation and conditioning are general means of activation of different networks. Future directions for placebo research can be summarized as: 1- to study the networks operating in different pathological conditions, emphasising their similarities and differences and the possible role of common denominators such as the reward mechanism; 2- to exploit recent technological advances in neuroimaging and electrophysiology to design new placebo studies to detail the mechanisms of action of cognitive factors. 3- to elucidate how the psychosocial variables (patient's and clinician's personality, cultural characteristics, affective states...) interact to produce the psychophysiological changes typical of placebo effects. This can be best accomplished by integrating physiology and neurobiology with disciplines as diverse as sociology, anthropology and psychology. Most importantly, the knowledge gained in the laboratory must be applied in clinical practice. In this respect, only first tentative steps have been taken, and much remains to be done to fruitfully exploit and maximize the placebo effects, while minimizing nocebo effects: among the lines to follow, context optimization, improvement of the patient-clinician relationship, and development of specifically designed clinical trials, which take cognitive factors into account.

References

Ader, R. (1997). The role of conditioning in pharmacotherapy. In: Harrington, A. (Ed.). *The placebo effect: An interdisciplinary exploration* (pp. 138–165). Cambridge, MA: Harvard University Press.

Ader, R., & Cohen, N. (1982). Behaviorally conditioned immunosuppression and murine systemic lupus erythematosus. *Science, 215*:1534–1536.

Amanzio, M., & Benedetti, F. (1999). Neuropharmacological dissection of placebo analgesia: Expectation-activated 7/26/2008 3:28AMopioid systems versus conditioning-activated specific sub-systems. *Journal of Neuroscience, 19*:484–494.

Amanzio, M., Pollo, A., Maggi, G., & Benedetti, F. (2001). Response variability and to analgesics: A role for non-specific activation of endogenous opioids. *Pain, 90*:205–215.

Andre, J., Zeau, B., Pohl, M., Cesselin, F., Benoliel, J. J., & Becker, C. (2005). Involvement of cholecystokininergic systems in anxiety-induced hyperalgesia in male rats: behavioural and biochemical studies. *Journal of Neuroscience. 25*:7896–7904.

Bausell, R. B., Lao, L., Bergman, S., Lee, W. L., & Berman, B. M. (2005). Is acupuncture analgesia an expectancy effect? *Evaluation and The Health Professions, 215*:9–26.

Bencherif, B., Fuchs, P. N., Sheth, R., Dannals, R. F., Campbell, J. N., & Frost, J. J. (2002). Pain activation of human supraspinal opioid pathways as demonstrated by [11C]-carfentanil and positron emission tomography (PET). *Pain, 215*:589–598.

Benedetti, F. (1996). The opposite effects of the opiate antagonist naloxone and the cholecystokinin antagonist proglumide on placebo analgesia. *Pain, 215*:535–543.

Benedetti, F. (2002). How the doctor's words affect the patient's brain. *Evaluation and The Health Professions, 215*:369–386.

Benedetti, F., Amanzio, M., & Maggi, G. (1995). Potentiation of placebo analgesia by proglumide. *Lancet, 215*:1231.

Benedetti, F., Amanzio, M., Casadio, C., Oliaro, A., & Maggi, G. (1997). Blockade of nocebo hyperalgesia by the cholecystokinin antagonist proglumide. *Pain, 215*:135–140.

Benedetti, F., Arduino, C., & Amanzio, M. (1999a). Somatotopic activation of opioid systems by target-directed expectations of analgesia. *Journal of Neuroscience, 215*:3639–3648.

Benedetti, F., Amanzio, M., Baldi, S., Casadio, C., & Maggi, G. (1999b). Inducing placebo respiratory depressant responses in humans via opioid receptors. *European Journal of Neuroscience, 215*:625–631.

Benedetti, F., Maggi, G., Lopiano, L., Lanotte, M., Rainero, I., Vighetti, S., et al. (2003). Open versus hidden medical treatments: The patient's knowledge about a therapy affects the therapy outcome. *Prevention and Treatment*. http://content2.apa.org/journals/pre/6/1/1

Benedetti, F., Pollo, A., Lopiano, L., Lanotte, M., Vighetti, S., & Rainero, I. (2003). Conscious expectation and unconscious conditioning in analgesic, motor and hormonal placebo/nocebo responses. *Journal of Neuroscience, 23*:4315–4323.

Benedetti, F., Amanzio, M., Vighetti, S., & Asteggiano, G. (2006) The biochemical and neuroendocrine bases of the hyperalgesic nocebo effect. *Journal of Neuroscience*, *215*:12014–12022.

Benedetti, F., Arduino, C., Costa, S., Vighetti, S., Tarenzi, L., Rainero, I., et al. (2006). Loss of expectation-related mechanisms in Alzheimer's disease makes analgesic therapies less effective. *Pain*, *215*:133–144.

Benedetti, F., Lanotte, M., Lopiano, L., & Colloca, L. (2007) When words are painful: unraveling the mechanisms of the nocebo effect. *Neuroscience*, *215*:260–271.

Bingel, U., Lorenz, J., Schoell, E., Weiller, C., & Büchel, C. (2006). Mechanisms of placebo analgesia: rACC recruitment of a subcortical antinociceptive network. *Pain*, *215*:8–15.

Brody, H. (2000). *The placebo response*. New York. Harper Collins.

Charron, J., Rainville, P., & Marchand, S. (2006). Direct comparison of placebo effects on clinical and experimental pain. *Clinical Journal of Pain* 22:204–211.

Colloca, L., & Benedetti, F. (2005). Placebos and painkillers: is mind as real as matter? *Nature Reviews Neuroscience*, *215*:545–552.

Colloca, L., Lopiano, L., Lanotte, M., & Benedetti, F. (2004). Overt versus covert treatment for pain, anxiety, and Parkinson's disease. *Lancet Neurology*,*3*:679–684.

Davis, C. E. (2002). Regression to the mean or placebo effect? In: Guess, H. A., Kleinman, A., Kusek, J. W., & Engel, L. W. (Eds.), *The science of the placebo: Toward an interdisciplinary research agenda* (pp. 158–166). London: BMJ Books.

Di Blasi, Z., Harkness, E., Ernst, E., Georgiou, A., & Kleijnen, J. (2001). Influence of context effect on health outcomes: A systematic review. *Lancet* 357:757–762.

Dworkin, S. F., Chen, A. C., LeResche, L., & Clark, D. W. (1983). Cognitive reversal of expected nitrous oxide analgesia for acute pain. *Anesthesia and Analgesia*, *215*:1073–1077.

Fields, H. (2004). State-dependent opioid control of pain. *Nature Reviews Neuroscience*, *215*:565–575.

Fields, H. L., & Levine, J. D. (1984). Placebo analgesia – a role for endorphins? *Trends Neuroscience*, *215*:271–273.

Giang, D. W., Goodman, A. D., Schiffer, R. B., Mattson, D. H., Petrie, M., Cohen, N., et al. (1996). Conditioning of cyclophosphamide-induced leukopenia in humans. *Journal of Neuropsychiatry and Clinical Neurosciences*, *215*:194–201.

Goebel, M. U., Trebst, A. E., Steiner, J., Xie, Y. F., Exton, M. S., Frede, S., et al. (2002). Behavioral conditioning of immunosuppression is possible in humans. *FASEB Journal*, *215*:1869–1873.

Gracely, R. H., Dubner, R., Wolskee, P. J., & Deeter, W. R. (1983). Placebo and naloxone can alter post-surgical pain by separate mechanisms. *Nature*, *215*:264–265.

Gracely, R. H., Dubner, R., Deeter, W. D., & Wolskee, P. J. (1985). Clinician's expectations influence placebo analgesia. *Lancet*, *215*:43.

Grevert, P., Albert, L. H., & Goldstein, A. (1983). Partial antagonism of placebo analgesia by naloxone. *Pain*, *215*:129–143.

Hahn, R. A. (1985). A sociocultural model of illness and healing. In: White, L., Tursky, B., & Schwartz, G. E. (Eds.), *Placebo: Theory, research and mechanisms* (pp.167–195). New York: Guilford.

Hebb, A. L. O., Poulin, J. F., Roach, S. P., Zacharko, R. M. & Drolet, G. (2005). Cholecystokinin and endogenous opioid peptides: Interactive influence on pain, cognition and emotion. *Progress in Neuropsychopharmacology and Biological Psychiatry*, *215*:1225–1238.

Hrobjartsson, A., & Gotzsche, P. C. (2001). Is the placebo powerless? An analysis of clinical trials comparing placebo with no treatment. *New England Journal of Medicine*, *215*:1594–1602.

Hughes, J. (1975). Search for the endogenous ligand of the opiate receptor. *Neuroscience Research Program Bulletin*, *215*:55–58.

Keltner, J. R., Furst, A., Fan, C., Redfern, R., Inglis, B., & Fields, H. L. (2006). Isolating the modulatory effect of expectation on pain transmission: a functional magnetic imaging study. *Journal of Neuroscience*, *215*:4437–4443.

Kirsch, I. (1985). Response expectancy as a determinant of experience and behavior. *American Psychological*, 40:1189–1202.

Kirsch, I. (1990). *Changing expectations: A key to effective psychotherapy*. Pacific Grove, CA: Brooks-Cole.

Kirsch, I. (Ed) (1999). *How expectancies shape experience*. Washington, DC: American Psychological Association.

Kissel, P., & Barrucand, D. (1964). Placébos et effet-placébo en médicine. Paris: Masson.

Kong, J., Gollub, R. L., Rosman, I. S., Webb, J. M., Vangel, M. G., Kirsch, I., et al. (2006). Brain activity associated with expectancy-enhanced placebo analgesia as measured by functional magnetic resonance imaging. *Journal of Neuroscience*, 215:381–388.

Koyama, T., Tanaka, Y. Z., & Mikami, A. (1998). Nociceptive neurons in the macaque anterior cingulate activate during anticipation of pain. *Neuroreport*, 9:2663–2667.

Koyama, T., McHaffie, J. G., Laurienti, P. J., & Coghill, R. C. (2005). The subjective experience of pain: Where expectations become reality. *Proceedings of National Academy of Science*, 215:12950–12955.

Levine, J. D., & Gordon, N. C. (1984). Influence of the method of drug administration on analgesic response. *Nature*, 215:755–756.

Levine, J. D., Gordon, N. C., & Fields, H. L. (1978). The mechanisms of placebo analgesia. *Lancet*, 2:654–657.

Linde, K., Witt, C. M., Streng, A., Weidenhammer, W., Wagenpfeil, S., Brinkhous, B., et al. (2007). The impact of patient expectations on outcomes in four randomized controlled trials of acupuncture in patients with chronic pain. *Pain*, 215:264–271.

Lipman, J. J., Miller, B. E., Mays, K. S., Miller, M. N., North, W. C., & Byrne, W. L. (1990). Peak B endorphin concentration in cerebrospinal fluid: reduced in chronic pain patients and increased during the placebo response. *Psychopharmacology*, 102:112–6.

Lorenz, J., Hauch, M., Paur, R. C., Nakamura, Y., Zimmermann, R., Bromm, B., et al. (2005). Cortical correlates of false expectations during pain intensity judgments – A possible manifestation of placebo/nocebo cognitions. *Brain Behavior, and Immunity*, 19:283–295.

Lydiard, R. B. (1994). Neuropeptides and anxiety: Focus on cholecystokinin. *Clinical Chemistry*, 215:315–318.

Matre, D., Casey, K. L., & Knardahl, S. (2006). Placebo-induced changes in spinal cord pain processing. *Journal of Neuroscience*, 215:559–63.

Millan, M. J. (2002). Descending control of pain. *Progress in Neurobiology*, 215:355–474.

Moerman, D. E. (2002). *Meaning, medicine and the placebo effect*. Cambridge, MA. Cambridge University Press.

Montgomery, G. H., & Kirsch, I. (1997). Classical conditioning and the placebo effect. *Pain*, 215:107–113.

Noble, F., & Roques, B. P. (2003). The role of CCK2 receptors in the homeostasis of the opioid system. *Drugs Today*, 215:897–908.

Pacheco-López, G., Engler, H., Niemi, M. B., & Schedlowski, M. (2006). Expectations and associations that heal: Immunomodulatory placebo effects and its neurobiology. *Brain Behavavior, and Immunity*, 20:430–446.

Pariente, J., White, P., Frackowiak, R. S. J., & Lewith, G. (2005). Expectancy and belief modulate the neuronal substrates of pain treated by acupuncture. *NeuroImage*, 215:1161–1167.

Pert, C. B., & Snyder, S. H. (1973). Opiate receptor: Demonstration in nervous tissue. *Science*, 215:1011–1013.

Petrovic, P., Kalso, E., Petersson, K. M., & Ingvar, M. (2002). Placebo and opioid analgesia-Imaging a shared neuronal network. *Science*, 215:1737–1740.

Pollo, A., Amanzio, M., Arslanian, A., Casadio, C., Maggi, G., & Benedetti, F. (2001). Response expectancies in placebo analgesia and their clinical relevance. *Pain*, 215:77–83.

Pollo, A., Vighetti, S., Rainero, I., & Benedetti, F. (2003). Placebo analgesia and the heart. *Pain*, 215:125–133.

Porro, C. A., Baraldi, P., Pagnoni, G., Serafini, M., Facchin, P., Maieron, M., et al. (2002). Does anticipation of pain affect cortical nociceptive systems? *Journal of Neuroscience*, *215*:3206–3214.

Porro, C. A., Cettolo, V., Francescano, M. P., & Baraldi, P. (2003). Functional activity mapping of the mesial hemispheric wall durino anticipation of pain. *Neuroimage*, *215*:1738–1747.

Price, D. D., Milling, L. S., Kirsch, I., Duff, A., Montgomery, G. H., & Nicholls, S. S. (1999). An analysis of factors that contribute to the magnitude of placebo analgesia in an experimental paradigm. *Pain*, *215*:147–156.

Price, D. D., Craggs, J., Verne, G. N., Perlstein, W. M., & Robinson, M. E. (2007). Placebo analgesia is accompanied by large reductions in pain-related brain activity in irritable bowel syndrome patients. *Pain*, *215*:63–72.

Reiss, S. (1980). Pavlovian conditioning and human fear: An expectancy model. *Behavior Therapy*, *215*:380–396.

Rescorla, R. A. (1988). Pavlovian conditioning: it is not what you think it is. *American Psychologist*, *215*:151–160.

Reynolds, D. V. (1969). Surgery in the rat during electrical analgesia induced by focal brain stimulation. *Science*, *215*:444–445.

Sawamoto, N., Honda, M., Okada, T., Hanakawa, T., Kanda, M., Fukuyama, H., et al. (2000). Expectation of pain enhances responses to nonpainful somatosensory stimulation in the anterior cingulated cortex and parietal operculum/posterior insula: an event-related functional magnetic resonance imaging study. *Journal of Neuroscience*, *215*:7438–7445.

Siegel, S. (1985). Drug anticipatory responses in animals. In: White, L., Tursky, B., & Schwartz, G. E. (Eds.) *Placebo: Theory, research and mechanisms* (pp. 288–305). New York: Guilford Press.

Siegel, S. (2002). Explanatory mechanisms for placebo effects: Pavlovian conditioning. In: Guess, H. A., Kleinman, A., Kusek, J. W, & Engel, L. W. (Eds.), *The Science of the Placebo: Toward an Interdisciplinary Research Agenda* (pp. 133–157). London: BMJ Books.

Thorn, B. (2007). Commentaries on the placebo concept in psychotherapy. *Journal of Clinical Psychology*, *215*:371–372.

Vase, L., Riley, J. L. 3rd, & Price, D. D. (2002). A comparison of placebo effects in clinical analgesic trials versus studies of placebo analgesia. *Pain*, *215*:443–452.

Vase, L., Robinson, M. E., Verne, G. N., & Price, D. D. (2005). Increased placebo analgesia over timein irritable bowel syndrome (IBS) patients is associated with desire and expectation but not endogenous opioid mechanisms. *Pain*, *215*:338–347.

Voudouris, N. J., Peck, C. L., & Coleman, G. (1985). Conditioned placebo responses. *Journal of Personality and Social Psychology*, *215*:47–53.

Voudouris, N. J., Peck, C. L., & Coleman, G. (1989). Conditioned response models of placebo phenomena: further support. *Pain*, *215*:109–116.

Voudouris, N. J., Peck, C. L., & Coleman, G. (1990). The role of conditioning and verbal expectancy in the placebo response. *Pain*, *215*:121–128.

Wager, T. D., Rilling, J. K., Smith, E. E., Sokolik, A., Casey, K. L., Davidson, R. J., et al. (2004). Placebo-induced changes in fMRI in the anticipation and experience of pain. *Science*, *215*:1162–1166.

Wager, T. D., Matre, D., & Casey, K. L. (2006). Placebo effects in laser-evoked pain potentials. *Brain Behavior, and Immunity*, *215*:219–230.

Wampold, B. E., Minami, T., Callen Tierney, S., Baskin, T. W., & Bhati, K. S. (2005). The placebo is powerful: Estimating placebo effects in medicine and psychotherapy from randomized clinical trials. *Journal of Clinical Psychology*, 61:835–854.

Wikramasekera, I. (1985). A conditioned response model of the placebo effect: predictions of the model. In: White, L., Tursky, B., & Schwartz, G. E. (Eds.), *Placebo: Theory, research and mechanisms*. New York: Guilford Press.

Zubieta, J. K., Bueller, J. A., Jackson, L. R., Scott, D. J., Xu, Y., Koeppe, R. A., et al. (2005). Placebo effects mediated by endogenous opioid activity on μ-opioid receptors. *Journal of Neuroscience, 215*:7754–7762.
Zubieta, J. K., Yau, W. Y., Scott, D. J., & Stohler, C. S. (2006). Belief or need? Accounting for individual variations in the neurochemistry of the placebo effect. *Brain Behavior, and Immunity, 215*:15–26.

The Narrative Approach to Pain

Howard M. Spiro

Introduction: Narrative

Narrative- framing the patient's story as important- has become attractive to medical practitioners who worry about the growing dominance of "images" in medical diagnosis. "Images" has proven to be the right term for the x-ray/computer generated illustrations which call up the reverence of icons begun in the Byzantine Empire. What patients have to say—how they feel—gets less attention from physicians than the images of their organs. Physicians are so pressed for time that they quickly interrupt their patients, to give the impression they are not listening. And often, they are not! Aggrieved, many patients have turned to alternative practitioners who show more interest in people than in their parts, and who spend more time than mainstream physicians in discussing how their patients feel, and what they want.

Oncologists are well acquainted with the pathos of patients' stories, for they deal with primal issues daily, sharing the suffering of patients fighting cancer. This brief commentary is intended to be an account of what one old doctor thinks about it all. Rita Charon, one of narrative's foremost proponents, defines narrative competence as "recognizing the predicament of others." She is right, of course, but that may reflect no more than empathy, feeling what another feels. The emotion of stories can recall to physicians hardened by experience the passion of their earlier "pre-med" years.

History: Changes in the Clinical Focus

Narrative is the trendy word for telling a story. In oncologic practice, narrative calls the physician back to the story the patient tells, shoves attention from the cancer/tumor back to the patient, moves the physician focus from the statistics of the controlled clinical trial to the pains of the subjects/patients, from

H.M. Spiro (✉)
Yale University of Medicine, New Haven, CT, USA

R.J. Moore (ed.), *Biobehavioral Approaches to Pain*,
DOI 10.1007/978-0-387-78323-9_5, © Springer Science+Business Media, LLC 2009

considering only their survival to enhancing their comfort and their way of life and, sometimes, death.

In the 1940s when I was in medical school, medical practice was slouching slowly towards uniformity: doctors had learned to evaluate patients in a formalized progression through the bodily systems. Patients came to their doctors with a problem, the doctors listened patiently to what they had to say, asked a lot of questions in the "system review" and then carried out a ritual bodily examination searching for deviations from the normal. Only after that "physical" did mid -20thCentury physicians think about a diagnosis. Sometimes treatment without diagnosis seemed appropriate, but that was usually derided as something that only family docs got away with. The telephone could elide all steps but therapy, famously "Take two aspirin and call me in the morning," or the ubiquitous antibiotic for a common cold. But patients remained the focus of physicians' attention.

In growing distrust of the general practitioner, each consultant to whom the patient came carried out the physical examination very precisely—at least that was the rule. Academic physicians demonstrated their unique skills by repeating the "complete physical," from eye movements to dorsalis pedis pulse, regardless of how often and how skillfully others had done the same. During their first few days in a teaching hospital, patients could be thoroughly examined three or four times. It was a reaffirmation of his prowess (few women then) for an attending physician to find something that the house staff in training had missed.

That has all changed, as over the past few decades CAT scans and PET scans, MRIs and ultrasounds which display so much to the physician have put the physical examination into the shadows, so to speak. Surgeons, who had prided themselves on nice discrimination about the cause of an "acute belly," came to rely more on the "scans" than on their fingers. They trained their medical students and graduate physicians in this new approach, with the result that very quickly looking at images supplanted the physical examination. Some internists admitted that the "physical" gave them a chance to establish the dominance that might make patients do what they were told, but that was meager praise for the now archaic skills of middle-aged doctors. Only elderly cardiologists listen to the sounds of a heart through the stethoscope, still on the shoulders of younger colleagues, covered in metaphorical dust.

To tell the truth, not much was lost in that exchange, except that going to the physician came to seem something like taking your car in for repairs. My worries about the rattles in my Volkswagen, for example, cut very little ice with a mechanic who has instruments to display their origin. "Truth" became what the doctor could find, not what the patient said. And doctors could find more and more by their diagnostic machinery.

Before that, available diagnostic studies had been helpful but not always persuasive, unless they displayed something as obvious as a broken leg. Suggestive shadows required the radiologist to let the clinicians put everything together, by taking into account what the patients had told them. But physicians have always felt on stronger ground with some visible abnormality on which they can blame the complaint.

Even though the 1940s and 1950s had been the heyday of psychosomatic medicine, physicians preferred seeing/finding anatomic abnormalities. A gastroenterologist told me that as a young man he had been asked to see the wife of a doctor who was a close friend of a senior clinician. He early concluded that her problems stemmed from a tormented relationship with her physician-husband that she could never talk about to his colleagues. A diagnostic "workup" finding nothing awry, the young man hoped that his senior would be relieved to hear that troubles at home were the problem, but found him quietly skeptical The divorce that followed two years later may have raised his standing some, but finding something "physical" has always been rated higher than what remains hidden in mind or spirit.

Curiously, the resurgence of "psychosomatic" medicine in the 21st century as "mind-body" medicine (why not "brain-body?" or even "brain-gut" given the identity of so many hormones in them both?) reflected in the chiaroscuro of PET scans and fMRI has done little to change that predilection. Thoughts may reflect brain-events, but only those deviations that can be displayed on a computer screen avoid disavowal.

Devotion to the Images

The focus on images has been reflected in the way clinical problems are now presented in teaching conferences. Previously, a physician would describe the patient's complaints and the physical findings. Then the doctors in attendance would discuss the possibilities in a "differential diagnosis." Only after that would participants hear about the laboratory studies and the x-ray findings. Finally, a senior physician would try to put together what was going on, in a sequence that tied together the clinical aspects with the radiologic findings.

Visual diagnostics make what the patient has to say seems less important than what the images have shown. Now most current presentations link the laboratory and the imaging studies with the history and the physical examination before any diagnosis is attempted. So persuasive are the images that it is hard for clinicians to discount what is seen for what is heard. And such conferences make the "narrative" seem superfluous.

"Images" was always the right term. The purpose of the icons that so bedeviled the iconoclasts of the Byzantine era was to turn the mind of the observers to the Reality they represented. In our secular era physicians take the images for the patients' problem. Vigilance against a malpractice suit enhances this pursuit of detectable abnormalities. The bell-shaped curve of normal values brings with it 5% of "high" normal areas and 5% of ones "too low", but "outliers" get further study.

That "the eye is for accuracy, and the ear for truth" is lost in a time of visual evidence. It is far quicker to glimpse a tumor on a scan than to hear about troubles, and even harder for physicians in their triumphant thirties to pay attention to the anxieties of a 70-year-old woman reluctantly moving into a retirement center. Physicians have less time to talk to patients anyway.

The revolutions of the 1960s which brought opportunity for all, brought along derogation of expertise and authority, raising the unexamined predilections of the patients to the same level as the knowledge of their physicians. That patient "Autonomy" trumped everything but the power of images, and still does.

Narrative Brings Empathy

Attention to the patient's story, the Narrative, restores some balance to the science of diagnosing disease, the art of interpreting maladies even if stories vary with who tells them, who listens and why, the context of the clinical meeting. Some patients, of course, are reluctant to talk about anything but their symptoms, and then doctors must rely on their intuition and their experience. The physical examination may prove mainly symbolic in recalling the patient, but attention to narrative demands it, and the retelling of the story may bring healing comfort with it.

Narrative helps physicians to understand the stories that their patients can tell, gives meaning to illness and provides the narrative competence to grasp the needs of the sick and how they vary with age and culture and much else. Understanding begets creativity, and that in turn aids understanding, as psychoanalysts know. These stories teach physicians to be human, not just scientific. They help the sick to come to terms with the betrayal of the body, with the dreadful metamorphosis that has taken place. Obviously, physicians interpret illness differently from their patients, but when physicians are patients, their common humanity becomes evident, however much diluted by knowledge and concentrated by fear.

Narrative in Oncology

Patients with cancer need more than guidance to surgery, radiation, or chemotherapy. They need help in coming to terms with their disease which, no matter its cure, will forever change their lives. "Why me?" is a common question in that quest for meaning. Anne Hawkins, who terms the narratives of the sick "pathography," calls attention to how reading stories of illness and disease help other patients to cope, to express their anger, and to search for alternative approaches. She relates how some accounts bring "healing", where others are cathartic.

In extolling what she calls "narrative oncology," Rita Charon describes how she gets oncology physicians and nurses to write down what they do and what they worry about. At Yale some years ago the GI Tumor Study Group physicians and nurses grew depressed at treating so many dying patients little helped by their studies. A divinity student recruited to let the doctors and nurses talk together about their frustrations and their real sadness at so much death led discussions about their travails. Those "T-sessions" worked as well for them as writing things down, which suggests that there are many different roads to catharsis for medical care workers and their patients. One method may be no better than the other, but what counts is the interest, the empathy, the fellow-feeling that is revealed. It is very hard, however, not be overcome by numbness on walking into an infusion- treatment room as large as a waiting room at the railroad station to see everyone receiving an infusion.

There is, understandably, little humor in most stories of cancer, although I admire Aldous Huxley's celebration of his colostomy for rectal cancer, "Now I am like the great God Janus, the only God who could see his anus." Empathy, feeling what the patient feels, develops when physicians sensitive to their patient's concerns, take the time to listen. That's an old saw now, but reliance on images for diagnosis makes it more fundamental than ever.

Pain and Suffering in Oncology

Regardless of any hiccups in the projected number of physicians needed to care for the growing population of the United States, practicing physicians have grown ever busier after the mid-century, and they have less "face time" with patients. Pain is one of the few complaints which gets their full attention even now, but all of us need to remember that acute pain is quite different from that more chronic.

Acute pain triggers an immediate response, where chronic pain calls for more deliberation. Chronic pain finds many different descriptions, because it is often a stand-in for something else, and far more than what comes traveling up the C-fibers . A complaint yes, but it is also a metaphor and it may be a cry for help, sometimes without words. Chronic pain is mysterious, sometimes coming from anguish, sorrow or tribulation, and sometimes from sadness at the loss of health or fear for life. " The sorrow that has no vent in tears makes other organs weep" holds as true for people with cancer as for those in health. "Sometimes, chronic pain seems to bring meaning to a life that has been without events, a friend come at last, a reason to get out of the house, to visit the doctor and find a friend." Jeffrey Borkan makes the telling point that sometimes the only witness of the patient's life is the hospital record .

For chronic pain, then, physicians should supplement opiates and anodynes by consolation, rhetoric, comfort, the relief of spiritual faltering by religion and prayer. The clergy should be involved lest "spiritual aridity", as it is called, bring suffering when there seems no logic, nor reason to the question, "Why me?" Narrative brings religion back into the medical fold, and nowhere more than in oncology, where death and dying loom so near. Stories of believing Christians show how faith brings relief, turns suffering into witnessing the sacrifice of the Savior, and so makes pain more bearable for them. For many, suffering and isolation are relieved by the doctor's being there, listening and even keeping silent. Yet, catharsis, the relief that comes from talk, is crucial. Suffering is so often intertwined with chronic pain.

Sometimes numbness can be mistaken for depression, but it is the opposite of pain. It comes as withdrawal, giving up, and it is difficult to recognize without conversation. Only a little empathy is needed to share the sorrow of young woman or young man, cut down before accomplishment. Cancer like any other disease changes the image we have, destroys our possibilities, turns the body long unheeded into a challenge. Can this be me?

Context Counts in Cancer

Context counts: cancer afflicts the young more intensely than the old, for the young have not finished living. They can be blamed for getting cancer: before age 50 cancer is often deemed a fault of the patient, a secular sin by one who has worried too much, worked too hard, or eaten the wrong foods. "Why has this happened to you?" finds a secular response as well as one religious. To the 35-year-old mother with breast cancer, pain comes from radiation, the aftermath of surgery, the torment of chemotherapy accepted as a duty, but it may stem as much from sorrow, anguish at not being there for the children and their joy, for the husband bereft and lost, for hope and dreams unfulfilled.

For the old, cancer is different. We see death on our horizon, come close without our knowing, near enough to touch. Like *The Wonderful "One- hoss" Shay* of Holmes, our parts fail in tandem. Livers and kidneys can be replaced, but who can trace new arteries, and even so, who will save the mind, the spirit lived so long? We old are encompassed and defined by loss: men and women loved for years are gone; friends seem players at a masquerade where all are made up to look like death. Fortitude has replaced duty; more and more, life reminds us of death. We who survive for a while are lucky to have paid our civic debts and we hope we have settled all our accounts. Serenity enfolds us like a shroud, and cancer comes as only one of many ways to die. Who will long weep for an 80 year old? Pain from cancer is no metaphor, and it should be treated by narcotics. Our addictions will not endure. Yet, where we may lose ourself in pain, we may lose our selves even more in opiates.

The elderly tell us they die without regret and more than rarely with relief, where the young yearn for the shore but cannot swim. Physicians can help with conversation and with a rhetoric that does not lie, but in the 21st-century even, faith and belief in something greater than humanity is essential for most people. Pierced by arrows, St Sebastian looks towards heaven with serenity that affirms his faith.

When to Emphasize Narrative/Empathy

The relief from placebos reminds physicians who treat patients with cancer something doctors used to know about pain, that it can be mollified by reassuring companionship. More than a third of healthy people find relief from a sugar pill, the placebo given by a doctor trying to help. But anecdotes teach generalities and possibilities, and they can widen the outlook of physicians who take the time to listen or to read the stories of great writers and the tales of small people. Empathy is turned off by medical training, but the legends of our childhood, the stories we have been told, and also important, the stories we read when young remain.

Medical students will learn from talking about matters that lie far from science but close to their patients. Reading a story takes time, pictures can be grasped at a glance. To train their pattern recognition I used to run the residents in gastroenterology by the x-ray view-box to take a quick glance at what they showed. But to listen to the patient is not so quick, they have to listen, to concentrate, and they must focus on what they hear. Free-floating attention, some call it, but receptive in a way that is only possible when the physician is not in a hurry. The "listening healer" is possible only when a physician is ready to receive, it is no fax machine and no voice recorder.

All clinicians need more skilled sympathy. When and how should medical students who will care for patients get training to expand their horizons beyond science and measuring and seeing? Working with college students, many of them premedical, I am sure that the time for expanding their minds is when they are avid for learning. That time lies in college, before minds are filled up by so much science and knowledge. "Heaven lies about us in our infancy" when students are still open to the world . But Wordsworth goes on to warn that "shades of the prison-house begin to close upon the growing boy." Medical school may be too late, and there is much to learn.

Practicing physicians need to be like a chameleon, changing attitudes, gestures, and manner to bring out the story the patients have to tell. Receptivity to the patient's narrative may be genetic, but it comes partly from training and culture. Some doctors are "people-people," while others are better with distance. Clinicians have different aptitudes from research people. Not all the reading in the world— nor all the rhetoric—will change them. If there is any best time to insert the "milk of human kindness" into the genome of medical students, it is in college. The problem comes in how students are chosen for medical school, nowadays by criteria for technical expertise and scientific know how, more than on human understanding. That goes back a hundred years; Harvard's Dean in the 1920s wondered whether the blossoming of science in the 20th Century led medical schools to build their reputation on science and research too enthusiastically.

How one listens changes what the doctor hears, what the patient says. Physicians really do take the history from a patient, shaping it by what and when they write, drawing it out by gesture or body language, and by that ineffable communion that Martin Buber called I and Thou. "Being there" can be described but it is so hard to teach. Doctors have to be able to put themselves in the right mood.

Final Remarks

Clinicians know that not all the sick are willing to talk about more than their complaints, and find it an intrusion to be asked. Indeed, some might wonder whether emphasis n narrative could overbalance the physician-patient relationship. Uncomfortable physicians will quickly turn to diagnostic studies, or the prescription pad. Sensitivity is not encouraged in medical students and yet it is so important for practicing physicians to understand, and empathize with, the patient's concerns. Patients with cancer are often difficult, sometimes very difficult. And narrative gives the doctor clues about the psychic and social aspects of what is going on. How else will you know if you do not ask?

While I was writing out these thoughts, I went to hear the research reports of the Yale gastrointestinal fellows. There was jubilation at a new endoscope through which doctors can look beyond even the mucosa into the very cells to evaluate their internal mechanisms! "Through the gut with gun and camera" has become "Into the cell with cannula and camera" to record broken lysosomes or, someday, to mend a limping cytokine.

Narrative medicine acts as a supplement, a stimulant one hopes, to these quantitative technical approaches to frightened human beings. One shares the joy doctors feel in seeing what has been hidden; but in the last decades understanding the biology of disease has moved far ahead of understanding the mind .For observations from the past help a lot more, for several thousand years has already plumbed deeply into the human psyche and dilemmas. What our predecessors have pondered, and recorded, the story of Philoctetes alone with his stinking leg on a deserted island, for example, helps doctors to understand the loneliness of the sick, Kafka's tale of a man turned into a bug helps us to feel the horror at the betrayal of disease.

Emphasis on narrative writing has proved a wonderful stimulus to empathy and relief, but not all professionals are good at writing , and many patients might prove equally inept at being asked to write. But they can feel and they can suffer just as much. We owe much to Rita Charon for uncovering what has been hidden, but each of us must get at it in his or her own way. But for some, it may be best to remain hidden. Not everyone can read Henry James: I did not read him until past 70 years of age. Gothic architecture has little to say to someone growing up in the Bauhaus era, in modernism. You only like details when you have the time to appreciate them. Roy Schaffer, a psychoanalyst, is certain that empathy turns into altruism when it is truly felt.

A psychiatrist I know very well, however, has suggested that writing narrative is not for him. "I prefer talking, and obviously, so do my patients." The narrative impetus may apply mainly to middle-class students and physicians, as self-absorbed- as most patients have to be. Narrative as a way of analysis may parallel the Freudian therapy which worked for middle-class Jews in German-speaking Europe, but which did not long prevail after the destruction of that society. It is not easy to imagine an illiterate patient with alcoholism responding to a request for his written story.

Physicians may remain skeptically cautious about enthusiasm for any single approach to our patients. Narrative provides a powerful counter-influence to evidence-based medicine in our medical schools, but it is after all only one new way of looking at matters. Claims of its effectiveness may not last longer than its novelty, like so much in teaching methods. After all, most arguments come down to whether "truth" is an absolute eternal or whether it varies with context, with culture and era the times, the old discourse about whether medical practice is a science or an art. Of course, it is both.

Like Sisyphus, in a sense, practitioners roll the stone up the hill, only to find it, instead,rolling down the other side, as victory over one problem brings an unexpected new one. Who in the 1970s would have foreseen the resurgence of bacterial diseases in so many new forms? Just as each generation must work out its ideals and its goals, so too each generation finds its own work and in our imperfect world, work will always be abounding.

One suggestion for the selection of physicians and other care-takers, nurses, physician-assistants, and all the rest. Practitioners do not need so much science to care for the sick, as much as they need character, compassion, and empathy. Medical school admission committees might reconsider how they select students for clinical medicine.

References

Broyard A: Intoxicated by My Illness. New York, Clarkson Potter, 1992.

Charon R. Narrative Medicine: Form, Function, and Ethics. Ann Intern Med. 2001; 134:83–87.

Charon R. Narrative Medicine: Attention, Representation, Affiliation. Narrative 2005; 13: 261–270.

Hawkins AH: Reconstructing Illness: Studies in Pathography. West Lafayette, Indiana, Purdue University Press, 1999.

Jackson SW: Care of the Psyche: A History of Psychological Healing. New Haven, Connecticut, Yale University Press, 1999.

Switankowsky I: Empathy as a Foundation for the Biopsychosocial Model of Medicine. Hum Health Care 2004; 4:21–34.

Verghese A: The physician as storyteller. Ann Intern Med; 2001; 135:1012–1017.

Understanding and Enhancing Patient and Partner Adjustment to Disease-Related Pain: A Biopsychosocial Perspective

Tamara J. Somers, Francis J. Keefe, and Laura Porter

Persistent, disease-related pain is a challenge not only for patients who experience it, but also for their loved ones. There is growing interest in involving partners and caregivers in pain management efforts. The purpose of this chapter is to discuss factors that influence patient and partner adjustment to disease-related pain within a biopsychosocial framework and provide an overview of biopsychosocial approaches involving partners in pain management. The chapter is divided into three sections. In the first section, we present a biopsychosocial model that can be used to understand how patients and their partners adjust to disease-related pain. In the second section, we discuss factors that influence patient and partner adjustment to both arthritis pain and cancer pain and how these factors are influenced by patient and partner pain management interventions. Finally, we highlight important future directions for clinical and research efforts in this area.

A Biopsychosocial Model of Adjustment to Pain

Over the past decade, the biopsychosocial model has emerged as one of the most useful models in understanding how individuals adjust to disease-related pain. A major tenet of this chapter is that this model can also be applied to understanding the adjustment of partners to the challenges of living with someone with persistent pain. In this section, we briefly consider the history of the biospsychosocial model and its applications to pain. We then describe how this model can be applied to understand the patient's adjustment and the partner's adjustment to pain. We also discuss how the biopsychosocial model can be used to guide interventions for enhancing patient and partner adjustment to persistent pain.

George Engel, a pioneer in psychosomatic medicine, developed the biopsychoscial model in the 1960s to assist clinicians in understanding the complex

T.J. Somers (✉)
Duke University Medical Center, Durham, NC, USA

R.J. Moore (ed.), *Biobehavioral Approaches to Pain*,
DOI 10.1007/978-0-387-78323-9_6, © Springer Science+Business Media, LLC 2009

problems experienced by patients with chronic diseases. The hallmark of Engel's model was its insistence that biological factors, psychological factors, and social factors almost always had direct and interacting influences on how persons adjusted to chronic diseases such as asthma, hypertension, back pain, and heart disease. Although this model was used by psychosomatic medicine practitioners and researchers, it was not widely adopted by pain clinicians until the 1980s. Prior to that time, the practice of pain management was dominated by the biomedical model of pain. The biomedical model maintains that pain is due to underlying tissue damage or injury. The model also assumes that pain is proportional to the extent of underlying tissue damage/injury. According to this model, pain is best managed by first identifying through careful history taking and diagnostic evaluation the underlying cause of pain and then eliminating that cause through medical or surgical intervention.

With the emergence of specialized pain clinics and pain management programs came increasing dissatisfaction with the biomedical model. This model was not very useful in understanding the pain experience of many patients with chronic pain treated in these settings. The model had some major limitations. First, many patients who report chronic pain do not show evidence of underlying tissue damage/injury that might explain the persistence of their pain. Second, in persons with chronic pain, pain severity often fails to match underlying tissue damage/injury with some patients reporting much more than would be expected. Third, the majority of patients with persistent pain are not successfully treated with conventional medical and surgical interventions. Finally, the biomedical model ignores important factors other than biology, such as psychological, existential or social factors that might influence the experience and meaning of pain. By the mid 1980s, an increasing body of clinical observations as well as psychosocial research provided strong evidence for the role that psychological factors and social factors can play in the pain experience.

Figure 1 illustrates how a biopsychosocial model can be applied to understand patient adjustment to pain. As can be seen in the left hand side of this figure, this model maintains that patient adjustment to pain is determined by the separate and combined effects of biological, psychological, and social factors. In persons with disease-related pain, biological factors that influence adjustment to pain often include the disease process itself, side effects of treatment, or biological changes related to the stress of living with a chronic disease (e.g. sleep disturbance, fatigue). Psychological factors influencing adjustment often include general psychological distress (e.g. depression, anxiety), pain or disease-related distress (e.g. fear of pain, uncertainty, loss of control), behavioral and cognitive pain coping strategies (both adaptive and maladaptive), and pain beliefs and attitudes. Social factors influencing adjustment often include perceptions of support from one's partner or family members, the quality of pain-related interactions with others, changes in social roles or functioning (e.g. inability to fulfill responsibilities as a parent or spouse, work-related problems), and cultural and economic factors (e.g. socioeconomic status, race, or ethnicity).

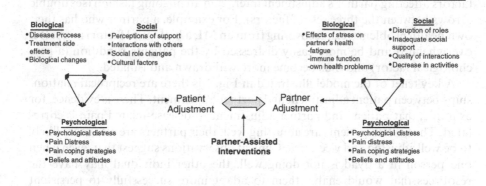

Fig. 1 Patient and partner adjustment to pain

A key tenet of the biopsychosocial model of patient adjustment to pain is that biological, psychological, and social factors interact in an ongoing fashion. This is illustrated by the double arrows between the three sets of factors. Interaction may take several forms. Thus, a patient whose pain interferes with sleep (a biological factor) may be more psychologically distressed (a psychological factor) and less able to fulfill social responsibilities (a social factor.) A patient who is unable to continue working (a social factor) may become depressed (a psychological factor) and adopt an overly sedentary lifestyle that contributes to physical deconditioning (a biological factor). A patient who anxiously ruminates about an uncertain future with persistent pain (a psychological factor) may discount others attempts to support them or place excessive demands on family members (a social factor) and may rely excessively on pain medications and/or anxiolytic medications (a biological factor).

As depicted in Fig. 1, the biopsychosocial model can also be applied to understanding how partners adjust to living with someone with persistent pain. Biological factors that could influence a partner's adjustment include effects of stress associated with caregiving (e.g. fatigue, decreases in immune functioning, or worsening of their own pre-existing health problems). Interestingly, the psychological factors that might influence partner adjustment are often quite similar to those influencing patient adjustment. These psychological factors include the partner's own general psychological distress, distress related to the patient's pain or disease-related symptoms, their own strategies for coping with the patient's pain, and their own beliefs and attitudes about pain and illness. The social factors influencing partner adjustment often include disruption in roles (e.g. disruptions in work or leisure activities), inadequate social support, and the quality of interactions with the patient around both pain/disease, and the resultant decrease in mutually enjoyable activities and interests. As with patient's adjustment, the biological, psychological, and social factors affecting partner's adjustment interact in an ongoing fashion (see double arrows between the three sets of factors). For example, a partner who has their own health problems (e.g. recovering from an MI, a biological factor) might feel overwhelmed and be more easily distressed by the patients condition (a psychological factor) and thus become more withdrawn and isolated.

A key tenet of the model illustrated in Fig. 1 is there are reciprocal relationships between patient adjustment and partner adjustment. There is evidence, for example, that patient and partner adjustment to disease-related pain is correlated. Thus, when patients are adjusting well, their partners are also more likely to be well adjusted and vice versa. Clinical observations suggest that, even when one person in a dyad is not doing well, the other individual may have the resources that would enable them to adapt more successfully to persistent pain. For example, a patient who is confident in their own abilities to cope with and control pain may reassure their partner in ways that reduce the partner's distress and enable the partner to more effectively cope with their own concerns about the patient's pain. Researchers working from the biopsychosocial perspective are just beginning to explore the specific ways in which patient adjustment and partner adjustment influence each other.

The model depicted in Fig. 1 not only can be used to understand patient and partner adjustment to disease-related pain, it can also be used to inform various treatment interventions. For instance, over the past 20 years, a number of efficacious biopsychosocial interventions for helping patients manage pain have been identified (e.g. cognitive behavioral treatments, imagery/hypnosis-based interventions, biofeedback). The growing recognition of the role that partners play has led to increased interest in involving partners in pain management efforts. There are two major approaches that can be used to integrate partners into psychosocial interventions for controlling pain or other symptoms (Epstein & Baucom, 2002). First, in a partner-assisted approach, the focus is clearly the patient; the partner's role is an ancillary one, i.e. to serve as a coach who assists the patient in learning symptom management skills. There have been several studies testing partner-assisted interventions for pain which are described below. A second approach to involving partners in psychosocial interventions is a couples-based disorder specific approach (Epstein & Baucom, 2002). In this couple-based approach, the focus is on the couple and the role of the partner is that of an equal participant with the patient. The target of such a couples-based approach is improving couples' interactions around a specific problem or disorder, e.g. pain. Couple-based interventions have been shown to be effective for treating a number of individual disorders including agoraphobia, depression, alcohol abuse and dependence (Baucom et al., 1998), but have received limited attention in regard to pain.

The following sections first present unique factors that influence patient and partner adjustment to arthritis pain and arthritis pain interventions that address some of these factors. Next, unique factors that influence patient and partner adjustment to cancer pain and cancer pain interventions that address some of these factors are summarized. Finally, future directions in this field are described.

Arthritis

Unique Demands of Patient Adjustment to Arthritis

Biological. Studies of patient adjustment to arthritis have focused on two of the most common forms of arthritis: rheumatoid arthritis (RA) and osteoarthritis (OA). Although rheumatoid arthritis (RA) is a systemic inflammatory disease that can affect many organ systems, its major symptom is pain and inflammation in the joints. One of the challenges of RA pain is that it can vary substantially both within and across patients. Many RA patients report unpredictable flares in RA pain. Another challenge of RA pain is that it is usually more severe than OA pain. In a daily diary study conducted in our lab (Affleck et al., 1999) we found that RA patients report over 40% higher levels of daily joint pain than patients having osteoarthritis. A third challenge for RA patients is that, in light of recent evidence of the benefits of early medical intervention, the medical treatment for RA has become much more aggressive. Patients are now treated much earlier in the disease course with disease modifying drugs that were once reserved as a last resort. Although this approach is effective in preventing joint damage, the drugs used may also have major side effects. Use of these drugs presents several challenges. First, RA patients are often asked to go on the drugs before they develop full blown symptoms of RA. Second, some patients find adherence with long-term use of these medications to be difficult, particularly when patient's symptoms are minimal. Even with optimal treatment some RA patients experience significant joint damage and are then candidates for surgical interventions such as joint replacement. The timing for joint replacement is based in large part on the patient reaching the point where they can no longer tolerate pain in that joint. Thus, another challenge for RA patients is communicating to physicians when they have reached the point of pain tolerance and are ready to undergo joint replacement surgery.

OA, a progressive disease, is a much more common source of arthritis pain than RA. It is estimated that over 80% of adults over the age of 65 experience pain due to OA. OA affects joint cartilage causing it to breakdown and produces pain and inflammation. OA typically affects the major weight bearing joints (e.g. knees and hips) and produces pain that is increased with weight bearing activities (e.g. walking, standing, transferring from sitting to standing). Because of its relationship to activity, the pain of OA is more predictable than that of RA. However, because their pain increases with activity many OA patients learn to reduce activity to minimize their pain. The sedentary lifestyle that results is problematic since it leads to weight gain (a factor known to increase OA pain) and reduces the strength of muscles around joints (another factor that can increase OA pain). Medical treatments for OA pain also present challenges. Because OA pain is chronic, many patients must take analgesics or nonsteroidal anti-inflammatory drugs (NSAIDS) for months or years. Unfortunately, older adults (many of whom have OA) have difficulty tolerating prolonged use of these medications and may develop ulcers or other gastro-intestinal problems. Exercise is often recommended for patients having OA pain, yet patients often report increased pain when starting an exercise program causing them to discontinue an intervention that might have long-term benefits. Like RA, surgical joint replacement is another treatment option, but is usually reserved as a last resort. Many OA patients experience significant weight gain over the course of their disease and obesity may make them poor candidates for surgery.

Psychological. There is a growing body of literature on the relationship of patient psychological adjustment to arthritis pain (Keefe, Abernethy, & Campbell, 2005; Keefe et al., 2002). Many studies have examined pain coping strategies in patients with RA and OA. These studies have shown that both behavioral and cognitive pain coping strategies can be measured in a sensitive and reliable fashion in arthritis patients. However, in general, these studies have not found consistent relationships between specific coping strategies and pain-related outcomes. Research assessing patient's appraisals of their pain coping efforts, in contrast, have shown more consistent results. Several types of appraisals have been studied. First, studies of RA patients, for example, have shown that those who report a sense of helplessness in dealing with their disease are much more likely to report higher levels of pain (Smith & Wallston, 1992; Nicassio et al. 1993). It is interesting that findings regarding helplessness have been reported primarily in RA patients, rather than OA patients given that RA is more unpredictable and more likely to foster a sense of helplessness. Second, studies of both RA and OA have underscored the importance of self-efficacy appraisals about pain control in understanding arthritis pain. Self-efficacy refers to the belief that one has in their ability to successfully execute behavior to control pain. Research has shown that RA patients who report high self-efficacy report much lower levels of pain, physical disability, and psychological distress (Lorig et al., 1989). In a laboratory study of OA patients we found that those who reported high self-efficacy judged laboratory pain stimuli (thermal pain stimuli) as much less unpleasant and showed a higher pain tolerance for these stimuli. Changes in self-efficacy that occur over the course of educational or psychosocial protocols for OA and RA pain management also have been found to relate to long-term improvements in pain and other important out-comes (Lorig et al., 1993; Smarr et al, 1997).

Social. Arthritis pain occurs in a social context and patient's adjustment is often influenced by social factors. A number of studies have examined the influence of social support on adjustment. Arthritis patients who have larger social networks show a significantly higher level of mobility than those with small social networks (Evers et al., 1998). Research also has shown that RA patients who report receiving higher levels of daily emotional support are much less likely to be depressed and more likely to report high levels of psychological well being (Doeglas et al., 1994). Social support seems to have particularly beneficial effects in individuals with more severe disease. Penninx et al.

(1997), for example, found that high levels of social support served as a buffer against depression in persons with severe arthritis.

There is also growing recognition that socioeconomic status is related to poor adjustment and related morbidity in patients with arthritis. RA patients with low levels of formal education are not only at increased risk for higher levels of RA morbidity, but also for early mortality (Pincus & Callahan, 1985). Persons having RA living in less affluent areas also have been found to report significantly lower health status and self-efficacy than those living in affluent areas, even though their levels of joint damage are similar (Brekke et al., 1999). There are a variety of reasons that low socioeconomic status might be associated with poor RA outcomes. These include social factors (low literacy, minority status, environmental stress), economic factors (unemployment / underemployment, reliance on inexperienced, or poorly trained health care providers), cultural factors (cultural beliefs about illness, cultural mores regarding symptom expression such as stoicism), care seeking factors (a preference for natural remedies), behavioral factors (lower rates of care seeking), poor health behaviors (poor nutrition and exercise habits, increased smoking/drinking) and psychological factors (helplessness, distrust of the healthcare system) (e.g., Anderson et al., 2000, 2002; Brekke et al., 1999; Pincus & Callahan, 1985; Ward et al., 1993).

Unique Demands of Partner Adjustment to Arthritis

Biological. Pain due to arthritis not only can affect the patient but also the patient's partner. The stress of caring for a person having RA can be considerable, particularly given the uncertain course of this disease and the need to adjust one's caregiving efforts in response to ongoing changes in medication regimens and side effects. Partners of arthritis patients often report that they must take on physical tasks, chores, and responsibilities that the patient can no longer do. The physical strain of caring for a partner having arthritis can be significant. This is especially true for partners of OA patients who may suffer from OA themselves or may have other co-morbid medical conditions (e.g. heart disease, chronic obstructive pulmonary disease, cancer) that limit their ability to assist with the physical aspects of caregiving.

Psychological. The psychological impact of providing care to an arthritis patient can be profound. Walsh, Blanchard, Kremer, & Blanchard (1999) examined depression in couples in which one member suffered from RA and found that 35.7% of persons with RA and 23.3% of their partners would be classified as depressed. The actual levels of depression reported in patients and partners did not differ significantly suggesting the psychological impact of RA is experienced not only by the patient, but also by the partner. Partners of patients who report low self-efficacy might be at risk for negative psychological outcomes. Beckham, Burker, Rice, & Talton (1995) reported that RA patients' reports of self-efficacy were one of the strongest predictors of their partners' reports of caregiver burden.

When arthritis patients express pain, partners may experience an increase in their own negative emotions such as depression, anxiety, or guilt. Partners of arthritis patients report that seeing their loved one suffering from pain is one of the most stressful aspects of the partner's illness (Revenson, 1994). One of the fundamental challenges for partners is differentiating his/her sense of the patient's pain from their own personal affective response to their partner's distress (Cano et al., 2005; Goubert et al., 2005). One might expect partners who are successful in this task of experiencing more other-oriented emotions (e.g. increases in intimacy, closeness), whereas those who are not may experience even more psychological distress and helplessness (Goubert et al., 2005).

Social. There is growing evidence that partner's own negative thoughts and beliefs about the patient's pain, such as *partner's level of pain catastrophizing* can influence how they evaluate and respond to pain (Cano et al., 2005). Partners of arthritis patients who catastrophize about the patient's pain, may tend to view the patient as having much more pain and are more hypervigilant to pain displays (Cano et al., 2005; Leonard & Cano, 2006; Sullivan et al., 2006). Partners often have difficulty estimating pain in the patient and may over-estimate or underestimate it. For example, underestimations and overestima-tions of patient's pain have been described in spouses of OA patients (Beaupre et al., 1997; Creamins-Smith et al., 2003) and both have been associated with poor outcomes. When the partner underestimates pain their experience of pain, the patient may feel misunderstood and devalued (Creamins-Smith et al., 2003; Miaskowski et al., 1997). Indeed, overestimations of pain may also lead to overly solicitous and protective partner responses that foster a sedentary and dependent lifestyle (Martire et al., 2005). Finally, despite their best intentions, spouses may respond to patients in ways that the patient perceives as unhelpful. In a study of women with RA and their husbands, Manne and Zautra (1990) showed that in couples where husbands were more likely to make critical remarks about the patient the patient experienced higher levels of pain and disability, whereas in couples where husbands were more likely to be supportive the patient exhibited better psychological adjustment. These findings, along with those of other studies, suggest that when partners are overprotective, overly solicitous, critical or punishing, that arthritis patients experience increased pain, distress, and higher levels of physical disability which may develop into a lower sense of confidence in their own abilities to manage their problems (Beaupre et al., 1997; Creamins-Smith et al., 2003).

Intervention Studies

There is growing interest in involving partners and caregivers in psychosocial interventions for managing arthritis pain. One of the earliest studies to explore this approach was a study of 65 RA patients conducted by Radojevic, Nicassio, and Weisman (1992). In this study patients were randomly assigned to one of four conditions: behavior therapy with a family support component, behavior therapy alone, arthritis education with a family support component, or a no treatment control condition. This study showed that behavior therapy either with a family component or alone produced significant improvements in joint swelling and pain as compared to the arthritis education and no treatment control conditions. This was one of the first studies to support the utility of involving family members in psychosocial pain management efforts.

In our lab at Duke University, we have conducted several studies of spouse-assisted pain coping skills training (CST) in patients with OA of the knee(s). In our first study, 88 patients were randomly assigned pain coping skills training, conventional coping skills training without spouse involvement, or an arthritis education-spousal support control condition (Keefe et al., 1996). Individuals assigned to the conventional coping skills training received a 10 week protocol that provided a rationale for coping skills training along with training in how to use attention diversion, activity pacing, and cognitive coping strategies to control pain. Individuals assigned to the spouse-assisted coping skills training condition received training in pain coping skills with their spouses and also received training in couples skills (i.e. communication, behavioral rehearsal, mutual goal setting, joint home and in vivo practice sessions) to enhance the acquisition and maintenance of pain coping skills. Data analyses revealed a consistent pattern in which patients in the spouse-assisted CST condition showed the best outcome, those in the conventional CST condition the next best outcomes, and those in the arthritis education with spousal support control condition showed the worst outcomes.

We subsequently reported on 6- and 12-months follow-up data on these study participants (Keefe et al., 1999). Interestingly, patients in the spouse-assisted CST condition showed the best maintenance of therapeutic improvements in coping and self-efficacy. Those patients who showed the largest pre- to post-treatment increases in marital adjustment over the course of spouse-assisted CST showed the best long-term outcomes. Taken together, these findings underscore the importance of increases in self-efficacy and marital adjustment in understanding long-term outcomes in OA patients undergoing spouse-assisted CST.

In our most recent study, we conducted a randomized clinical trial testing separate and combined effects of spouse-assisted pain coping skills training and exercise training (ET). In this study, we randomly assigned OA patients having knee pain to one of four conditions: spouse-assisted coping skills training alone, spouse-assisted coping skills training plus exercise, exercise alone, or standard care. Several major findings were obtained. First, significant improvements in physical fitness were obtained in patients who received the exercise intervention (either alone or combined with spouse-assisted coping skills training). Second, patients who received coping skills training either by itself or in combination with exercise showed significant improvements in the frequency of pain coping attempts. Third, patients who received the combination of spouse-assisted coping skills training and exercise training showed the largest improvements in self-efficacy. These findings suggest that, in OA patients, the combination of spouse-assisted coping skills training and exercise may lead to a broader range of outcome improvements than either treatment alone (Keefe et al., 2004).

Patients who have OA or RA experience significant pain that influences their life as well as the lives of those around them. Several studies have demonstrated the efficacy of patient and partner interventions that target improving biological, psychological, and social aspects of pain. Current evidence provides us with a solid base for applying patient and partner interventions and suggests several areas where we could improve our understanding to provide maximum benefit to arthritis patients and their partners.

First, although OA and RA are quite different diseases, clinical research studies have not systematically examined what psychosocial treatment components might be most beneficial for patients and their partners with these two different disease types. To date, most of studies of partner-based approaches have focused on patients with OA. Interestingly, there is evidence that RA patients are more reactive to interpersonal stress than OA patients (Zautra & Smith, 2001). This suggests partner-assisted protocols that teach couples how to better deal with interpersonal stress potentially could be more useful for RA patients than OA. RA patients report higher levels of daily joint pain than OA patients (Affleck et al., 1999), are more likely to have organ systems other than their joints affected by disease than OA patients, and take medications that have more potential side effects than OA patients. As a result, RA patients and their partners are usually coping with higher demands in terms of pain and other symptoms. Partner-based interventions for RA thus may need to be more intensive than those used in managing OA.

Second, pain communication with physicians is very important if arthritis patients are to receive appropriate medical management. Partner-based protocols provide an opportunity for patients to learn to effectively communicate about pain and pain-related concerns to another person (i.e., the partner). Future studies need to examine whether training in pain communication skills offered in the context of partner-based protocols can enhance arthritis patients abilities to communication with members of their health care team. Future studies should also examine how to best coach patients and their partners in communication skills specific for interacting with physicians and other health-care professionals. Work from other areas has shown that coaching patients about communicating with their physicians has increased their communication and improved health outcomes (Ashton et al., 2003).

In addition, one of the most important directions for future development is the dissemination of partner-based protocols for managing arthritis pain. The studies we have reviewed demonstrate that, particularly in OA patients, partner-assisted approaches to pain management can be effective when applied in state-of-the art research settings. Yet these studies focus on carefully screened patients, highly trained and supervised therapists, and intensive monitoring of treatment effects. Moreover, research needs to examine whether the protocols used in these studies can be effective when applied to patients who are more typical of primary care settings (i.e. not as highly screened and having multiple comorbidities) and when delivered by therapists who are not as highly trained and supervised. This approach is particularly important in OA pain because such a large portion (approximately 80%) of individuals over 65 experiences OA related pain and are treated in primary care settings.

Finally, as patient and partner arthritis pain interventions are more widely applied, it will be important to investigate the "dosage" of the intervention required to obtain clinical or therapeutic benefit. How many treatment sessions are needed to obtain improvement in pain and other outcomes? To date, no studies have investigated this question. Such studies are essential, though, if partner-assisted pain management protocols are to be considered a cost-effective adjunct to medical treatments for arthritis.

Cancer Pain

Unique Demands of Patient Adjustment to Cancer Pain

Biological. Pain due to cancer is major source of suffering and disability for patients. Cancer pain comes from a variety of cancer-related sources including tumor site, progression, and invasion, cancer treatments including surgery and therapies (e.g., antineoplastic chemotherapy, hormone therapy, or radiotherapy), cancer related infections, and musculoskeletal complaints related to inactivity and fatigue. For example, patients with head and neck, gynecological, and prostate cancer tend to report more cancer related pain than patients with cancer at other primary sites (Vainio & Auvinen, 1996). Patients with advanced disease experience increased pain. Other biological factors such as comorbid illnesses, age, and cognitive functioning and dementia can also influence cancer pain (i.e., Sutton, Porter, & Keefe, 2002). Not surprisingly, a higher number of medical comorbidities are related to increased cancer pain (Meuser et al., 2001). Partially due to increased comorbidities, older cancer patients tend to experience more pain than their younger counterparts (Crook et al., 1984). Poor cognitive functioning and dementia, particularly in older populations, can also adversely impact pain communication which can then affect pain management decisions (Landi et al., 2001). Last, medical management of cancer pain impacts the degree of cancer pain that the patient experiences. Physicians and patients are often reluctant to use effective analgesics due to fear of undesirable side-effects, addictions, or stigmatizations (Meuser et al., 2001; Anderson et al., 2002; See also Heit and Lipman, this volume). Meuser et al. (2001) demonstrated that if established guidelines (e.g., WHO-recommendations) for medical management of cancer pain are followed, patient pain and subsequent distress can be decreased.

Psychological. A recent review of the literature on cancer pain and psychological factors (Zaza & Baine, 2002) identified 19 studies examining associations between cancer pain and psychological distress, including mood disturbance, emotional distress, psychological well being, depression, anxiety, and worry. Fourteen of the 19 studies found a significant association with cancer pain and psychological distress, with correlations ranging from r = .019 to r = 0.51 and OR ranging from 1.2 to 6.0. The authors conclude that these studies provide strong evidence for an association between cancer pain and psychological distress due to the high quality of the studies, the consistency across studies, and the number of studies available.

More recent studies also support this association. Keefe et al. (2005) showed that cancer patients with pain report higher levels of depression, fatigue, anxiety, fear and worry, and mood disturbance than patients without pain. Some preliminary data from our lab also suggest that that there may be links between emotional regulation and cancer pain. One way of characterizing emotional regulation style is ambivalence over emotional expression, defined by conflict between wanting to express one's feelings yet fearing the consequences of such expression (King & Emmons, 1990). In a study of Gastrointestinal (GI) cancer patients and their caregivers, we showed that patients who were ambivalent about expressing their emotions reported higher levels of pain, pain catastrophizing, and pain behaviors (Porter et al., 2005). Another study found that cancer patients who have pain experience greater difficulty identifying their feelings than those who do not have pain (Porcelli et al., 2007). Due to the common co-occurrence of cancer pain and distress (e.g., depression), investigators have suggested that to optimize patient care providers consider using treatments that simultaneously address both pain and distress.

Cancer patients and their family members often view a cancer diagnosis and accompanying symptoms as indicative of disease progression, uncertainty, and loss of control (Turk, 2002). Pain related to cancer is unique because of beliefs that cancer patients and their family members often hold. Although many cancer patients experience pain even after successful treatment of disease, any new pain is often interpreted as disease recurrence or progression. In addition, patients often have concerns and misconceptions about pain and pain medications that serve as barriers to effective treatment. For instance, many patients report fears of addiction, concerns about side effects, the idea that "good" patients do not complain about pain, and fears that discussion of pain distracts the physician from focusing on curing the cancer (Sutton et al., 2002; Ward et al., 2000).

Self-efficacy, or the confidence in one's ability to perform a specific behavior or task (Bandura, 1997), is another psychological factor that has been associated with adjustment to pain in a variety of patient populations (Bandura, 1997; Keefe et al., 1997; Lorig et al., 1989). With regard to cancer pain, there is some preliminary evidence that self-efficacy for managing pain is associated with patient adjustment. In a recent study, we found that, among patients with lung cancer those who reported low self-efficacy for managing pain reported significantly higher levels of pain, fatigue, lung cancer symptoms, depression, and anxiety, and significantly worse physical and functional well being. In addition, the caregivers' ratings of their own self-efficacy for helping the patient manage symptoms were significantly related to patients' ratings of symptoms and distress (Porter et al., in press). Similar findings were obtained in a study of African American prostate cancer survivors: Survivors who reported higher self-efficacy for symptom control also reported better quality of life related to urinary, bowel, and hormonal symptoms as well as better physical functioning and better mental health. Higher self-efficacy in partners was also associated with better adjustment to bowel and hormonal symptoms and better mental health in patients (Campbell et al., 2004). Finally, in a study examining self-efficacy in caregivers (90% spouses or intimate partners) of patients with cancer pain at the end of life, caregivers with higher self-efficacy reported lower levels of caregiver strain, decreased negative mood, and increased positive mood. Interestingly, caregiver self-efficacy was not related to patient pain, but was positively associated with patient's physical well-being. In dyads where the caregiver reported high self-efficacy the patient reported having more energy, feeling less ill, and spending less time in bed (Keefe et al., 2003).

A number of recent studies suggest that pain catastrophizing may play an important role in the experience of cancer pain. Among breast cancer patients with chronic pain due to either cancer or cancer-related treatment, catastrophizing was associated with higher levels of anxiety and depression (Bishop & Warr, 2003). In two preliminary studies of GI cancer patients, we have found that patients who catastrophize report higher levels of pain and psychological distress (Keefe et al., 2002; Porter et al., 2005). Interestingly, patient catastrophizing was also associated with caregiver adjustment. Caregivers of patients who catastrophized also reported increased levels of caregiver stress and critical behaviors towards the patient (Keefe et al., 2002). Catastrophizing has also been associated with greater postoperative pain and more analgesic use following breast cancer surgery (Jacobsen & Butler, 1996).

Social. Social support provided by partners of cancer patients is one of the strongest predictors of psychological adaptation to the diagnosis and treatment of cancer (e.g., Helgeson & Cohen, 1996; Manne, 1998). Support from loved ones can predict physical well-being for cancer patients (Ell et al., 1992). An unsupportive social environment can be detrimental to patients' adjustment to disease and illness (Lepore, Ragan, & Jones, 2000).

There may be particular aspects of social support that are relevant to the pain experience. For instance, Miaskowski and colleagues (1997) investigated the possible implications of differing perceptions of patient pain by patients and caregivers. They found that, when caregivers overestimated or underestimated the patient's pain, patients reported significantly higher levels of anger and fatigue, poorer psychological and interpersonal well being, and lower overall quality of life. When the partner underestimates pain the patient may feel misunderstood and devalued, while overestimations of pain may lead to overly solicitous or protective behavior. Similarly, caregivers may be inaccurate in their perceptions about the patient's self-efficacy for managing pain. Caregivers who overestimate the patient's ability to manage his/her symptoms and continue daily activities may not recognize the extent of the patient's needs, while those who underestimate the patient's ability to manage his/her disease may unwittingly foster sick-role behavior and over-dependency. In a recent study, we examined the degree of correspondence between lung cancer patients and their family caregivers in their perceptions of the patient's self-efficacy for managing pain and other symptoms of lung cancer and found that patients in non-congruent dyads tended to report more pain and more psychological distress (Porter et al., 2002).

The broader social context may also influence the way cancer pain is treated. Cancer pain is often under managed in minority populations and in female patient populations (Cleeland et al., 1997). Physician and patient variables impact cancer pain mismanagement. One study found that physicians of Hispanic and African-American patients underestimated their patient's pain severity and may have prescribed inadequate analgesic dosages (Anderson et al., 2000). It is also possible that when appropriate dosages are prescribed, patients may not adhere to the suggested medication regimen. Patients who are less educated or who have lower incomes are more likely to be non-adherent to their medication because of have concerns about the potential side-effects of pain medication regimens (Ward et al., 1993). Health literacy, which is defined as "the capacity of an individual to obtain, interpret, and understand basic health information and services and the competence to use such information and services in ways which are health enhancing" (Joint Committee on National Health Education Standards, 1995) can impact adherence to medication regimens. Adherence may also be influenced by a lack of appropriate education about side-effects from healthcare providers. Anderson et al. (2002) found that among a group of Hispanic and African-American cancer patients, no patient reported receiving dietary recommendations on how to decrease constipation which is the most common side effect of analgesics. Minority patients with cancer also face barriers to appropriate pain control including limited financial resources, lack of health insurance, pharmacies with inadequate analgesic supplies, transportation issues, and childcare issues (i.e., Anderson et al., 2002).

Unique Demands of Partner Adjustment to Cancer Pain

Biological. Pain due to cancer has a profound effect on both the patient and the patient's partner. Partners of cancer patients often take on the roles of attending to changes in patient's pain status, delivering medication, and organizing rehabilitation and prevention efforts (e.g., exercise, regular movement, activities of daily living, diet changes). These new responsibilities can often lead to fatigue for the caregiver which has been linked to several negative health consequences (Alattar et al., 2007). There is evidence that caregivers of patients with chronic illnesses are also at risk of suffering from poorer immune responses, slower wound healing, greater risk of hypertension, and premature aging of the immune system (Kiecolt-Glaser et al., 2003). Partners of cancer patients worry not only about the biological processes involved in the patients' disease, but they also often have significant concerns about their own biological vulnerability to a cancer diagnosis. Caregivers who appraise their role as caregiver as highly stressful have a higher risk of mortality than noncaregivers and caregivers who do not report burden in caregiving (Schultz & Beach, 1999).

Psychological. Cancer and cancer pain have an adverse psychological impact on patients and their caregivers. Caregivers of patients with cancer pain experience higher levels of tension, depression, and overall mood disturbance than caregivers of pain-free patients (Miaskowski et al., 1997). Partners of patients with cancer often worry about their ability to help patients manage their pain (Keefe, Ahles, et al., 2003). Partners of cancer patients must adjust to changes and disruptions of their daily life brought on by the patient's disease as well as cope with increases in their own emotional strain, fatigue, depression, and stress (Haley et al., 2001, Nijboer et al., 1998, Raveis et al., 1998). Partners of chronically ill patients can experience high levels of stress, loneliness and isolation (Blanchard, Albrecht, & Ruckdeschel, 1997; Blanchard et al., 1997; Walsh, Estrada, et al., 2004), and report as much distress, if not more, than patients (Baider & Kaplan De-Nour, 1988). Partners of patients with cancer often live with a sense of uncertainty and fear the death of their partner (Toseland et al., 1995).

The partner's thoughts and beliefs about the patient's pain, including misconceptions about pain medications and pain catastrophizing, can also influence how the partner responds to the patient's pain (Cano et al., 2005). For example, many partners have misconceptions regarding pain medications, which can serve as barriers to the patient receiving adequate treatment. To date, there has been little empirical research on partner catastrophizing in response to cancer pain, however it seems likely that partners who believe that the pain in unmanageable, or that it is a sign of cancer progression, will be more hyper vigilant to pain displays and more personally distressed in response to pain (Cano et al., 2005). Similarly, partners who lack confidence in their ability to help the patient manage pain are likely to be more negatively affected by the patient's pain. For instance in a recent study, we found that partner self-efficacy for helping the patient manage pain was negatively correlated with caregiver strain and mood disturbance (Porter et al., in press).

Social. The social impact of a cancer diagnosis and cancer pain is felt by parents, partners, children, and other loved ones of cancer patients. The partner of the cancer patient is often the patient's key source of social support. Partners take on new social roles such as facilitating activities of daily living for the cancer patient , often serving as a liaison between the patient and their medical team of professionals. This is particularly true when the patient is experiencing chronic pain. For the partner, the demands associated with caregiving often result in the elimination or minimization of former social roles or activities which can then lead to increased stress and decreased social interactions and social support. Studies have shown that spouses of cancer patients report lower levels of perceived social support than both cancer patients and community dwelling adults (Baron et al., 1990; Northouse et al., 2007). Low perceived social support in spouses of cancer patients has also been associated with markers of poor immune function (Baron et al., 1990).

Intervention Studies

Psychosocial interventions that include the cancer patient's partner may provide benefits to the patient and partner through biological pathways (e.g., reduction in pain and physiological arousal, stress hormones, muscle tension), through psychological pathways (e.g., changes in thoughts, attitudes, or beliefs), or social changes (e.g., alterations in the way the partner interacts with the patient and others) (Keefe et al., 2005). In addition, there is a growing interest in the benefits of partner-assisted cancer pain interventions and a limited number of studies have shown initial support for these interventions.

Keefe and colleagues (2005) tested a feasibility study of a partner-assisted pain management protocol in terminally ill cancer patients that integrated information about cancer pain with systematic training of patients and partners (N = 78) in cognitive and behavioral pain coping skills. Couples received three sessions over two weeks that lasted approximately an hour each or usual care. There were no reported differences in the patient's pain as a result of the intervention. However, partners receiving the intervention reported higher self efficacy in helping the patient control their pain and other symptoms and lower levels of caregiver strain. Caregiving can lead to negative physiological and psychological outcomes and these results suggest that partner-assisted pain management training may buffer the stressful impact of caregiving at the end of life (Keefe et al., 2005).

Another study investigated the effects of partner-assisted reflexology for cancer pain and anxiety in patients with metastatic cancer (N = 86; Stephenson et al., 2007). Reflexology is a manual technique based that involves massaging specific areas in the hands and feet to provide pain relief. In this study partners were taught to massage the outer edges of the patient's metatarsals. Partners of cancer patients were taught the reflexology techniques, practiced the techniques, and were provided with feedback at a hospital based teaching session. When compared with a control group, patients who received partner-delivered reflexology reported decreases in pain levels and anxiety levels. Partners of patients who delivered reflexology also reported feeling increased closeness with their partners and increased self-efficacy for helping their partner control their pain.

Campbell et al. (2007) explored the feasibility and efficacy of coping skills training (CST) in a sample of African American prostate cancer survivors and their intimate partners. This study addressed issues in a group of individuals (i.e., African-American men) who have been significantly underrepresented in the cancer literature. CST included six sessions and was designed to train prostate survivors and their partners in skills for managing symptoms experienced after cancer treatment. Study results suggested that telephone based CST can successfully enhance coping in African-American prostate cancer survivors and their partners. Cancer survivors who received CST reported significant improvements in quality of life related to bowel, urinary, sexual, and hormonal symptoms compared to the control group. The effects for partners approached conventional levels of statistical significance with partners who received CST reporting less caregiver strain, depression, and fatigue, and more vigor than partners who did not receive CST.

We are currently conducting a study examining the efficacy of a partner-assisted coping skills training protocol for patients with early stage lung cancer. In this study, lung cancer patients and their family caregivers are randomly assigned to coping skills training, which systematically trains caregivers in methods for guiding the patient in the use of coping skills for managing symptoms such as pain and fatigue (i.e. relaxation training, imagery, activity pacing, and communication skills), or to an education/support condition. All intervention sessions will be conducted over the telephone. Primary outcome measures include pain, fatigue, self-efficacy, depression, and anxiety. With approximately 300 dyads, this will be one of the largest partner-assisted interventions conducted to date, and the results will add to the literature regarding the efficacy of these partner-assisted interventions for decreasing pain and other cancer-related symptoms as well as psychological distress among both patients and their partners.

Cancer pain is one of the most feared and burdensome symptoms of the disease. The majority of individuals who have cancer will experience moderate to severe cancer pain during the course of their disease and into survivorship (Mantyh, 2006). Partners and caregivers of patient with cancer pain often worry about and lack confidence in their ability to help the patient manage cancer pain (Keefe, Ahles, et al., 2003). Further, partners of cancer patients are at risk of increased physical illness and psychological distress. Caregiving for cancer patients can be extremely stressful and interventions that help partners with caregiving skills (e.g., pain management) may decrease the stressful impact of caregiving while simultaneously providing positive benefits for the cancer patient (Keefe et al., 2005).

In sum, there have been a limited number of studies that have examined the impact of partner-assisted interventions for cancer pain. Available studies suggest that partner-assisted interventions have beneficial effects for both cancer patients and their partners. There are several ways that we can increase our understanding about the benefits of partner-assisted pain management for cancer pain. First, future design of intervention protocols should consider the biopsychosocial model of cancer pain and begin testing the efficacy of strategies that will address components of this model. For example, incorporating progressive muscle relaxation into treatments cancer have positive biological effects by decreasing muscle tension, positive psychological effects by decreasing stress, and positive social effects by providing a coping strategy that can have positive effects on patients and their partners. Likewise, incorporating communication training into intervention protocols can have positive biological (e.g., better medical management of pain), psychological (e.g., decreased distress), and social (e.g., increased feelings of patient/partner closeness) benefits.

Next, intervention strategies that decrease patient and partner burden should also be explored. Partners of cancer patients may feel overwhelmed by their daily caregiving responsibilities and be resistant to participating in a psychosocial intervention that might be perceived as additional responsibility (Keefe et al., 2005). It is important that interventions are not so brief that they are not beneficial, nor any longer than necessary to present skills for pain reduction. Work in our lab has suggested that interventions protocols that include 4 to 6 sessions are sufficient to present pain coping skills and allow the participants to practice and incorporate these skills into their daily life. Another way to decease patient/partner burden is to examine the efficacy of alternative delivery methods for intervention. For example, work in other pain management areas has tested the use of audiotape, telephone, printed material, internet, or some combination of these methods with face-to-face interventions.

Last, it will be important to develop and test partner-assisted cancer pain interventions with large, randomized controlled clinical trials. To date, few studies have tested the efficacy of partner-assisted interventions for cancer pain in randomized controlled trials. A randomized trial would allow for the implementation of appropriate control groups and sample sizes, standardized intervention protocols and assessment measures, and other research quality control issues (e.g., appropriate training of interventionist).

Future Directions for Clinical and Research Efforts in Disease Related Pain

It is clear that having pain influences not only the individual with pain, but also those who are close to the person experiencing pain. Partners of individuals with pain can influence the individual's responses to pain and are themselves impacted by their loved ones pain. As research and clinical application related to addressing patient and partner adjustment to disease related pain advances, there are several important areas to be considered. We comment on several of these areas below.

Focus on Partner's Experience

Understandably, the focus of pain research has traditionally been on the individual experiencing pain, and there has been relatively little attention to the partner's experience. For instance, while the importance of patient pain catastrophizing is well-established, research on partner pain catastrophizing is in its infancy with less than a handful of published studies. Clearly, more research is needed to better understand the partner's experience of pain, in terms of how this is affected by and influences the patient's experience, and how partners can be supportive to the patient while also maintaining their own quality of life. In addition to longitudinal studies mentioned above, qualitative studies may be particularly useful to identify distinct constructs that are central to the partner's experience, as well as to identify partner's needs and how they might best be met. It is also likely that new measures, such as the partner version of the pain catastrophizing scale (Cano et al., 2005), will also need to be developed in order to move this area of research forward.

Individual Differences in Response to Couples Interventions

In addition to developing and testing partner-assisted and couple-based interventions, it is also important to determine when and with whom it is most beneficial as the focus of these intervention efforts. For instance, it may be possible to identify circumstances (e.g. at the end-of-life), or patient characteristics (e.g. extremely high levels of psychological distress) that make it more effective to intervene with a caregiver as opposed to a patient. Alternatively, it may be possible to identify high-risk dyads (e.g. those in which both individuals are low in self-efficacy or high in catastrophizing) that are most likely to benefit from a joint intervention.

Disease-Specific Couples Interventions

While there are some potential targets for interventions that are likely to be relevant regardless of disease (e.g. self-efficacy, social support), there are also pain-related challenges that may be unique to specific diseases such as arthritis or cancer. For instance, the meaning of pain may be quite different to couples dealing with osteoarthritis, a chronic but non-life threatening condition, than to couples facing advanced cancer, where chronic unremitting pain may signal disease progression and impending death. Thus, the goals of treatment may ultimately differ not only based on the disease; but also on the stage of the disease . For arthritis patients and their partners, the goal may be to minimize the impact that pain has on their everyday lives and to increase or maintain levels of activity, while for cancer patients and their partners, the goal may be to prevent pain from escalating and to help the couple find meaning in the shared activities that are realistic for them as the patient's health potentially declines. Researchers designing couples interventions for pain management should pay particular attention to specific disease-related challenges, modify their intervention protocols accordingly, and measure whether these modifications have their desired effect. Future research could also examine whether different intervention components are more or less useful for couples with different diseases. Measuring the frequency of use and perceived helpfulness of various coping skills would enable researchers to evaluate which strategies are most effective for couples dealing with specific diseases.

Couple Based Interventions

To date, interventions for pain that include partners have almost exclusively been partner-assisted, that is, focusing primarily on the patient with the partner serving as a coach who assists the patient in learning pain management skills. As noted in the beginning of this chapter, an alternative method of involving a partner is through couple-based interventions in which the focus is on the couple and the target is improving couples' interactions around pain. To date, this approach has received very little attention as a treatment strategy for pain management. There have been applications of couple-based interventions to cancer (e.g. Manne et al., 2005), with primary outcomes focused on psychological distress and relationship functioning. However, the effects of such interventions on pain have not been examined. We recently conducted a small pilot study focused on couples' communication regarding osteoarthritis pain (Keefe, 2007). Findings suggested that patients and partners who were low in self-efficacy for communicating with each other regarding pain, and who reported that they held back from discussing pain-related issues, also reported higher levels of pain and psychological distress. Based on these findings, we are currently in the process of developing a couple-based intervention focused on pain communication which is designed to educate couples about pain and pain communication and train them in specific couples communication skills (skills for sharing thoughts and feelings and problem solving skills) to increase the effectiveness of their pain communication.

Depression in Chronic Pain

Rates of diagnosable clinical depression in chronic pain patients range from 30 to 54% (Banks & Kerns, 1996). Partners of individuals with chronic pain are also susceptible to high levels of depression. Walsh et al. (1999) reported that among individuals with chronic RA pain, 38% of individuals with RA met were depressed and 23% of their partners were depressed. It is important that depression be addressed within the context of psychosocial pain interventions as it is likely to be a barrier to treatment benefit if not adequately addressed. There are two ways that depression could be addressed within psychosocial interventions for pain. First, the interventionist should be aware of the high levels of clinical depression in chronic pain patients and their partner. If a clinician suspects that the patient or partner is depressed, appropriate referrals for treatment of depression should be made. Alternatively, given the high rates of clinical depression in patients with chronic pain and their partners, future work should also investigate the benefits of specifically addressing depression within psychosocial interventions for pain. Several components that are already included in psychosocial pain interventions could be dually applied to address issues of depression in both patients and partners. For example, cognitive restructuring is often used to reorganize patient's negative thoughts about their pain and limitation and could also be employed to address depressive thought patterns. Relaxation techniques, such as hypnosis and guided imagery, can also be used as part of pain interventions to decrease tension related pain and could also be used as a coping technique to interrupt depressive thoughts (e.g., Murphy et al., 1995).

Family Intervention

The approaches outlined in this chapter have focused on the patient-partner dyad. An important future direction for research is to explore these effects, involving a broader range of significant others in psychosocial interventions for pain management. For example, a patient who has pain in the context of advanced cancer may rely on support not only from their partner but also from their children, friends, and co-workers. Training these individuals in methods for assisting and guiding the patient in pain management techniques could potentially be quite beneficial. Such training could help these individuals better understand the goals of pain management and prevent them from unwittingly interfering with the patients efforts to remain active or take their pain medications on a time contingent schedule. Once trained these individuals could provide a skilled support team that could provide more consistent prompting and reinforcement of pain coping skills.

Pain Patients Without an Intimate Partner

To date, most research examining the use of partner-based interventions for chronic pain have included the patient and their intimate partner. However, approximately half of the US population is unmarried and single (US Census, 2004) which suggest that many individuals who suffer from chronic pain do not have an intimate partner and may have to cope with their pain alone. The benefits of social support for patients with pain have been well demonstrated. Future research should examine the feasibility and benefits of designing psychosocial pain interventions that include a support person other than an intimate partner. Patients with pain may elect to have a non-intimate family member (e.g., parent, child, aunt, uncle, cousin, friend, church member, or other support person) participate with them in a partner-based pain intervention. It is possible that interventions could also be designed to include a more formal patient partner such as a hospital volunteer or patient advocate that could attend session with the pain patient and provide social support. One model that might prove useful for designing this type of intervention is birthing classes that incorporate a patient coach when a partner is not available (Oster, 1994).

More Behavioral Intervention

Partner-assisted and couples-based interventions for pain management need to place greater emphasis on the importance of behavioral interventions. Descriptions of these interventions often tend to highlight the utility of cognitive interventions designed to alter thoughts, beliefs, expectations, and feelings in patients and partners. However, couples who live together have many opportunities to do activities together. By exercising together, taking regular rest breaks, and setting aside time to talk together and set reasonable goals, couples may be able to prevent the patient from developing pain flares and setbacks in their coping efforts. Practicing with learned pain control skills such as imagery can be especially helpful at times of severe pain when patients may become overwhelmed and benefit from active guidance and support in their pain management efforts.

Positive Emotions

All too often, patients and partners who are faced with the task of managing pain in the context of life limiting illness report their emotional lives dominated by negative emotions (Glover et al., 1995; Miaskowski et al., 1997).Training in coping skills (e.g. hypnosis, guided imagery, relaxation, pleasant activity scheduling) is important because it can provide patients and partners with opportunities to experience a decrease in negative emotions along with an increase in positive emotions during a stressful and demanding time. The broaden and build theory developed by Barbara Fredrickson (2001) recognizes that stressful life events (such as dealing with a life limiting illness) can increase negative and decrease positive emotions. Yet individuals who are able to nurture and sustain positive emotion in the face of these stressful circumstances can show much better outcomes. There is evidence that positive emotions can quell or undo the lingering physiological effects of negative emotion (e.g. by reducing autonomic arousal) and thereby potentially provide a psychological break or respite to restore and replenish resources that have been depleted by pain or stress. Such a respite might be particularly beneficial for patients and partners who are coping with pain in the context of life limiting illness. Fredrickson has argued that, over time, the broadening triggered by positive emotions can build a range of social resources (e.g. social closeness), psychological resources (e.g. resilience, optimism) and physical resources (e.g. improved sleep quality) that can have enduring effects on patients' and partners' psychological and physical outcomes. Future studies need to explore how the increases in positive emotion that often occur over the course of partner-assisted and couples-based interventions relate to patient and partner outcomes.

Physiological Mechanisms

Interactions that occur over the course of partner-assisted and couples-based interventions could alter physiological responses in patients and their partners in ways that are beneficial. Previous studies have found evidence that, among women with metastatic breast cancer, social support and emotional expression are associated with diurnal cortisol slopes (Giese-Davis et al., 2004; Turner-Cobb et al.,2000), which in turn are associated with mortality (Sephton et al., 2000; Antoni et al., 2006).

To our knowledge, however, no studies have examined physiological mechanisms in the context of partner-assisted interventions. Patients who experience a sense of support and understanding from their partner may show reductions in physiological arousal and muscle tension. Increased physical intimacy and physical contact may lead to release of oxytocin in patients and partners that may promote a greater sense of calm and relaxation in the face of pain. Finally, it is possible that the increased sense of self-efficacy patients report following partner-assisted interventions (Keefe et al., 2005) may be linked to the enhancement of endogenous pain regulatory systems (e.g. release of endorphins).

Acceptability of Psychosocial Pain Treatment

Although the benefits of treating chronic pain within the context of the biopsychosocial model have been well documented, many providers, patients, and family members continue to approach the problem of chronic pain using the biomedical model (e.g., pain is proportionate to physical damage or injury and should be treated with pharmacology and procedures). Patients who can benefit from psychosocial pain interventions are rarely offered these treatments (Keefe, Abernethy, & Campbell, 2005). It continues to be imperative that physicians and other healthcare providers be made aware of empirical work that suggests the benefits of psychosocial treatments for pain. Patients and partners will be influenced by the suggestions and opinions of their physicians. It is also necessary that behavioral health professionals continue to work toward increasing the availability of psychosocial pain interventions for patients and partners. Further, when employing partner-based treatment for pain, it is important that both the patient and partner are concordant in their beliefs about the benefits of psychosocial interventions. If either the patient or the partner holds attitudes or beliefs that a psychosocial treatment for pain will not be beneficial, the treatment is likely to be undermined and not as useful as possible for the couple. In addition, educational and informational programs targeted at healthcare professionals and patient populations should address the unique benefits of psychosocial interventions for disease-related pain.

Delivery Methods of Partner-Based Interventions

Psychosocial interventions have traditionally been delivered in a face-to-face format at the workplace of the intervention provider. There are several barriers to traditional face-to-face patient-partner psychosocial interventions for disease-related pain. First, patients who are in considerable or unpredictable pain may be physically unable to keep scheduled intervention appointments. Interventions that are not delivered in a timely manner or where session are missed or delayed are also not as effective as more consistent interventions. Next, partners of patients with pain may feel overwhelmed by their daily caregiving activities and may be resistant to scheduling a traditional face-to-face sessions. There are also several logistical barriers that arise when scheduling face-to-face medical setting based session. These include availability of provider, patient, and partner to meet at the same time, physical disability (e.g., patient or partner), travel distance, time, or cost, and the availability of transportation and childcare. Several options exist as alternative methods of delivery including telephone, audiotape, internet, printed materials, in-home sessions, and combinations of these methods with face-to-face sessions. Studies have started to examine the utility of some alternative delivery methods (e.g., telephone, printed materials, internet) and the results are promising (Donnelly, Kornblith, Fleischman, et al., 2000; Sandgren & McCaul, 2007). Partner-assisted psychosocial interventions for disease related pain should also be designed using the results of rigorous clinical trials to best understand their benefit.

Longitudinal Studies

To date, the vast majority of research on couples' adaptation to arthritis and cancer pain has been cross-sectional, limiting our ability to identify causal effects and understand how patient and partner experiences unfold and influence each other over time. Longitudinal studies based on the biopsychosocial model of pain and involving multiple assessments from both patients and partners would be particularly valuable in identifying key variables influencing each person's adjustment. For instance, longitudinal studies of patient and partner self-efficacy could examine whether each partner's level of self-efficacy tends to remain stable over time, or if having a partner who is high in self-efficacy can lead to increases in the other partner's self-efficacy over time. Studies could also examine congruence between patients and partners in their perceptions of the patient's pain and self-efficacy for managing pain, how this may change over time, and what impact congruence has on outcome variables such as the patient's symptom distress and medical management, the patient's psychological distress, the caregiver's level of psychological distress and caregiver strain, and the quality of the relationship between the patient and caregiver. Data from such longitudinal studies could provide valuable insight for couple-based and partner-assisted interventions.

Increasing Diversity

As in many areas of research, examining patient and partner adjustment to pain would benefit from inclusion of more culturally and ethnically diverse participants. Specifically, research in this area has tended to include a predominance of white, well educated participants, limiting the generalizability of the findings to ethnic minorities and to individuals/couples of lower socioeconomic status. As noted earlier, there has been some research demonstrating that patients who are ethnic minorities or of low SES face additional barriers to adequate medical treatment of pain. However, there has been less attention to the ways in which social context factors such as minority status or SES influence other aspects of the pain experience. Moreover, despite the strain that persistent pain can put on relationships, research that is focused on partners or couples tends to attract participants with high levels of marital satisfaction. Thus relatively little is known about adjustment to pain in couples who are maritally distressed. Future research should specifically target maritally distressed couples as participants to provide a more comprehensive portrait of the ways couples interact around pain, and to develop interventions which may potentially be helpful to a broad range of couples.

Conclusions

As discussed in this chapter, there is growing evidence that a biopsychosocial approach can be helpful in understanding and enhancing the adjustment of patient-partner dyads to disease-related pain. Although the findings already obtained in this area are promising, research and clinical efforts are still in the early stages. Additional research studies must be completed before the promise of this field can be fully realized. Such work is extremely important because it has the potential of reducing the suffering experienced by many patients and their caregivers.

Acknowledgments Preparation of this chapter was supported by grants from the National Institutes of Health (NR01 CA107477-01, R01 CA100743-01, R01 CA91947-01, AR47218). We would also like to thank members of our laboratory (Paul Riordan, Yelena Riordan, Rebecca Shelby, Chante Wellington) who gave helpful feedback on an early draft of this chapter.

References

Affleck, G., Tennen, H., Keefe, F.J., Lefebvre, J.C., Kashikar-Zuck, S., Wright, K., et al. (1999). Everyday life with osteoarthritis or rheumatoid arthritis: Independent effects of disease on daily pain, mood, and coping. *Pain, 83,* 601–609.
Alattar, M., Harrington, J.J., Mitchell, M., & Sloan, P. (2007). Sleep problems in primary care: A North Carolina family practice research network (NC-FP-RN) study. *Journal of the American Board of Family Medicine, 20,* 365–374.
Anderson, K.O., Mendoza, T.R., Valero, V., Richman, S.P., Russell, C., Hurley, J., et al. (2000). Minority cancer patients and their providers. *Cancer, 88,* 1929–1938.
Anderson, K.O., Richman, S.P., Hurley, J., Palos, G., Valero, V., Mendoza, T.R., et al. (2002). Cancer pain management among underserved minority outpatients. *Cancer, 94,* 2295–2304.

Antoni, M.H., Lutgendorf, S.K., Cole, S.W., Dhabhar, F.S., Sephton, S.E., McDonald, P.G., et al. (2006). The influence of bio-behavioural factors on tumour biology: Pathways and mechanisms. *Nature Review Cancer, 6*(3):240–8.

Ashton, C., Haidet, P., Paterniti, D.A., Collins, T.C., Gordon, H., O'Malley, K., et al. (2003). Racial and ethnic disparities in the use of healthcare services. *Journal of General Internal Medicine, 18*, 146–152.

Baider, L., & Kaplan De-Nour, A. (1988). Adjustment to cancer: Who is the patient—the husband or the wife? *Israel Journal of Medical Sciences, 24*, 631–636.

Bandura, A. (1997). The anatomy of stages of change. *American Journal of Health Promotion, 12*, 8–10.

Banks, S.M. & Kerns, R.D. (1996). Explaining high rates of depression in chronic pain: A diathesis-stress framework. *Psychological Bulletin, 119*, 95–110.

Baron, R.S., Cutrona, C.E., Hicklin, D., Russell, D.W., & Lubaroff, D.M. (1990). Social support and immune function among spouses of cancer patients. *Journal of Personality and Social Psychology, 59*, 344–352.

Baucom, D.H., Shoham, V., Mueser, K.T., Daiuto, A.D., & Stickle, T.R. (1998). Empirically supported couples and family therapies for adult problems. *Journal of Consulting and Clinical Psychology, 66*, 53–88.

Beaupre, P., Keefe, F.J., Lester, N., Affleck, G., Frederickson, B, & Caldwell, D.S. (1997). A Computer-assisted observational method for assessing spouses' judgments of osteoarthritis patients' pain. *Psychology, Health, & Medicine, 2*, 99–108.

Beckham, J.C., Burker, E.J., Rice, J.R., & Talton, S.L. (1995). Patient predictors of caregiver burden, optimism, and pessimism in rheumatoid arthritis. *Behavioral Medicine, 20*, 171–178.

Bishop, S.R., & Warr, D. (2003). Coping, catastrophizing, and chronic pain in breast cancer. *Journal of Behavioral Medicine, 26*, 265–281.

Blanchard, C.G., Albrecht, T.L., & Ruckdeschel, J.C. (1997). The crisis of cancer: Psychological impact on family caregivers. *Oncology, 11*, 189–194.

Brekke, M., Hjortdahl, P., Thelle, D.S., & Kvien, T.K. (1999). Disease activity and severity in patients with rheumatoid arthritis: Relations to socioeconomic inequality. *Social Sciences Medicine, 48*, 1743–1750.

Campbell, L.C., Keefe, F.J., McKee, D.C., Edwards, C.L., Herman, S.H., Johnson, L.E., et al. (2004). Prostate cancer in African-Americans: Relationship to patient and partner self-efficacy to quality of life. *Journal of Pain and Symptom Management, 28*, 433–444.

Campbell, L.C., Keefe, F.J., Scipio, C., McKee, D.C., Edwards, C.L., Herman, S.H., et al. (2007). Facilitating research participation and improving quality of life for African American prostate cancer survivors and their intimate partners. A pilot study of telephone-based coping skills training. *Cancer, 109*, 414–424.

Cano, A., Leonard, M.T., & Franz, A. (2005). The significant other version of the Pain Catastrophizing Scale (PCS-S): Preliminary validation. *Pain, 119*, 26–37.

Cleeland, C.S., Gonin, R., Baez, L., Loehrer, P., & Pandva, K.J. (1997). Pain and treatment of pain in minority patients with cancer. The Eastern Cooperative Oncology Group Minority Outpatient Pain Study. *Annals of Internal Medicine, 127*, 813–816.

Creamins-Smith, J.K, Stephens, M.A.P., Franks, M.M., Martire, L.M., Druley, J.A., & Wojno, W.C. (2003). Spouses' and physicians' perceptions of pain severity in older women with osteoarthritis: Dyadic agreement and patients' well being. *Pain. 106*: 27–34.

Crook, J., Rideout, E., & Brown, E (1984). The prevalence of pain complaints in a general population. *Pain, 18*, 299–314.

Doeglas, D., Suurmeijer, T., Krol, B., Sanderman, R., van Rijswijk, M., & van Leeuwen, M. (1994). Social support, social disability, and psychological well-being in rheumatoid arthritis. *Arthritis Care Research, 7*, 10–15.

Donnelly, J.M., Kornblith, A.B., Fleishman, S., Zuckerman, E., Raptis, G., Hudis, C.A., et al. (2000). A pilot study of interpersonal psychotherapy by telephone with cancer patients and their partners. *Psycho-Oncology, 9*, 44–56.

Ell, K., Nishimoto, R., Mediansky, L., Mantell, J., & Hamovitch, M. (1992). Social relations, social support, and survival among patients with cancer. *Journal of Psychosomatic Research*, *36*, 531–541.

Epstein, N.B., & Baucom, D.H. (2002). Enhanced cognitive-behavioral therapy for couples: A contextual approach. *American Psychological Association*. Washington, D.C.

Evers, A.W., Kraaimaat, F.W., Geenen, R., & Bijlsma, J.W. (1998). Psychosocial predictors of functional change in recently diagnosed rheumatoid arthritis patients. *Behavioral Research and Therapy*, *36*, 179–193.

Fredrickson, B.L. (2001). The role of positive emotions in positive psychology. The broaden-and-build theory of positive emotions. *American Psychologist*, *56*(3), 218–26.

Giese-Davis, J., Sephton, S.E., Abercrombie, H.C., Durán, R.E., & Spiegel, D. (2004). Repression and high anxiety are associated with aberrant diurnal cortisol rhythms in women with metastatic breast cancer. *Health Psychology*, *23*(6), 645–50.

Glover, J., Dibble, S., Dodd, M.J., & Miaskowski, C. (1995). Mood states of oncology outpatients: Does pain make a difference. *Journal of Pain and Symptom Management*, 10, 120–128.

Goubert, L., Craig, K.D., Vervoort, T., Morley, S., Sullivan, M.J.L., Williams, A.C., et al. (2005). Facing others in pain: The effects of empathy. *Pain*, *188*, 285–288.

Haley, W.E., LaMonde, L.A., Han, B., Narramore, S., & Schonwetter, R. (2001). Family caregiving in hospice: Effects on psychological and health functioning among spousal caregivers of hospice patients with lung cancer or dementia. *Hospice Journal*, *15*, 1–18.

Helgeson, V.S. & Cohen, S. (1996). Social support and adjustment to cancer: Reconciling descriptive, correlational, and intervention research. *Health Psychology*, *15*, 135–148.

Jacobsen, P.B. & Butler, R.W. (1996). Relation of cognitive coping and catastrophizing to acute pain and analgesic use following breast cancer surgery. *Journal of Behavioral Medicine*, *19*, 17–29.

Joint Committee on National Health Education Standards. (1995). National health education standards: Achieving health literacy. Reston, VA: Association for the Advancement of Health Education.

Keefe, F.J. (2007). Pain catastorphizing in the context of satisfaction with spousal respones: New perspectives and new opportunities. *Pain, 131*, 1–2.

Keefe, F.J., Abernethy, A.P., & Campbell, L.C. (2005). Psychological approaches to understanding and treating disease-related pain. *Annual Review of Psychology*, *56*, 601–630.

Keefe, F.J., Ahles, T., Porter, L., Sutton, L., McBride, C., Pope, M.S., et al. (2003). The self-efficacy of family caregivers for helping cancer patients manage pain at end-of-life. *Pain*, *103*, 157–162.

Keefe, F.J., Ahles, T.A., Sutton, L., Daton, J., Baucom, D., Pope, M.S., et al. (2005). Partner-guided cancer pain management at the end-of-life: A preliminary study. *Journal of Pain and Symptom Management*, *29*, 263–272.

Keefe, F.J., Blumenthal, J. A., Baucom, D., Affleck, G., Waugh, R., Caldwell, D.S., et al. (2004). Effects of spouse-assisted coping skills training and exercise training in patients with osteoarthritic knee pain: A randomized controlled study. *Pain*, *100*, 539–549.

Keefe, F.J., Caldwell, D.S., Baucom, D., Salley, A., Robinson, E., Timmons, K., et al. (1996). Spouse-assisted coping skills training in the management of osteoarthritis knee pain. *Arthritis Care and Research*, *9*, 279–291.

Keefe, F.J., Caldwell, D.S., Baucom, D., Salley, A., Robinson, E., Timmons, K., et al. (1999). Spouse-assisted coping skills training in the management of knee pain in osteoarthritis: Long-term follow-up results. *Arthritis Care and Research*, *12*, 101–111.

Keefe, F.J., Kashikar-Zuck, S., Robinson, E., Salley, A., Beaupre, P., Caldwell, D., et al. (1997). Pain coping strategies that predict patients' and spouses' ratings of patients' self-efficacy. *Pain*, *73*, 191–199.

Keefe, F.J., Smith, S.J., Buffington, A.L., Gibson, J., Studts, J.L., & Caldwell, D.S. (2002). Recent advances and future directions in the biopsychosocial assessment and treatment of arthritis. *Journal of Consulting and Clinical Psychology*, *70*, 640–655.

Kiecolt-Glaser, J.K., Preacher, K.J., MacCallum, R.C., Atkinson, C., Malarkey, W.B., & Glaser, R. (2003). Chronic stress and age-related increases in the proinflammatory cytockine IL-6. *Proceedings of the National Academy of Sciences, 100,* 9090–9095.

King, L.A., & Emmons, R.A. (1990). Conflict over emotional expression: Psychological and physical correlates. *Journal of Personality and Social Psychology, 58,* 864–877.

Landi, F., Onder, G., Cesari, M., Gambassi, G., Steel, K., Russo, A., et al. (2001). Pain management in frail, community-living elderly patients. *Archives of Internal Medicine, 161,* 2721–2724.

Leonard, M.T., & Cano, A. (2006). Pain affects spouses too: Personal experience with pain and catastrophizing as correlates of spouse distress. *Pain, 126,* 139–146.

Lepore, S.J., Ragan, J.D., & Jones, S. (2000). Talking facilitates cognitive-emotional processes of adaptation to an acute stressor. *Journal of Personality and Social Psychology, 78,* 499–508.

Lorig, K., Chastain, R.L., Ung, E., Shoor, S., & Holman, H.R. (1989). Development and evaluation of a scale to measure perceived self-efficacy in people with arthritis. *Arthritis and Rheumatology, 32,* 37–44.

Lorig, K.R., Mazonson, P.D., & Holman, H.R. (1993). Evidence suggesting that health education for self-management in patients with chronic arthritis has sustained health benefits while reducing health care costs. *Arthritis and Rheumatology, 36,* 439–446.

Manne, S.L., Ostroff, J.S., Winkel, G., Fox, K., Grana, G., Miller, E., et al. (2005). Couple-focused group intervention for women with early stage breast cancer. *Journal of Consulting and Clinical Psychology, 73(4),* 634–646.

Manne, S.L. & Zautra, A.J. (1990). Couples coping with chronic illness: Women with rheumatoid arthritis and their healthy husbands. *Journal of Behavioral Medicine, 13,* 327–342.

Manne, S.L. (1998). Cancer in the marital context: A review of the literature. *Cancer Investigations, 16,* 188–202.

Mantyh, P.W. (2006). Cancer pain and its impact on diagnosis, survival and quality of life. *Nature, 7,* 797–809.

Martire, L.M., Keefe, F.J., Schultz, R. Ready, R., Beach, S.R., Rudy, T.E., et al. (2005). Older spouses' perceptions of partners' chronic arthritis pain: Implications for spousal responses, support provision, and caregiver experiences. *Psychology and Aging, 21,* 222–230.

Meuser, T., Pietruck, C., Radbruch, L., Stute, P., Lehmann, K.A., & Grond, S. (2001). Symptoms during cancer pain treatment following WHO-guidelines: A longitudinal follow-up study of symptom prevalence, severity, and etiology. *Pain, 93,* 247–257.

Miaskowski, C., Kragness, L., Dibble, S., & Wallhagen, M. (1997). Differences in mood states, health status, and caregiver strain between family caregivers of oncology outpatients with and without cancer-related pain. *Journal of Pain and Symptom Management, 13,* 138–47.

Miaskowski, C., Zimmer, E.F., Barrett, K.M., Dibble, S.L., & Wallhagen, M. (1997). Differences in patients' and family caregivers' perceptions of the pain experience and caregiver outcomes. *Pain, 72,* 217–226.

Murphy, G.E., Carney, R.M., Knesevich, M.A., Wetzel, R.D., & Whitworth, P. (1995). Cognitive behavior therapy, relaxation training, and tricyclic antidepressant medication in the treatment of depression. *Psychological Report, 77,* 403–420.

Nicassio, P.M., Radojevic, V., Weisman, M.H., Culbertson, A.L., Lewis, C., & Clemmy, P. (1993). The role of helplessness in the response of disease modifying drugs in rheumatoid arthritis. *Journal of Rheumatology, 20,* 1114–1120.

Nijboer, C., Tempelaar, R., Sanderman, R., Triemstra, M., Spruijt, R.J., & van den Bos, G.A. (1998). Cancer and caregiving: The impact on the caregiver's health. *Psycho-Oncology, 7,* 3–13.

Northouse, L.L., Mood, D.W., Montie, J.E., Sandler, H.M., Forman, J.D., Hussain, M., et al. (2007). Living with prostate cancer: Patients' and spouses' psychosocial status and quality of life. *Journal of Clinical Oncology, 25*, 1–7.

Oster, M.I. (1994). Psychological preparation for labor and delivery using hypnosis. *American Journal of Clinical Hypnosis, 37*, 12–21.

Penninx, B.W., van Tilburg, T., Deeg, D.J., Kriegsman, D.M., Boeke, & van Eijk, J.T. (1997). Direct and buffer effects of social support and personal coping resources in individuals with arthritis. *Social Science and Medicine, 44*, 393–402.

Pincus, T. & Callahan, L.F. (1985). Formal education as a marker for increased mortality and morbidity in rheumatoid arthritis. *Journal of Chronic Disease, 38*, 973–984.

Porcelli, P., Tulipani, C., Maiello, E., Cilenti, G., & Todarello, O. (2007). Alexithymia, coping, and illness behavior correlates of pain experience in cancer patients. *Psycho-Oncology, 16*, 644–650.

Porter, L.A., Keefe, F.J., McBride, C.M., Pollack, K., Fish, L., & Garst, J. (2002). Perceptions of patients' self-efficacy for managing pain and lung cancer symptoms: Correspondence between patients and family caregivers. *Pain, 98*, 169–178.

Porter, L.S., Keefe, F.J., Lipkus, I., & Hurwitz, H. (2005). Ambivalence over emotional expression in patients with gastrointestinal cancer and their caregivers: Associations with patient pain and quality of life. *Pain, 177*, 340–348.

Porter, L.S., Keefe, F.J., Garst, J., McBride, C.M., Baucom, D. (2008). Self-efficacy for managing pain, symptoms, and function in patients with lung cancer and their informal caregivers: Associations with symptoms and distress. *Pain, 137*, 306–315.

Radojevic, V., Nicassio, P.M., & Weisman, M.H. (1992). Behavioral intervention with and without family support for rheumatoid arthritis. *Behavior Therapy, 23*, 13–30.

Raveis, V.H., Karus, D.G., & Siegel, K. (1998). Correlates of depressive symptomatology among adult daughter caregivers of a parent with cancer. *Cancer, 83*, 1652–1663.

Revenson, T.A. (1994). Social support and marital coping with chronic illness. *Annals of Behavioral Medicine, 16(2)*, 122–130.

Sandgren, A.K., & McCaul, K.D. (2007). Long-term telephone therapy outcomes for breast cancer patients. *Psycho-Oncology, 16*, 38–47.

Schultz, R. & Beach, S.R. (1999). Caregiving as a risk factor for mortality. *Journal of the American Medical Association, 282*, 2215–2219.

Sephton, S.E., Sapolsky, R.M., Kraemer, H.C., Spiegel, D. (2000). Diurnal cortisol rhythm as a predictor of breast cancer survival. *Journal of the National Cancer Institute, 92(12)*, 994–1000.

Smarr, K.L., Parker, J.C., Wright, G.E., Stucky-Ropp, R.C., Buckelew, S.P., Hoffman, R.W., et al. (1997). The importance of enhancing self-efficacy in rheumatoid arthritis. *Arthritis Care and Research, 10*, 18–26.

Smith, C.A. & Wallston, K.A. (1992). Adaptation in patients with chronic rheumatoid arthritis: Application of a general model. *Health Psychology, 11*, 151–162.

Stephenson, N.L., Swanson, M., Dalton, J., Keefe, F.J., & Engelke, M. (2007). Partner-delivered reflexology: Effects on cancer pain and anxiety. *Oncology Nursing Forum, 34*, 127–132.

Sullivan, M.J.L., Martel, M.O., Tripp, D.A., Savard, A., & Crombez, G. (2006). Catastrophic thinking and heightened perception of pain in others. *Pain, 123*, 37–44.

Sutton, L.M., Porter, L.S., & Keefe, F.J. (2002). Cancer pain at the end of life: A biopsychosocial perspective. *Pain, 99*, 5–10.

Toseland, R.W., Blanchard, C.G., & McCallion, P. (1995). A problem solving intervention for caregivers of cancer patients. *Social Science and Medicine, 40*, 517–528.

Turner-Cobb, J.M., Sephton, S.E., Koopman, C., Blake-Mortimer, J., Spiegel, D. (2000). Social support and salivary cortisol in women with metastatic breast cancer. *Psychosomatic Medicine, 62(3)*, 337–45.

Turk, D.C. (2002). A diathesis-stress model of chronic pain and disability following traumatic injury. *Pain Research and Management, 7*, 9–19.

Vainio, A. & Auvinen, A. (1996). Prevalence of symptoms among patients with advanced cancer: An international collaborative study. *Journal of Pain and Symptom Management*, *12*, 3–10.

Walsh, J.D., Blanchard, E.B., Kremer, J.M., & Blanchard, C.G. (1999). The psychosocial effects of rheumatoid arthritis on the patient and the well partner. *Behavior Research and Therapy*, *37*, 259–271.

Walsh, S.M., Estrada, G.B., & Hogan, N. (2004). Individual telephone support for family caregivers of seriously ill cancer patients. *Medical-Surgical Nursing*, *13*, 181–189.

Ward, S.E., Goldberg, N., Miller-McCauley, V., Mueller, C., Nolan, A., Pawlik-Plank, D., et al. (1993). Patient-related barriers to management of cancer pain. *Pain*, *52*, 319–324.

Ward, S., Donovan, H.S., Owen, B., Grosen, E., & Serlin, R. (2000). An individualized intervention to overcome patient-related barriers to pain management in women with gynecologic cancers. *Research in Nursing Health*, *23*, 393–405.

Zautra, A.J. & Smith, B.W. (2001). Depression and reactivity to stress in older women with rheumatoid arthritis and osteoarthritis. *Psychosomatic Medicine*, *63*, 687–696.

Zaza, C., & Baine, N. (2002). Cancer pain and psychosocial factors: A critical review of the literature. *Journal of Pain and Symptom Management*, *24(5)*, 526–542.

Sex Differences in Pain

Edmund Keogh

Introduction

It is now generally acknowledged that sex and gender are important factors in
the perception and experience of pain (Berkley, 1997; Berkley, Hoffman,
Murphy, & Holdcroft, 2002; Bernardes, Keogh, & Lima, 2008; Dao &
LeResche, 2000; Fillingim, 2000; Holdcroft & Berkley, 2005; Keogh, 2006;
LeResche, 1999; Rollman & Lautenbacher, 2001; Wiesenfeld-Hallin, 2005).
The focus of this chapter will be to review the evidence for variability in
human pain experiences, as ascribed to the sex of the individual, as well as
considering some of the reasons why such differences exist. As will become
apparent, not only are there important biological differences that help to
explain why men and women may differ, but there are a range of psychological
and socio-cultural factors that need to be considered when attempting to
account for sex-specific variation in pain and analgesia.

Evidence for Sex Differences in Pain and Analgesia

Sex Differences in Prevalence of Pain Experience

Evidence for sex differences in pain can be found in surveys of pain experiences
(e.g., Bingefors & Isacson, 2004; Gran, 2003; Isacson & Bingefors, 2002;
Robinson, Wise, Riley, & Atchison, 1998; Schneider, Randoll, & Buchner,
2006; Von Korff, Dworkin, Le Resche, & Kruger, 1988). Such studies suggest
greater pain prevalence in women when compared to men. For example, in a
review of a wide range of different studies Unruh (1996) concluded that, when
compared to men, women are more likely to experience recurrent pain, more
severe and frequent pain, and pain which last for longer duration. Similarly,

E. Keogh (✉)
Centre for Pain Research & Department of Psychology, University of Bath,
Claverton Down, Bath BA2 7AY, UK
e-mail: e.m.keogh@bath.ac.uk

R.J. Moore (ed.), *Biobehavioral Approaches to Pain*,
DOI 10.1007/978-0-387-78323-9_7, © Springer Science+Business Media, LLC 2009

Robinson et al. (1998) found that in five different chronic pain samples, women generally report higher levels of pain than men. Such studies also suggest that there are sex differences in the type and location of pain experienced. For example, in a study of 1500 adults in a health maintenance organization, Von Korff et al. (1988) not only confirmed that women reported more pain than men, but that such differences were more likely to be found in head, facial and abdominal locations. The general conclusion, therefore, is that women seem to suffer from more pain when compared to men.

Alongside investigating the general prevalence of pain, there have also been investigations into disorders that may have a sex-specific bias. Greater female pain prevalence has been found for musculoskeletal pain (Rollman & Lautenbacher, 2001; Wijnhoven, de Vet, & Picavet, 2006), rheumatoid arthritis (Theis, Helmick, & Hootman, 2007), gastrointestinal pain (Mayer, Berman, Lin, & Naliboff, 2004), facial pain and headache (Cairns, 2007; Shinal & Fillingim, 2007). However, there are also painful conditions where men seem to dominate. For example, cluster headache shows a male prevalence, although it has been noted that the differences between the sexes has been reducing (Dodick, Rozen, Goadsby, & Silberstein, 2000; Manzoni, 1998). When these sex differences in the prevalence of painful conditions are examined, it seems that there are more where females dominate, than where males dominate (Berkley, 1997; Holdcroft & Berkley, 2005). Thus one reason why women report more pain overall could be due to the fact that there are more painful conditions that they suffer from.

Although women generally seem to report more pain than men, there is still some degree of variability within the sexes that needs to be explained. For example, LeResche (1999) notes that although both migraine headache and temporomandibular disorder exhibit higher female prevalence, this difference is most pronounced during the reproductive years e.g., from puberty to menopause. She also notes that female prevalence of abdominal pain declines with age. It also seems that race and cultural differences may moderate some of the sex differences in pain (Weisse, Foster, & Fisher, 2005; Weisse, Sorum, & Dominguez, 2003; Weisse, Sorum, Sanders, & Syat, 2001). Contextual factors also produce variability in male and female pain reports. For example, in a systematic review into occupational risk factors involved in musculoskeletal complaints, men were found to be more vulnerable to back problems due to lifting, and neck-shoulder related complaints due to hand-arm vibration, whereas women were more vulnerable to neck-shoulder complaints, related to arm posture (Hooftman, van Poppel, van der Beek, Bongers, & van Mechelen, 2004). The authors suggests that although sex differences exist in work-related complaints, the direction of the effect depends on the type of occupation involved, which in turn is likely to reflect different types of risk exposure.

Thus it seems that while there is good evidence for general sex differences in pain, there is variability that needs to be considered.

Sex Differences in Health Care Utilization, Analgesic Use and Analgesic Effectiveness

If women experience more pain than men, then we might also expect to see sex differences in pain-related behaviors, such as health care utilization and medication use. Since women are generally more likely to make use of health care services than men (Green & Pope, 1999; Koopmans & Lamers, 2007; Redondo-Sendino, Guallar-Castillon, Banegas, & Rodriguez-Artalejo, 2006), it perhaps comes as no surprise to see a similar pattern in the use of pain services (Eriksen, Sjogren, Ekholm, & Rasmussen, 2004; Kaur, Stechuchak, Coffman, Allen, & Bastian, 2007; Weir, Browne, Tunks, Gafni, & Roberts, 1996). For example, in a large scale Danish sample, women were found to have more contact with primary health care than men (Eriksen et al., 2004), and in a recent study on veterans with pain, Kaur et al. (2007) found that women had a 27% higher rate of healthcare visits. In a study on patients referred to a chronic pain clinic, Weir et al. (1996) not only found that women used more health care services than men who were judged to have similar needs, but that psychological factors played a role in this increased use.

Sex differences have also been reported in the use of pain medications, with women tending to report greater use of prescription and non-prescription based analgesics (Antonov & Isacson, 1996, 1998; Isacson & Bingcfors, 2002; Paulose-Ram et al., 2003; Porteous, Bond, Hannaford, & Sinclair, 2005; Redondo-Sendino et al., 2006; Sihvo, Klaukka, Martikainen, & Hemminki, 2000; Turunen, Mantyselka, Kumpusalo, & Ahonen, 2005). For example, Antonov and Isacson report responses from 12,781 Swedish adults who were asked about drug usage over two weeks prior to interview. They found sex differences in analgesic use, in that 42.4% of women reported using analgesics at least once in comparison to 26.8% of men. In a second Swedish study, Antonov and Isacson found a similar sex bias for both prescription (females = 12.2%; males = 7.2%) and non-prescription analgesics (females = 30.4%; males = 20.0%), with the sex difference in non-prescription analgesic use being particularly pronounced for musculoskeletal pain. In a US sample of just over 20,000 US adults, Paulose-Ram et al. (2003) not only found that females were more likely to use prescription (females = 11%; males = 7%) and non-prescription analgesics (females = 81%; males = 71%), but that women were more likely to use multiple analgesics over a one-month period (females = 35%; males = 25%). There are examples, however, where such sex differences have not been found (e.g., Turunen et al., 2005).

Alongside analgesic use, some have examined whether there are sex differences in the effectiveness that these analgesics have in clinical settings (Craft, 2003; Craft, Mogil, & Aloisi, 2004; Fillingim & Gear, 2004; Giles & Walker, 2000; Holdcroft, 2002; Holdcroft & Berkley, 2005; Kest, Sarton, & Dahan, 2000; Miaskowski, Gear, & Levine, 2000; Miaskowski & Levine, 1999; Pleym, Spigset, Kharasch, & Dale, 2003). Although findings are mixed, a number of studies conclude that women receive greater opioid analgesia when compared to men (Aubrun, Salvi, Coriat, & Riou, 2005; Cepeda & Carr, 2003; Gear et al., 1999, 2006; Logan & Rose, 2004; Miaskowski et al., 2000; Ochroch, Gottschalk, Troxel, & Farrar, 2006; Rosseland & Stubhaug, 2004). For example, in a sample of patients undergoing dental surgery, Gear et al. (1996) found that women experienced greater analgesia when compared to men. In their review of analgesic responses to kappa-like opioids, Miaskowski et al. also concluded that such studies tend to show that women exhibit greater analgesia to post-operative pain, but also noted that were some exceptions to this general pattern. More recent studies also report discrepancies. For example, Cepeda and Carr report a prospective study in which 700 patients (38.6% male) were examined in terms of their pain report and morphine consumption following surgery requiring general anaesthetic. Even when controlling for the type of operation and age, women reported more pain and required more morphine than men. Similarly, Aubrun et al. (2005) report a large study in which post-operative pain and morphine consumption was examined in 4317 patients (54% male) from a post-anaesthesia care unit. Females had higher initial pain, and required a higher dose of morphine than men. Interestingly, this sex difference was not found in older patients (75 years and older), suggesting that age may moderate such effects.

Reasons for such discrepancies might be partially due to sex differences in side effects (Ciccone & Holdcroft, 1999; Pleym et al., 2003; Wu et al., 2006). For example, in a review of drug effects, Pleym et al. found that women were more sensitive to some drugs, especially some muscle relaxants and opioids, whereas for other drugs, males showed greater sensitivity. Furthermore, a meta-analysis into sex differences in post-dural puncture headache, which examined 18 clinical trials, incorporating 2163 males and 1917 females, concluded that women were more susceptible than men (Wu et al.). It therefore seems that while there is evidence for sex differences in analgesia, the general pattern is not clear at the present time.

Sex Difference in Pain Sensitivity to Experimental Stimuli

Experimental approaches have also been used to examine sex differences in pain (Fillingim, 2002; Rollman, Lautenbacher, & Jones, 2000). The advantage of this approach is the controlled use of standardized methods and stimulus intensities, which can not easily be achieved in the clinical setting. There are a range of different methods used to induce pain, which include thermal stimuli (heat and cold), pressure pain, ischemic pain and electrical stimulation. These techniques generally require participants to indicate the point at which the pain is first detected (pain threshold), and the point at which the sensation becomes unbearable (pain tolerance). When the sexes are compared, the typical finding is that women exhibit lower pain threshold and tolerance when compared to men

(Fillingim & Maixner, 1995; Riley, Robinson, Wise, Myers, & Fillingim, 1998). In a meta-analysis of 22 studies of sex differences in experimental pain, Riley et al. (1998) found effect sizes were of moderate to large in magnitude.

As with the epidemiological studies reported above, although general sex differences in experimental pain are found, there is variability that needs to be accounted for. The type of stimulus is also considered to be an important factor, in that some types of pain induction produce stronger effects that others. Indeed, in the Riley et al. (1998) meta-analysis, the strongest sex differences were found for pressure pain and electrical stimulation. Fillingim (2002) also reports variability in sex difference effects based on stimulus type, even within the same laboratory. He found that effect sizes associated with sex differences in pain threshold and tolerance were of moderate to large magnitude, with the smallest effects being found for ischemic pain. There are also a range of psychosocial factors that moderate sex differences in experimental pain, some of which will be considered later in this chapter (Rollman et al., 2000).

Pain induction methods have also been used in combination with drugs to examine sex differences in pain and analgesia (Fillingim, 2002; Fillingim & Gear, 2004). Unfortunately, results are mixed, in that some studies report finding sex differences in analgesia, whereas others have not (Fillingim et al., 2005a, 2005c, 2004; Olofsen et al., 2005; Sarton et al., 2000). For example, when Fillingim et al. (2005c) exposed a group of men and women in terms of morphine analgesia to a range of different experimental pain stimuli, no differences were found between the sexes in terms of pain. Others showed that sex differences in analgesia may depend on the type of pain induction method used (e.g., Fillingim, 2002). Therefore, it seems that although there is good evidence that there are sex differences in experimental pain sensitivity, at present, there are too few studies to draw any firm conclusions about sex differences in analgesia using such methods.

Sex Differences in Non-pharmacological Treatment

The possibility that there are differences in how men and women respond to pharmacological treatments for pain has also led some to ask whether there are sex differences non-pharmacological interventions (Burns, Johnson, Devine, Mahoney, & Pawl, 1998; Edwards, Augustson, & Fillingim, 2003a; Edwards, Doleys, Lowery, & Fillingim, 2003b; Hansen et al. 1993; Jensen, Bergstrom, Ljungquist, Bodin, & Nygren, 2001; Keogh, McCracken, & Eccleston, 2005b; Krogstad, Jokstad, Dahl, & Vassend, 1996; Lund, Lundeberg, Kowalski, & Svensson, 2005; McGeary, Mayer, Gatchel, Anagnostis, & Proctor, 2003). There are a few studies conducted on healthy individuals, which show that pain sensitivity can be moderated by interventions in a sex-specific manner, although such effects are mixed (Keogh, Bond, Hanmer, & Tilston, 2005a; Keogh, Hatton, & Ellery, 2000; Keogh & Herdenfeldt, 2002; Lund et al.,

2005). For example, Keogh et al. (2000) found that a psychological manipulation of attentional instructions revealed that men benefited from focusing on experimental pain when compared to women. However, others find greater benefits in women (Keogh et al., 2005a; Lund et al., 2005). For example, in a study using transcutaneous electrical nerve stimulation (TENS), Lund et al. found that although both men and women demonstrated increases in sensory thresholds, only women displayed increases in pain thresholds. Differences between the interventions may help explain the variability in study findings, and it is certainly possible that men and women may benefit in different ways.

Investigations into non-pharmacological pain interventions within a clinical treatment context have also been conducted. For example, Burns et al. (1998) report a study in which 101 chronic pain patients were followed through a multidisciplinary pain management programme. They found that anger expression and suppression were negatively related, respectively, to effective lifting capacity improvements and improvements in depression. However, these relationships were only found in men. In a second study, McGeary et al. (2003) examined a group of patients with chronic musculoskeletal disorder before and following a functional restoration programme, which consisted of guided exercises and multimodal disability management (counselling, stress management etc.). At 1-year follow-up, men were more likely than women to return to work (men= 87%, women = 81%), and less likely to seek help from new health providers (men= 25%, women = 31%). Keogh et al. (2005b) examined sex differences in a range of outcomes related to pain and disability following multidisciplinary chronic pain management. They compared pain reports at the start of the intervention, at the end, and then at 3-months follow-up. Both men and women were found to show an initial improvement immediately following the intervention, with reductions reported in pain, disability and negative mood. However, between the end of the intervention and 3-months follow-up men maintained this improvement, whereas in women there were significant increases in self-report pain, pain-related catastrophizing and distress. Interestingly, both sexes maintained improvements in disability, suggesting that careful attention to the outcome measures used is important when considering sex-specific effects.

Unfortunately, there are also examples of clinical interventions that find different patterns to those just reported (Jensen et al., 2001; Krogstad et al., 1996). For example, Jensen et al. assessed the impact of four different treatment conditions – a treatment as usual control, physical therapy, cognitive-behavioral therapy, and a combination of the two – on a group of patients with chronic non-specific spinal pain. Although improvements in outcome where generally found for those in the treatment groups (e.g., lower risk of early retirement, better health-related quality of life), these benefits were limited to females, and were not found for all treatment conditions. As with the healthy volunteer studies, male and female patients may benefit in different ways from pain interventions. One study found that the degree of treatment success depends on both the type of intervention and sex of the patient (Hansen et al.,

1993), whereas another reported sex-related differences in how patients bene-fited from a treatment intervention (Edwards et al., 2003b).

Taken together, these studies suggest that while sex differences may exist in the effects of some non-pharmacological treatment interventions, the paucity of studies, and variability in treatment approaches and findings in those that have been conducted, mean that no definite conclusions can be made at present. However, this is an exciting area for development, and the emergence of more studies should hopefully help address the interesting possibility that the type of treatment approach adopted may need to depend on the sex of the individual.

Explanations for Sex Differences in Pain

The evidence presented in the first section of this chapter indicates that men and women differ with respect to pain and analgesia. The second half of this chapter will outline some of the explanations that have been proposed to account for why sex differences in pain exist. Although these explanations are presented separately, it is assumed that there are important interactions between them, and that no one explanation totally accounts for the differences between men and women in pain.

Emotions and Pain: The Role of Depression, Anxiety and Anger

Emotions have been proposed as a possible explanation as to why there is a sex difference in pain. The rationale for this is based partly on the fact that pain is both a sensory and an emotional experience, and partly because sex differences exist in the expression and experience of both emotions and pain (Jones & Zachariae, 2002; Rhudy & Williams, 2005). Indeed, sex differences in pain and emotions manifest at an early age, in that they are more readily expressed by females when compared to males (Hamann & Canli, 2004; McClure, 2000; Wager & Ochsner, 2005). As adults, there is also evidence that women may be more vulnerable to emotional disorders such as anxiety and depression, both of which are known to be important in clinical pain (Kessler et al., 1994; Linzer et al., 1996; Weissman et al. 1996). There is also a suggestion that the co-morbidity between pain and emotional disorders may be stronger in women than men (Bingefors & Isacson, 2004; Meana, 1998; Rethelyi, Berghammer, & Kopp, 2001). In terms of research, a few studies have examined sex differences in the relationship between general negative affect and pain (Hirsh, Waxenberg, Atchison, Gremillion, & Robinson, 2006; Riley, Robinson, Wade, Myers, & Price, 2001). For example, Hirsh et al. (2006) examined a group of chronic pain patients and found a direct relationship between disability and pain in men, whereas in women this relationship was mediated by negative mood. However, since most studies tend to examine specific states, such as depression, anxiety and anger, the remainder of this section will focus on these.

A number of studies have examined whether depression impacts on pain in a sex-specific manner. The general finding is that a stronger relationship tends to be found between pain and depression in women (Haley, Turner, & Romano, 1985; Keogh, McCracken, & Eccleston, 2006b; Novy, Nelson, Averill, & Berry, 1996; Tsai, 2005). For example, within a group of chronic pain patients, Keogh et al. (2006b) found a stronger relationship between depression and pain-related disability in females, when compared to males. However, there are examples where a stronger relationship is found in men. Indeed, even within the Keogh et al. study just mentioned, a stronger relationship was found in men between the number of pain medications used and depression. This is interesting, not only in light of the potential sex differences reported earlier relating to analgesic effectiveness, but in that it also highlights that careful consideration of the measurement tools is required. This latter point is further underlined by a study by Haley et al. (1985) who found that whereas depression was related to pain reports in women, it was related to physical impairment in men. Together these studies suggest that there is a sex-specific relationship between pain and depression. While women tend to show a stronger relationship, this may depend on the pain measures taken.

Given that depression is closely related to anxiety, it is perhaps not surprisingly to also find that anxiety is related to pain, and possibly in a sex-specific manner (Keogh & Asmundson, 2004). A number of studies have found that anxiety is more strongly related to pain in men, when compared to women (Edwards et al., 2003a; Edwards, Augustson, & Fillingim, 2000; Elklit & Jones, 2006; Frot, Feine, & Bushnell, 2004; Jones, Zachariae, & Arendt-Nielsen, 2003; McCracken & Houle, 2000; Morin, Lund, Villarroel, Clokie, & Feine, 2000). For example, Frot et al. (2004) report an experimental study on healthy volunteers, who were exposed to pain using a capsaicin model. They found that anxiety was positively related to pain reports in men, but not women. Furthermore, this sex-specific relationship remained when the capsaicin was removed, and residual sensation assessed. Within a clinical context, McCracken and Houle found that within a group of chronic pain patients, males showed stronger relationships between anxiety and pain-related sensations than females. However, there are inconsistencies in the literature, in that others have failed to find sex differences in the relationship between anxiety and pain (Keogh et al., 2006b; Lautenbacher & Rollman, 1993). There are also examples where anxiety is more strongly related to pain in women than men (Keogh & Birkby, 1999; Keogh, Hamid, Hamid, & Ellery, 2004; Thompson, Keogh, French, & Davis, 2008). A number of possible reasons may account for these differences, including how anxiety is measured (Keogh, 2006; Rhudy & Williams, 2005). For example, in the studies that show stronger relationships between pain and anxiety in women, the type of anxiety under investigation is anxiety sensitivity, which is conceptualized as general fear of bodily sensations that includes, but is not limited to, pain. Thus like depression, anxiety does seem to be related to pain in a sex-specific manner, although the specific direction may depend on the measure used.

Anger and aggression are another set of emotional experiences that are related to pain (Bruehl, Chung, & Burns, 2006). It is important to differentiate anger from aggression, especially when considering sex differences, since it has been found that although aggression is higher in males than females, anger frequency occurs to a similar degree in both sexes (Campbell, 2006). However, there maybe sex differences in how anger is expressed, with men being more likely to make direct confrontations. Unfortunately, only a few studies have examined whether anger impacts on pain and disability in a sex-specific way (Bruehl et al., 2007; Burns et al., 1998; Burns, Johnson, Mahoney, Devine, & Pawl, 1996). For example, Bruehl et al. examined the role of anger management style on experimental pain responses following either a placebo or opioid drug. They found that in women, the tendency to manage anger through direct expression was associated with a relative reduction in opioid analgesia, whereas in men such overt anger expression was related to a relative increase in analgesia. Sex differences in the effect of anger on pain have also been examined in the context of patient-spouse interactions. Burns et al. (1996) examined whether spouse support would impact on the expression of anger in 54 female and 73 male chronic pain patients. They found that negative spouse behaviors (punishing responses) accounted for the relationship between high anger/hostility expression and poor adjustment to pain. However, this was only found for male patients, and no such relationship was found in females. Thus, although research into sex-specific differences in the relationship between anger and pain is still in its infancy, it certainly seems as if further research is warranted.

Health Cognitions, Beliefs and Expectations

Given that there are important links between what we think and feel, explanations for sex differences have also focused on cognitive factors. For example, it has been suggested that one reason why men do not seek out health care resources as frequently as women, which may include pain services, is less to do with better health, and more to do with health beliefs (Galdas, Cheater, & Marshall, 2005; Moller-Leimkuhler, 2002). Indeed, it is possible that men and women may differ in their pain and healthcare beliefs, which may in turn affect pain behaviors. This section will explore the evidence for sex differences in health cognitions, beliefs and expectations.

One line of research has examined the concept of self efficacy, which is the belief that one has in being able to successfully perform behaviors. Self-efficacy can be seen as a secondary, higher-order, appraisal process, and there is good evidence to suggest that it is related to the experience of pain (Bandura, O'Leary, Taylor, Gauthier, & Gossard, 1987; Jackson, Iezzi, Gunderson, Nagasaka, & Fritch, 2002). In terms of sex differences it has been suggested that men and women might differ in such self-efficacy beliefs, which in turn accounts for differences in pain (Miller & Newton, 2006). For example, Jackson et al. (2002) report an experimental study in which they found that self-efficacy beliefs mediated the relationship between gender and cold pressor pain reports. This suggests that the reason why women might be more sensitive to pain is due to lower self-efficacy beliefs in their ability to deal with pain.

Another health belief that is used to explain sex differences in pain is pain-related catastrophizing, which is defined as tendency to negatively ruminate, worry over pain and exaggerate the possible negative outcomes from a given situation. It is closely related to anxiety, and occurs to a greater degree in women when compared to men (Osman et al., 2000, 1997; Sullivan, Bishop, & Pivik, 1995). Most importantly, however, is that catastrophizing has also been found to play a role in explaining some of the sex differences in pain experiences, in both the laboratory and the clinic (Dixon, Thorn, & Ward, 2004; Edwards, Haythornthwaite, Sullivan, & Fillingim, 2004; Keefe et al., 2000; Keogh & Eccleston, 2006; Keogh et al., 2005b; Sullivan, Tripp, & Santor, 2000). For example, Sullivan et al. (2000) found that pain catastrophizing accounted for women's pain, but not men's. Keefe et al. also found that pain catastrophizing mediated sex differences in pain within a group of osteoarthritis patients. Keogh and Eccleston found that pain catastrophizing mediated sex differences in adolescents with chronic pain, whereas Keogh et al. found catastrophizing mediated sex differences in the pain reports of adult patients following a multidisciplinary pain management intervention. Taken together it certainly seems as if catastrophizing about painful events is an important belief mechanism that helps to explain sex differences in pain.

Another factor that has been strongly correlated with belief, attitudes and behaviors, and which has been proposed as a possible explanation for sex differences in pain is that of gender roles. Here it is assumed that gender is socially constructed, and we learn stereotypical gender-roles that influence our beliefs and expectations about how the typical man and women should act when in pain, which in turn, influences how we behave, as well as how we perceive pain in others. Evidence for the significance of gender-roles on a range of pain-related behaviors is accumulating (Myers et al., 2006; Pool, Schwegler, Theodore, & Fuchs, 2007; Robinson, Gagnon, Riley, & Price, 2003b; Robinson et al., 2003a, 2004a, 2001; Robinson & Wise, 2003, 2004; Robinson, Wise, Gagnon, Fillingim, & Price, 2004b; Sanford, Kersh, Thorn, Rich, & Ward, 2002; Wise, Price, Myers, Heft, & Robinson, 2002). For example, Robinson et al. found that while both males and females believed that women are more sensitive to pain, men are less willing to report pain. A study by Pool et al. (2007) found that both men and women possessed the view that ideal man should tolerate more pain than the ideal woman. Gender-roles have also been found to account for sex differences in experimental pain reports (Robinson et al., 2004b; Sanford et al., 2002). For example, Robinson et al. found that stereotypical willingness to report pain mediated sex differences in pain. Interestingly it also seems that gender-role expectations can be experimentally manipulated to vary pain reports (Robinson et al., 2003a), and such expectations can also impact on how men and women perceived pain in others (Robinson & Wise, 2003). Such studies highlight the need to consider how beliefs about men and women's pain behaviors contribute to how pain is both expressed and perceived by others.

Together health cognitions are important in helping to account for sex differences in pain. However, there are few studies that have directly compared these different beliefs to see which provides the strongest explanation for such differences.

Coping Behaviors

As outlined above, it is assumed that emotions, beliefs and expectations have an impact on pain behaviors. It may come as no surprise to discover, therefore, that another possible reason why there are differences between men and women in terms of pain is due to differences in the coping behaviors used to deal with pain. Coping is usually defined as a set of strategies and behaviors that are used following the initial appraisal of a challenging event or situation. Coping strategies are wide ranging, and can include specific behaviors (distraction, praying, use of social support), through to more general behavior patterns (approach vs. avoidance, illness vs. wellness focused, passive vs. active). There are general differences between the sexes in type of coping strategy used when in challenging situations (Nolen-Hoeksema, 2001; Nolen-Hoeksema, Larson, & Grayson, 1999; Tamres, Janicki, & Helgeson, 2002). For example, Tamres et al. (2002) found that women reported engaging in support seeking, especially emotional support, whereas men reported using problem focused coping strategies. If there are differences the effectiveness of some strategies over others, then it possible that coping may partly account for why there are differences between the sexes in pain and pain-related behaviors.

Sex differences have been found in the reported use of pain coping strategies (Smith, Lumley, & Longo, 2002; Unruh, 1996; Unruh, Ritchie, & Merskey, 1999). In her review, Unruh concluded that that women not only reported making use of more coping strategies, but that there were differences in the type of strategies typically used, with women making greater use of social support networks than men. In two separate studies on adolescent pain, Keogh and Eccleston (2006) found that females reported making greater use of social support than males, and Lynch, Kashikar-Zuck, Goldschneider, and Jones (2007) found that boys engaged in more behavioral distraction and girls in social support strategies.

It has also emerged that the same coping strategy might have different benefits for men and women. Smith et al. (2002) found that emotional-focused coping was related to lower pain reports in men, whereas it was related to lower depression in women. However, the differential effectiveness of coping strategies in men and women has been most directly examined in studies that experimentally manipulate coping instruction, and measure the effect this has on pain (Keogh, Barlow, Mounce, & Bond, 2006a; Keogh et al., 2005a; 2000; Keogh & Herdenfeldt, 2002). For example, Keogh et al. (2000) asked healthy men and women to use either avoidance or focused instruction whilst completing a cold pressor pain task. They found that within men focusing on the pain resulted in lower sensory pain ratings than when asked to avoid it. No such benefit was found within women. In a follow-up study Keogh and Herdenfeldt compared emotion-focused and sensory-focused coping instructions. They also found that focusing on the sensory qualities of pain was of benefit for men. For women, however, focusing on the emotional side of pain seemed to increase affective pain responses, suggesting that this type of focusing is not beneficial. This is interesting in light of the results reported above by Smith et al., who found a benefit with emotion-focused coping in pain patients. More recently, Keogh et al. (2005a) compared acceptance and cognitive control performance on cold pressor pain. They found that the acceptance approach was more beneficial for women, in that they reported lower affective pain.

It therefore seems that men and women adopt different strategies, and that there may be differences in how effective they are. However, more research is required to see whether different coping strategies have a differential effect on pain, and if this works in a sex-specific manner.

Interpersonal Interactions

The above section on gender-roles, beliefs and attitudes draws attention to the fact that pain and pain-behaviors can be shaped and influenced by others. This section will focus on interpersonal interactions and social context as potential factors in explaining sex differences in pain (Robinson, Riley, & Myers, 2000). Indirect evidence for the role of social interaction includes experimental research that demonstrates that the sex of an observer can influence pain experiences and reporting behaviors of men and women (Kallai, Barke, & Voss, 2004; Levine & Desimone, 1991; Weisse et al., 2005). For example, Levine and Desimone report an experimental pain study in which both the sex of the experimenter and the participant was examined to see whether differences would be found in pain. The general finding was that for men pain reports were lower if the experimenter was female. Others have found a similar pattern in women i.e., that when the experimenter is male, females exhibited greater pain tolerance (Kallai et al., 2004).

More direct evidence for the role of social interactions on sex differences in pain also exists. For example, Jackson et al. (2005) allowed some participants to engage in spoken interactions during an experimental pain task. When allowed to engage in transactions with an experimenter, women exhibited lower pain tolerance levels when compared to men. The authors note that their findings are similar to those found in a previous study on children

(Chambers, Craig, & Bennett, 2002) that examined the role of maternal behavior on children's responses to experimental pain, and showed that type of social interaction had an effect on girl's pain responses, but not boys. Others examples where interpersonal interactions have been examined are in studies that examine spousal support on patient's pain. For example, Smith et al. (2004) examined the role of spouse behaviors on male and female pain patients with osteoarthritis, by videoing couple's behaviors when patients were asked to engaging in a series of everyday household tasks. In terms of spouse effects, there were differences between husbands and wives in facilitative, rather than solicitous behaviors. Wives were found to engage in more facilitative behaviors before and after the task when compared to husbands (see also Keefe, This Volume).

Together this work suggests that social interactions and context may be important in helping to understanding some of the differences in the pain behaviors of men and women.

Biological Factors

Alongside psychosocial factors there are also a range of biological mechanisms that may potentially account for some of the sex differences in pain (Berkley et al., 2002; Holdcroft & Berkley, 2005). Such factors include cardiovascular and immunological functions (Fillingim & Maixner, 1996; Keogh & Witt, 2001; Levine, Khasar, & Green, 2006). There also seem to be genetic factors that account for some of the variation in pain within human males and females (Fillingim et al., 2005b; Kim et al., 2004; Mogil et al., 2003; Wellcome Trust Case Control Consortium, 2007; Devor et al., 2007; See also MacGregor, this volume), and imaging studies suggest that there may be sex differences in the regions of the brain associated with pain (Berman et al., 2006; Derbyshire, Nichols, Firestone, Townsend, & Jones, 2002; Paulson, Minoshima, Morrow, & Casey, 1998; See also Matre and Tuan, This Volume). However, the area that seems to have been most extensively developed in terms of biological mechanisms for sex differences in pain is that of sex hormones (Aloisi, 2003; Aloisi & Bonifazi, 2006; Cairns, 2007; Craft et al., 2004; Fillingim & Ness, 2000b). The reasoning for this stems partly from the finding that a number of sex differences in pain occur during the reproductive years, and partly from differences that stem from circulating levels of sex hormones such as estrogen, progesterone and testosterone.

If sex hormones do mediate sex differences in pain then variation in such hormones might be related to changes in pain sensitivity (Fillingim & Ness, 2000a, 2000b). One method employed to examine this has been to use a menstrual cycle paradigm, to see whether cycle-related changes in pain occur in clinical groups (LeResche, Mancl, Sherman, Gandara, & Dworkin, 2003; LeResche et al., 2005; Sherman et al., 2004, 2005). When LeResche et al. (2003)

examined temporomandibular disorder-related pain across the menstrual cycle, they found that pain reports were highest when estrogen levels were low, and when there were sudden changes in estrogen concentration i.e., around ovulation and menstruation. There have also been studies, mostly conducted on healthy adults, which examine whether there is greater sensitivity to experimental pain at different phases of the menstrual cycle (Bajaj, Arendt-Nielsen, Bajaj, & Madsen, 2001; Fillingim et al., 1997; Giamberardino, Berkley, Iezzi, deBigontina, & Vecchiet, 1997; Pfleeger, Straneva, Fillingim, Maixner, & Girdler, 1997). For example, Fillingim et al. (1997) tested 11 healthy women on days corresponding to the follicular, ovulatory and luteal phases of the cycle using an ischemic pain task. They found greater pain sensitivity during the luteal phase compared to follicular phase. However, since inconsistent findings have also been reported (Giamberardino et al., 1997), Riley at al. (1999) conducted a review and meta-analysis of the evidence for menstrual cycle-related changes in sensitivity to experimental pain in healthy women. They concluded that whereas pain sensitivity does vary across the menstrual cycle, effect sizes range from low to moderate magnitude depending on the type of pain induction method used. Greater sensitivity was found within the luteal phase when compared to follicular phase for most forms of pain induction method, with the exception of electrical stimulation, which showed the opposite pattern. Clinical studies that employ experimental pain induction methods have also found that phase effects may depend on the type of pain induction method used (Sherman et al., 2005). Alongside type of stimulus, other methodological differences between studies include stimulation site, definition of menstrual cycle phase, inclusion of males as controls, and inclusion of women taking oral contraceptives (Fillingim & Ness, 2000a; Sherman & LeResche, 2006).

A second method that has been used to examine hormonal factors in pain sensitivity has been to consider other periods of hormonal change, such as pregnancy and the menopause (LeResche et al., 2005). Not only does pain sensitivity change during pregnancy, but some painful conditions, such as rheumatoid arthritis and temporomandibular disorder, are temporarily alleviated during this period (Drossaers-Bakker, Zwinderman, van Zeben, Breedveld, & Hazes, 2002; Hazes, 1991; Hazes, Dijkmans, Vandenbroucke, de Vries, & Cats, 1990; LeResche et al., 2005). Pharmacological manipulation of sex hormones can affect pain, in that oral contraceptive use mediates pain, as does hormone-replacement therapy (LeResche, Saunders, Von Korff, Barlow, & Dworkin, 1997). One study found that headaches are more likely to occur in post-menopausal women taking hormone-replacement therapy than those who are not (Aegidius, Zwart, Hagen, Schei, & Stovner, 2007).

Most pain-related studies have focused on females and/or sex hormones that occur to a greater extent within females e.g., estrogen. Only a few have examined testosterone within the context of pain. For example, a study on a group of male patients with Irritable Bowel Syndrome found that testosterone levels were negatively related to sensory thresholds during a rectal sensitivity test (Houghton, Jackson, Whorwell, & Morris, 2000). It has also been noted that long term use of opioids for chronic pain can result in opioid-induced androgen deficiency syndrome (Daniell, 2002), which can in turn be reduced through testosterone therapy (Daniell, Lentz, & Mazer, 2006; Malkin et al., 2004). Testosterone therapy has also found to reduce exercise-induced ischemia in a group of men with angina (English, Steeds, Jones, Diver, & Channer, 2000). Finally, there is also a suggestion that sex hormones affect pain reports in transsexuals (Aloisi et al., 2007). More research is clearly required examining the effects of androgens on pain.

Summary and Conclusions

The above review suggests that being male or female can impact on how pain is perceived and experienced. Although it seems women report more pain across a range of different situations and conditions, other factors affect this relationship e.g., age, type of condition etc. It also seems as if differences exist in responses to pharmacological and non-pharmacological pain management. This is important in that it may mean that different treatment approaches, or at least a different emphasis in treatment, may be required when dealing with male and female pain. However, such a proposal is only speculative at present since there are few treatment-outcome studies that explicitly consider sex. That said, progress is being made in terms of understanding why sex differences in pain occur. Although still far from completely understanding these various mechanisms, it seems likely that a multidisciplinary approach is required in order to fully understand the similarities and differences in the pain experiences of men and women.

In terms of future directions, it would be helpful if treatment-outcome studies examine and report on sex-specific effects, rather than simply statistically controlling for them. Given the wide range of treatment approaches, we need to know whether different approaches produce similar responses in men and women, or whether the sexes benefit in different ways. At present, there has been good progress into the biological, and to some extent the psychosocial factors, in explaining this phenomenon. However, there is still room for development. For example, within the psychological arena, there is still relatively little known about possible differences in health beliefs. Social and contextual factors have also received relatively little attention, although we are beginning to see an emergence of research in this area (see, Bernardes et al., 2008). This work is important, as it is only when these separate biological, psychological and social factors have been identified as possible explanations for sex differences in pain will it be possible to consider interactions between these variables. Although it is generally assumed that sex and gender interact (Holdcroft & Berkley, 2005), to date very few studies consider these potential interactive effects. In time, we should have a much better understanding as to how and why differences between the sexes in pain experiences occur, and in doing so be in a better position to treat people more effectively.

References

Aegidius, K. L., Zwart, J. A., Hagen, K., Schei, B., & Stovner, L. J. (2007). Hormone replacement therapy and headache prevalence in postmenopausal women. The Head-HUNT study. *European Journal of Neurology, 14,* 73–78.

Aloisi, A. M. (2003). Gonadal hormones and sex differences in pain reactivity. *Clinical Journal of Pain, 19,* 168–174.

Aloisi, A. M., Bachiocco, V., Costantino, A., Stefani, R., Ceccarelli, I., & Bertaccini, A., et al. (2007). Cross-sex hormone administration changes pain in transsexual women and men. *Pain, 132,* Suppl 1, S60–67.

Aloisi, A. M., & Bonifazi, M. (2006). Sex hormones, central nervous system and pain. *Hormones & Behavior, 50,* 1–7.

Antonov, K. I., & Isacson, D. (1996). Use of analgesics in Sweden–the importance of socio-demographic factors, physical fitness, health and health-related factors, and working conditions. *Social Science & Medicine, 42,* 1473–1481.

Antonov, K. I., & Isacson, D. G. (1998). Prescription and nonprescription analgesic use in Sweden. *The Annals of Pharmacotherapy, 32,* 485–494.

Aubrun, F., Salvi, N., Coriat, P., & Riou, B. (2005). Sex- and age-related differences in morphine requirements for postoperative pain relief. *Anesthesiology, 103,* 156–160.

Bajaj, P., Arendt-Nielsen, L., Bajaj, P., & Madsen, H. (2001). Sensory changes during the ovulatory phase of the menstrual cycle in healthy women. *European Journal of Pain, 5,* 135–144.

Bandura, A., O'Leary, A., Taylor, C. B., Gauthier, J., & Gossard, D. (1987). Perceived self-efficacy and pain control: Opioid and nonopioid mechanisms. *Journal of Personality & Social Psychology, 53,* 563–571.

Berkley, K. J. (1997). Sex differences in pain. *Behavioral & Brain Sciences, 20,* 371–380.

Berkley, K. J., Hoffman, G. E., Murphy, A. Z., & Holdcroft, A. (2002). Pain: Sex/gender differences. In D. Pfaff, A. Arnold, A. Etgen, S. Fahrbach & R. Rubin (Eds.), *Hormones, brain & behavior* (Vol. 5, pp. 409–442). London: Academic Press.

Berman, S. M., Naliboff, B. D., Suyenobu, B., Labus, J. S., Stains, J., & Bueller, J. A., et al. (2006). Sex differences in regional brain response to aversive pelvic visceral stimuli. *American Journal of Physiology-Regulatory Integrative and Comparative Physiology, 291,* R268–R276.

Bernardes, S. F., Keogh, E., & Lima, M. L. (2008). Bridging the gap between pain and gender research: A selective literature review. *European Journal of Pain, 12,* 427–440.

Bingefors, K., & Isacson, D. (2004). Epidemiology, co-morbidity, and impact on health-related quality of life of self-reported headache and musculoskeletal pain – a gender perspective. *European Journal of Pain, 8,* 435–450.

Bruehl, S., Al'absi, M., France, C. R., France, J., Harju, A., & Burns, J. W., et al. (2007). Anger management style and endogenous opioid function: Is gender a moderator? *Journal of Behavioral Medicine, 30,* 209–219.

Bruehl, S., Chung, O. Y., & Burns, J. W. (2006). Anger expression and pain: An overview of findings and possible mechanisms. *Journal of Behavioral Medicine, 29,* 593–606.

Burns, J. W., Johnson, B. J., Devine, J., Mahoney, N., & Pawl, R. (1998). Anger management style and the prediction of treatment outcome among male and female chronic pain patients. *Behaviour Research & Therapy, 36,* 1051–1062.

Burns, J. W., Johnson, B. J., Mahoney, N., Devine, J., & Pawl, R. (1996). Anger management style, hostility and spouse responses: Gender differences in predictors of adjustment among chronic pain patients. *Pain, 64,* 445–453.

Cairns, B. E. (2007). The influence of gender and sex steroids on craniofacial nociception. *Headache, 47,* 319–324.

Campbell, A. (2006). Sex differences in direct aggression: What are the psychological mediators? *Aggression & Violent Behavior, 11,* 237–264.

Cepeda, M. S., & Carr, D. B. (2003). Women experience more pain and require more morphine than men to achieve a similar degree of analgesia. *Anesthesia & Analgesia, 97,* 1464–1468.

Chambers, C. T., Craig, K. D., & Bennett, S. M. (2002). The impact of maternal behavior on children's pain experiences: An experimental analysis. *Journal of Pediatric Psychology, 27,* 293–301.

Ciccone, G. K., & Holdcroft, A. (1999). Drugs and sex differences: A review of drugs relating to anaesthesia. *British Journal of Anaesthesia, 82,* 255–265.

Craft, R. M. (2003). Sex differences in opioid analgesia: "From mouse to man". *Clinical Journal of Pain, 19,* 175–186.

Craft, R. M., Mogil, J. S., & Aloisi, A. M. (2004). Sex differences in pain and analgesia: The role of gonadal hormones. *European Journal of Pain, 8,* 397–411.

Daniell, H. W. (2002). Hypogonadism in men consuming sustained-action oral opioids. *The Journal of Pain, 3,* 377–384.

Daniell, H. W., Lentz, R., & Mazer, N. A. (2006). Open-label pilot study of testosterone patch therapy in men with opioid-induced androgen deficiency. *The Journal of Pain, 7,* 200–210.

Dao, T. T., & LeResche, L. (2000). Gender differences in pain. *Journal of Orofacial Pain, 14,* 169–184.

Devor, M., Gilad, A., Arbilly, M., Nissenbaum, J., Yakir, B., & Raber, P., et al. (2007). Sex-specific variability and a "cage effect" independently mask a neuropathic pain quantitative trait locus detected in a whole genome scan. *European Journal of Neuroscience, 26,* 681–688.

Derbyshire, S. W. G., Nichols, T. E., Firestone, L., Townsend, D. W., & Jones, A. K. P. (2002). Gender differences in patterns of cerebral activation during equal experience of painful laser stimulation. *The Journal of Pain, 3,* 401–411.

Dixon, K. E., Thorn, B. E., & Ward, L. C. (2004). An evaluation of sex differences in psychological and physiological responses to experimentally-induced pain: A path analytic description. *Pain, 112,* 188–196.

Dodick, D. W., Rozen, T. D., Goadsby, P. J., & Silberstein, S. D. (2000). Cluster headache. *Cephalalgia, 20,* 787–803.

Drossaers-Bakker, K. W., Zwinderman, A. H., van Zeben, D., Breedveld, F. C., & Hazes, J. M. (2002). Pregnancy and oral contraceptive use do not significantly influence outcome in long term rheumatoid arthritis. *Annals of the Rheumatic Diseases, 61,* 405–408.

Edwards, R. R., Augustson, E. M., & Fillingim, R. B. (2000). Sex-specific effects of pain-related anxiety on adjustment to chronic pain. *Clinical Journal of Pain, 16,* 46–53.

Edwards, R. R., Augustson, E., & Fillingim, R. B. (2003a). Differential relationships between anxiety and treatment-associated pain reduction among male and female chronic pain patients. *Clinical Journal of Pain, 19,* 208–216.

Edwards, R. R., Doleys, D. M., Lowery, D., & Fillingim, R. B. (2003b). Pain tolerance as a predictor of outcome following multidisciplinary treatment for chronic pain: Differential effects as a function of sex. *Pain, 106,* 419–426.

Edwards, R. R., Haythornthwaite, J. A., Sullivan, M. J., & Fillingim, R. B. (2004). Catastrophizing as a mediator of sex differences in pain: Differential effects for daily pain versus laboratory-induced pain. *Pain, 111,* 335–341.

Elklit, A., & Jones, A. (2006). The association between anxiety and chronic pain after whiplash injury – Gender-specific effects. *Clinical Journal of Pain, 22,* 487–490.

English, K. M., Steeds, R. P., Jones, T. H., Diver, M. J., & Channer, K. S. (2000). Low-dose transdermal testosterone therapy improves angina threshold in men with chronic stable angina: A randomized, double-blind, placebo-controlled study. *Circulation, 102,* 1906–1911.

Eriksen, J., Sjogren, P., Ekholm, O., & Rasmussen, N. K. (2004). Health care utilisation among individuals reporting long-term pain: An epidemiological study based on Danish National Health Surveys. *European Journal of Pain, 8,* 517–523.

Fillingim, R. B. (Ed.). (2000). *Sex, gender, & pain* (Vol. 17). Seattle, WA: IASP Press.

Fillingim, R. B. (2002). Sex differences in analgesic responses: evidence from experimental pain models. *European Journal of Anaesthesiology, 19*, 16–24.

Fillingim, R. B., & Gear, R. W. (2004). Sex differences in opioid analgesia: Clinical and experimental findings. *European Journal of Pain, 8*, 413–425.

Fillingim, R. B., Hastie, B. A., Ness, T. J., Glover, T. L., Campbell, C. M., & Staud, R. (2005a). Sex-related psychological predictors of baseline pain perception and analgesic responses to pentazocine. *Biological Psychology, 69*, 97–112.

Fillingim, R. B., Kaplan, L., Staud, R., Ness, T. J., Glover, T. L., & Campbell, C., et al. (2005b). The A118G single nucleotide polymorphism of the mu-opioid receptor gene (OPRM1) is associated with pressure pain sensitivity in humans. *The Journal of Pain, 6*, 159–167.

Fillingim, R. B., & Maixner, W. (1995). Gender differences in the responses to noxious stimuli. *Pain Forum, 4*, 209–221.

Fillingim, R. B., & Maixner, W. (1996). The influence of resting blood pressure and gender on pain responses. *Psychosomatic Medicine, 58*, 326–332.

Fillingim, R. B., Maixner, W., Girdler, S. S., Light, K. C., Harris, M. B., & Sheps, D. S., et al. (1997). Ischemic but not thermal pain sensitivity varies across the menstrual cycle. *Psychosomatic Medicine, 59*, 512–520.

Fillingim, R. B., & Ness, T. J. (2000a). The influence of menstrual cycle and sex hormones on pain responses in humans. In R. B. Fillingim (Ed.), *Sex, gender & pain* (pp. 191–207). Seattle, WA: IASP Press.

Fillingim, R. B., & Ness, T. J. (2000b). Sex-related hormonal influences on pain and analgesic responses. *Neuroscience & Biobehavioural Reviews, 24*, 485–501.

Fillingim, R. B., Ness, T. J., Glover, T. L., Campbell, C. M., Hastie, B. A., & Price, D. D., et al. (2005c). Morphine responses and experimental pain: Sex differences in side effects and cardiovascular responses but not analgesia. *The Journal of Pain, 6*, 116–124.

Fillingim, R. B., Ness, T. J., Glover, T. L., Campbell, C. M., Price, D. D., & Staud, R. (2004). Experimental pain models reveal no sex differences in pentazocine analgesia in humans. *Anesthesiology, 100*, 1263–1270.

Frot, M., Feine, J. S., & Bushnell, M. C. (2004). Sex differences in pain perception and anxiety. A psychophysical study with topical capsaicin. *Pain, 108*, 230–236.

Galdas, P. M., Cheater, F., & Marshall, P. (2005). Men and health help-seeking behaviour: Literature review. *Journal of Advanced Nursing, 49*, 616–623.

Gear, R. W., Lee, J. S., Miaskowski, C., Gordon, N. C., Paul, S. M., & Levine, J. D. (2006). Neuroleptics antagonize nalbuphine antianalgesia. *The Journal of Pain, 7*, 187–191.

Gear, R. W., Miaskowski, C., Gordon, N. C., Paul, S. M., Heller, P. H., & Levine, J. D. (1996). Kappa-opioids produce significantly greater analgesia in women than in men. *Nature Medicine, 2*, 1248–1250.

Gear, R. W., Miaskowski, C., Gordon, N. C., Paul, S. M., Heller, P. H., & Levine, J. D. (1999). The kappa opioid nalbuphine produces gender- and dose-dependent analgesia and antianalgesia in patients with postoperative pain. *Pain, 83*, 339–345.

Giamberardino, M. A., Berkley, K. J., Iezzi, S., deBigontina, P., & Vecchiet, L. (1997). Pain threshold variations in somatic wall tissues as a function of menstrual cycle, segmental site and tissue depth in non-dysmenorrheic women, dysmenorrheic women and men. *Pain, 71*, 187–197.

Giles, B. E., & Walker, J. S. (2000). Sex differences in pain and analgesia. *Pain Reviews, 7*, 181–193.

Gran, J. T. (2003). The epidemiology of chronic generalized musculoskeletal pain. *Best Practice & Research Clinical Rheumatology, 17*, 547–561.

Green, C. A., & Pope, C. R. (1999). Gender, psychosocial factors and the use of medical services: a longitudinal analysis. *Social Science & Medicine, 48*, 1363–1372.

Haley, W. E., Turner, J. A., & Romano, J. M. (1985). Depression in chronic pain patients: relation to pain, activity, and sex differences. *Pain, 23*, 337–343.

Hamann, S., & Canli, T. (2004). Individual differences in emotion processing. *Current Opinions in Neurobiology, 14*, 233–238.

Hansen, F. R., Bendix, T., Skov, P., Jensen, C. V., Kristensen, J. H., & Krohn, L., et al. (1993). Intensive, dynamic back-muscle exercises, conventional physiotherapy, or placebo-control treatment of low-back pain. A randomized, observer-blind trial. *Spine, 18*, 98–108.

Hazes, J. M. (1991). Pregnancy and its effect on the risk of developing rheumatoid arthritis. *Annals of the Rheumatic Diseases, 50*, 71–72.

Hazes, J. M., Dijkmans, B. A., Vandenbroucke, J. P., de Vries, R. R., & Cats, A. (1990). Pregnancy and the risk of developing rheumatoid arthritis. *Arthritis & Rheumatism, 33*, 1770–1775.

Hirsh, A. T., Waxenberg, L. B., Atchison, J. W., Gremillion, H. A., & Robinson, M. E. (2006). Evidence for sex differences in the relationships of pain, mood, and disability. *The Journal of Pain, 7*, 592–601.

Holdcroft, A. (2002). Sex differences and analgesics. *European Journal of Anaesthesiology Supplement, 26*, 1–2.

Holdcroft, A., & Berkley, K. J. (2005). Sex and gender differences in pain and its relief. In S. B. McMahon, M. Koltzenburg, P. D. Wall & R. Melzack (Eds.), *Wall & Melzack's textbook of pain* (5th ed., pp. 1181–1197). Edinburgh: Elsevier Churchill Livingstone.

Hooftman, W. E., van Poppel, M. N., van der Beek, A. J., Bongers, P. M., & van Mechelen, W. (2004). Gender differences in the relations between work-related physical and psychosocial risk factors and musculoskeletal complaints. *Scandinavian Journal of Work, Environment & Health, 30*, 261–278.

Houghton, L. A., Jackson, N. A., Whorwell, P. J., & Morris, J. (2000). Do male sex hormones protect from irritable bowel syndrome? *American Journal of Gastroenterology, 95*, 2296–2300.

Isacson, D., & Bingefors, K. (2002). Epidemiology of analgesic use: A gender perspective. *European Journal of Anaesthesiology, 19*, 5–15.

Jackson, T., Iezzi, T., Chen, H., Ebnet, S., & Eglitis, K. (2005). Gender, interpersonal transactions, and the perception of pain: An experimental analysis. *Journal of Pain, 6*, 228–236.

Jackson, T., Iezzi, T., Gunderson, J., Nagasaka, T., & Fritch, A. (2002). Gender differences in pain perception: The mediating role of self-efficacy beliefs. *Sex Roles, 47*, 561–568.

Jensen, I. B., Bergstrom, G., Ljungquist, T., Bodin, L., & Nygren, A. L. (2001). A randomized controlled component analysis of a behavioral medicine rehabilitation program for chronic spinal pain: Are the effects dependent on gender? *Pain, 91*, 65–78.

Jones, A., & Zachariae, R. (2002). Gender, anxiety, and experimental pain sensitivity: an overview. *Journal of American Medical Women's Association, 57*, 91–94.

Jones, A., Zachariae, R., & Arendt-Nielsen, L. (2003). Dispositional anxiety and the experience of pain: Gender-specific effects. *European Journal of Pain, 7*, 387–395.

Kallai, I., Barke, A., & Voss, U. (2004). The effects of experimenter characteristics on pain reports in women and men. *Pain, 112*, 142–147.

Kaur, S., Stechuchak, K. M., Coffman, C. J., Allen, K. D., & Bastian, L. A. (2007). Gender differences in health care utilization among veterans with chronic pain. *Journal of General Internal Medicine, 22*, 228–233.

Keefe, F. J., Lefebvre, J. C., Egert, J. R., Affleck, G., Sullivan, M. J., & Caldwell, D. S. (2000). The relationship of gender to pain, pain behavior, and disability in osteoarthritis patients: The role of catastrophizing. *Pain, 87*, 325–334.

Keogh, E. (2006). Sex and gender differences in pain: A selective review of biological and psychosocial factors. *The Journal of Men's Health & Gender 3*, 236–243.

Keogh, E., & Asmundson, G. J. G. (2004). Negative affectivity, catastrophizing and anxiety sensitivity. In G. J. G. Asmundson, J. W. Vlaeyen & G. Crombez (Eds.), *Understanding & treating fear of pain* (pp. 91–115). Oxford: Oxford University Press.

Keogh, E., Barlow, C., Mounce, C., & Bond, F. W. (2006a). Assessing the relationship between cold pressor pain responses and dimensions of the anxiety sensitivity profile in healthy men and women. *Cognitive Behaviour Therapy*, *35*, 198–206.

Keogh, E., & Birkby, J. (1999). The effect of anxiety sensitivity and gender on the experience of pain. *Cognition & Emotion*, *13*, 813–829.

Keogh, E., Bond, F. W., Hanmer, R., & Tilston, J. (2005a). Comparing acceptance- and control-based coping instructions on the cold-pressor pain experiences of healthy men and women. *European Journal of Pain*, *9*, 591–598.

Keogh, E., & Eccleston, C. (2006). Sex differences in adolescent chronic pain and pain-related coping. *Pain*, *123*, 275–284.

Keogh, E., Hamid, R., Hamid, S., & Ellery, D. (2004). Investigating the effect of anxiety sensitivity, gender and negative interpretative bias on the perception of chest pain. *Pain*, *111*, 209–217.

Keogh, E., Hatton, K., & Ellery, D. (2000). Avoidance versus focused attention and the perception of pain: Differential effects for men and women. *Pain*, *85*, 225–230.

Keogh, E., & Herdenfeldt, M. (2002). Gender, coping and the perception of pain. *Pain*, *97*, 195–201.

Keogh, E., McCracken, L. M., & Eccleston, C. (2005b). Do men and women differ in their response to interdisciplinary chronic pain management? *Pain*, *114*, 37–46.

Keogh, E., McCracken, L. M., & Eccleston, C. (2006b). Gender moderates the association between depression and disability in chronic pain patients. *European Journal of Pain*, *10*, 413–422.

Keogh, E., & Witt, G. (2001). Hypoalgesic effect of caffeine in normotensive men and women. *Psychophysiology*, *38*, 886–895.

Kessler, R. C., McGonagle, K. A., Zhao, S., Nelson, C. B., Hughes, M., & Eshleman, S., et al. (1994). Lifetime and 12-month prevalence of DSM-III-R psychiatric disorders in the United States. Results from the National Comorbidity Survey. *Archives of General Psychiatry*, *51*, 8–19.

Kest, B., Sarton, E., & Dahan, A. (2000). Gender differences in opioid-mediated analgesic – Animal and human studies. *Anesthesiology*, *93*, 539–547.

Kim, H., Neubert, J. K., San Miguel, A., Xu, K., Krishnaraju, R. K., & Iadarola, M. J., et al. (2004). Genetic influence on variability in human acute experimental pain sensitivity associated with gender, ethnicity and psychological temperament. *Pain*, *109*, 488–496.

Koopmans, G. T., & Lamers, L. M. (2007). Gender and health care utilization: the role of mental distress and help-seeking propensity. *Social Science & Medicine*, *64*, 1216–1230.

Krogstad, B. S., Jokstad, A., Dahl, B. L., & Vassend, O. (1996). The reporting of pain, somatic complaints, and anxiety in a group of patients with TMD before and 2 years after treatment: Sex differences. *Journal of Orofacial Pain*, *10*, 263–269.

Lautenbacher, S., & Rollman, G. B. (1993). Sex differences in responsiveness to painful and non-painful stimuli are dependent upon the stimulation method. *Pain*, *53*, 255–264.

LeResche, L. (1999). Gender considerations in the epidemiology of chronic pain. In I. K. Crombie, P. R. Croft, S. J. Linton, L. LeResche & M. Von Korff (Eds.), *Epidemiology of Pain* (pp. 43–52). Seattle, WA: IASP Press.

LeResche, L., Mancl, L., Sherman, J. J., Gandara, B., & Dworkin, S. F. (2003). Changes in temporomandibular pain and other symptoms across the menstrual cycle. *Pain*, *106*, 253–261.

LeResche, L., Saunders, K., Von Korff, M. R., Barlow, W., & Dworkin, S. F. (1997). Use of exogenous hormones and risk of temporomandibular disorder pain. *Pain*, *69*, 153–160.

LeResche, L., Sherman, J. J., Huggins, K., Saunders, K., Mancl, L. A., & Lentz, G., et al. (2005). Musculoskeletal orofacial pain and other signs and symptoms of temporomandibular disorders during pregnancy: A prospective study. *Journal of Orofacial Pain*, *19*, 193–201.

Levine, F. M., & Desimone, L. L. (1991). The effects of experimenter gender on pain report in male and female subjects. *Pain, 44*, 69–72.

Levine, J. D., Khasar, S. G., & Green, P. G. (2006). Neurogenic inflammation and arthritis. *Annals of the New York Academy of Sciences, 1069*, 155–167.

Linzer, M., Spitzer, R., Kroenke, K., Williams, J. B., Hahn, S., & Brody, D., et al. (1996). Gender, quality of life, and mental disorders in primary care: Results from the PRIME-MD 1000 study. *The American Journal of Medicine, 101*, 526–533.

Logan, D. E., & Rose, J. B. (2004). Gender differences in post-operative pain and patient controlled analgesia use among adolescent surgical patients. *Pain, 109*, 481–487.

Lund, I., Lundeberg, T., Kowalski, J., & Svensson, E. (2005). Gender differences in electrical pain threshold responses to transcutaneous electrical nerve stimulation (TENS). *Neuroscience Letters, 375*, 75–80.

Lynch, A. M., Kashikar-Zuck, S., Goldschneider, K. R., & Jones, B. A. (2007). Sex and age differences in coping styles among children with chronic pain. *The Journal of Pain Symptom Management, 33*, 208–216.

Malkin, C. J., Pugh, P. J., Morris, P. D., Kerry, K. E., Jones, R. D., & Jones, T. H., et al. (2004). Testosterone replacement in hypogonadal men with angina improves ischaemic threshold and quality of life. *Heart, 90*, 871–876.

Manzoni, G. C. (1998). Gender ratio of cluster headache over the years: A possible role of changes in lifestyle. *Cephalalgia, 18*, 138–142.

Mayer, E. A., Berman, S., Lin, C., & Naliboff, B. D. (2004). Sex-based differences in gastrointestinal pain. *European Journal of Pain, 8*, 451–463.

McClure, E. B. (2000). A meta-analytic review of sex differences in facial expression processing and their development in infants, children, and adolescents. *Psychological Bulletin, 126*, 424–453.

McCracken, L. M., & Houle, T. (2000). Sex-specific and general roles of pain-related anxiety in adjustment to chronic pain: A reply to Edwards et al. *Clinical Journal of Pain, 16*, 275–276.

McGeary, D. D., Mayer, T. G., Gatchel, R. J., Anagnostis, C., & Proctor, T. J. (2003). Gender-related differences in treatment outcomes for patients with musculoskeletal disorders. *The Spine Journal, 3*, 197–203.

Meana, M. (1998). The meeting of pain and depression: Comorbidity in women. *Canadian Journal of Psychiatry, 43*, 893–899.

Miaskowski, C., Gear, R. W., & Levine, J. D. (2000). Sex-related differences in analgesic responses. In R. B. Fillingim (Ed.), *Sex, gender, & pain* (pp. 209–230). Seattle, WA: IASP Press.

Miaskowski, C., & Levine, J. D. (1999). Does opioid analgesia show a gender preference for females? *Pain Forum, 8*, 34–44.

Miller, C., & Newton, S. E. (2006). Pain perception and expression: The influence of gender, personal self-efficacy, and lifespan socialization. *Pain Management Nursing, 7*, 148–152.

Mogil, J. S., Wilson, S. G., Chesler, E. J., Rankin, A. L., Nemmani, K. V., & Lariviere, et al. (2003). The melanocortin-1 receptor gene mediates female-specific mechanisms of analgesia in mice and humans. *Proceedings of the National Academy of Sciences of the United States of America, 100*, 4867–4872.

Moller-Leimkuhler, A. M. (2002). Barriers to help-seeking by men: A review of sociocultural and clinical literature with particular reference to depression. *Journal of Affective Disorders, 71*, 1–9.

Morin, C., Lund, J. P., Villarroel, T., Clokie, C. M., & Feine, J. S. (2000). Differences between the sexes in post-surgical pain. *Pain, 85*, 79–85.

Myers, C. D., Tsao, J. C. I., Glover, D. A., Kim, S. C., Turk, N., & Zeltzer, L. K. (2006). Sex, gender, and age: Contributions to laboratory pain responding in children and adolescents. *The Journal of Pain, 7*, 556–564.

Nolen-Hoeksema, S. (2001). Gender differences in depression. *Current Directions in Psychological Science, 10*, 173–176.

Nolen-Hoeksema, S., Larson, J., & Grayson, C. (1999). Explaining the gender difference in depressive symptoms. *Journal of Personality and Social Psychology, 77*, 1061–1072.

Novy, D. M., Nelson, D. V., Averill, P. M., & Berry, L. A. (1996). Gender differences in the expression of depressive symptoms among chronic pain patients. *Clinical Journal of Pain, 12*, 23–29.

Ochroch, E. A., Gottschalk, A., Troxel, A. B., & Farrar, J. T. (2006). Women suffer more short and long-term pain than men after major thoracotomy. *Clinical Journal of Pain, 22*, 491–498.

Olofsen, E., Romberg, R., Bijl, H., Mooren, R., Engbers, F., & Kest, B., et al. (2005). Alfentanil and placebo analgesia – No sex differences detected in models of experimental pain. *Anesthesiology, 103*, 130–139.

Osman, A., Barrios, F. X., Gutierrez, P. M., Kopper, B. A., Merrifield, T., & Grittmann, L. (2000). The pain catastrophizing scale: Further psychometric evaluation with adult samples. *Journal of Behavioral Medicine, 23*, 351–365.

Osman, A., Barrios, F. X., Kopper, B. A., Hauptmann, W., Jones, J., & O'Neill, E. (1997). Factor structure, reliability, and validity of the pain catastrophizing scale. *Journal of Behavioral Medicine, 20*, 589–605.

Paulose-Ram, R., Hirsch, R., Dillon, C., Losonczy, K., Cooper, M., & Ostchega, Y. (2003). Prescription and non-prescription analgesic use among the US adult population: Results from the third National Health and Nutrition Examination Survey (NHANES III). *Pharmacoepidemiology & Drug Safety, 12*, 315–326.

Paulson, P. E., Minoshima, S., Morrow, T. J., & Casey, K. L. (1998). Gender differences in pain perception and patterns of cerebral activation during noxious heat stimulation in humans. *Pain, 76*, 223–229.

Pfleeger, M., Straneva, P. A., Fillingim, R. B., Maixner, W., & Girdler, S. S. (1997). Menstrual cycle, blood pressure and ischemic pain sensitivity in women: A preliminary investigation. *International Journal of Psychophysiology, 27*, 161–166.

Pleym, H., Spigset, O., Kharasch, E. D., & Dale, O. (2003). Gender differences in drug effects: Implications for anesthesiologists. *Acta Anaesthesiologica Scandinavica, 47*, 241–259.

Pool, G. J., Schwegler, A. F., Theodore, B. R., & Fuchs, P. N. (2007). Role of gender norms and group identification on hypothetical and experimental pain tolerance. *Pain, 129*, 122–129.

Porteous, T., Bond, C., Hannaford, P., & Sinclair, H. (2005). How and why are non-prescription analgesics used in Scotland? *Family Practice, 22*, 78–85.

Redondo-Sendino, A., Guallar-Castillon, P., Banegas, J. R., & Rodriguez-Artalejo, F. (2006). Gender differences in the utilization of health-care services among the older adult population of Spain. *BMC Public Health, 6*, 155.

Rethelyi, J. M., Berghammer, R., & Kopp, M. S. (2001). Comorbidity of pain-associated disability and depressive symptoms in connection with sociodemographic variables: Results from a cross-sectional epidemiological survey in Hungary. *Pain, 93*, 115–121.

Rhudy, J. L., & Williams, A. E. (2005). Gender differences in pain: Do emotions play a role? *Gender Medicine, 2*, 208–226.

Riley, J. L., Robinson, M. E., Wade, J. B., Myers, C. D., & Price, D. D. (2001). Sex differences in negative emotional responses to chronic pain. *The Journal of Pain, 2*, 354–359.

Riley, J. L., Robinson, M. E., Wise, E. A., Myers, C. D., & Fillingim, R. B. (1998). Sex differences in the perception of noxious experimental stimuli: A meta-analysis. *Pain, 74*, 181–187.

Riley, J. L., Robinson, M. E., Wise, E. A., & Price, D. D. (1999). A meta-analytic review of pain perception across the menstrual cycle. *Pain, 81*, 225–235.

Robinson, M. E., Gagnon, C. M., Dannecker, E. A., Brown, J. L., Jump, R. L., & Price, D. D. (2003a). Sex differences in common pain events: Expectations and anchors. *The Journal of Pain, 4*, 40–45.

Robinson, M. E., Gagnon, C. M., Riley, J. L., & Price, D. D. (2003b). Altering gender role expectations: Effects on pain tolerance, pain threshold, and pain ratings. *The Journal of Pain, 4*, 284–288.

Robinson, M. E., George, S. Z., Dannecker, E. A., Jump, R. L., Hirsh, A. T., & Gagnon, C. M., et al. (2004a). Sex differences in pain anchors revisited: Further investigation of "most intense" and common pain events. *European Journal of Pain, 8*, 299–305.

Robinson, M. E., Riley, J. L., & Myers, C. D. (2000). Psychsocial contributions to sex-related differences in pain responses. In R. B. Fillingim (Ed.), *Sex, gender & pain* (pp. 41–68). Seattle, WA: IASP Press.

Robinson, M. E., Riley, J. L., Myers, C. D., Papas, R. K., Wise, E. A., & Waxenberg, L. B., et al. (2001). Gender role expectations of pain: Relationship to sex differences in pain. *The Journal of Pain, 2*, 251–257.

Robinson, M. E., & Wise, E. A. (2003). Gender bias in the observation of experimental pain. *Pain, 104*, 259–264.

Robinson, M. E., & Wise, E. A. (2004). Prior pain experience: Influence on the observation of experimental pain in men and women. *The Journal of Pain, 5*, 264–269.

Robinson, M. E., Wise, E. A., Gagnon, C., Fillingim, R. B., & Price, D. D. (2004b). Influences of gender role and anxiety on sex differences in temporal summation of pain. *The Journal of Pain, 5*, 77–82.

Robinson, M. E., Wise, E. A., Riley, J. L., & Atchison, J. W. (1998). Sex differences in clinical pain: A multisample study. *Journal of Clinical Psychology in Medical Settings, 5*, 413–424.

Rollman, G. B., & Lautenbacher, S. (2001). Sex differences in musculoskeletal pain. *Clinical Journal of Pain, 17*, 20–24.

Rollman, G. B., Lautenbacher, S., & Jones, K. S. (2000). Sex and gender differences in response to experimentally induced pain in humans. In R. B. Fillingim (Ed.), *Sex, gender, & pain* (pp. 165–190). Seattle, WA: IASP Press.

Rosseland, L. A., & Stubhaug, A. (2004). Gender is a confounding factor in pain trials: Women report more pain than men after arthroscopic surgery. *Pain, 112*, 248–253.

Sanford, S. D., Kersh, B. C., Thorn, B. E., Rich, M. A., & Ward, L. C. (2002). Psychosocial mediators of sex differences in pain responsivity. *The Journal of Pain, 3*, 58–64.

Sarton, E., Olofsen, E., Romberg, R., den Hartigh, J., Kest, B., & Nieuwenhuijs, D., et al. (2000). Sex differences in morphine analgesia – An experimental study in healthy volunteers. *Anesthesiology, 93*, 1245–1254.

Schneider, S., Randoll, D., & Buchner, M. (2006). Why do women have back pain more than men? A representative prevalence study in the federal republic of Germany. *Clinical Journal of Pain, 22*, 738–747.

Sherman, J. J., & LeResche, L. (2006). Does experimental pain response vary across the menstrual cycle? A methodological review. *American Journal of Physiology – Regulatory, Integrative & Comparative Physiology, 291*, R245–R256.

Sherman, J. J., LeResche, L., Huggins, K. H., Mancl, L. A., Sage, J. C., & Dworkin, S. F. (2004). The relationship of somatization and depression to experimental pain response in women with temporomandibular disorders. *Psychosomatic Medicine, 66*, 852–860.

Sherman, J. J., LeResche, L., Mancl, L. A., Huggins, K., Sage, J. C., & Dworkin, S. F. (2005). Cyclic effects on experimental pain response in women with temporomandibular disorders. *Journal of Orofacial Pain, 19*, 133–143.

Shinal, R. M., & Fillingim, R. B. (2007). Overview of orofacial pain: epidemiology and gender differences in orofacial pain. *Dental Clinics of North America, 51*, 1–18.

Sihvo, S., Klaukka, T., Martikainen, J., & Hemminki, E. (2000). Frequency of daily over-the-counter drug use and potential clinically significant over-the-counter-prescription drug interactions in the Finnish adult population. *European Journal of Clinical Pharmacology*, *56*, 495–499.

Smith, S. J., Keefe, F. J., Caldwell, D. S., Romano, J., & Baucom, D. (2004). Gender differences in patient-spouse interactions: A sequential analysis of behavioral interactions in patients having osteoarthritic knee pain. *Pain, 112*, 183–187.

Smith, J. A., Lumley, M. A., & Longo, D. J. (2002). Contrasting emotional approach coping with passive coping for chronic myofascial pain. *Annals of Behavioral Medicine, 24*, 326–335.

Sullivan, M. J. L., Bishop, S. R., & Pivik, J. (1995). The pain catastrophizing scale: Development and validation. *Psychological Assessment, 7*, 524–532.

Sullivan, M. J. L., Tripp, D. A., & Santor, D. (2000). Gender differences in pain and pain behavior: The role of catastrophizing. *Cognitive Therapy & Research, 24*, 121–134.

Tamres, L. K., Janicki, D., & Helgeson, V. S. (2002). Sex differences in coping behavior: A meta-analytic review and an examination of relative coping. *Personality & Social Psychology Review, 6*, 2–30.

Theis, K. A., Helmick, C. G., & Hootman, J. M. (2007). Arthritis burden and impact are greater among U.S. women than men: Intervention opportunities. *Journal of Women's Health, 16*, 441–453.

Thompson, T., Keogh, E., French, C. C., & Davis, R. (2008). Anxiety sensitivity and pain: Generalisability across noxious stimuli. *Pain, 134*, 187–196.

Tsai, P. F. (2005). Predictors of distress and depression in elders with arthritic pain. *Journal of Advanced Nursing, 51*, 158–165.

Turunen, J. H., Mantyselka, P. T., Kumpusalo, E. A., & Ahonen, R. S. (2005). Frequent analgesic use at population level: Prevalence and patterns of use. *Pain, 115*, 374–381.

Unruh, A. M. (1996). Gender variations in clinical pain experience. *Pain, 65*, 123–167.

Unruh, A. M., Ritchie, J., & Merskey, H. (1999). Does gender affect appraisal of pain and pain coping strategies? *Clinical Journal of Pain, 15*, 31–40.

Von Korff, M., Dworkin, S. F., Le Resche, L., & Kruger, A. (1988). An epidemiologic comparison of pain complaints. *Pain, 32*, 173–183.

Wager, T. D., & Ochsner, K. N. (2005). Sex differences in the emotional brain. *Neuroreport, 16*, 85–87.

Weir, R., Browne, G., Tunks, E., Gafni, A., & Roberts, J. (1996). Gender differences in psychosocial adjustment to chronic pain and expenditures for health care services used. *Clinical Journal of Pain, 12*, 277–290.

Weisse, C. S., Foster, K. K., & Fisher, E. A. (2005). The influence of experimenter gender and race on pain reporting: Does racial or gender concordance matter? *Pain Medicine, 6*, 80–87.

Weisse, C. S., Sorum, P. C., & Dominguez, R. E. (2003). The influence of gender and race on physicians' pain management decisions. *The Journal of Pain, 4*, 505–510.

Weisse, C. S., Sorum, P. C., Sanders, K. N., & Syat, B. L. (2001). Do gender and race affect decisions about pain management? *Journal of General Internal Medicine, 16*, 211–217.

Weissman, M. M., Bland, R. C., Canino, G. J., Faravelli, C., Greenwald, S., & Hwu, H. G., et al. (1996). Cross-national epidemiology of major depression and bipolar disorder. *Journal of the American Medical Association, 276*, 293–299.

Wellcome Trust Case Control Consortium. (2007). Genome-wide association study of 14,000 cases of seven common diseases and 3,000 shared controls. *Nature, 447*, 661–678.

Wiesenfeld-Hallin, Z. (2005). Sex differences in pain perception. *Gender Medicine, 2*, 137–145.

Wijnhoven, H. A. H., de Vet, H. C. W., & Picavet, H. S. J. (2006). Prevalence of musculoskeletal disorders is systematically higher in women than in men. *Clinical Journal of Pain, 22*, 717–724.

Wise, E. A., Price, D. D., Myers, C. D., Heft, M. W., & Robinson, M. E. (2002). Gender role expectations of pain: Relationship to experimental pain perception. *Pain, 96*, 335–342.

Wu, C. L., Rowlingson, A. J., Cohen, S. R., Michaels, R. K., Courpas, G. E., & Joe, E. M., et al. (2006). Gender and post-dural puncture headache. *Anesthesiology, 105*, 613–618.

Pain in Children

Giovanni Cucchiaro

The systematic approach to management of acute and chronic pain in children is a relatively new concept [1]. One reason for the neglect of pain management in children in general, and in neonates in particular is that pain is quite difficult to assess, and even more challenging when its victims are very young or preverbal. Another reason is historical, as old anatomy studies proposed that the brain's key development finished within the first few years of life. At the time, this view led the medical community to believe that since the central nervous system of the neonate and child was not fully developed, and that neonates were not capable of perceiving pain. This often resulted in conducting invasive procedures without analgesic or anesthesia [1–4].

Anatomical studies and experimental evidence published in the seventies and eighties confirmed that the neuronal pathways responsible for pain transmission are already present in neonates [5, 6], and that the cerebral cortex is also functional at that age in terms of pain perception [7, 8]. Current understandings of the neurobiology of brain development support these points and further suggest that the mechanisms by which infants and children process pain should be viewed within the context of a developing sensory nervous system [9]. After birth, many regions of the somatosensory nervous system continue to undergo changes in connectivity, leading to transient functional stages before the adult pattern is finally achieved. Such changes are also likely to determine perceptions and responses to pain and sensory processing at each developmental stage, as well as, later in life. Additional studies also suggest that tissue injury at a young age may contribute long-lasting somatosensory sequelae including central sensitization [10].

Similar to the history of pain management in infants, pain management in older children has suffered a similar neglect that has also afflicted early studies on adult pain management. The most obvious causes include: low priority, failure to routinely assess and document pain, lack of protocols and accountability for poor pain management, and a lack of pain education programs for health care

G. Cucchiaro (✉)
Department of Anesthesia and Critical Care Medicine, The Children's Hospital of Philadelphia, 34th. St and Civic Center Blvd., Philadelphia, PA 19104, USA

R.J. Moore (ed.), *Biobehavioral Approaches to Pain*,   149
DOI 10.1007/978-0-387-78323-9_8, © Springer Science+Business Media, LLC 2009

professionals. In an attempt to remedy this problem, The Joint Commission on Accreditation of Healthcare Organizations (JCAHO) approved new pain assessment and management standards in 1999, which include recognition of patients' right to pain control, barriers to the effective evaluation and treatment of pain, the need for screening and assessing patients for pain, set standard for monitoring and intervention, and education of health care providers, patients and families [11]. Moreover, despite reports of a considerable variability in the application of JCAHO standards amongst different hospital, these standards have still had a significant impact on clinician behaviors, and encouraged evidence based best pain practice and appropriate use of analgesics, particularly in children.

The goals of this chapter are to discuss the assessment, management and treatment of pain in children. First, we define the neurobiology of pain in children. Then we proceed to describe the epidemiology of acute and chronic pain in several clinical pain populations including headache, central regional pain syndrome (CPRS), and abdominal pain. We then evaluate the different factors that directly impact acute and chronic pain management in these previously mentioned populations. Finally, we describe evidence based best practices for the effective assessment, management and treatment of pain in children.

Neurobiology of Pain Pathways in Children

Current understandings of the neurobiology of brain development suggest that the mechanisms by which infants and children process pain should be viewed within the context of a developing sensory nervous system [9]. Free nerve endings, responsible for sensing pain stimuli begin to develop at about seven weeks' gestation [12, 13] and projections from the spinal cord to the brain, can reach the thalamus at seven weeks' gestation [14]. Although present, these spinothalamic projections, which are the minimal necessary anatomical structures to initiate pain transmission, are in reality ineffective because the central nervous system has yet to fully mature. No laminar structure is evident in the thalamus or cortex, which is a defining feature of maturity [15, 16]. Without thalamic projections, the cortical outer layer neurons cannot process noxious information from the periphery [17]. At the 12th–16th week of gestation, it is possible to begin to identify thalamic projections into the cortex [18]. By this stage the brain's outer layer has split into an outer cortical rim, with a subplate developing below. Pain transmitting fibers (thalamocortical, basal forebrain, and corticocortical) can wait in the subplate for several weeks, before they penetrate and form synapses within the cortical plate from 23 to 25 weeks' gestation. Again, although these spinothalamic projections into the subplate may provide the minimal anatomy necessary for pain perception and experience, the subplate is still developing and its functional capabilities, as we intend in an adult, are questionable. For instance, a lack of functional neuronal activity within the subplate calls into question the pain experience of a fetus before the penetration of spinothalamic fibers into the cortical plate.

It is finally by the 26th gestational week that the characteristic layers of the thalamus and cortex become visible, with obvious similarities to the adult brain [18, 19]. Physiologic data confirm that the anatomic structures necessary for pain are intact and functional from around 26 weeks' gestation. Noxious stimulation can evoke hemodynamic changes in the somatosensory cortex of premature babies from a gestational age of 25 weeks [9] and the hormonal stress response of adults or older infants, required for pain reporting is present in fetuses at 18 weeks' gestation [20]. Although the anatomic basis for pain transmission and perception are present at birth, they are by no means mature and over the postnatal period and the life course undergo substantial alterations at the spinal and cerebral level. For instance, the descending pathway with which the brain inhibits pain transmission at the level of the dorsal horn, although anatomically intact, is still not functional at birth and descending stimulation begins to resemble that of adult animals only by the 19th day of life in rats [21], which corresponds to the developmental age of a 3–4 years old child. It is important at this point to remember that many aspects of pain pathways that develop are activity dependent, which implies that excessive sensory or pain activity early in development as may occur in infant surgery and intensive care may alter their maturation. Examples of these postnatal changes are those that occur in the dorsal horn of the spinal cord, where sensory inputs are topographically orga- nized. These are initially diffuse projections that are fine-tuned postnatally, when [22, 23] layer/laminar specific changes occur. In other work, experimental evi- dence from animal and human studies also indicates that acute stress and anxiety alter GI function and animal studies show that stress such as maternal separation in childhood can lead to visceral hypersensitivity in adult life [24, 25]

The development in later phases of life of the central nervous system involved in pain transmission and processing remains unclear. However, it is reasona- ble to assume that, given the tremendous neuroplasticity in brain function, the areas of the brain involved with pain processing continue to evolve through life and change through life experience similar to other brain regions [26],

What Is a Child: Towards a Definition

In this text, the term "neonate" is applied to infants in the first 28 days (month) of life [27] and the term "infant" includes the neonatal period and extends to the age of 1 year (12 months). Children between 1 and 3 years of age are called toddler, while children ages 12 through 18 are called adolescents.

Epidemiology

Despite an extensive literature focused on pain in children, there is still limited data regarding the prevalence of pain in this population.

Neonates

There is no valid data on the epidemiology of acute pain in the newborn. The major difficulty in collecting this data is that newborn infants depend on caregivers for the interpretation of their feelings and needs. It is now accepted that all newborn babies experience pain immediately after birth, if not before or during delivery [28]. Intramuscular vitamin K and the Guthrie test are almost invariable painful stimuli during the 1st week of life and immunizations are given over the first few months at regular intervals. Some newborns, such as those requiring intensive care may receive a multitude of such small yet obviously painful stimuli and a further subgroup may need operative procedures complicated by painful postoperative courses. More distressing is that in the treatment of neonates, the clinician still does not have reliable methods to identify or quantify chronic pain in this age group.

Acute Pain in Children

A recent study that targeted Dutch children between the age of 1 and 18 showed that 15.6% of children and adolescents had experienced episodes of acute pain (pain lasting less than 3 months) within 3 months from the initial interview, with no significant difference between boys and girls. Acute pain was more common in children aged 8–11 (27%), and less common in neonates and toddlers (7.5%) [29]. Similar data were obtained in a Canadian study that reported a prevalence of acute pain of 96% in a group of children 9–13 years of age. However, when analyzing the severity of their symptoms, pain was secondary to a severe trauma or disease in only 35% of the cases, and the majority of the pain episodes were secondary to minor events. Headache was by far the most commonly reported type of pain in this population [30, 31].

The prevalence of acute episodes of pain seems to increase slightly with age, being more common in adolescents (17% in the 14–16 years of age range) compared to younger children (11% in the 5–7 years of age range) [31]

Chronic Pain in Children

A review of the published data on the prevalence of pain in children and adolescents in different countries showed that despite significant differences in the socio-economic development, including cultural and religious background there are surprising similarities with respect to the prevalence of chronic pain in children, the type of symptoms reported and the gender distribution [30, 32–35]. A recent study on US patients reported a prevalence of chronic pain (pain lasting more than 3 months)[36] in approximately 25% in children, with a significantly higher presence of pain in girls (30%) compared to boys (19%)($p<0.001$), and in teenagers compared to younger children (35% versus 19%). Another study conducted in Germany [37] showed that 38.9% of the children reported at least one episode of acute pain in the previous three months, while 40.4% of the children had experienced episodes of chronic pain lasting more than one year. The most commonly reported type of pain was headache (60.5%) followed by abdominal pain (43.3%) and sore throat (35%). Approximately 50% of these children sought medical care (occasional or repeated) to manage their symptoms. A study on the prevalence of headache, stomach ache and back pain conducted in a group of children age 6–13 in Sweden showed that 2/3 of the children had experienced at least one of these types of pain in the previous 6 months [38]. More significant was the fact that 29% of these children experienced pain monthly and 35% experienced pain at least once a week. Co-occurring pain symptoms were present in at least 50% of the children and 9% had pain related to all three body locations. In a study limited to adolescents in the US, headache was the most commonly reported chronic symptom (29%), closely followed by musculoskeletal pain (27%), fatigue (21%), and stomach ache (18%) [39]. Approximately one third of the adolescents reported multiple symptoms. In another study on chronic pain in Canadian children age 5–16, arthritis was the most common cause of chronic pain, followed by cancer related pain and headache [31] Similar to previously published studies on sex differences in pain, the prevalence based on self-report was higher in girls for the majority of symptoms, except for musculoskeletal pain [39]. What these data underscore is the importance of pain in children and the need to adequately assess and manage children's acute and chronic pain. Health care professionals, parents and teachers should be trained to recognize pain in children and direct those patients in need to proper facilities that specialize in the management of acute and chronic pain in young patients.

Headache

Recurrent headache is the most common type of chronic pain found in children and adolescents. These include migraine, tension-type, cervicogenic, a mix of migraine and tension-type, and post-traumatic headache. The exact prevalence of these different types of headache is actually difficult to discern from the literature because of the differences, study design, inclusion criteria in the studied populations and the non-uniform use of the International Headache Society (IHS.) criteria to classify headache [40].

Migraine is the most common type of headache, with a prevalence of 2–3% in young children (3–7 years old) and 10–23% in older children [41–43]. In younger children, boys seem to be more affected than girls. However, this observed trend is reversed by the age of 11, when girls are almost three times more likely to develop migraine and to report symptoms than boys.

Chronic Tension-Type Headache

Chronic tension-type headache is characterized by spells of almost daily attacks of headache and is the most common cause of chronic daily headache. It is described as mild to moderate in severity, pressing or tightening in nature, bilateral and does not worsen on physical activities. Symptoms include nausea, photophobia or phonophobia. Tension-type headache is as prevalent as migraine in children, ranging between 10 and 73% [44, 45] and approximately 30% of these children suffer also from migraine, which may be a predisposing factor towards the development of chronic headache [46]. The relatively recent recognition that chronic tension-type headache affects also children and adolescents and the consequent lack of definitions applicable to children, can explain the significant differences in the reported prevalence. Cultural factors and differences in adherence to the HIS criteria may also explain apparently contradictory data. There is also a significant difference between migraine and tension-type headache: children rarely complain of excruciating pain, and more often they describe their headache as mild. The pain usually does not affect their daily activities. It is also possible to identify predisposing risk factors in the majority of cases. Over half of the children in a recent study reported that they were exposed to stressful events around the time of onset of headache [46].

Chronic Post-Traumatic Headache

Chronic Post-Traumatic headache has now been described in full detail and is recognized as a disease entity [47] rather than merely a psychological disorder of non-organic origin affecting only the adult population [48]. Post-traumatic headache is defined by the IHS as recurrent headaches occurring within 14 days after an injury to the head and lasting for at least 8 weeks. The number of people who develop chronic post-traumatic headache after mild or severe head injury ranges between 30 and 90%. If organic factors were the predominant mechanism of post-traumatic neck and head pain, one would expect that the degree of trauma would commensurate with the incidence and prevalence of the pain syndromes. Yet there is no consistent pattern and the incidence of headache and other features of the post-concussion syndrome have been shown to be unrelated to the severity of the head injury [49–51].

Complex Regional Pain Syndrome

CRPS is a relatively new diagnostic entity in pediatrics. Complex regional pain syndrome (CRPS) is clinically characterized by pain, abnormal regulation of blood flow and sweating, edema of skin and subcutaneous tissues, trophic changes of skin, appendages of skin and subcutaneous tissues, and active and passive movement disorders. Historically, CRPS has been classified into type I (previously reflex sympathetic dystrophy) and type II (previously causalgia). Central mechanisms are almost always involved but peripheral pain mechanisms may also be secondarily involved in the etiology of CRPS. There is debate as to what constitutes the most effective treatment for pediatric CRPS since it is quite rare in children and more common in adolescents [52]. Pediatric CRPS tends to be under-recognized by clinicians. However it should be suspected in the presence of the following:

- an injury or trauma
- continuing pain where normal light touch or temperature change leads to pain (allodynia), or an increased response to pain after the event (hyperalgesia)
- abnormal sweating at some point in the painful region
- no other coexisting conditions or diseases that could explain the cause of the pain.

CRPS-I consists of post-traumatic limb pain and autonomic abnormalities that continue despite apparent healing of the inciting injuries. The cause of symptoms is unknown and objective findings are few, making diagnosis and treatment controversial, and research difficult. CRPS type I (children experience spontaneous pain, increased response to pain after the initial event (hyperalgesia), pain following temperature changes (allodynia) *plus* at least two of the above elements) is more common in girls with incidence raising at the time of puberty [53, 54]. It also appears to be more common in non-Hispanic white children than in children of other ethnicities [55].

CRPS II is diagnosed when pain can be traced to an identifiable nerve injury. The incidence of CRPS type II (children experience an injury or trauma, abnormal sweating, and there are not other diseases or conditions that could explain the pain) is similar in both girls and boys and can be found in children as young as 3 years of age [56]. One frustrating issue is the relatively high incidence of recurrence. Despite a high immediate success rate after 1–2 weeks of intensive physical and occupational therapy (92%), 12% of children experienced recurrent, persistent pain, occasionally with functional limitations, within 6 months after treatment [53]. The reasons for the relatively high incidence of recurrence are unclear, although it is often possible to identify significant emotional stressors in these children's history. The most common psychosocial event identified in children with CRPS is the high prevalence of relatives in the same family with chronic pain conditions or psychiatric conditions, approximately 70% in a recent study [57]. This high incidence of chronic illness within the family is likely to have influences on children understanding of pain and have a significant impact upon the pain experiences of the young person and their uptake of the "sick-role." Many of these children have also previous history of sleep disorders, anxiety or other pain, such as headaches [58].

Abdominal Pain

Chronic abdominal pain is another common complaint in children and adolescents. Pain can be secondary to functional or organic diseases. The prevalence of chronic abdominal pain in community based studies ranges between 0.5 and 19% [59, 60],and it varies according to age and definitions used (Table 1).There

Table 1 Dose conversion guidelines

Current analgesic daily dosage (mg/day)				
Oral morphine	60–134	135–224	225–314	315–404
IM/IV morphine	10–22	23–37	38–52	53–67
Oral oxycodone	30–67	67.5–112	112.5–157	157.5–202
IM/IV oxycodone	15–33	33.1–56	56.1–78	78.1–101
Oral codeine	150–447	448–747	748–1047	1048–1347
Oral hydromorphone	8–17	17.1–28	28.1–39	39.1–51
IV hydromorphone	1.5–3.4	3.5–5.6	5.7–7.9	8–10
IM meperidine	75–165	166–278	279–390	391–503
Oral methadone	20–44	45–74	75–104	105–134
IM methadone	10–22	23–37	38–52	53–67
DURAGESIC®Dose	25 mcg/h	50 mcg/h	75 mcg/h	100 mcg/h

are two age peaks; the first at 4–6 years of age and the second at 7–12 years of age. The predominance of girls is controversial.

The classification of chronic abdominal pain has evolved since the original classification by Apley and Naish in 1958 [61]. The most recent classification (the Rome III criteria) describes five different functional gastrointestinal disorders related to abdominal pain [62]: functional dyspepsia, irritable bowel syndrome, functional abdominal pain, functional abdominal pain syndrome and abdominal migraine. The usefulness of this classification in the daily practice is however unclear, mostly because it does not clearly demarcate abdominal pain secondary to an organic cause from everything else, which is, according to a few gastroenterological studies, simply functional in origin.

Recent advances have helped to identify organic causes for what was once considered functional abdominal pain [63]. Abnormal small-bowel transit, constipation and food allergies have been recently identified as possible sources of abdominal pain in children [64, 65]. Hence, transit studies and dietary restrictions have been recommended in case of chronic abdominal pain. Abdominal migraine has also been recognized as a potential cause of recurrent pain in approximately 2% of children [66], a finding confirmed by the good response to anti-migraine treatments. Helicobacter pylori (*H pylori*) infection is commonly found in children with abdominal pain [67, 68]. This pathogen infects at least 50% of the world's population and causes gastritis and peptic ulcer disease in children. The prevalence of *H pylori* in children ranges between 15 and 48% with higher prevalence in those living in low socioeconomic status and poor hygienic conditions [69–72]. The prevalence in subpopulations of Native Americans or select ethnic populations within the United States (African-Americans and Hispanics) approaches that seen in developing nations [73]. Untreated, *H pylori* infection may result in gastric adenocarcinoma and lymphoma in adults [74, 75].

It is commonly held in pediatric gastroenterologist practice that the majority of chronic abdominal cases that come to their attention are functional in origin, and studies have consistently shown that only 5–10% of children with recurrent abdominal pain have an underlying organic process that contributes to chronic pain [76]. However, the diagnosis is often complicated by the fact that symptoms reported by children are not useful to discriminate between these two conditions. The history and physical examination are inconclusive because the frequency and severity of pain is similar in both clinical scenarios as well as the reported incidence of anorexia, nausea, and vomiting. Only the presence of severe symptoms such as prolonged vomiting and diarrhea, gastrointestinal bleeding, persistent fever, weight loss and family history of inflammatory bowel disease increase the probability of an organic disease and warrant additional laboratory and radiologic testing [77]. Detecting recent stressful events in patients' lives does not help either in differentiating between the two types of pain. Moreover, it is often unclear whether children are anxious because of pain or developed pain because of psychological disorders [77]. As a consequence, in chronic or recurrent pain patients, a psychological assessment of pain might also be warranted as it may provide additional information regarding the origin of the pain.

Diagnosing and Measuring Pain in Children

A pain history is essential for the timely identification of the primary, secondary and tertiary sources of pain. This also includes the appropriate documentation of the physical examination as well as documenting physical, psychosocial, biologic and emotional variables associated with the onset, course, status and duration of pain.

Taking a Pain History

The assessment of acute and chronic pain and the determination of its severity in children can be a challenge. Effective pain management is based on proper evaluation of patients and requires assessment of pain intensity and treatment efficacy using reliable and valid clinical tools. However, in addition to the usual difficulties encountered in the adult population, children, and neonates in particular, present specific difficulties due to their inability to properly express the severity of their symptoms. As a consequence, establishing trust during the first medical encounter with a child who is experiencing pain and his/her family is essential because it is at this time that the foundations for a trustworthy relationship are created. Effective communication has been recently identified as the key element for a successful relationship between clinicians and patients [78]. There is clear documentation that parents expectations do not match physicians approach to effective communication [79]; also, children, who are the main target of any intervention, are usually not actively involved in the encounter [80] and are rarely asked to describe their experience with pain [81, 82].

Acute Pain

The diagnosis of acute pain in children is relatively straightforward in the great majority of cases. The medical history obtained from the child and/or the parents will assist in the identification of the source of an acute episode of pain, which is commonly trauma, surgery or associated with an acute inflammatory process. The severity of pain can be determined by the use of different pain scales (see below). Most of them are age specific and have been designed to evaluate acute pain. The use of these pain scales will also help clinician's determine the effectiveness of the treatment during their medical follow up.

Chronic Pain

The assessment of recurrent or chronic pain in children is more complex. Complicating these treatment scenarios is the fact that clinicians can face several scenarios that range from pain due to chronic disease such as cystic fibrosis and juvenile arthritis to terminal cancer, migraine, or inflammatory bowel disease. The diagnosis and treatment of these patients can be relatively straightforward most of the time. However, the clinician may face more challenging scenarios, including those where children and adolescents complain of "functional" chronic pain, like chronic headache, chronic abdominal pain, or other scenarios (total body pain) where it is impossible to recognize an obvious triggering event. The apparent lack of objective findings in this group of patients can lead clinicians to dismiss these patients as "fakers", "crazy" or depending on the context or the patient's clinical history, as "drug seekers" (See also, Heit and Lipman, This Volume). In addition, it may also be challenging to obtain an appropriate medical history from individuals in this patient population because of the known problems that children have in reporting their symptoms. Moreover despite efforts to establish a supportive clinician-patient relationship based on trust, the fact remains that parents may still be an unreliable source of information in terms of reporting their children's symptoms. Several studies have shown significant discrepancies between parents and children when parents are asked to report their children level of pain and the severity of their functional disability [83–85]. In addition, it is not unusual to find parents who show signs of anger and hostility towards the medical profession [86]. This behavior should not be surprising because these patients have often visited a great number of specialists before arriving in the pediatric pain specialist's office, after an unsuccessful quest for a diagnosis and effective treatment. This lengthy and frustrating process can contribute to anxiety, anger and distrust of the medical profession.

An accurate medical history is essential to better understand and appropriately assess the type of pain that children experience. This should not only focus on physical signs and symptoms and history of previous medical treatments, but should also look at the social and emotional impact that pain has on these children and their families [87]. Changes are more obvious in children with chronic pain. Their behavior may be inappropriate, like showing a flat affect in response to pain or an exaggerated response to light touch often signs of learned behavior, which is related to emotional factors or anxiety [88]. Children may have sleep problems and changes in their appetite and mood, which may be indicative of depression. Their school attendance and/or performance may be compromised as well as their involvement in social activities, including sports. Families' dynamics should be investigated along with the child's medical history. For instance, it is also not unusual to find dysfunctions in families of children with chronic pain (recent divorces, the arrival of a new child, abuse, a move to a different town, financial difficulties). Also, family members may provide inadequate or inappropriate models for coping with pain [89]. In other instances, one of the parents might suffer from chronic pain and share his/her medications with the child, or may, for complex psychological reasons, exaggerate the child's symptoms and reports of pain [90].

Acute Pain Assessment

Three methods to evaluate pain have been identified in the literature: self-report, behavioral observation and physiological changes [91]. The correlation between these approaches is quite low, indicating that they probably measures different aspects of pain experience.

Self Report

Theoretically self-report scales are the best method to adequately assess pain. However, children's self reports of pain intensity might be misleading and ratings need to be interpreted in light of information from other sources such as direct observation of behavior, knowledge of the circumstances of the pain and parents' reports [92]. Visual analogue scales (VAS) and numeric scales have also been used to assess pain in adults and children of school age, who have limited verbal and cognitive skills. When using a visual analogue scale, children are shown a scale graduated from 0 (no pain) to 100 mm (worst possible pain) and are then asked to indicate on this scale where they rate their pain (Fig. 1).

Several modifications of the visual analogue scale have been proposed (i.e. vertical or horizontal; feeling thermometer tool) [93, 94], with good correlation between the different techniques. When using the numeric scale a respondent is asked to estimate the severity of his/her pain and rate it verbally on a scale from 0 to 10. The major limitation of both these techniques is that they are based on the assumption that a pain coded as 7 has the same intensity for all the respondents.

Physiologic

There is limited data on the physiologic measure of pain in children. The use of physiological changes such as respiratory and heart rate are only loosely correlated with the intensity of pain experienced by children and may be secondary to other clinical conditions such as fever, hypovolemia, and hypoxemia [95].

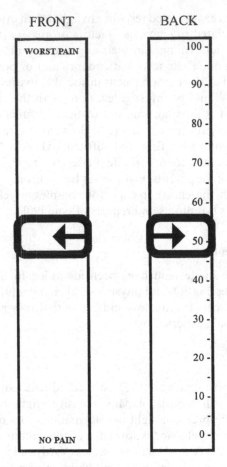

Fig. 1 VAS tool for self report of pain severity

Behavioral Observation

Observational assessment of pain is also needed for children who are too young to understand and use self-report scales [95]. For example, pain evaluation in preschool children or in children who are cognitive impaired because of illness or medications is based on behavioral scales. Although not suitable for use in older children (i.e., children older than 3 years of age) due to a lack of correlation between self-report and behavioral pain measures [96, 97], non-verbal behavioral information is required in this population. Several behavioral scales have been described in the literature. Some of them are lengthy and difficult to use. The CHEOPS scale (Children's Hospital of Eastern Ontario Pain Scale) is one of the first and widely used scales (Table 2) [98]. However, it requires a fairly complex scoring of six different variables. Other commonly used scales are the OPS (Objective Pain Scale) [99] and the TPPPS (Toddler Preschool

Table 2 CHEOPS pain scale: a score greater than 4 indicates pain. Recommended for children 1–7 years of age

Item	Behavioral		Definition	Score
Cry	No cry	1	Child is not crying.	
	Moaning	2	Child is moaning or quietly vocalizing silent cry.	
	Crying	2	Child is crying, but the cry is gentle or whimpering.	
	Scream	3	Child is in a full-lunged cry; sobbing; may be scored with complaint or without complaint.	
Facial	Composed	1	Neutral facial expression.	
	Grimace	2	Score only if definite negative facial expression.	
	Smiling	0	Score only if definite positive facial expression.	
Child Verbal	None	1	Child not talking.	
	Other complaints	1	Child complains, but not about pain, e.g., "I want to see mommy" of "I am thirsty".	
	Pain complaints	2	Child complains about pain.	
	Both complaints	2	Child complains about pain and about other things, e.g., "It hurts; I want my mommy".	
	Positive	0	Child makes any positive statement or talks about others things without complaint.	
Torso	Neutral	1	Body (not limbs) is at rest; torso is inactive.	
	Shifting	2	Body is in motion in a shifting or serpentine fashion.	
	Tense	2	Body is arched or rigid.	
	Shivering	2	Body is shuddering or shaking involuntarily.	
	Upright	2	Child is in a vertical or upright position.	
	Restrained	2	Body is restrained.	
Touch	Not touching	1	Child is not touching or grabbing at wound.	
	Reach	2	Child is reaching for but not touching wound.	
	Touch	2	Child is gently touching wound or wound area.	
	Grab	2	Child is grabbing vigorously at wound.	
	Restrained	2	Child's arms are restrained.	
Legs	Neutral	1	Legs may be in any position but are relaxed; includes gentle swimming or separate-like movements.	
	Squirm/ kicking	2	Definitive uneasy or restless movements in the legs and/or striking out with foot or feet.	
	Drawn up/ tensed	2	Legs tensed and/or pulled up tightly to body and kept there.	
	Standing	2	Standing, crouching or kneeling.	
	Restrained	2	Child's legs are being held down.	

Postoperative Pain Scale) [100]. The FLACC scale (Face, Legs, Activity, Cry, Consolability) [101] has been shown to provide a simple framework to assess pain in children 2 months to 7 years of age (Table 3). The FLACC offers two

Table 3 FLACC pain scale: a score greater than 3 indicates pain. Recommended for children 2 months to 7 years of age

	Scoring		
Categories	0	1	2
FACE	No particular expression or smile	Occasional grimace or frown, withdrawn, disinterested.	Frequent to constant quivering chin, clenched jaw.
LEGS	Normal position or relaxed.	Uneasy, restless, tense.	Kicking, or legs drawn up.
ACTIVITY	Lying quietly, normal position moves easily.	Squirming, shifting back and forth, tense.	Arched, rigid or jerking.
CRY	No cry, (awake or asleep)	Moans or whimpers; occasional complaint	Crying steadily, screams or sobs, frequent complaints.
CONSOLABILITY	Content, relaxed.	Reassured by occasional touching hugging or being talked to, distractable.	Difficulty to console or comfort

main advantages compared to other scales. It is easier to use and the final score ranges between 0 and 10, making comparisons between the FLACC and the VAS and numeric scales easier [102, 103]. Yet, researchers have cautioned against correlating FLACC and VAS scores since it cannot be assumed that the 0–10 scale of the FLACC is psychometrically equivalent to an ideal or self-report 0–10 scale [95]. The CRIES (Crying, Requires oxygen, Increased vital signs, Expression, Sleeplessness) scale is a common used scale for neonates, in their first month of life [104]. CRIES is an acronym of five physiological and behavioral variables shown to be associated with neonatal pain (Table 4). The most obvious limitations of this scale is the dependence on vital signs for interpretation of pain, because elevated blood pressure and heart rate could be caused by other factors besides pain. Because of this limitation, the Neonatal Infant Pain Scale (NIPS) scale (Table 5), which is purely based on infants behaviors, is preferred at some institutions [105]

Chronic Pain Assessment

The measurement of chronic pain adds additional complexity to the task of identifying the ideal tools for the measurement of pain intensity in children. While self-report methods may be still representing the individual perception of pain intensity, scales based on behavioral measurements tend to lose their validity because behavioral signs and symptoms of pain tend to dissipate or habituate with time [95]. In younger patients with chronic pain, the usual signs observed during the acute phase or re-exacerbation episodes (grimacing, crying) are

Table 4 CRIES pain scale: a score greater than 3 indicates pain. Recommended for neonates in their first month of life

Crying –
0 – No cry or cry that is not high-pitched
1 – Cry high pitched but baby is easily consolable
2 – Cry high pitched but baby is inconsolable

Requires O2 for SaO2 < 95% -
0 – No oxygen required
1 – < 30% oxygen required
2 – > 30% oxygen required

Increased vital signs (BP and HR) -
0 – Both HR and BP unchanged or less than baseline
1 – HR or BP increased but increase in < 20% of baseline
2 – HR or BP is increased > 20% over baseline.

Expression -
0 – No grimace present
1 – Grimace alone is present
2 – Grimace and non-cry vocalization grunt is present

Sleepless -
0 – Child has been continuously asleep
1 – Child has awakened at frequent intervals
2 – Child has been awake constantly

lost and the observer should look for other signs like rigidity, guarding and silence. When examining older children, a more complex examination is required and other signs besides the common indicators of pain. Changes in sleep pattern as well as mood changes, irritability, changes is eating habits and school performance may all be indicators of chronic pain. The Douleur Enfant Gustave Roussy (DEGR) is a scale validated for evaluation of chronic pain in children [106]. The main characteristic of this scale is that it incorporates items that evaluate depression-like symptoms and anxiety in addition to behavior typical of pain. Although there has been important discussions about what we really measure in patients with chronic pain [107], anxiety and depression can be two common and important indicators of pain in both children and adults [108, 109].

Disability is a common finding in children who present to hospital outpatient pain clinics or to tertiary pain clinics [110, 111]. Intuitively, it might seem that worse disability might stem from greater pain, and that poorer social/adaptive functioning might be a function of greater pain and disability [112]. While this paradigm might hold true in adults, other factors such as depression [113], anxiety or parental behavior [114] should also be considered besides pain as the cause of functional disability. A recent study cautioned against attributing functional disability exclusively to pain, and highlighted depression and parental stress as other independent factors [112]. Other studies have shown that direct treatment of depression and disability in addition to pain relief can be

Table 5 NIPS pain scale: a score greater than 3 indicates pain. Recommended for neonates and infants in their first year of life

	Pain assessment	Score
Facial expression		
0 – Relaxed muscles	Restful face, neutral expression	
1 – Grimace	Tight facial muscles; furrowed brow, chin, jaw, (negative facial expression – nose, mouth and brow)	
Cry		
0 – No Cry	Quiet, not crying	
1 – Whimper	Mild moaning, intermittent	
2 – Vigorous Cry	Loud scream; rising, shrill, continuous (Note: Silent cry may be scored if baby is intubated as evidenced by obvious mouth and facial movement.)	
Breathing patterns		
0 – Relaxed	Usual pattern for this infant	
1 – Change in Breathing	Indrawing, irregular, faster than usual; gagging; breath holding	
Arms		
0 – Relaxed/Restrained	No muscular rigidity; occasional random movements of arms	
1 – Flexed/Extended	Tense, straight legs; rigid and/or rapid extension, flexion	
Legs		
0 – Relaxed/Restrained	No muscular rigidity; occasional random leg movement	
1 – Flexed/Extended	Tense, straight legs; rigid and/or rapid extension, flexion	
State of arousal		
0 – Sleeping/Awake	Quiet, peaceful sleeping or alert random leg movement	
1 – Fussy	Alert, restless, and thrashing	

effective [115]. Other important studies strongly support the use of a multi-disciplinary approach to the management of chronic pain in children.

Several scales have been proposed to assess emotional functioning in the adult population; however, none have been validated in children. The Beck Depression Inventory(BPI) [116] and the Profile of Mood States (POMS) [117] have been used in the assessment and management of patients with chronic pain. They provide a well accepted measure of the level of depressed mood and response to treatment. The most updated version of the BPI is a self-administered 21 item self-report scale measuring supposed manifestations of depression, including sadness, insomnia, guilt, loss of appetite, weight, suicidal ideation, irritability, fatigability [118]. The POMS assesses six mood states—tension–anxiety, depression–dejection, anger–hostility, vigor–activity, fatigue–inertia, and confusion–bewilderment—and also provides a summary measure of total mood disturbance. It also has the three most important dimensions of emotional functioning in chronic pain patients (depression, anxiety, anger) and also assesses three other dimensions that are very relevant to chronic pain and its treatment, including a positive mood scale of vigor–activity [119].

Medications: Evidence-Based Best Practices

Before describing the different options available to manage acute and chronic pain, it is important to realize that historically pain has been under treated in children as compared to adults [120, 121]. The most common explanations for this kind of approach to pain in children is fear of adverse reactions, side-effects like over sedation or drug dependency. Another possible reason why infants are usually under treated is that they can not verbalize pain. Use of single words does not start until children are at least 12–18 months old and we have to wait until the age of 2 years for the child to verbalize two-word sentences [122]. Previous clinical studies support this trend and have shown that children younger than 2 years of age were less likely to receive pain medications compared to older children (17 vs 38%) [120, 123]. More recent studies have shown an improvement in this trend, with no significant differences between infants and older children [124, 125]. These changes are due to increased education and awareness amongst clinicians, pointing out that type of practice (academic versus general practice), education and training of the care providers [124] are now a major determinant of the type of management offered to children.

The "science" on which acute pain management in children is based is empirical. Classical methodologies (type of intravenous medications; techniques, including PCA or continuous intravenous infusions; regional anesthesia) are derived from the adult practice. For instance, there is no firm data on which opioid to choose in order to prevent opioid-induced side-effects and there is no clear data on whether regional anesthesia offers better outcomes compared to intravenous analgesia in children.

Acute Pain

Intravenous Medications: The management of acute pain, independent of the nature of the acute injury, relies on two main lines of treatment: intravenous medication or regional anesthesia. Intravenous medications include opioids and non-steroidal anti-inflammatory drugs (NSAIDS).

Opioids

An opioid is a chemical substance that has a morphine-like action in the body. The main use is for pain relief. These agents work by binding to opioid receptors, which are found principally in the central nervous system and the gastrointestinal tract. The receptors in these two organ systems mediate both the beneficial effects, and the undesirable side effects. There are five broad classes of narcotics: endogenous opioid peptides (opioids produced naturally in the body); opiates, such as naturally occurring morphine and codeine, and heroin (processed morphine); semi-synthetic opioids, created from the natural opioids, such as hydromorphone and oxycodone; fully synthetic opioids, such as fentanyl, pethi-dine, methadone, and tramadol.

Opioids are the most commonly used medications in acute settings when managing pain secondary to surgery and trauma. They include fentanyl, mor-phine and hydromorphone. The use of fentanyl, a highly liphophilic drug, is limited by its pharmacodynicamics. Its onset of action after intravenous admin-istration (1–2 mcg/kg) is almost immediate, and the usual duration of action is of approximately 30 min [126]. This makes it suitable for rapid control of acute pain in emergency room situations (i.e. contusions, bone fractures), for pain after short operations (dental extraction, closed reduction of bone fractures) or for sedation to facilitate endoscopic and radiologic procedures (CT scan, MRI). Repeated doses of fentanyl may lead to accumulation because of its lipophilicity and delayed respiratory depression. Morphine and hydromorphone are two hydrophilic drugs with longer onset and duration of action and do not carry the risk of accumulation. They are better suited for repeated administration and management of patients who may experience prolonged pain.

These drugs can be administered intermittently, or, depending on the child's age, using a continuous infusion or a PCA (Patient Controlled Analgesia) device. It has been shown in multiple studies that when using a PCA to administer morphine and provide analgesia patients require significant lower amounts of opioids and are less sedated compared to those patients who receive preset amounts of morphine via a continuous intravenous infusion [127]. The use of a PCA is limited by the mental and health status of the child and on his/her level of comprehension of the proper use of the device. Children as young as 6 years have been shown to safely and effectively use a PCA [128, 129]. The parameters used to program a morphine PCA are usually 20–30 mcg/kg as a bolus, 7–8 min as interval between boluses, 0–10 mcg/kg as continuous infusion, 150–200 mcg/kg as a maximum hourly dose. When PCA devices were first used in children, physicians discussed the safety of adding a continuous infusion. Multiple studies have shown that it is safe to add a small continuous infusion to the demand doses [130, 131] in children. The most common side effects of intrave-nous morphine are (1) itching, which can be controlled with intravenous nal-buphine (50 mcg/kg IV), (2) vomiting, which can be controlled with intravenous ondansetron (50 mcg/kg, max 4 mg IV) and metoclopramide (200 mcg/kg, max 12 mg IV), and, (3) respiratory depression with hypoxemia, which rarely requires reversal with naloxone (1–5 mcg/kg IV). Hydromorphone, a semi synthetic derivative of morphine, is 3–4 times more potent than morphine [132]. Although it was initially thought to have a better side-effect profile than morphine, with a lower incidence of itching and nausea and vomiting [133], subsequent studies have failed to confirm these earlier findings [134, 135]. That said, despite the lack of firm evidence, the current practice is to switch children to hydromorphone when they experience significant side-effects from morphine. The same drug used in the PCA can be used for break-thru pain control. The recommended dose of morphine for break-thru pain control is approximately 100 mcg/kg (max

4–5 mg), for fentanyl it is of 0.5–1 mcg/kg (max 50 mcg) and hydromorphone is 10 mcg/kg (max 1 mg).

Non-steroidal Anti-inflammatory Drugs (NSAIDS)

Acetylsalicylic acid (Aspirin) is the most commonly used NSAID in the adult population. However, because of its association with Reye's syndrome, a severe acute form of encephalopathy, current recommendations are to avoid aspirin in children and adolescents less than 18 years old [136]. Acetaminophen and ibuprofen are the most commonly prescribed over-the-counter analgesic and antipyretic in children [137]. The intravenous preparation of acetaminophen is only available in a few countries. Although some studies have concluded that ibuprofen is a better analgesic and antipyretic drug [138, 139] a recent meta-analysis of the evidence published in the pediatric literature comparing these two drugs came to the conclusion that oral ibuprofen (4–10 mg/kg) is as effective as acetaminophen (7–15 mg/kg) [140]. There is no evidence that the safety profile of these two drugs is different. However, ibuprofen is a non-selective inhibitor of both constitutive and inducible cyclooxygenase (COX-1 and COX-2), which results in a diminished synthesis of prostacyclin [141]. Endothelial prostacyclin has antithrombogenic properties [142], while gastric mucosal prostacyclin is cytoprotective [143]. Renal prostacyclin reduce renal vascular resistance and consequently increase the renal blood flow and glomerular filtration rate [144]. Long-term use of ibuprofen may also have adverse effects on bone healing [145]. Henceforth, ibuprofen should be used with caution in children who are at risk for bleeding (spontaneous or post-surgical), with acute or chronic gastritis, borderline renal function and bone fractures. Ketorolac is the only parenteral NSAID available in the Unites States. Although probably less effective than intravenous opioids, it may offer some advantages compared to intravenous opioids, particularly when trying to avoid respiratory depression in specific groups of patients like neonates [146] and obese patients [147]. Ketorolac may also offer the advantage of reducing the morphine requirements when used in combination with opioids, hence lowering the incidence of opioid-related side-effects [148].

Acute Pain: Regional Anesthesia

The benefit of using regional anesthesia as an alternative to intravenous medications for the treatment of acute pain has not been demonstrated [149, 150]. Recent reports in the adult literature have suggested that regional anesthesia may offer great advantages compared to intravenous opioids in term of patients comfort [151], duration of hospital stay [152] and improved functional outcome [153]. More recent evidence from studies conducted in the pediatric population suggest that regional anesthesia can provide advantages compared to intravenous medications because it prevents opioid induced side-effects [154], or can facilitate the resolution of acute sickle cell crisis [155, 156].

Epidural catheters can also be useful in managing acute pain secondary to trauma. Although epidural catheters appear to offer advantages compared to intravenous opioids in any type of trauma, they have been shown to be particularly useful in patients with chest trauma complicated by multiple ribs fractures, where they seem to help in decreasing the rate of nosocomial pneumonia, shorten the duration of mechanical ventilation [157] and overall reduction in mortality [158]. Since epidurals, spinals and peripheral nerve blocks are usually performed in anesthetized children, one common myth in pediatric regional anesthesia is that there is a potential high risk for nerve injuries. However, multiple studies have failed to confirm this hypothesis [159–161]. In addition, in many instances, children do not cooperate with physicians and this makes it impossible to perform regional anesthesia in an awake or only mildly sedated child. In those cases where it is possible to obtain the child and parents' cooperation it is possible to perform these blocks under sedation. Midazolam and morphine are the two drugs most commonly used for sedation. Unfortunately, Midazolam (starting with 0.5 mg/kg orally or 50 mcg/kg intravenously) often produces the opposite effect because of disinhibition, which will make the child agitated and restless making the placement of the block impossible. Morphine (100 mcg/kg) may have better sedative effects and may deliver in a more cooperative child. The risks involved with performing regional anesthesia in an anesthetized child are twofold: (1) the potential risk of missing an intravascular injection of local anesthetic with catastrophic cardiovascular consequences, (2) the inability of anesthetized children to report pain in case of intraneural injection, which may result in a long-lasting nerve injury. The use of a test dose, which combines a local anesthetic with an appropriate dose of epinephrine (0.25–0.5 mcg/kg) [162], will allow for a prompt detection of accidental intravascular injections because of significant electrocardiographic changes (tachycardia, peeked T-waves) [163, 164]. With respect to the potential increased risk of nerve injury because of the general anesthesia, as mentioned before, multiple studies have failed to confirm this hypothesis [159–161]. Major progress has been made in the last few years with the use of peripheral nerve blocks in the management of acute postoperative pain and post-trauma pain. The introduction of stimulating nerve catheters and elastomeric pumps for continuous delivery of local anesthetics has allowed anesthesiologists to replace epidural catheters with peripheral nerve catheters. The management of epidural catheters is more complex than that of peripheral nerve catheters from a clinical perspective.

Chronic Pain

The management of chronic pain in children and adolescents is an extremely difficult task. The importance of a proper management of chronic or recurrent pain in this group of patients has been highlighted by experimental data, which indicate that prolonged exposure to pain can have significant effects on patients' psychological, physiological, and emotional development. However, there is a lack in the literature of uniform benchmark criteria that the clinicians should adopt when treating children with chronic pain. The Initiative on Methods, Measurement, and Pain Assessment in Clinical Trials (IMMPACT) issued six recommendations on core outcome measures to be followed in chronic pain clinical trials. These criteria should be incorporated into our daily clinical practice: (1) level of pain; (2) physical functioning; (3) emotional functioning; (4) children ratings of improvement and satisfaction with the treatment; (5) adverse events; and (6) participant disposition [165].

Other additional factors should be considered in the management of children with chronic pain. The clinician should also take in consideration the age, language, education and cultural background of patients and their families. Hence, treatment options should be tailored in terms of the individual patients, since they have to be accepted in order to achieve good adherence and compliance. The clinician should also evaluate the availability of specific treatments, and the equivalence of alternative managements. There are very few clinical reports or trial examining the efficacy of complementary and alternative medicine for chronic pain in children. Acupuncture for instance is a well accepted technique in the management of chronic pain in adults. However, the few trials describing the use of acupuncture, hypnosis and biofeedback in children are inconclusive, mainly because of methodology problems and small number of children recruited in each study [166, 167]. It is also difficult to convince parents of children with chronic pain to accept alternative treatments such hands-on or distance healing, meditation, yoga, Traditional Chinese Medicine, and Ayurveda, let alone to participate in clinical trials.

Chronic Pain and Development

Pain is a complex phenomenon that requires two different processes: the ability to sense and transmit painful stimuli at the peripheral level (nociception), and the ability of central pain processing of these stimuli, which is a cortical event [168] There is clear clinical and experimental evidence to support the fact that early pain experiences have long-term sequelae: as shown by the long-term perseverance of central nervous system changes following painful insults in the very young organism and, similarly, long-term changes in responsiveness of the neuroendocrine and immune systems to stress at maturity [169, 170].

Once we accept the idea that neonates and infant, independent of their gestational age can not only sense pain but can also emotionally process these stimuli, it is logical to take into consideration the consequences that the experience of chronic pain has on child development.

For instance, injury in the rat pup has been shown to have profound effects on both peripheral and central neuronal circuits. Full-thickness skin wounding of the hind paw during the first 21 postnatal days was shown to result in local

hyperinnervation associated with healing of the wound. This translates clinically in prolonged local hypersensitivity as demonstrated by the fact that the
mechanical flexion reflex threshold remained markedly lower in these compared to non-wounded animals [169]. Similarly, plantar skin wounding on the
day of birth has been recently shown to modify the organization of receptive
fields in the dorsal horn later in life, finding that is consistent with hypersensitivity to pain [170].

There is also clear evidence from human studies that the adverse effects of the
early pain experience may extend into infancy and perhaps beyond. Studies on
the effects of early pain exposure in newborn infants, have shown a sensitization
to repeated noxious stimuli (heelstick-induced pain) [171]. In an often cited
study on the effects of circumcision pain in term-born infants, it has been shown
that infants circumcised without anesthesia had a greater pain response to
subsequent immunizations than uncircumcised infants [172]. Also, the pain
response was attenuated in infants pretreated with eutectic mixture of local
anesthetics. Repeated exposure to pain in premature babies has also been
associated with down-regulation of the hypothalamic-pituitary-adrenal axis
(HPAA) [173]. Reduced HPAA activity is characteristic of a number of stress-
related disorders later in life, including posttraumatic stress disorder; chronic
pain; fatigue; and atypical, melancholic depression [174].

There is also indirect evidence which indicates that the effects of early pain
extend beyond infancy into childhood in former extremely low birth weight
(ELBW) infants. Parent ratings of child sensitivity to everyday pain at 18 months
of age showed they regarded their ELBW premature toddlers (birth weight
<1000 g) as significantly less sensitive than heavier preterm (1500–2499 g) and
full birth weight (FBW) toddlers [175]. However, when these children were
examined later in life, 25% at age 4.5 years showed clinically higher ratings of
physical complaints of no known medical cause when compared to full term
children [176]. At 8–10 years of age, former ELBW children rated the pictures of
painful events in recreational settings higher than FBW children and the emotional responses ascribed to the children in the pictures was correlated with time
spent in the NICU [177].

Chronic Pain Management

When managing chronic pain in children, the clinician must not only focus on
the sensory aspects of the pain experience, but also on the affective components
of pain. Whereas pain intensity may provide some indication about the overall
severity of pain, management of pain per-se often fails to take into consideration the effects of pain on the child's affective status. Physical functioning is
almost invariably compromised in the presence of chronic pain and one of
the goals of chronic pain management is to restore normal activity. However,
in many chronic pain conditions, increased activity is also accompanied by
increased pain. Some children, particularly in the youngest age groups, will tend
to limit their physical functioning until a proper control of their symptoms is

obtained. Others will tolerate increased pain to maintain a desired level of function if proper supportive treatments are provided. With respect to emotional functioning, chronic pain is often accompanied by symptoms such as psychological distress and other psychiatric disorders, including depression, anxiety, and anger [178]. Disturbed sleep is a major disruption of children physical functioning, and a major objective of chronic pain management should be to improve the child's sleep pattern [179]. Thus, psychosocial, emotional, pharmacologic assessment, management and treatment of these issues are also essential for the successful management of chronic pain in children.

The Process

Before taking charge of a child with chronic pain, the clinician must understand the potential source of pain. The most common scenarios include: (1) cancer pain, (2) headache, (3) neuropathic pain, (4) recurrent abdominal pain (5) post-traumatic chronic pain, and (6) pain secondary to other chronic diseases.

Managing chronic pain is based on three major modes of treatment [180, 181]:

1) Pharmacological. The pharmacological treatment should then be focused on at least three different targets: pain, sleep and mood disorders.
2) Psychological. Psychological pain management methods should be directed towards increasing the child's and family's understanding of the child's pain and its treatment, and enhancing their cognitive and behavioral coping skills.
3) Rehabilitation. Rehabilitation, including occupational and physical therapy, are essential components of the child's recovery towards a normal life.

Cancer Pain

Pharmacological

Opioids

Opioids are probably the more effective medication for treatment of children with cancer pain. Opioids can be delivered orally, intravenously, transdermally or intrathecally. While the intravenous route is the most commonly used method of giving opioids in hospitalized patients, the oral and transdermal route are the easiest and most commonly used ways of giving opioids when patients are discharged home.

When transitioning patients from intravenous to oral opioids the clinician might consider that oral opioids will have different pharmacokinetics compared to intravenous opioids, mainly because of the intestinal absorption factor. It is difficult to exactly calculate the conversion factor from parenteral into oral morphine. The daily oral dose of morphine in children is usually three times less than (or 1/3 less than) the total dose of parenteral daily dose of morphine. Patients should be started on immediate-release oral morphine every 4 h. Patients are then transitioned to longer acting morphine (MS CONTIN®) in either of two ways: (1) by administering one-half of the patient's 24-hour requirement as MS CONTIN on an every 12-hour schedule; or, (2) by administering one-third of the patient's daily requirement as MS CONTIN on an every eight hour schedule. Usually, in case of severe or breakthrough pain, patients can still receive immediate-release morphine as a rescue, in between the doses of MS CONTIN. Occasionally, clinicians use Oxycodone, a drug in a similar class, for rescue purposes.

Methadone

Methadone is another option when considering oral opioids for treatment of cancer patients. Methadone's properties of high oral bioavailability, rapid onset of analgesic effect, long half-life (resulting in infrequent dosing schedules), lack of active metabolites, low rate of induction of tolerance and low cost are characteristics that result in its use in the management of profoundly ill patients [182]. The clinical scenarios where methadone has been used include: morphine allergy, during rotation of opioids because of side-effects, renal failure, situations in health economics where there is a demand for cheap, safe and effective analgesics, in pain with a neuropathic component and pain that is non responsive to opioids.

Although effective in controlling pain, there is no obvious advantage in using methadone over morphine in this patient population [183, 184] from efficacy and side-effects point of view.

Fentanyl

Fentanyl is the only opioid that can be administered transdermally. It comes in a patch (Duragesic®) delivering 12.5-25-50-75-100 mcg per hour. It takes anywhere between 12 and 24 h to reach a peak and 72 h to have a steady plasma concentration of fentanyl. The patch has to be usually replaced every 72 h. Transdermal fentanyl is indicated in children who are already receiving opioid medications, most often given intravenously, as the sole drug or in combination with oral opioids. It also represents an easy way to transition patients from intravenous opioids when they are discharged home. Transdermal fentanyl ideally replaces the continuous intravenous administration or high intermittent doses of opioids by providing a constant plasma concentration of drug overtime. Table 1 shows the recommended conversion doses when going from intravenous or oral opioids to transdermal Fentanyl.

Implanted Infusion Pumps

A potential and still underutilized route for administration of opioids in children with advanced, metastatic cancer is their delivery into the subarachnoid space via implanted infusion pumps. While the intrathecal drug delivery via external catheters in children with cancer is well established [185], and implanted intrathecal pumps are used to infuse baclofen in children with intractable spasticity [186], there are very few reports on children with cancer pain treated with intrathecal infusions via an implanted pump [187]. This technique offers a few advantages compared with the intravenous, oral or transdermal administration of opioids. In particular, the quality of the pain control is superior, as pain coming from multiple processes almost anywhere in the body below the cervical dermatomes can be controlled simultaneously, and the doses needed are minimal compared to what would be needed in a systemic administration. This significantly reduces the incidence of opioid-related side-effects, and allows children to have an acceptable social life until the end of life. The most common indications for intrathecal administration of opioids include refractory pain, diminished performance status, poor tolerability of oral-intravenous medications, polyanalgesia for complex pain, and inadequate dosing due to addiction concerns. Intrathecal catheters can be connected to an external pump in patients with short life expectancy or to an implantable pump, which is placed subfascially with a simple operation [188]. There are potential mechanical complications (catheter dislodgement or disconnection), and side-effects which include infection (from meningitis to subcutaneous abscesses), and granulomas, which can cause spinal cord compression with new neurological deficits, myelopathy, or radiculopathy [189]. These types of complications are seen mostly in patients receiving opioid infusions over long period of time (years), and are unlikely to happen in this type of short duration palliative care.

Headache

There are a various types of headache that typically affect children. In this section we will briefly discuss migraine, tension-type headache, post-traumatic headache, and cervicogenic headache. There is no clear data on the typical management of chronic headache in children. There are several headache treatment approaches. Often, headaches are treated pharmacologically in addition to various forms of physical treatment. A review of the pharmacological management of children with chronic headache shows that analgesic overuse is a common pattern in the management of these patients. In a recent study conducted in a tertiary care center, frequent analgesic use occurred in 38.5% of the children with chronic headache, with 61.0% using analgesics daily and 71.4% using analgesics five or more times per week [190]. Data from the adult literature show that overuse of acute headache medication is the most frequent cause of recurrent chronic headache in adults. Headache frequency may increase in headache-prone patients with intake of ergotamine or triptans ≥10 days/month, or analgesics, opioids or combination medication ≥15 days/month [191]. However, it has been shown that when patients with chronic headache and analgesic overuse successfully discontinue their analgesics, the mean headache frequency is reduced from 27.5 to 5.4 episodes days/month (a reduction of 80%) [192]

Migraine

Pharmacologic interventions include the use of symptomatic medication such as analgesics (acetaminophen, ibuprofen, ketorolac), and non-analgesic such as nasal-spray sumatriptan, oral sumatriptan, oral rizatriptan, oral dihydroergotamine, intravenous prochlorperazine, antiemetics (prochlorperazine) and the use of prophylactic medications.

Several randomized clinical trials comparing acetaminophen, ibuprofen and placebo have shown that analgesic drugs are more effective in reduction of symptoms 1 and 2 h after intake than placebo, with minor adverse effects [193, 194]. No clear differences in effect were found between acetaminophen and ibuprofen or nimesulide [195]. Oral triptans do not appear to offer any benefit compared to placebo [196], and only nasal triptan offers significantly better pain relief [197, 198]. However, the number of adverse effects was significantly higher after sumatriptan, and these include nausea and vomiting, dizziness and photophobia. Oral rizatriptan and dihydroergotamine failed to offer any benefit compared to placebo [199, 200]. The reasons for the poor results offered by triptan in children and adolescents may be due to the fact that migraine episodes are usually shorter in children compared to adults and generally resolve spontaneously within 2 h [201]. Nasal administration of triptans could also be more effective due to the lower incidence of nausea and vomiting. Also, pharmacokinetic data after oral administration in patients suffering from migraine has shown that the absorption from an oral tablet is often delayed during a migraine attack because of gastric stasis, nausea, and vomiting [202].

Given the natural history of migraine and the social and medical costs of recurrent migraine, it seems appropriate to consider prophylactic management of migraine in children with recurrent episodes. The goals of prophylactic therapy should include reducing attack frequency, severity, and duration; improving responsiveness to treatment of acute attacks; improving function and quality of life; and reducing disability [203]. A multitude of drugs and combination of drugs have been tested. However, none are FDA approved for the prophylaxis of migraine in children.

a. *Antihistamines*: Cyproheptadine, which possesses antiserotonergic and calcium-channel blocking properties, has been shown to be effective in more than 80% of children and reduce the incidence of monthly episodes of headache by approximately 55% [204, 205]. The reported side-effects include drowsiness, sleep disturbance, weight gain and fatigue.

b. *Antidepressants*: Amitriptyline, a tricyclic antidepressant, is one of the most widely used prophylactic agents for migraines in children, despite the lack of proper randomized trial data supporting its use. The specific mechanism for prophylaxis is unknown; however, the drug does inhibit reuptake of serotonin and norepinephrine in the central nervous system. Amitriptyline has been shown to be effective in more than 80% of the treated patients, with significant reduction in the recurrence and severity of headache episodes [204, 206].

c. *Antihypertensive*: Amongst the different classes of antihypertensive medications tested, only the calcium channel blocker flunarizine, which is not available in the US, significantly improved children symptoms [207, 208]. Surprisingly, other calcium channel blockers like nimodipine had no effect [209] compared to placebo. Multiple studies on the β-blocker propranolol and the α2-agonist clonidine have also failed to show any advantage compared to placebo [210]. The results of recent studies are reassuring in terms of relative safety of different antidepressant medications, in particular with respect to their association to an increased risk of suicide [211, 212]. An electrocardiogram to verify the QT interval is recommended before starting children on psychotropic medications. Secondary (nortriptyline) and tertiary tryciclic antidepressants (amitriptyline) have been shown to prolong the QT interval, which is a risk factor for developing Torsades des points and sudden death.

d. *Antiepileptic*: Antiepileptic drugs, as a group, have been shown to be the most effective medication in decreasing the frequency, duration and severity of migraine episodes. Divalproex sodium, gabapentin, topiramate, zonisamide and levetiracetam have been shown in multiple studies to be effective [210].

e. *Non-pharmacological interventions*: Non-pharmacologic preventive measures such as sleep hygiene, psychosocial interventions, diet, and exercise may reduce headache frequency; however, these measures have not been studied in children. Lack of sleep can be a significant trigger for many children. An alteration of sleep behavior such as going to bed late or sleeping late can precipitate headaches [213]. Keeping a regular and balanced diet it is also beneficial. Also, although rare, identification of potential food triggers like cheese and chocolate could help reducing the number of migraine episodes [213]. While relaxation techniques (including progressive muscle relaxation, autogenic training and self hypnosis), biofeedback (EMG feedback, hand temperature feedback, vasomotor feedback, neuro-feedback) and cognitive behavioral interventions have been show to be effective in adults, there is no clear evidence regarding the efficacy of these psychological techniques in children. Recent meta-analysis have shown that psychological treatments, principally relaxation and cognitive behavioral therapy, can significantly lower the number migraine episodes in children compared to control groups [214, 215]. The analysis showed a significant improvement also for intensity and duration of headache. However it is still unclear whether these improvements in symptoms parallel a decrease in medication consumption.

Tension-Type Headache

Initial pharmacological treatment is, for the most part, based on the appropriate use of acetaminophen and ibuprofen. A neurological examination and occasionally neuroimaging studies are warranted to exclude anatomic basis for the tension-type headache (i.e. increased intracranial pressure, chronic sinusitis), which may require surgical intervention [216]. Meningismus (presence of meningeal signs on physical examination) must also be ruled out. Other studies highlight the possible role of chronic inflammatory diseases, especially in the otolaryngologic region, in the etiology of meningismus [217]. The finding of a high frequency of positive Epstein-Barr virus serology in children with chronic headache [218, 219] confirms this assumption. In addition, insignificant traumas of the head or back and perhaps severe coughing or lifting a heavy weight might also play a role. Thus, it is important to exclude from the potential causes of headache the so-called analgesia- induced headaches, which can be treated with a slow withdrawal of analgesics [220]. A multidisciplinary approach is often helpful. For example, a psychologist should focus on biofeedback, mental and physical relaxation. This multidisciplinary approach should also involve the patients' family because this type of headache is often an index of family related problems, particularly in younger patients [221].

Post-Traumatic Headache

Independent from the cause of the trauma, minor fall at the playground, or a concussion following a car accident, once major cranial injuries are rule out, the outcome of post-traumatic headache is benign. Observation or routine management with analgesic results in resolution of the symptoms within a few weeks from the trauma [222].

Cervicogenic Headache

Cervicogenic headache is a chronic headache where the source of pain is located in the cervical spine or soft tissues of the neck but the sensation of pain is referred to the head. Neural networks between upper cervical nuclei (i.e. trigeminal nucleus) and sensory fibers from the upper cervical roots allows the referral of pain signals from the neck to the trigeminal sensory receptive fields of the face and head. This may be the basis for the well- recognized patterns of referred pain from the trapezius and sternocleidomastoid muscles to the face and head [223].Congenital or traumatic laxness of the transverse ligament of atlas is a common cause of headache in children [224]. The dens-atlas distance is greater than 5 mm, while the dens-clivus angle is decreased on a lateral x-ray involving flexion of the cervical spine. Pain occurs typically following the second or third hour of school, as the head is bent forward for ever longer periods. Mechanical stretching of the transverse ligament could be pain-generating mechanism [225]. Sometimes compression of the diencephalons by the dens can result in headache. A comprehensive program including pharmacologic, non-pharmacologic, anesthetic, and rehabilitative interventions are recommended when treating individuals from these patient populations.

Neuropathic Pain

Neuropathic pain is chronic pain that results from injury to the nervous system. The injury can be to the central nervous system (brain and spinal cord) or the peripheral nervous system (nerves outside the brain and spinal cord). Neuro-pathic pain can occur after trauma and many diseases such as multiple sclerosis and stroke. It is common and affects more than 2 million people in the US alone. This type of pain is often difficult to treat. The approach to the treatment of neuropathic pain in children is often quite different from that of adult patients, mainly because the causes of neuropathic pain are different in these two populations. With the term neuropathic pain we actually include diff-erent groups of diseases: (1) peripheral neuropathy (2) trigeminal neuralgia, (3) central pain (4) complex regional pain syndrome (type I and II).

Peripheral neuropathy is rare in children. Post-herpetic and trigeminal neur-algia, diabetic neuropathy and phantom-limb pain are more common in adults. In those exceptional cases involving children and adolescents, the current recommendations include three categories of drugs: (1) tricyclic antidepressants (2) anticonvulsant medications (3) opioids.

Peripheral and Trigeminal Neuropathy

Based on the location (proximal or distal to the central neuraxis) and the structure (axon or myelin) it is possible to identify different types of peripheral neuropathies. Distal lesions of the axon (distal axonopathies) can be caused by diabetes, alcoholism, malnutrition and renal insufficiency. Myelinopathies result in the damage of the myelin and disruption of the nerve conductivity. The most common causes are acute inflammatory demyelinating polyneuro-pathy (Guillain-Barré syndrome), chronic inflammatory demyelinating poly-neuropathy, or genetic metabolic disorders (e.g., leukodystrophy), or toxins. Neuronopathies are the result of destruction of peripheral nervous system neurons. They may be caused by motor neuron diseases, sensory neuronopa-thies (Herpes zoster), autonomic dysfunction or neurotoxins such as vincris-tine or genetic (Charcot-Marie-Tooth disease) [226]. Trigeminal neuralgia, also called *tic douloureux*, is a chronic pain condition that causes extreme, sporadic, sudden burning or shock-like face pain that lasts anywhere from a few seconds to as long as 2 min per episode. The causes of trigeminal neuralgia are unclear, and can sometimes be attributed to loss of myelin such as in multiple sclerosis, neuronal compression by vessels, tumors, or aging [227].

Tricyclic Antidepressants

The rationale for using tricyclic antidepressants, the most commonly used being amitriptyline, is that these medications inhibit the re-uptake of biogenic amines and are also strong sodium-channel modulators [228, 229]. These act by enhancing dorsal horn inhibition and diminishing peripheral sensitisation. Data from meta-analysis studies conducted in adults show clear benefits from treating patients with peripheral neuropathic pain with tricyclic antidepressants [230, 231]. The initial low dose (at bedtime) of 10–25 mg, can be gradually increased on a weekly schedule to a maximum of 150 mg.

Anticonvulsants

Anticonvulsants act on neuropathic pain, probably by reducing central sensitization [232]. Gabapentin is an anticonvulsant that has antinociceptive and anti-hyperalgesic properties [233]. It has a well-established role in the treatment of chronic pain with particular efficacy in the treatment of neuropathic pain syndromes including [234] diabetic neuropathy [235], peripheral and trigeminal neuropathies, postherpetic neuralgia [119] and complex regional pain syndrome [236] It works by binding the α-2-δ subunits of voltage-dependent calcium ion channels and blocks the development of hyperalgesia and central sensitization [237]. Gabapentin, for which there is the most convincing evidence of efficacy in managing peripheral neuropathy, binds to the alpha2-delta sub-unit of a voltage-dependent calcium channel in laminae I and II, the termination sites of the nociceptors [238]. Multiple randomized trials conducted in adults have demonstrated the efficacy of gabapentin in managing neuropathic pain [119, 239–241]. The initial dosage should be 100 mg three times a day, or even lower in case of side-effects (dizziness and somnolence), which are quite common in children. Doses are then gradually increased every two to three days to a max of 3600 mg in three divided doses a day [242]. Carbamazepine is the only anticonvulsant drug that has been repeatedly shown in multiple randomized studies to be effective in treating symptomatic trigeminal neuralgia. The initial response is quite fast with significant reduction in the spontaneous high-frequency firing only after a few days of treatment [243, 244]. The doses need to be gradually increased up to 500 mg twice a day with time, because of the side-effects, which include sedation, blurred vision, diplopia, dizziness, ataxia, gait disturbance, nausea and vomiting. Also, hematological and hepatic functions should be monitored during carbamazepine administration. Oxcarbazepine, although as effective as carbamazepine, also has a better side-effect profile [228].

Opioids

Opioids, including oxycodone, morphine and methadone, have been shown to be more effective than placebo in managing neuropathic and phantom-limb pain [245].

Central neuropathic pain: Patients who suffer from spinal cord injury or stroke can experience severe neuropathic pain. There is no data in the literature reporting the treatment experience in children. There is some evidence from small trials conducted in adults that the usual pharmacological treatments (antidepressants and anticonvulsants) are more effective than placebo [246, 247] and can significantly improve patients quality of life.

Complex Regional Pain Syndrome

Pharmacological management of complex regional pain syndrome in children is generally considered ineffective. Although a few sporadic studies have reported success with the use of opioids, steroids, anticonvulsants and antidepressants, there is no convincing data in the literature supporting the pharmacological approach to CPRS in children. The role of regional anesthesia is also unclear. Although peripheral nerve blocks seem to be the logical treatment of CRPS symptoms, there is no data on their long-term effects in children. Repeated peripheral nerve blocks have been shown to be effective in adults; however, regional anesthesia can only be performed in heavily sedated children most of the times, causing significant organizational and psychological issues. Selected groups of patients may rather benefit from placing indwelling catheters, which can allow for a prolonged nerve block [54, 248]. Because of the current trends, which mainly focus on physical therapy and rehabilitation, few clinicians recommend the use of peripheral nerve catheters to provide continuous pain control and facilitate more intensive physical therapy [54, 249]. Recent reports have emphasized the success of the physical therapy approach in managing children with CPRS [53, 248, 250, 251]. Most of these practitioners have eliminated every pharmacological intervention and completely rely on daily, intense physical therapy, to achieve a functional recovery within 2–3 weeks from the beginning of the therapy. Some authors recommend against the use of treatments that could facilitate the therapy (i.e. peripheral nerve blocks), emphasizing the importance of patients' motivation as a tool towards improvements [53, 252, 253]. The literature is not clear on the importance of psychological dysfunctions in originating or maintaining CRPS symptoms. Emotional dysfunction, including unsolved fears of early childhood [254], conflict between parents, sexual abuse and school problems [255] have been described in children with CPRS, to such an extent that there are suggestions that a psychological treatment should be taken in consideration every time we take care of these patients. Cognitive and behavioral therapies are now part of the armamentarium utilized in the management of children with CPRS [55].

Abdominal Pain

Management of chronic abdominal pain in children and adolescents can be an extremely frustrating. In the presence of an organic cause, i.e. inflammatory bowel disease, H. Pylori, the management of the underlying disease offers the best chance of resolving the pain issues. Data from a few randomized trials support the bio-psycho-social approach to recurrent abdominal pain in children and adolescents with significant improvements in the duration of symptoms, incidence of relapses, number of children responding to treatment and long-term results [76, 256, 257]. Behavioral changes may therefore be as effective as pharmacological interventions. Moreover, the pharmacological treatment of pain is not only ineffective but opioids and NSAIDS are often contraindicated.

Early studies have described episodes of relapsing colitis in patients taking non-steroidal anti-inflammatory drugs [258–260]. Recent studies confirmed these findings and extended the warning to patients diagnosed with Crohn's disease [261]. The management of functional abdominal pain relies on both pharmacological and psychological approach. The only pharmaceutical options found to be effective are pizotifen for abdominal migraine [262] and famotidine for children with dyspepsia [263]. The use of opioids can greatly magnify behavioral issues that often are associated with recurrent abdominal pain. Several psychological studies have shown that pain behaviors produce secondary gain (i.e. school avoidance, special attention) which reinforce pain behaviors [257, 264]. In addition, clinical studies conducted in adults have consistently shown that considerable number of adults with irritable bowel syndrome report histories of physical, emotional, and sexual abuse [265]. The relatively few studies conducted in children seem to indicate a higher incidence and longer lasting symptoms in children with history of sexual and physical abuse [266, 267]. As a consequence and given this environmental influence the role of the parents and family background should also be evaluated. Parental anxiety and approach towards their children's symptoms has a significant impact on the child's behavior and may increase the risks of developing and prolonging episodes of abdominal pain, particularly in young children [268, 269]. Similarly, the presence of abdominal symptoms in one of the parents increases the risk of the child's development of chronic abdominal pain [270]. Cognitive behavioral therapy directed towards children includes relaxation training, self-management techniques, and coping skills. Parents should also be included in the intervention plan and offered enhanced support, as well as training in distraction techniques and care-giving strategies [76].

Conclusion

A great deal of progress has been made in the last 20 years in the management of acute and chronic pain in children. The most significant advancement has been the recognition from the medical community of the fact that neonates and children feel pain and the government mandate to consider pain as the "fifth vital sign", with the implication that clinicians and nurses should be trained to recognize and treat pain [271]. Several major obstacles have also been overcome during this period of time. In particular, technological progress has provided clinicians with new tools to address pain in a safer and more effective way. Regional anesthesia and implantable devices have changed the way acute, chronic, and cancer pain are managed in many centers around the US and globally. New radiologic and endoscopic techniques have made it possible to identify the organic cause of several types of chronic pain, once considered merely as functional. Unfortunately these advancements have not been followed by a similar progress in the pharmacology field. We are still essentially dealing with a limited choice of medications, with all of their limitations.

Similarly, there are clear deficiencies in the psychological and psychiatric support of children with chronic pain. Many children are still treated with high doses narcotics rather than being evaluated for social and psychological issues which also contribute to the experience and perpetuation of pain states. The alleged undertreatment of pain as a major health problem in the United States has led to the development of initiatives to begin to address the multiple barriers responsible for the undertreatment of pain. Patient advocacy groups and professional organizations have been formed with a focus on improving the management of pain [272]. Consequently, numerous clinical guidelines, mainly based on prescription drugs, have been developed, even though very few have been developed using evidence-based medicine for the treatment of pain in children [273]. That said, the effectiveness of prescription opioids for chronic non-malignant pain is limited and the value of supportive treatments such as acupuncture, rehabilitation and psychologic interventions are still often ignored by clinicians. Recognition of psycho-social problems and prescription pain medication abuse is an additional, essential component of the assessment, management and treatment of pain in children and adolescents. A closer relationship between general practitioners and pain specialists is important because an early and accurate diagnosis of the cause of pain is essential to prevent long-term physical, emotional, and psychological consequences in children. Moreover, while the approach to acute pain management is established by well codified protocols, the management of chronic pain is often quite complex and requires a multifaceted and multidisciplinary approach.

Future Perspectives

Despite the significant progress made in the last few years, we are still far from offering an ideal treatment for the child who suffers from chronic pain. The limited choice of medications available constitutes probably the major obstacle. Although effective, they are often not specific for types and mechanism of pain and do not provide continuous coverage because their effects fluctuate with the plasma concentrations. Their side-effects profile is problematic and patients often refuse analgesic treatment out of fear of these side-effects. Pharmaceutical companies should encourage research on new categories of drugs, although the recent problems with COX-2 inhibitors (e.g., VIOXX) have caused severe set backs in this field. Efforts should also be directed towards filling the gap between basic and clinical research because animal models of pain can not completely represent the complex reality of human pain.

The future, particularly of chronic pain management, should also emphasize the design and development of new methods of delivering drugs. Traditionally, analgesics are mainly introduced by enteral, parenteral, intrathecal, peridural, or transdermal routes. These routes are known to have significant limitations due to the intermittent drug administration that leads to a fluctuation in plasma concentration. This fluctuation often results in either high or low drug blood levels and thus in toxicity or sub-therapeutic levels. Technology development should focus on controlled drug delivery systems where a carrier is combined with a selected drug in such a way that the selected drug is released from the carrier material in a pre-designed manner. Nanotechnology may offer even more sophisticated solutions, with targeted delivery of medications to selected areas of the body.

In addition to these much needed progress in type of drugs and delivery systems, the political and administrative ends of the medical care should focus not only on the standardization of clinical protocols that take a multidisciplinary approach to the assessment, management and treatment of pain in children; but also emphasize the creation of an organizational support structure for children with chronic pain. Pediatric pain clinics are rare in the United States, and often lack of the necessary structure required to offer a comprehensive approach to the problem of pain in children. An ideal team should include pain specialist, health educators, general practitioners [internists], social workers, psychologists, psychiatrists, neurologists, physical and occupational therapists. This approach will offer the possibility of treating not only pain symptoms but also the behavioral and psychological consequences of chronic pain and offer complementary treatments. In many cases, it should be possible to extend psychological and psychiatric support also to the families. Another major problem clinician's face when managing chronic pain in children is the total lack of structure to facilitate the effective management of opioid dependence. There is also an additional need for adequate, qualified environments where children can be helped to exit the tunnel of drug dependence.

Finally, the financial aspects of pain management in children must also be addressed. There is a significant divide between the political pressures to address pain in children and the financial support that pain services receive from the government, insurance companies and hospitals. None of the pediatric pain services in the Unites States is financially self-supported because of the poor reimbursement rate. In addition to the limited quality of the available infrastructure, the financial limitations greatly affect the number of physicians and amount of time available to provide adequate care to children with acute and chronic pain.

References

1. Hatch DJ. Analgesia in the neonate. Br Med J (Clin Res Ed) 1987;294:920.
2. Wallerstein E. Circumcision. The uniquely American medical enigma. Urol Clin North Am 1985;12:123–32.
3. Shearer MH. Surgery on the paralyzed, unanesthetized newborn. Birth 1986;13:79.
4. Lippmann M, Nelson RJ, Emmanouilides GC et al. Ligation of patent ductus arteriosus in premature infants. Br J Anaesth 1976;48:365–9.
5. Destuynder R, Lassauge F, Menget A et al. Pain in newborn infants hospitalized in pediatric intensive care unit. Pediatrie 1991;46:535–9.
6. Johnston CC, Stevens BJ. Experience in a neonatal intensive care unit affects pain response. Pediatrics 1996;98:925–30.
7. Bartocci M, Bergqvist LL, Lagercrantz H, Anand KJ. Pain activates cortical areas in the preterm newborn brain. Pain 2006;122:109–17.
8. Slater R, Boyd S, Meek J, Fitzgerald M. Cortical pain responses in the infant brain. Pain 2006;123:332.
9. Slater R, Cantarella A, Gallella S et al. Cortical pain responses in human infants. J Neurosci 2006;26:3662–6.
10. Page GG. Are there long-term consequences of pain in newborn or very young infants? J Perinat Educ 2004;13:10–7.
11. JCAHO. Standards, intents, examples and scoring samples for pain assessment and management. Comprehensive accreditation manual for hospital Oakbrook Terrace, IL: JCAHO, Department of standards, 1999:1–11.
12. Fitzgerald M. Prenatal growth of fine-diameter primary afferents into the rat spinal cord: a transganglionic tracer study. J Comp Neurol 1987;261:98–104.
13. Fitzgerald M. Cutaneous primary afferent properties in the hind limb of the neonatal rat. J Physiol 1987;383:79–92.
14. Andrews K, Fitzgerald M. The cutaneous withdrawal reflex in human neonates: sensitization, receptive fields, and the effects of contralateral stimulation. Pain 1994;56:95–101.
15. Hevner RF. Development of connections in the human visual system during fetal midgestation: a DiI-tracing study. J Neuropathol Exp Neurol 2000;59:385–92.
16. Larroche JC. The marginal layer in the neocortex of a 7 week-old human embryo. A light and electron microscopic study. Anat Embryol (Berl) 1981;162:301–12.
17. Derbyshire SW. Can fetuses feel pain? BMJ 2006;332:909–12.
18. Ulfig N, Neudorfer F, Bohl J. Transient structures of the human fetal brain: subplate, thalamic reticular complex, ganglionic eminence. Histol Histopathol 2000;15:771–90.
19. Kostovic I, Judas M. Correlation between the sequential ingrowth of afferents and transient patterns of cortical lamination in preterm infants. Anat Rec 2002;267:1–6.
20. Giannakoulopoulos X, Sepulveda W, Kourtis P et al. Fetal plasma cortisol and beta-endorphin response to intrauterine needling. Lancet 1994;344:77–81.
21. Fitzgerald M, Koltzenburg M. The functional development of descending inhibitory pathways in the dorsolateral funiculus of the newborn rat spinal cord. Brain Res 1986;389:261–70.
22. Fitzgerald M, Butcher T, Shortland P. Developmental changes in the laminar termination of A fibre cutaneous sensory afferents in the rat spinal cord dorsal horn. J Comp Neurol 1994;348:225–33.
23. Fitzgerald M, Jennings E. The postnatal development of spinal sensory processing. Proc Natl Acad Sci U S A 1999;96:7719–22.
24. Anand P, Aziz Q, Willert R, van Oudenhove L. Peripheral and central mechanisms of visceral sensitization in man. Neurogastroenterol Motil 2007;19:29–46.
25. Coutinho SV, Plotsky PM, Sablad M et al. Neonatal maternal separation alters stress-induced responses to viscerosomatic nociceptive stimuli in rat. Am J Physiol Gastrointest Liver Physiol 2002;282:G307–16.

26. Fisher RS, Almli CR. Postnatal development of sensory influences on lateral hypothalamic neurons of the rat. Brain Res 1984;314:55–75.
27. Hoyert DL, Kochanek KD, Murphy SL. Deaths: final data for 1997. Natl Vital Stat Rep 1999;47:1–104.
28. Glover V. The fetus may feel pain from 20 weeks. Conscience 2004;25:35–7.
29. Perquin CW, Hazebroek-Kampschreur AA, Hunfeld JA et al. Pain in children and adolescents: a common experience. Pain 2000;87:51–8.
30. van Dijk A, McGrath PA, Pickett W, VanDenKerkhof EG. Pain prevalence in nine- to 13-year-old schoolchildren. Pain Res Manag 2006;11:234–40.
31. McGrath PA, Speechley KN, Seifert CE et al. A survey of children's acute, recurrent, and chronic pain: validation of the pain experience interview. Pain 2000;87:59–73.
32. Galal SB, Hamad S, Hassan N. Self-reported adolescents' health and gender: an Egyptian study. East Mediterr Health J 2001;7:625–34.
33. Taimela S, Kujala UM, Salminen JJ, Viljanen T. The prevalence of low back pain among children and adolescents. A nationwide, cohort-based questionnaire survey in Finland. Spine 1997;22:1132–6.
34. Lau JT, Yu A, Cheung JC, Leung SS. Studies on common illnesses and medical care utilization patterns of adolescents in Hong Kong. J Adolesc Health 2000;27:443–52.
35. Bejia I, Abid N, Ben Salem K et al. Low back pain in a cohort of 622 Tunisian schoolchildren and adolescents: an epidemiological study. Eur Spine J 2005;14:331–6.
36. McGrath P. Chronic pain in children. In: Krombie IK, Croft PR, Linton SJ et al., eds. Epidemiology of pain. Seattle, WA: IASP Press, 1999:81–101.
37. Roth-Isigkeit A, Thyen U, Stoven H et al. Pain among children and adolescents: restrictions in daily living and triggering factors. Pediatrics 2005;115:e152–62.
38. Petersen S, Brulin C, Bergstrom E. Recurrent pain symptoms in young schoolchildren are often multiple. Pain 2006;121:145–50.
39. Rhee H, Miles MS, Halpern CT, Holditch-Davis D. Prevalence of recurrent physical symptoms in U.S. adolescents. Pediatr Nurs 2005;31:314–9, 50.
40. Classification and diagnostic criteria for headache disorders, cranial neuralgias and facial pain. Headache Classification Committee of the International Headache Society. Cephalalgia 1988;8 Suppl 7:1–96.
41. Annequin D, Tourniaire B, Massiou H. Migraine and headache in childhood and adolescence. Pediatr Clin North Am 2000;47:617–31.
42. Guidetti V, Galli F, Fabrizi P et al. Headache and psychiatric comorbidity: clinical aspects and outcome in an 8-year follow-up study. Cephalalgia 1998;18:455–62.
43. Lewis D, Ashwal S, Hershey A et al. Practice parameter: pharmacological treatment of migraine headache in children and adolescents: report of the American Academy of Neurology Quality Standards Subcommittee and the Practice Committee of the Child Neurology Society. Neurology 2004;63:2215–24.
44. Laurell K, Larsson B, Eeg-Olofsson O. Prevalence of headache in Swedish schoolchildren, with a focus on tension-type headache. Cephalalgia 2004;24:380–8.
45. Barea LM, Tannhauser M, Rotta NT. An epidemiologic study of headache among children and adolescents of southern Brazil. Cephalalgia 1996;16:545–9; discussion 23.
46. Abu-Arafeh I. Chronic tension-type headache in children and adolescents. Cephalalgia 2001;21:830–6.
47. Speed WG, 3rd. Closed head injury sequelae: changing concepts. Headache 1989;29:643–7.
48. Miller H. Accident neurosis. Br Med J 1961;1:919–25.
49. Solomon S. Chronic post-traumatic neck and head pain. Headache 2005;45:53–67.
50. McCrory PR, Berkovic SF. Concussion: the history of clinical and pathophysiological concepts and misconceptions. Neurology 2001;57:2283–9.
51. Couch JR, Bearss C. Chronic daily headache in the posttrauma syndrome: relation to extent of head injury. Headache 2001;41:559–64.

52. Low AK, Ward K, Wines AP. Pediatric complex regional pain syndrome. J Pediatr Orthop 2007;27:567–72.
53. Sherry DD, Wallace CA, Kelley C et al. Short- and long-term outcomes of children with complex regional pain syndrome type I treated with exercise therapy. Clin J Pain 1999;15:218–23.
54. Wilder RT, Berde CB, Wolohan M et al. Reflex sympathetic dystrophy in children. Clinical characteristics and follow-up of seventy patients. J Bone Joint Surg Am 1992;74:910–9.
55. Wilder RT. Management of pediatric patients with complex regional pain syndrome. Clin J Pain 2006;22:443–8.
56. Kozin F, Haughton V, Ryan L. The reflex sympathetic dystrophy syndrome in a child. J Pediatr 1977;90:417–9.
57. Maillard SM, Davies K, Khubchandani R et al. Reflex sympathetic dystrophy: a multi-disciplinary approach. Arthritis Rheum 2004;51:284–90.
58. Karakaya I, Coskun A, Agaoglu B et al. Psychiatric approach in the treatment of reflex sympathetic dystrophy in an adolescent girl: a case report. Turk J Pediatr 2006;48:369–72.
59. Chitkara DK, Rawat DJ, Talley NJ. The epidemiology of childhood recurrent abdominal pain in western countries: a systematic review. Am J Gastroenterol 2005;100:1868–75.
60. Ramchandani PG, Hotopf M, Sandhu B, Stein A. The epidemiology of recurrent abdominal pain from 2 to 6 years of age: results of a large, population-based study. Pediatrics 2005;116:46–50.
61. Apley J, Naish N. Recurrent abdominal pains: a field survey of 1,000 school children. Arch Dis Child 1958;33:165–70.
62. Rasquin A, Di Lorenzo C, Forbes D et al. Childhood functional gastrointestinal disorders: child/adolescent. Gastroenterology 2006;130:1527–37.
63. Plunkett A, Beattie RM. Recurrent abdominal pain in childhood. J R Soc Med 2005;98:101–6.
64. Chitkara DK, Delgado-Aros S, Bredenoord AJ et al. Functional dyspepsia, upper gastrointestinal symptoms, and transit in children. J Pediatr 2003;143:609–13.
65. Stordal K, Bentsen BS. Recurrent abdominal pain in school children revisited: fitting adverse food reactions into the puzzle. Acta Paediatr 2004;93:869–71.
66. Rasquin-Weber A, Hyman PE, Cucchiara S et al. Childhood functional gastrointestinal disorders. Gut 1999;45 Suppl 2:II60–8.
67. Ashorn M, Maki M, Ruuska T et al. Upper gastrointestinal endoscopy in recurrent abdominal pain of childhood. J Pediatr Gastroenterol Nutr 1993;16:273–7.
68. Hyams JS, Davis P, Sylvester FA et al. Dyspepsia in children and adolescents: a prospective study. J Pediatr Gastroenterol Nutr 2000;30:413–8.
69. Braga AB, Fialho AM, Rodrigues MN et al. Helicobacter pylori colonization among children up to 6 years: results of a community-based study from Northeastern Brazil. J Trop Pediatr 2007; 53:393–7.
70. Lin DB, Lin JB, Chen CY et al. Seroprevalence of Helicobacter pylori infection among schoolchildren and teachers in Taiwan. Helicobacter 2007;12:258–64.
71. Langat AC, Ogutu E, Kamenwa R, Simiyu DE. Prevalence of Helicobacter pylori in children less than three years of age in health facilities in Nairobi Province. East Afr Med J 2006;83:471–7.
72. Raymond J, Kalach N, Bergeret M et al. Prevalence of Helicobacter pylori infection in children according to their age. A retrospective study. Arch Pediatr 1998;5:617–20.
73. Malaty HM, Graham DY. Importance of childhood socioeconomic status on the current prevalence of Helicobacter pylori infection. Gut 1994;35:742–5.
74. Ernst PB, Gold BD. Helicobacter pylori in childhood: new insights into the immuno-pathogenesis of gastric disease and implications for managing infection in children. J Pediatr Gastroenterol Nutr 1999;28:462–73.
75. Asaka M, Takeda H, Sugiyama T, Kato M. What role does Helicobacter pylori play in gastric cancer? Gastroenterology 1997;113:S56–60.

76. Weydert JA, Ball TM, Davis MF. Systematic review of treatments for recurrent abdominal pain. Pediatrics 2003;111:e1–11.
77. Chronic abdominal pain in children. Pediatrics 2005;115:e370–81.
78. Carter B. Chronic pain in childhood and the medical encounter: professional ventriloquism and hidden voices. Qual Health Res 2002;12:28–41.
79. Worchel FF, Prevatt BC, Miner J et al. Pediatrician's communication style: relationship to parent's perceptions and behaviors. J Pediatr Psychol 1995;20:633–44.
80. van Dulmen AM. Children's contributions to pediatric outpatient encounters. Pediatrics 1998;102:563–8.
81. Pantell RH, Stewart TJ, Dias JK et al. Physician communication with children and parents. Pediatrics 1982;70:396–402.
82. Shiminski-Maher T. Physician-patient-parent communication problems. Pediatr Neurosurg 1993;19:104–8.
83. Palermo TM, Zebracki K, Cox S et al. Juvenile idiopathic arthritis: parent-child discrepancy on reports of pain and disability. J Rheumatol 2004;31:1840–6.
84. Parsons SK, Gelber S, Cole BF et al. Quality-adjusted survival after treatment for acute myeloid leukemia in childhood: A Q-TWiST analysis of the Pediatric Oncology Group Study 8821. J Clin Oncol 1999;17:2144–52.
85. Cremeens J, Eiser C, Blades M. Factors influencing agreement between child self-report and parent proxy-reports on the Pediatric Quality of Life Inventory 4.0 (PedsQL) generic core scales. Health Qual Life Outcomes 2006;4:58.
86. Liakopoulou-Kairis M, Alifieraki T, Protagora D et al. Recurrent abdominal pain and headache–psychopathology, life events and family functioning. Eur Child Adolesc Psychiatry 2002;11:115–22.
87. Eccleston C, Jordan A, McCracken LM et al. The Bath Adolescent Pain Questionnaire (BAPQ): development and preliminary psychometric evaluation of an instrument to assess the impact of chronic pain on adolescents. Pain 2005;118:263–70.
88. Eccleston C, Bruce E, Carter B. Chronic pain in children and adolescents. Paediatr Nurs 2006;18:30–3.
89. Gil KM, Williams DA, Thompson RJ, Jr., Kinney TR. Sickle cell disease in children and adolescents: the relation of child and parent pain coping strategies to adjustment. J Pediatr Psychol 1991;16:643–63.
90. Garber J, Van Slyke DA, Walker LS. Concordance between mothers' and children's reports of somatic and emotional symptoms in patients with recurrent abdominal pain or emotional disorders. J Abnorm Child Psychol 1998;26:381–91.
91. Walco GA, Conte PM, Labay LE et al. Procedural distress in children with cancer: self-report, behavioral observations, and physiological parameters. Clin J Pain 2005;21:484–90.
92. von Baeyer CL. Children's self-reports of pain intensity: scale selection, limitations and interpretation. Pain Res Manag 2006;11:157–62.
93. Scott J, Huskisson EC. Vertical or horizontal visual analogue scales. Ann Rheum Dis 1979;38:560.
94. Choiniere M, Amsel R. A visual analogue thermometer for measuring pain intensity. J Pain Symptom Manage 1996;11:299–311.
95. von Baeyer CL, Spagrud LJ. Systematic review of observational (behavioral) measures of pain for children and adolescents aged 3 to 18 years. Pain 2007;127:140–50.
96. Beyer JE, McGrath PJ, Berde CB. Discordance between self-report and behavioral pain measures in children aged 3–7 years after surgery. J Pain Symptom Manage 1990;5:350–6.
97. Vetter TR, Heiner EJ. Discordance between patient self-reported visual analog scale pain scores and observed pain-related behavior in older children after surgery. J Clin Anesth 1996;8:371–5.
98. McGrath PJ, Johnston J, Goodman J, et a. CHEOPS: a behavioral scale for rating postoperative pain in children. In: HL F, ed. New York: Raven Press, 1985:395–402.

99. Wilson GA, Doyle E. Validation of three paediatric pain scores for use by parents. Anaesthesia 1996;51:1005-7.
100. Tarbell SE, Cohen IT, Marsh JL. The Toddler-preschooler postoperative pain scale: an observational scale for measuring postoperative pain in children aged 1–5. Preliminary report. Pain 1992;50:273–80.
101. Merkel SI, Voepel-Lewis T, Shayevitz JR, Malviya S. The FLACC: a behavioral scale for scoring postoperative pain in young children. Pediatr Nurs 1997;23:293-7.
102. Manworren RC, Hynan LS. Clinical validation of FLACC: preverbal patient pain scale. Pediatr Nurs 2003;29:140–6.
103. Suraseranivongse S, Santawat U, Kraiprasit K et al. Cross-validation of a composite pain scale for preschool children within 24 hours of surgery. Br J Anaesth 2001;87:400–5.
104. Krechel SW, Bildner J. CRIES: a new neonatal postoperative pain measurement score. Initial testing of validity and reliability. Paediatr Anaesth 1995;5:53–61.
105. Suraseranivongse S, Kaosaard R, Intakong P et al. A comparison of postoperative pain scales in neonates. Br J Anaesth 2006;97:540–4.
106. Gauvain-Piquard A, Rodary C, Rezvani A, Serbouti S. The development of the DEGR(R): a scale to assess pain in young children with cancer. Eur J Pain 1999;3:165–76.
107. Shacham S, Daut R. Anxiety of pain: what does the scale measure? J Consult Clin Psychol 1981;49:468–9.
108. Wall PD. On the relation of injury to pain. The John J Bonica lecture Pain 1979;6:253–64.
109. Taylor PL. Post-operative pain in toddler and pre-school age children. Matern Child Nurs J 1983;12:35–50.
110. Konijnenberg AY, Uiterwaal CS, Kimpen JL et al. Children with unexplained chronic pain: substantial impairment in everyday life. Arch Dis Child 2005;90:680–6.
111. Eccleston C, Crombez G, Scotford A et al. Adolescent chronic pain: patterns and predictors of emotional distress in adolescents with chronic pain and their parents. Pain 2004;108:221–9.
112. Gauntlett-Gilbert J, Eccleston C. Disability in adolescents with chronic pain: Patterns and predictors across different domains of functioning. Pain 2007.
113. Kashikar-Zuck S, Vaught MH, Goldschneider KR et al. Depression, coping, and functional disability in juvenile primary fibromyalgia syndrome. J Pain 2002;3:412–9.
114. Peterson CC, Palermo TM. Parental reinforcement of recurrent pain: the moderating impact of child depression and anxiety on functional disability. J Pediatr Psychol 2004;29:331–41.
115. Eccleston C, Malleson PN, Clinch J et al. Chronic pain in adolescents: evaluation of a programme of interdisciplinary cognitive behaviour therapy. Arch Dis Child 2003;88:881–5.
116. Beck AT, Ward CH, Mendelson M et al. An inventory for measuring depression. Arch Gen Psychiatry 1961;4:561–71.
117. McNair D, Lorr M, Droppleman L. Profile of Mood States. San Diego, CA, Educational and Industrial Testing Service, 1971.
118. Beck AT, Steer RA, Ball R, Ranieri W. Comparison of beck depression inventories -IA and -II in psychiatric outpatients. J Pers Assess 1996;67:588–97.
119. Rowbotham M, Harden N, Stacey B et al. Gabapentin for the treatment of postherpetic neuralgia: a randomized controlled trial. JAMA 1998;280:1837–42.
120. Lewis LM, Lasater LC, Brooks CB. Are emergency physicians too stingy with analgesics? South Med J 1994;87:7–9.
121. Petrack EM, Christopher NC, Kriwinsky J. Pain management in the emergency department: patterns of analgesic utilization. Pediatrics 1997;99:711–4.
122. Kelly D, Sally J. Disorders of speech and language. In: Levine M, Carey W, Crocker A, eds. Development-behavioral pediatrics Philadelphia, PA: WB Saunders Company, 1999.
123. Selbst SM, Clark M. Analgesic use in the emergency department. Ann Emerg Med 1990;19:1010–3.

124. Alexander J, Manno M. Underuse of analgesia in very young pediatric patients with isolated painful injuries. Ann Emerg Med 2003;41:617–22.
125. Ngai B, Ducharme J. Documented use of analgesics in the emergency department and upon release of patients with extremity fractures. Acad Emerg Med 1997;4:1176–8.
126. Peng PW, Sandler AN. A review of the use of fentanyl analgesia in the management of acute pain in adults. Anesthesiology 1999;90:576–99.
127. Mackie AM, Coda BC, Hill HF. Adolescents use patient-controlled analgesia effectively for relief from prolonged oropharyngeal mucositis pain. Pain 1991;46:265–9.
128. Berde CB, Lehn BM, Yee JD et al. Patient-controlled analgesia in children and adolescents: a randomized, prospective comparison with intramuscular administration of morphine for postoperative analgesia. J Pediatr 1991;118:460–6.
129. Irwin M, Gillespie JA, Morton NS. Evaluation of a disposable patient-controlled analgesia device in children. Br J Anaesth 1992;68:411–3.
130. Trentadue NO, Kachoyeanos MK, Lea G. A comparison of two regimens of patient-controlled analgesia for children with sickle cell disease. J Pediatr Nurs 1998;13:15–9.
131. Doyle E, Harper I, Morton NS. Patient-controlled analgesia with low dose background infusions after lower abdominal surgery in children. Br J Anaesth 1993;71:818–22.
132. Dunbar PJ, Chapman CR, Buckley FP, Gavrin JR. Clinical analgesic equivalence for morphine and hydromorphone with prolonged PCA. Pain 1996;68:265–70.
133. Yaster M, Maxwell L. Opioid agonists and antagonists. In: Schechter N, Berde C, Yaster M, eds. Pain in infants, children and adolescents. Baltimore, MD: Williams & Wilkins:160
134. Collins JJ, Geake J, Grier HE et al. Patient-controlled analgesia for mucositis pain in children: a three-period crossover study comparing morphine and hydromorphone. J Pediatr 1996;129:722–8.
135. Quigley C, Wiffen P. A systematic review of hydromorphone in acute and chronic pain. J Pain Symptom Manage 2003;25:169–78.
136. Glasgow JF. Reye's syndrome: the case for a causal link with aspirin. Drug Saf 2006;29:1111–21.
137. Olive G. Analgesic/Antipyretic treatment: ibuprofen or acetaminophen? An update. Therapie 2006;61:151–60.
138. McGaw T, Raborn W, Grace M. Analgesics in pediatric dental surgery: relative efficacy of aluminum ibuprofen suspension and acetaminophen elixir. ASDC J Dent Child 1987;54:106–9.
139. Kauffman RE, Sawyer LA, Scheinbaum ML. Antipyretic efficacy of ibuprofen vs acetaminophen. Am J Dis Child 1992;146:622–5.
140. Perrott DA, Piira T, Goodenough B, Champion GD. Efficacy and safety of acetaminophen vs ibuprofen for treating children's pain or fever: a meta-analysis. Arch Pediatr Adolesc Med 2004;158:521–6.
141. Mitchell JA, Akarasereenont P, Thiemermann C et al. Selectivity of nonsteroidal anti-inflammatory drugs as inhibitors of constitutive and inducible cyclooxygenase. Proc Natl Acad Sci U S A 1993;90:11693–7.
142. Moncada S, Gryglewski R, Bunting S, Vane JR. An enzyme isolated from arteries transforms prostaglandin endoperoxides to an unstable substance that inhibits platelet aggregation. Nature 1976;263:663–5.
143. Whittle BJ. Role of prostaglandins in the defense of the gastric mucosa. Brain Res Bull 1980;5 Suppl 1:7–14.
144. Guignard JP. The adverse renal effects of prostaglandin-synthesis inhibitors in the newborn rabbit. Semin Perinatol 2002;26:398–405.
145. Leonelli SM, Goldberg BA, Safanda J et al. Effects of a cyclooxygenase-2 inhibitor (rofecoxib) on bone healing. Am J Orthop 2006;35:79–84.
146. Papacci P, De Francisci G, Iacobucci T et al. Use of intravenous ketorolac in the neonate and premature babies. Paediatr Anaesth 2004;14:487–92.

147. Govindarajan R, Ghosh B, Sathyamoorthy MK et al. Efficacy of ketorolac in lieu of narcotics in the operative management of laparoscopic surgery for morbid obesity. Surg Obes Relat Dis 2005;1:530–5; discussion 5–6.

148. Cepeda MS, Carr DB, Miranda N et al. Comparison of morphine, ketorolac, and their combination for postoperative pain: results from a large, randomized, double-blind trial. Anesthesiology 2005;103:1225–32.

149. Beattie WS, Badner NH, Choi P. Epidural analgesia reduces postoperative myocardial infarction: a meta-analysis. Anesth Analg 2001;93:853–8.

150. Wu CL, Naqibuddin M, Rowlingson AJ et al. The effect of pain on health-related quality of life in the immediate postoperative period. Anesth Analg 2003;97:1078–85.

151. Williams BA, Kentor ML, Vogt MT et al. Reduction of verbal pain scores after anterior cruciate ligament reconstruction with 2-day continuous femoral nerve block: a randomized clinical trial. Anesthesiology 2006;104:315–27.

152. Evans H, Steele SM, Nielsen KC et al. Peripheral nerve blocks and continuous catheter techniques. Anesthesiol Clin North America 2005;23:141–62.

153. Chelly JE, Greger J, Gebhard R et al. Continuous femoral blocks improve recovery and outcome of patients undergoing total knee arthroplasty. J Arthroplasty 2001;16:436–45.

154. Tran KM, Ganley TJ, Wells L et al. Intraarticular bupivacaine-clonidine-morphine versus femoral-sciatic nerve block in pediatric patients undergoing anterior cruciate ligament reconstruction. Anesth Analg 2005;101:1304–10.

155. Labat F, Dubousset AM, Baujard C et al. Epidural analgesia in a child with sickle cell disease complicated by acute abdominal pain and priapism. Br J Anaesth 2001;87:935–6.

156. Yaster M, Tobin JR, Billett C et al. Epidural analgesia in the management of severe vaso-occlusive sickle cell crisis. Pediatrics 1994;93:310–5.

157. Bulger EM, Edwards T, Klotz P, Jurkovich GJ. Epidural analgesia improves outcome after multiple rib fractures. Surgery 2004;136:426–30.

158. Flagel BT, Luchette FA, Reed RL et al. Half-a-dozen ribs: the breakpoint for mortality. Surgery 2005;138:717–23; discussion 23–5.

159. Giaufre E, Dalens B, Gombert A. Epidemiology and morbidity of regional anesthesia in children: a one-year prospective survey of the French-Language Society of Pediatric Anesthesiologists. Anesth Analg 1996;83:904–12.

160. Goldman LJ. Complications in regional anaesthesia. Paediatr Anaesth 1995;5:3–9.

161. Pietropaoli JA, Jr., Keller MS, Smail DF et al. Regional anesthesia in pediatric surgery: complications and postoperative comfort level in 174 children. J Pediatr Surg 1993;28:560–4.

162. Tanaka M, Kimura T, Goyagi T et al. Evaluating hemodynamic and T wave criteria of simulated intravascular test doses using bupivacaine or isoproterenol in anesthetized children. Anesth Analg 2000;91:567–72.

163. Freid EB, Bailey AG, Valley RD. Electrocardiographic and hemodynamic changes associated with unintentional intravascular injection of bupivacaine with epinephrine in infants. Anesthesiology 1993;79:394–8.

164. Mulroy MF. Systemic toxicity and cardiotoxicity from local anesthetics: incidence and preventive measures. Reg Anesth Pain Med 2002;27:556–61.

165. Dworkin RH, Turk DC, Farrar JT et al. Core outcome measures for chronic pain clinical trials: IMMPACT recommendations. Pain 2005;113:9–19.

166. Zeltzer LK, Tsao JC, Stelling C et al. A phase I study on the feasibility and acceptability of an acupuncture/hypnosis intervention for chronic pediatric pain. J Pain Symptom Manage 2002;24:437–46.

167. Pintov S, Lahat E, Alstein M et al. Acupuncture and the opioid system: implications in management of migraine. Pediatr Neurol 1997;17:129–33.

168. Simons SH, Tibboel D. Pain perception development and maturation. Semin Fetal Neonatal Med 2006;11:227–31.

169. Reynolds ML, Fitzgerald M. Long-term sensory hyperinnervation following neonatal skin wounds. J Comp Neurol 1995;358:487–98.
170. Torsney C, Fitzgerald M. Spinal dorsal horn cell receptive field size is increased in adult rats following neonatal hindpaw skin injury. J Physiol 2003;550:255–61.
171. Pineles BL, Sandman CA, Waffarn F et al. Sensitization of cardiac responses to pain in preterm infants. Neonatology 2007;91:190–5.
172. Taddio A, Katz J, Ilersich AL, Koren G. Effect of neonatal circumcision on pain response during subsequent routine vaccination. Lancet 1997;349:599–603.
173. Grunau RE, Holsti L, Haley DW et al. Neonatal procedural pain exposure predicts lower cortisol and behavioral reactivity in preterm infants in the NICU. Pain 2005;113:293–300.
174. Kajantie E. Fetal origins of stress-related adult disease. Ann N Y Acad Sci 2006;1083:11–27.
175. Grunau RV, Whitfield MF, Petrie JH. Pain sensitivity and temperament in extremely low-birth-weight premature toddlers and preterm and full-term controls. Pain 1994;58:341–6.
176. Grunau RV, Whitfield MF, Petrie JH, Fryer EL. Early pain experience, child and family factors, as precursors of somatization: a prospective study of extremely premature and fullterm children. Pain 1994;56:353–9.
177. Grunau RE, Whitfield MF, Petrie J. Children's judgements about pain at age 8–10 years: do extremely low birthweight (< or = 1000 g) children differ from full birthweight peers? J Child Psychol Psychiatry 1998;39:587–94.
178. Fernandez E. Anxiety, depression, and anger in pain: research findings and clinical options, Dallas, TX: Advanced Psychological Resources, Inc., 2002.
179. Casarett D, Karlawish J, Sankar P et al. Designing pain research from the patient's perspective: what trial end points are important to patients with chronic pain? Pain Med 2001;2:309–16.
180. Kashikar-Zuck S, Goldschneider KR, Powers SW et al. Depression and functional disability in chronic pediatric pain. Clin J Pain 2001;17:341–9.
181. Lynch AM, Kashikar-Zuck S, Goldschneider KR, Jones BA. Psychosocial risks for disability in children with chronic back pain. J Pain 2006;7:244–51.
182. Fainsinger R, Schoeller T, Bruera E. Methadone in the management of cancer pain: a review. Pain 1993;52:137–47.
183. Mercadante S, Casuccio A, Agnello A et al. Morphine versus methadone in the pain treatment of advanced-cancer patients followed up at home. J Clin Oncol 1998;16:3656–61.
184. Ventafridda V, Ripamonti C, Bianchi M et al. A randomized study on oral administration of morphine and methadone in the treatment of cancer pain. J Pain Symptom Manage 1986;1:203–7.
185. Collins JJ, Grier HE, Sethna NF et al. Regional anesthesia for pain associated with terminal pediatric malignancy. Pain 1996;65:63–9.
186. Albright AL, Ferson SS. Intrathecal baclofen therapy in children. Neurosurg Focus 2006;21:e3.
187. Galloway K, Staats PS, Bowers DC. Intrathecal analgesia for children with cancer via implanted infusion pumps. Med Pediatr Oncol 2000;34:265–7.
188. Vender JR, Hester S, Waller JL et al. Identification and management of intrathecal baclofen pump complications: a comparison of pediatric and adult patients. J Neurosurg 2006;104:9–15.
189. Miele VJ, Price KO, Bloomfield S et al. A review of intrathecal morphine therapy related granulomas. Eur J Pain 2006;10:251–61.
190. Hershey AD, Powers SW, Bentti AL et al. Characterization of chronic daily headaches in children in a multidisciplinary headache center. Neurology 2001;56:1032–7.
191. Wiendels NJ, van der Geest MC, Neven AK et al. Chronic daily headache in children and adolescents. Headache 2005;45:678–83.

192. Vasconcellos E, Pina-Garza JE, Millan EJ, Warner JS. Analgesic rebound headache in children and adolescents. J Child Neurol 1998;13:443–7.
193. Hamalainen ML, Hoppu K, Valkeila E, Santavuori P. Ibuprofen or acetaminophen for the acute treatment of migraine in children: a double-blind, randomized, placebo-controlled, crossover study. Neurology 1997;48:103–7.
194. Lewis DW, Kellstein D, Dahl G et al. Children's ibuprofen suspension for the acute treatment of pediatric migraine. Headache 2002;42:780–6.
195. Soriani S, Battistella P, Naccarella C et al. Nimesulide and acetaminophen for the treatment of juvenile migraine: a study for comparison of efficacy, safety, and tolerability. Headache Q 2001;12:233–6.
196. Hamalainen ML, Hoppu K, Santavuori P. Sumatriptan for migraine attacks in children: a randomized placebo-controlled study. Do children with migraine respond to oral sumatriptan differently from adults? Neurology 1997;48:1100–3.
197. Winner P, Rothner AD, Saper J et al. A randomized, double-blind, placebo-controlled study of sumatriptan nasal spray in the treatment of acute migraine in adolescents. Pediatrics 2000;106:989–97.
198. Ahonen K, Hamalainen ML, Rantala H, Hoppu K. Nasal sumatriptan is effective in treatment of migraine attacks in children: A randomized trial. Neurology 2004;62:883–7.
199. Winner P, Lewis D, Visser WH et al. Rizatriptan 5 mg for the acute treatment of migraine in adolescents: a randomized, double-blind, placebo-controlled study. Headache 2002;42:49–55.
200. Hamalainen ML, Hoppu K, Santavuori PR. Oral dihydroergotamine for therapy-resistant migraine attacks in children. Pediatr Neurol 1997;16:114–7.
201. Damen L, Bruijn JK, Verhagen AP et al. Symptomatic treatment of migraine in children: a systematic review of medication trials. Pediatrics 2005;116:e295–302.
202. Jhee SS, Shiovitz T, Crawford AW, Cutler NR. Pharmacokinetics and pharmacodynamics of the triptan antimigraine agents: a comparative review. Clin Pharmacokinet 2001;40:189–205.
203. Silberstein SD. Practice parameter: evidence-based guidelines for migraine headache (an evidence-based review): report of the Quality Standards Subcommittee of the American Academy of Neurology. Neurology 2000;55:754–62.
204. Lewis DW, Diamond S, Scott D, Jones V. Prophylactic treatment of pediatric migraine. Headache 2004;44:230–7.
205. Bille B, Ludvigsson J, Sanner G. Prophylaxis of migraine in children. Headache 1977;17:61–3.
206. Hershey AD, Powers SW, Bentti AL, Degrauw TJ. Effectiveness of amitriptyline in the prophylactic management of childhood headaches. Headache 2000;40:539–49.
207. Sorge F, Marano E. Flunarizine v. placebo in childhood migraine. A double-blind study. Cephalalgia 1985;5 Suppl 2:145–8.
208. Guidetti V, Moscato D, Ottaviano S et al. Flunarizine and migraine in childhood. An evaluation of endocrine function. Cephalalgia 1987;7:263–6.
209. Battistella PA, Ruffilli R, Moro R et al. A placebo-controlled crossover trial of nimodipine in pediatric migraine. Headache 1990;30:264–8.
210. Eiland LS, Jenkins LS, Durham SH. Pediatric Migraine: pharmacologic agents for prophylaxis (July/August). Ann Pharmacother 2007;41:1181–90.
211. Edwards JL, Kirk KK, Midha CK. Benefits and harms of pediatric antidepressant medications. Jama 2007;298:626–7.
212. Jick H, Kaye JA, Jick SS. Antidepressants and the risk of suicidal behaviors. JAMA 2004;292:338–43.
213. Wasiewski WW. Preventive therapy in pediatric migraine. J Child Neurol 2001;16:71–8.
214. Trautmann E, Lackschewitz H, Kroner-Herwig B. Psychological treatment of recurrent headache in children and adolescents–a meta-analysis. Cephalalgia 2006;26:1411–26.

215. Eccleston C, Yorke L, Morley S et al. Psychological therapies for the management of chronic and recurrent pain in children and adolescents. Cochrane Database Syst Rev 2003:CD003968.
216. Lewis DW, Dorbad D. The utility of neuroimaging in the evaluation of children with migraine or chronic daily headache who have normal neurological examinations. Headache 2000;40:629–32.
217. Almazov I, Brand N. Meningismus is a commonly overlooked finding in tension-type headache in children and adolescents. J Child Neurol 2006;21:423–5.
218. Diaz-Mitoma F, Vanast WJ, Tyrrell DL. Increased frequency of Epstein-Barr virus excretion in patients with new daily persistent headaches. Lancet 1987;1:411–5.
219. Mack KJ. What incites new daily persistent headache in children? Pediatr Neurol 2004;31:122–5.
220. Bahra A, Walsh M, Menon S, Goadsby PJ. Does chronic daily headache arise de novo in association with regular use of analgesics? Headache 2003;43:179–90.
221. Balottin U, Nicoli F, Pitillo G et al. Migraine and tension headache in children under 6 years of age. Eur J Pain 2004;8:307–14.
222. Callaghan M, Abu-Arafeh I. Chronic posttraumatic headache in children and adolescents. Dev Med Child Neurol 2001;43:819–22.
223. Biondi DM. Cervicogenic headache: diagnostic evaluation and treatment strategies. Curr Pain Headache Rep 2001;5:361–8.
224. Ormos G. Cervicogenic headache in children. Headache 2003;43:693–4.
225. Lewit K. Ligament pain and anteflexion headache. Eur Neurol 1971;5:365–78.
226. Vallat JM, Vallat-Decouvelaere AV. Histology and elementary pathology of the peripheral nerve. Rev Prat 2000;50:713–8.
227. Fromm GH, Terrence CF, Maroon JC. Trigeminal neuralgia. Current concepts regarding etiology and pathogenesis. Arch Neurol 1984;41:1204–7.
228. Beydoun A. Clinical use of tricyclic anticonvulsants in painful neuropathies and bipolar disorders. Epilepsy Behav 2002;3:S18–22.
229. Sanchez C, Hyttel J. Comparison of the effects of antidepressants and their metabolites on reuptake of biogenic amines and on receptor binding. Cell Mol Neurobiol 1999;19:467–89.
230. Sindrup SH, Jensen TS. Efficacy of pharmacological treatments of neuropathic pain: an update and effect related to mechanism of drug action. Pain 1999;83:389–400.
231. McQuay HJ, Tramer M, Nye BA et al. A systematic review of antidepressants in neuropathic pain. Pain 1996;68:217–27.
232. Gee NS, Brown JP, Dissanayake VU et al. The novel anticonvulsant drug, gabapentin (Neurontin), binds to the alpha2delta subunit of a calcium channel. J Biol Chem 1996;271:5768–76.
233. Rose MA, Kam PC. Gabapentin: pharmacology and its use in pain management. Anaesthesia 2002;57:451–62.
234. Bennett MI, Simpson KH. Gabapentin in the treatment of neuropathic pain. Palliat Med 2004;18:5–11.
235. Backonja M, Beydoun A, Edwards KR et al. Gabapentin for the symptomatic treatment of painful neuropathy in patients with diabetes mellitus: a randomized controlled trial. Jama 1998;280:1831–6.
236. van de Vusse AC, Stomp-van den Berg SG, Kessels AH, Weber WE. Randomised controlled trial of gabapentin in Complex Regional Pain Syndrome type 1 [ISRCTN84121379]. BMC Neurol 2004;4:13.
237. Ho KY, Gan TJ, Habib AS. Gabapentin and postoperative pain–a systematic review of randomized controlled trials. Pain 2006;126:91–101.
238. Beydoun A, Backonja MM. Mechanistic stratification of antineuralgic agents. J Pain Symptom Manage 2003;25:S18–30.

239. Caraceni A, Zecca E, Bonezzi C et al. Gabapentin for neuropathic cancer pain: a randomized controlled trial from the Gabapentin Cancer Pain Study Group. J Clin Oncol 2004;22:2909–17.

240. Rice AS, Maton S. Gabapentin in postherpetic neuralgia: a randomised, double blind, placebo controlled study. Pain 2001;94:215–24.

241. Bone M, Critchley P, Buggy DJ. Gabapentin in postamputation phantom limb pain: a randomized, double-blind, placebo-controlled, cross-over study. Reg Anesth Pain Med 2002;27:481–6.

242. Backonja M, Glanzman RL. Gabapentin dosing for neuropathic pain: evidence from randomized, placebo-controlled clinical trials. Clin Ther 2003;25:81–104.

243. Killian JM, Fromm GH. Carbamazepine in the treatment of neuralgia. Use of side effects. Arch Neurol 1968;19:129–36.

244. Nicol CF. A four year double-blind study of tegretol in facial pain. Headache 1969;9:54–7.

245. Beniczky S, Tajti J, Timea Varga E, Vecsei L. Evidence-based pharmacological treatment of neuropathic pain syndromes. J Neural Transm 2005;112:735–49.

246. Leijon G, Boivie J. Central post-stroke pain–a controlled trial of amitriptyline and carbamazepine. Pain 1989;36:27–36.

247. Levendoglu F, Ogun CO, Ozerbil O et al. Gabapentin is a first line drug for the treatment of neuropathic pain in spinal cord injury. Spine 2004;29:743–51.

248. Lee BH, Scharff L, Sethna NF et al. Physical therapy and cognitive-behavioral treatment for complex regional pain syndromes. J Pediatr 2002;141:135–40.

249. Matsui M, Ito M, Tomoda A, Miike T. Complex regional pain syndrome in childhood: report of three cases. Brain Dev 2000;22:445–8.

250. Bernstein BH, Singsen BH, Kent JT et al. Reflex neurovascular dystrophy in childhood. J Pediatr 1978;93:211–5.

251. Stanton-Hicks M, Baron R, Boas R et al. Complex Regional pain syndromes: guidelines for therapy. Clin J Pain 1998;14:155–66.

252. Stanton RP, Malcolm JR, Wesdock KA, Singsen BH. Reflex sympathetic dystrophy in children: an orthopedic perspective. Orthopedics 1993;16:773–9; discussion 9–80.

253. Murray CS, Cohen A, Perkins T et al. Morbidity in reflex sympathetic dystrophy. Arch Dis Child 2000;82:231–3.

254. Brommel B, Fialka V, Eschberger D et al. Personality markers in patients with Sudeck's disease. A psychoanalytic study. Z Psychosom Med Psychoanal 1993;39:346–55.

255. Sherry DD, Weisman R. Psychologic aspects of childhood reflex neurovascular dystrophy. Pediatrics 1988;81:572–8.

256. Huertas-Ceballos A, Macarthur C, Logan S. Pharmacological interventions for recurrent abdominal pain (RAP) in childhood. Cochrane Database Syst Rev 2002:CD003017.

257. Robins PM, Smith SM, Glutting JJ, Bishop CT. A randomized controlled trial of a cognitive-behavioral family intervention for pediatric recurrent abdominal pain. J Pediatr Psychol 2005;30:397–408.

258. Evans JM, McMahon AD, Murray FE et al. Non-steroidal anti-inflammatory drugs are associated with emergency admission to hospital for colitis due to inflammatory bowel disease. Gut 1997;40:619–22.

259. Walt RP, Hawkey CJ, Langman MJ. Colitis associated with non-steroidal anti-inflammatory drugs. Br Med J (Clin Res Ed) 1984;288:238.

260. Rampton DS, Sladen GE. Relapse of ulcerative proctocolitis during treatment with non-steroidal anti-inflammatory drugs. Postgrad Med J 1981;57:297–9.

261. Meyer AM, Ramzan NN, Heigh RI, Leighton JA. Relapse of inflammatory bowel disease associated with use of nonsteroidal anti-inflammatory drugs. Dig Dis Sci 2006;51:168–72.

262. Symon DN, Russell G. Double blind placebo controlled trial of pizotifen syrup in the treatment of abdominal migraine. Arch Dis Child 1995;72:48–50.

263. See MC, Birnbaum AH, Schechter CB et al. Double-blind, placebo-controlled trial of famotidine in children with abdominal pain and dyspepsia: global and quantitative assessment. Dig Dis Sci 2001;46:985–92.
264. Sanders MR, Shepherd RW, Cleghorn G, Woolford H. The treatment of recurrent abdominal pain in children: a controlled comparison of cognitive-behavioral family intervention and standard pediatric care. J Consult Clin Psychol 1994;62:306–14.
265. Koloski N, Talley N. Role of sexual and physical abuse in IBS. In: Camilleri M, Spiller R, eds. Irritable bowel syndrome. Diagnosis and treatment Oxford: WB Saunders, 2002:37–43.
266. Rimsza ME, Berg RA, Locke C. Sexual abuse: somatic and emotional reactions. Child Abuse Negl 1988;12:201–8.
267. Price L, Maddocks A, Davies S, Griffiths L. Somatic and psychological problems in a cohort of sexually abused boys: a six year follow up case-control study. Arch Dis Child 2002;86:164–7.
268. Ramchandani PG, Stein A, Hotopf M, Wiles NJ. Early parental and child predictors of recurrent abdominal pain at school age: results of a large population-based study. J Am Acad Child Adolesc Psychiatry 2006;45:729–36.
269. Walker LS, Williams SE, Smith CA et al. Parent attention versus distraction: impact on symptom complaints by children with and without chronic functional abdominal pain. Pain 2006;122:43–52.
270. Fitzpatrick KP, Sherman PM, Ipp M et al. Screening for celiac disease in children with recurrent abdominal pain. J Pediatr Gastroenterol Nutr 2001;33:250–2.
271. Joint Commission releases new pain management standards. Rep Med Guidel Outcomes Res 2000;11:7–10.
272. Fishman SM, Papazian JS, Gonzalez S et al. Regulating opioid prescribing through prescription monitoring programs: balancing drug diversion and treatment of pain. Pain Med 2004;5:309–24.
273. Manchikanti L. Prescription drug abuse: what is being done to address this new drug epidemic? Testimony before the Subcommittee on Criminal Justice, Drug Policy and Human Resources. Pain Physician 2006;9:287–321.

Pain in the Older Person

Bill McCarberg and B. Eliot Cole

Introduction

The US population is aging with those 65 years or older reaching 70 million (20% of the population) by the year 2030 [1]. Chronic conditions such as osteoarthritis, atherosclerosis, cancer, and diabetes prevalent in older Americans, will contribute to the increasing costs of health care. Today, $300 billion is spent annually for the healthcare needs of older patients, representing one third of total US health care costs. Among older patients, pain is the most common symptom noted when consulting a physician [2]. Common sources of pain in one study of 97 long-term care residents include lower back pain (40%), arthritis (24%), previous fractures (14%), and neuropathies (11%)[3].

Despite the frequency of pain and the suffering that occurs, it is often underreported and undertreated in older people. The incidence of undertreated pain ranges from 25 to 50% in adult communities [4, 5], from 45 to 80% in nursing homes [3, 4, 5, 6], and as high as 85% in long-term care facilities [7]. Patients often believe that pain is inevitable and that treatment is worse than the symptom. They fear underlying cancer and addiction to the analgesics. Health professionals lacking adequate pain management education may mistakenly believe that older patients have a higher pain tolerance [8]. Since cures for many of the chronic conditions manifesting in older patients are not always readily available, there must be a focus on the management of the pain associated with these conditions.

Several treatment guidelines for the assessment, treatment, and monitoring of chronic pain in older patients have been published, including recent guidelines from the American Geriatrics Society (AGS) and American Medical Directors Association (AMDA) [9,10]. These guidelines advocate individualized pain

B. McCarberg (✉)
Founder – Chronic Pain Management Program, Kaiser Permanente, Assistant Clinical Professor, University of California San Diego, 732 North Broadway, Escondido, CA 92025, USA
e-mail: bill.h.mccarberg@kp.org

R.J. Moore (ed.), *Biobehavioral Approaches to Pain*,
DOI 10.1007/978-0-387-78323-9_9, © Springer Science+Business Media, LLC 2009

management, vital to patients with multiple underlying chronic diseases. The AMDA guidelines state:

> In the long-term care setting, the comfort and well being of the individual patient must be paramount. This principal is the foundation for effective management of chronic pain. Neither resource constraints nor the perception of social disapproval ... must ever be an excuse for inadequate pain control [10].

There are multiple treatment modalities which have been shown to be effective for older people. Opioids are particularly useful in certain disease processes. Because the prevalence of abuse among older patients is low, treating chronic pain for these people should not be constrained by fears of, or misconceptions about drug dependency [11]. The choice of pharmacologic treatment for an individual patient will depend upon multiple factors, including the source and pathophysiology of the pain, and the presence of comorbid conditions. Older patients are more likely to have physiological or psychological factors that influence chronic pain treatment, but there are strategies available to address these factors. For example, combining pharmacologic and nonpharmacologic options help keep drug effects lower [12,13]. The growing number and types of analgesics available permit an individualized pharmacologic regimen that targets chronic pain while addressing the issues associated with treating older patients.

The goal of this chapter is to explore the topic of pain in the older person. First we cover the neurophysiology of aging in the older person. Then we proceed to discuss the following: the measurement of pain in the cognitively intact and non-intact patients; psychosocial issues associated with pain in this clinical population, including fatigue, the treatment of pain in the older person based upon diagnosis and physiology Complementary and alternative methods for treating pain; and pain at the end of life. Finally, we conclude this discussion of pain in the older person, and make some suggestions in terms of where the field might go from this point forward.

Neurophysiology of Aging

Functional, structural, and biochemical changes have been reported in aged subjects [14]. The experience of pain is dependent on a complex neural system incorporating excitatory and inhibitory mechanisms. Aging is associated with widespread changes in the cellular and neurochemical substrates of the nociceptive system. The functional consequences of structural age-related changes are difficult to extrapolate given the highly integrated nature of pain processing, but some definite patterns have emerged from the literature. Inferring from equivocal data of increased pain threshold that older people are marginally insensitive to pain is no longer sustainable. Under circumstances where pain is likely to persist, older people are especially vulnerable to the negative effect of chronic pain.

Peripheral nerves, both unmyelinated and myelinated, decrease with age. The magnitude of reduction is thought to be greater for unmyelinated fibers with an apparent loss of about 50% compared to a 35% loss in myelinated afferent fibers in people 65–75 years [14]. The number of sensory fibers with signs of damage or degeneration also shows a marked increase with advancing age [14, 15]. Neurotransmitters of primary sensory nerves, substance P and calcitonin gene related protein (CGRP), are found at lower levels with increasing age, reflecting a reduction in the density or functional integrity of nociceptive nerves.

The age-related nerve and neurotransmitter reduction described above also occurs in other nerves including sudomotor and sympathetic. The extent of age-related change in the human brain is known to be both sizable and ubiquitous, involving changes in structure, neurochemistry, and function. Widespread degenerative changes have been found in spinal dorsal horn sensory neurons of healthy older adults [16]. Decreased CGRP, substance P, and somatostatin levels in the cervical, thoracic, and lumbar dorsal horn of aged rats have been demonstrated [17, 18]. Strong evidence for progressive age-related loss of serotonergic and noradrenergic neurons in the dorsal horn [19, 20] indicating an impaired pain inhibitory system is known.

The pain threshold represents the acuity of pain as a warning system—the minimal stimulus that is sensed as noxious [21, 22]. The pain threshold is a convenient point to investigate aging effects upon pain function. Increased pain threshold to noxious thermal, mechanical, and electrical stimuli with age has been shown in over 40 studies, yet there was no unanimity among studies. Since pain threshold is the initiating event of the alerting system, an increased threshold results in less difference between the point of initial identification of pain and the onset of tissue injury. Thus, there are circumstances where decreased awareness for pain places older people at significant risk of sustaining tissue damage. However, aging does not appear to be associated with substantive functional change over much of the pain stimulus-response curve. Hyperalgesia results from damage or dysfunction of the peripheral or central nervous system, whereby nonpainful stimuli are perceived as painful. Hyperalgesia is maladaptive if the pain does not resolve in concert with tissue healing. Along with their prolonged time to heal, older people are more likely to demonstrate slower resolution of hyperalgesia [23, 24].

Assessing and Measuring Pain in Older People

Assessing and measuring the pain for the majority of older people is performed the same as it is for other patients–by having them provide self-reports [25]. The most direct method of pain assessment is to ask patients about pain's presence, and when pain is present to then ask about its precise location, intensity, duration, exacerbating and relieving factors, and associated interferences with their daily activities [26]. Since patients typically report pain with many common medical procedures (i.e., use of mechanical restraints, line placements, movement from bed to chair, transfers from stretchers or wheelchairs, being mechanically ventilated, having urinary catheters placed, having blood draws or IM/SC injections) [27], astute clinicians anticipate pain with these typical interventions, procedures, and situations, so intervene before, during, and after such events.

Assessing and Measuring Pain in Cognitively Intact Patients

Pain assessment for cognitively intact patients is relatively straightforward, with healthcare providers needing to address painful conditions more commonly seen with advancing age: post-herpetic neuralgia, diabetic peripheral neuropathies, temporal arteritis, osteoarthritis, angina, claudication and other ischemic pain due to occlusive vascular disease, and cancer. Beyond the obvious biomedical assessment, however, a more thorough and focused assessment is often needed to identify important pain-related issues: depression, functional impairment, social isolation and suffering [27].

Cognitively intact older patients should be able to report pain using a numerical scale, although a 5-point Likert scale likely will produce more reliable responses than a 10-point scale [28]. Asking older people to what degree their pain limits activities may be a more reliable guide for titration of medication than is pain severity level [29]. Age differences in pain intensity scores may be dependent upon the pain scale used: older men having significantly lower scores than younger men on the McGill Pain Questionnaire (MPQ) and Prospective Pain Inventory (PPI), while having no differences on the Visual Analog Scale (VAS) [30]. Other psychometric studies suggest that the Numeric Rating Scale (NRS) is the preferred pain intensity scale for older people because its properties are not age related; however, due to difficulties encountered when older patients use the VAS they should not be postoperatively assessed with it [31, 32].

Assessing and Measuring Pain in Cognitively Impaired Patients

It is relatively common for providers of care for older people to inaccurately assume that those who are cognitively impaired cannot be assessed for pain, or much worse, cannot have their pain meaningfully measured or managed. While some cognitively impaired patients may pose assessment challenges, it is reasonable to expect all but the most disabled to grimace, moan, wince, and demonstrate other automatic forms of pain expression [33]. This has led to the need to perform behavioral assessments instead of relying upon the typical self-report measures such as the numeric, descriptive, and visual analog scales. Instead, noting protective behaviors, posturing, unwillingness to engage in usually pleasurable activities, and impaired sleep may better signal the presence and severity of pain in cognitively impaired patients [33].

Pain is infrequently appreciated as an independent source of agitation in people with dementia; when pain is the source of agitation, treatment will be different [34]. Vexingly, pain is more poorly treated in patients with dementia [35]. Assuming that non-communicative patients do not have pain present when they are being quiet or are at rest does them equally a great disservice.

Psychosocial Issues Associated with Pain in the Older Person

Pain occurs for older people within the context of their advancing age –itself associated with social support system losses through death, illness, retirement, and relocation [36, 37].

Most Americans successfully age despite their underlying health issues; [38] contrary to popular misconceptions, older Americans are not commonly aban-doned by their families, and they do serve as significant resources for their families, providing meaningful economic and social support [36, 39]. Their well being is ultimately derived from the constellation of good health, adequate social support systems, and economic resources [40]. The implication for healthcare providers and concerned family members regarding psychosocial considerations for pain management is how to simultaneously respect autonomy while providing needed care [36, 41].

Older people may use less cognitive pain-coping strategies than younger people [42]; with coping efforts that appear maladaptive [43]. For those with osteoarthritis, their pain is linked to the activity limitations it produces [44]. However, the patient must be independently evaluated rather than being expected to display certain behaviors solely on the basis of their age.

Depression

Individuals who develop pain or depression are at risk for developing the other, with a spiraling risk of pain and depression. Because pain and depression share predictors, individuals who are at high risk of developing these two outcomes [45, 46].

Depression is a major comorbidity and significant risk factor for those with terminal illness, interfering with their end-of-life care. While diagnosing depres-sion remains clinical [47], interfering with its diagnostic determination is the fact that patients themselves often underestimate their own level of distress [48]. Trivializing or failing to recognize depression produces additional potentially lethal consequences other than just suicide. Medical inpatients with major depres-sive disorders and serious medical conditions are more likely to die while hospi-talized independent of the severity of their nonpsychiatric medical illnesses; having a past history of major depressive disorder or dysthymia increases the odds ratio of dying to 7.8 after controlling for illness severity [49].

Anxiety and alcoholism are other comorbidities for older people dealing with chronic pain, disease burden, and overall health decline [50]. Pain related anxiety is itself associated with depression, poorer coping, catastrophizing, and worsening health perception [51]. That said, older people do not routinely develop depressive disorders as part of their aging, even though disabled and medically ill people are at greater risk for depressive symptoms [52], as well as for those with persistent pain [53]. In general, late-life depression produces significant emotional distress and poorer quality of life [54] and is tragically associated with suicide completion [55] (suicide rates are 3 times greater than the general US population average for those 63–69 years of age and 5 times greater for men over the age of 85 years) [55].

Symptoms Associated with Depression

Clinicians should be suspicious about the possibility of depression when patients complain of fatigue, pain, sleep disturbances, anxiety, and irritability. Overlapping features of depression, pain, and the natural events associated with serious medical illness do make early depression recognition more difficult. To better identify depression in medically ill patients, nonsomatic symptoms may be substituted for the somatic symptoms associated with depression; tearfulness, appearing sad or depressed, social withdrawal, and pessimism may be more reliable markers of depression instead of anorexia, fatigue, insomnia, and impaired concentration. Excluding somatic symptoms and only considering psychological features (pervasive feelings of worthlessness, hopelessness, and helplessness) or including all somatic and psychological symptoms together, regardless of their source, may help clinicians recognize depression in the medically ill [56].

Fatigue

Over the past several years many authors have examined the relationship between pain, mood and fatigue. In the condition of fibromyalgia some studies have noted that between 78 and 94% of patients describe fatgiue, yet it was found in a survey of 105 adults with the condition that greater depression and lower sleep quality were associated with higher fatigue, but pain itself did not independently contribute to fatigue [57]. Another group using a structured, evidence-based review of 17 studies related to the coexistence of fatigue and pain found that 94.1% indicated that there was an association between fatigue and pain; a subgroup of 13 reports indicated there may be a cause and effect relationship between pain and fatigue [58]. The links between pain and fatigue included development of fatigue after the development of pain, and improvement in fatigue with lessening of pain; the longer pain was present the greater the likelihood of fatigue; the greater the pain experienced the more certain it was that fatigue occurred.

Confounding the relationship between pain and fatigue, mood was found to be a significant contributor in a study of 274 community-dwelling adults. Pain, mood, and sleep all were associated with fatigue. While pain accounted for the largest contribution to fatigue, mood modified the relationship between pain and fatigue [59]. The role of mood was further explored in a study of 175 people with chronic lower back pain and 33 with chronic neck pain. This study found fatigue was a significant problem for those with chronic lower back pain and chronic neck pain, noting that predictors for fatigue included the presence of neuropathic pain, female gender, presence of depression, and the total number of DSM-IV diagnoses [60]. Finally, the same authors of the previous study examined the role of multidisciplinary pain facility treatment on pain-associated fatigue and found that multidisciplinary multimodal treatment significantly improved fatigue for those with chronic lower back pain and chronic neck pain [61].

Treating Older People with Pain Based Upon Pathophysiology

There is no single guideline for the treatment of all types of pain in all older people. Comprehensive recommendations are available from the American Geriatric Society (AGS) [26], as well as guidelines for neuropathic pain in general [62] and for diabetic peripheral neuropathic pain (DPNP) in particular [63]. The AGS recommendations progress pharmacologically from nonopioid medications to neurotransmitter-modulating and membranes-stabilizing agents to opioid analgesics with the goal of balancing medical risks while addressing more severe pain. The AGS guidelines are a reworking of the cancer pain guidelines originally proposed by the World Health Organization, with a strong position taken that the use of placebos in the treatment of pain is unethical, and there is no role for them in the management of persistent pain. Nonpharmacological strategies include physical and psychological treatments that require varying degrees of active and passive participation, patient education programs perhaps being the most important aspect. Additionally, the AGS guidelines challenge practitioners to consider the possibility of coincident depression and anxiety that may modulate diagnosis and management, perhaps necessitating referral to a comprehensive, multidisciplinary pain program [26].

The *American Society of Pain Educators* (DPNP) guidelines developed by a consensus panel at the request of the American Society of Pain Educators (ASPE) looked at the strength of published articles and determined that based upon randomized controlled trials (RCTs) pharmacotherapeutic approaches could be classified as first-tier, second-tier, topical, and other. First-tier medications had two or more RCTs specifically in DPNP; second-tier agents had one Randomised Controlled Trial (RCT) in DPNP and one or more RCTs in other painful neuropathies (need citations) ; topicals were those medications whose mechanism of action would be beneficial when applied directly to the painful location (e.g. lidocaine); and other medications were those with one or more RCTs in other painful neuropathies or having evidence suggesting potential benefit (need citations). First-line therapies include duloxetine, oxycodone controlled-release (CR), pregabalin, and tricyclic antidepressants (TCAs) as a class; second-tier includecarbamazepine, gabapentin, lamotrigine, tramadol, and venlafaxine extended-release (ER); topicals included capsaicin and lidocaine; and others included bupropion, citalopram, methadone, paroxetine, phenytoin, and topiramate. Of note, the group had concerns about the use of tricyclics in older people, especially those with cardiovascular disease. Additionally, the use of selective serotonin reuptake inhibitors has not been shown to be particularly efficacious in older people unless clinical depression was also present [63].

Evidence Based Interventions

While not representing an evidence-based standard of care, the American Society of Interventional Pain Physicians (ASIPP) has recently developed interventional technique guidelines for chronic spinal pain [64]. Their 2007 version reports the diagnostic accuracy of facet joint nerve blocks is strong in the diagnosis of lumbar and cervical facet joint disease, but moderate in the diagnosis of thoracic facet joint disease. There is strong evidence for the use lumbar discography, but limited evidence for the use of cervical and thoracic discography. Evidence for diagnostic sacroiliac joint injections is moderate. Therapeutically, the ASIPP guidelines provides strong evidence for the use of caudal epidural steroid injections for chronic lower back pain and radicular pain, interlaminar epidural steroid injections for lumbar radiculopathy, transforaminal epidural steroid injections for lumbar nerve root pain, percutaneous epidural adhesiolysis, spinal endoscopic adhesiolysis, spinal cord stimulation for failed back surgery syndrome and complex region pain syndrome, and the use of implantable intrathecal infusions systems for chronic pain. Moderate evidence for the use of lumbar facet injections, lumbar and cervical medial branch blocks, medial branch neurotomy, interlaminar epidural steroid injections for cervical radiculopathy, transforaminal epidural steroid injections for cervical root pain, sacroiliac intraarticular injections, intradiscal electrothermal therapy for chronic discogenic low back pain, automated percutaneous lumbar discectomy and percutaneous laser discectomy, vertebroplasty, and kyphoplasty. Limited evidence for the use of cervical facet injections, caudal epidural steroid injections for post-lumbar laminectomy syndrome, transforaminal epidural steroid injections for pain secondary to lumbar post-laminectomy syndrome or spinal stenosis, radiofrequency neurotomy for sacroiliac joint pain, annuloplasty for chronic discogenic low back pain, nucleoplasty, and DeKompressor technology [65]. Taken as a whole, guidelines offer strategies for the management of pain.

Medications

Axiomatically, starting any new medication slowly, increasing dosages slowly, considering implications of cytochrome P-450 mediated oxidative metabolism when new medications are given to older people already taking a number of agents for their underlying medical conditions, and dealing with lower rates of elimination due to renal changes will make pain treatment more challenging and potentially less forgiving for older people [66, 67, 68, 69]. This is not to say that pain cannot be effectively managed, or that practitioners should be so conservative that undertreatment is acceptable, but to suggest that the management of pain in older people is not the same as it is for younger people, requiring more consideration, and more use of rational polypharmacy.

Complementary and Alternative Medicine (CAM)

Complementary and alternative (also described as integrative medicine) approaches to pain management play an especially important role in aging individuals worldwide. In the United States, the use of these modalities by patients of all age groups has significantly escalated over the past decade [70, 71, 72]. For instance, despite the fact that musculoskeletal disorders are commonplace and potentially disabling in older adults, safe, effective treatment may be elusive. Nonsteroidal antiinflammatory drugs (NSAIDs), the most common medications used to treat pain associated with arthritis, often lead to serious morbidity and mortality in older adults [73, 74]. Opioids, while effective analgesics, may also have hazardous side effects, including obstipation, delirium, impaired mobility, and falls [75, 76, 77, 78]..

Even when medications are tolerated, pain associated with fibromyalgia and myofascial pathology may be particularly recalcitrant to opioids [79]. When pharmacological options are not available or tolerated, the older adult often believes that suffering is inevitable. Recently, it has been estimated that two thirds of individuals suffering from pain associated with arthritis and other musculoskeletal disorders have used complementary and alternative treatments to control their symptoms [80]. Most third-party payers do not reimburse patients for the cost of many of these approaches [81, 82, 83, 84, 85].

Herbal medicines are among the most popular forms of complementary treatments. In the US, the herbal market's annual turnover exceeds $1.5 billion and grows each year by approximately 25% [86]. Between 1990 and 1997, the use of herbal remedies in the US increased by 380% with a large proportion used for musculoskeletal pain [87]. Many consumers believe that herbal medicines are natural and therefore safe. The truth is that all such treatments have been associated with numerous, diverse adverse effects. This is hardly surprising considering the fact that medicinal herbs contain pharmacologically active ingredients [88]. Since herbals are considered food additives, and thereby unregulated, suboptimal product quality may present a serious safety issue. For mild to moderate pain, herbals have shown benefit. Discussing the risks and knowing the herb-drug interactions will help patients decide about this therapy [89].

Acupuncture is one of the most enduring of all complementary medicine modalities. The precise mechanism of action of acupuncture is unknown. Human and animal studies utilizing functional imaging of the central nervous system indicate that acupuncture engages the descending inhibitory system affecting afferent pathways [90, 91]. Insufficient experimental evidence exists to definitively recommend the use of acupuncture over traditional treatment of persistent musculoskeletal pain. Many studies are difficult to control, and acupuncture remains a safe and very popular alternative for the older pain patient. Judicious support for a pain patient seeking advice on acupuncture is warranted, bearing in mind the burden of cost [92, 93].

Spinal manipulation is a popular form of treatment used by chiropractors, osteopathic physicians, allopathic physicians, physiotherapists, and other healthcare professionals to treat musculoskeletal problems [94, 95, 96, 97].

The Cochrane Review recommended manipulation for acute and chronic back pain in 2005 [98]. A review of manipulation for chronic neck pain failed to demonstrate efficacy to recommend this technique [99]. There are many treatment options for older adults with persistent pain, but often these therapies are poorly tolerated or not beneficial. Given the enduring nature of complementary forms of analgesia and their popularity with patients, the potential for efficacy seems considerable. Until more research is available, providers can help patients decide whether to invest the money and time in CAM therapy and discuss safety issues [100, 101, 102, 103, 104, 105].

Pain Management in Long-Term Care Facilities

The goals of nursing home care vary widely from short-term rehabilitation, to short-term hospice care, to long-term custodial care with an average length of stay of 2 years. This number is deceiving since large number of patients stay 6 months, approximately 20% stay longer than 5 years, and about 20% of discharges are ultimately secondary to death. Nursing homes account for more than twice as many beds as acute care hospitals, and there are more than 3 times as many facilities in the US [106, 107, 108, 109, 110, 111, 112, 113, 114, 115, 116, 117, 118].

Residents of nursing homes are typically poor, very disabled, and funded with Medicaid providing more than 50% of the reimbursement and 45% of care is paid for out of the pockets of these residents. It has also been estimated that for every resident in nursing homes, there are 3 disabled persons living at home, or in other long-term care facilities, relying on family caregivers and community resources for their dependency needs [119].

Barriers

While the effective assessment and management of pain should be a clinical priority; the improvement of pain management in long-term care facilities presents unique barriers. Most of the care is delivered by nurses' aides with little or no formal medical education and no formal training in pain management. Staffing turnover can be more than 150% per year. Physicians play a minor role in directing resources and quality improvement in many facilities since they see patients only every 30 days and with no organized medical staff [120].

Unique challenges for optimal pain management are present for providers of older long term care residents. The spectrum of complaints, manifestations of disease and distress, and determination of differential diagnoses are often difficult. Older persons present with multiple medical problems, many of which are irreversible, and expectations for cure or recovery are disappointing. Unlike a younger population, aggressive testing for a definitive diagnosis or implementation of complicated treatment protocols is less important than providing comfort and effective symptom management, especially near the end of life [121].

The initial assessment may also be difficult since medical records may be incomplete, and consultants are not accessible; diagnostic laboratories, radiographs, or other resources are commonly not available. Transportation to needed services results in missed meals, missed medications, and diagnostic records that are misplaced [120].

Assessing pain can also be a problem with a high incidence of vision and hearing impairments and more than 50% of people having significant cognitive impairment or psychological illness [124]. However, even moderate cognitively impaired residents can provide meaningful and reliable information if given the time and consideration of a sensitive clinician. If questions are concrete with yes or no answers, even the severe impaired can make their needs known. Pain experiences often wax and wane requiring frequent assessments instead of relying on memory [122]. Sometimes observation of behavior, information from caregivers, and other signs of distress may be needed when communication skills are lacking.

For example, cancer is a source of severe pain and distress among patients and staff, yet it is not nearly as prevalent an etiology of pain as arthritis. Pain is common among nursing home residents. Up to 80% of residents have substantial pain that may affect their functional status and quality of life [123].] Despite the prevalence, pain often is undertreated: Medicare and Medicaid data indicated that more than a quarter of nursing home residents with severe cancer pain did not receive any analgesic medication [124]. Pain for older people often leads to depression, decreased ability to socialize, sleep disturbance, decreases in ambulation, slow rehabilitation, and adverse effects from multiple drug prescriptions [125].

Medications for Pain

All long-term care residents with pain that compromises function or quality of life are candidates for analgesic medications, keeping in mind the inherent added risks in this population [126]. Non-opioid analgesics have high rates of side effects for frail long-term care residents. These patients have multiple risk factors and are sensitive to gastrointestinal bleeding from long-term use of nonsteroidal antiinflammatories. These agents should not be used in this population, especially in high doses for long periods [26, 127, 128, 129, 130].

Adjuvant analgesic medications such as tricyclic antidepressants, anticonvulsants, and other agents, also have an increased rate of side effects. More is known about tricyclic antidepressants for chronic pain than other adjuvants, yet most frail older patients exhibit substantial anticholinergic side effects from these medications, so should not take them. Newer antidepressants and anticonvulsants medications (eg, duloxetine, pregabalin) may be as effective for neuropathic pain problems with fewer overall side effects [9, 131]. Most nursing homes provide substantial exercise, recreation, and rehabilitation resources for their residents and should be part of the treatment plan [132]. Physical activities are vital to deconditioned older people with mobility deficits [133, 134, 135].

Providers of long-term care services must help establish a treatment plan that is reasonable given the limited resources and skills available. Medication regimens should be simplified when possible using long-acting medications whenever possible for better comfort and fewer doses for nurses to administer. Contingency plans for pain management are needed, taking into account delays in pain care during medication changes or dosage adjustments. Long-term care facilities also need substantial support from physicians and other pain experts for education to continuously update their skills and knowledge [136, 137].

Pain at the End of Life

Preparing for death is very important work for those providing care to dying people. Focus group participants noting preferences about their end-of-life care agree on the importance of naming someone to make medical decisions for them if they are not capable of making their own decisions, knowing what to expect about their physical condition, having their financial affairs in order, having their treatment preferences in writing, and knowing that their physicians are comfortable talking about death and dying [138, 139, 140, 141, 142, 143].

Patients, more so than their physicians, are interested in funeral planning and knowing the timing of their deaths, but are less likely than family members or physicians in wanting to discuss personal fears about dying [144, 145, 146, 147, 148, 149, 150].

This is mainly because death in America has mostly occurred within institutional settings, generally without the benefit of meaningful psychiatric, psychological, and social services [151, 152, 153, 154, 155].

The Study to Understand Prognoses and Preferences for Outcomes and Risks of Treatments (SUPPORT) found that more than half of American patients suffered from inadequate pain control, a quarter from emotional distress, and almost a quarter from social isolation and feelings of abandonment. Their family members perceived that health care providers did not seem to listen to them or to relieve the suffering of their loved ones. Patients and loved ones alike wanted enhanced quality of life, not extended quantity, as death approached [156]. Chart reviews in 1 study noted that only 46% had comfort care plans (when present they were initiated 15 days after admission on average); those having such comfort care plans in place were often still receiving antibiotics (41%) and blood draws (30%) [157]. Many things done for hospitalized patients, especially those who were terminally ill, were very painful; why such things were done to these people was not clear or perhaps not even warranted.

Evaluating the quality of dying and death relative to what experience is desired leads to an appreciation of certain key domains: symptom management and personal care, preparation for death, moment of death, family involvement, treatment preferences, and other "whole person" concerns [158]. Other factors defining quality end-of-life care include providing desired physical comfort, helping patients control decisions about medical care and daily routines, relieving family members of the burden of being present at all times, educating family members so they feel confident to care for their loved ones, and providing emotional support for family members before and after the patient's death [159]. Addressing these patient and family expectations necessitates a team approach more than a single well-intentioned practitioner, no matter how well-trained the practitioner might be. Psychological support along with top notch medical and nursing care, pharmacological consultation, and spiritual service truly make for successful outcome in the care of patients facing the end of their lives.

A 5-step adaptational process has been described for patients learning they are terminally ill: shock and denial, anger, bargaining, depression, and acceptance. This formulation assumes that patients work through the steps without necessarily moving through them in a linear sequence. The goals of treatment for these people include addressing their unfinished life's business while simultaneously helping them maintaining hope [160].

Seven themes characteristics about dying come from interviews with terminally ill people: struggle (living and dying are difficult), dissonance (dying is not living), endurance (triumph of inner strength), coping (finding a new balance), incorporation (belief system accommodates death), quest (seeking meaning in death), and volatile (unresolved and unresigned) [161]. Exploring these perspectives gives powerful evidence that dying itself must be integrated into the lives of the terminally ill, along with all of their other experiences, suggesting that more effective interventions are possible with these people.

Considerations for patients with potentially terminally diagnoses usually center on telling them exactly what is happening to them (delivering the "bad news"), maintaining the truth about the situation despite the discomfort it often produces for everyone involved, not being pushed off of truth by patients demanding other explanations and prognoses, and preserving hope while helping families prepare for the worst [162]. These challenges require effective communication between caregivers, patients and family members. With bothersome symptoms occurring during dying process, preserving emotional well being may be one of the most critical tasks for the caregivers providing end-of-life care.

Consideration may be given for a variety of therapeutic interventions early on in a patient's end-of-life care; many things may be tried, often rather quickly, to improve the overall quality of life. The treatment goal is to provide care consistent with the overall care plan established with the patient, family and professional caregivers. Patients may need to undergo medical and behavioral assessments, with these assessments leading to patient categorizations such as having no contraindications to the therapy proposed, having contraindications due to behavioral issues, having relative contraindications but still being considered for having a trial, or being completely unsuitable [163].

The experience of pain in older dying patients is multifactorial. Factors contributing to the pain experienced by older dying people include the nature of their underlying medical conditions, the adverse pathophysiology of their terminal disease, causes for breakthrough pain, impact of care procedures, numerous emotional and cognitive states, and the response of others to their pain. To alleviate pain the caregivers must provide optimal analgesic management using around-the-clock dosing for constant pain, backed up by breakthrough medications, while providing much needed comfort measures, attempting treatment for underlying causes, anticipating future pain occurrences and preemptively addressing them, using nonpharmacological interventions along with medications, correcting depression and anxiety, maintaining hope, and giving compassionate and respectful care [164].

Hospice Versus Palliative Care

With the majority of US hospice care provided in patients' own homes [165], and with other forms of end-of-life care (palliative care) provided in long-term care facilities and specialized inpatient acute care hospitals, access to specialized routes of administration and technology for the safest delivery of analgesics and anesthetics may not be available (see also Hallenbeck and McDaniel, this volume). These circumstances lead to the belief that oral or transdermal routes of administration are more desirable for most terminally patients. Once we understand what patients are telling us about their pain, moving through some process leads to better overall pain management. The schema of the former Agency for Health Care Policy and Research (AHCPR), incorporates recommendations of the World Health Organization, and advocates for a step-by-step approach to pain relief beginning with antiinflammatory and mild analgesics (aspirin, acetaminophen and non-steroidal agents), progressing to combinations involving opioids and the previously tried medications, moving on to single-entity opioids, employing selective neurodestructive or neurostimulatory procedures, novel routes of administration, and the considerable use of many adjuvant medications [166, 167]. Other key aspects of controlling pain in end-of-life care include using oral medications whenever possible, giving these medications around the clock and from the appropriate step of the so called "WHO analgesic ladder," providing adequate "rescue doses" for breakthrough pain, effectively converting medications and routes of administration using equianalgesic dosing, anticipating and treating side effects early, continuing to modify the disease process, and offering simple-to-follow instructions [168].

Adjuvant medications (anticonvulsants, antidepressants, antipsychotics, anxiolytics, and stimulants) are remarkable agents modulating the release and presence of neurotransmitters and influencing binding at their receptor sites [169]. Of the adjuvants, anticonvulsants, older tricyclic antidepressants, and newer serotonin and norepinephrine reuptake inhibitors (more than the pure selective serotonin reuptake inhibitors) have been quite effective in the management of cancer pain whether patients are depressed or not [170].

Providing the Best Care at the End of Life

Dying in pain is not a natural consequence of the dying process, but it is common for older people with advanced diseases to experience moderate to severe levels of pain. Not relieving pain is recognized as more than just medical failure; it is now viewed as an ethical and legal failure [171]. (see also Rich, This volume) The belief that physicians are obligated to relieve human suffering [172], coupled with decisions in Oregon and California (medical board disciplinary action in California and a monetary judgment by an Oregon jury against physicians undertreating pain associated with terminal illness), makes it very clear that Americans are no longer tolerant of practitioners who under treat pain, especially when it is part of the suffering of dying family members.

To better care for older people in pain near the end of their lives practitioners must think beyond the use of the 3 well-described analgesic steps (anti-inflammatory analgesics for mild pain, lower potency combinations with acetaminophen or ibuprofen plus opioid analgesics for moderate pain, and high-potency, single-entity opioid analgesics backed up with adjuvants for severe pain). Physicians caring for these people must receive proper clinically oriented education to enable them to accurately determine the causes for pain, improve their evaluation strategies to identify pain syndromes, and make the adequate amount of time available to conduct the evaluations properly [173]. Education, evaluation, and taking sufficient time make the accuracy of the diagnosis and the effectiveness of pain treatments using the analgesic steps more likely.

Conclusions

Pain in older patients is often underreported, underdiagnosed, under evaluated and consequently, undertreated. While significant barriers exist, clinicians have a duty to relieve pain and suffering even when unable to cure the underlying pathology. Pain and suffering are feared most at the end of life [156]. Dying in pain, filled with depression, being afraid of abandonment, and wishing death would come sooner, should be understood to reflect unrecognized and untreated pain and/or psychiatric co-morbidities. The majority do not chose to become palliative care experts, yet elements of palliative care must be provided by nearly all clinicians for their patients.

An enhanced understanding of the experience of pain in older persons, strategies for assessment and appropriate use of pharmacologic and non-pharmacologic approaches (including complementary and alternative thera-pies as an adjuvant to conventional treatments) are necessary to improve management of pain in this population. More valid and reliable pain measures are necessary as are new drugs with milder side effects. Nondrug strategies require further investigation for this highly disabled population. These regimens should also be simplified as much as possible. Long-acting medications are often best to provide longer durations of comfort and fewer doses for nurses or other caregivers to administer. As the need for health systems for frail older persons continues to grow, it is our most important obligation to provide comfort and effective pain control appro-priate for these new settings.

Future Directions

Nowhere in pain management is there such an acute need as in the care of the older person. Myths and biases, from providers and patients, persist and the consequence is needless suffering that occurs daily under the label of "nothing can be done", or "I am old and should feel this pain". The aging baby boomers will force a change in this attitude resulting in needed research and more clinical studies. For example, the 85 year and older population has very few pharmacologic trials yet is one of the fasting growing populations sectors in society. As a consequence, there is limited data to provide answers to the following questions if an elderly patient responds the same to combination drug therapy; are complimentary and alternative therapies effective; does side effects outweigh benefits for treatment; and, are behavioral and lifestyle interventions as effective as in a younger population? These are just a few of the questions which desperately need outcomes research in order to provide the required therapy for our geriatric patients. Since the majority will be spending some time in a nursing home, how will pain care improve since it is poorly managed now?

The future always holds uncertainty except that pain will be undertreated and that quality of life will be impacted unless there is more research and aggressive management strategies. We should all be lobbying for this informa-tion for your patients, our families and ourselves.

References

1. Centers for Disease Control. *Healthy Aging: Preventing Disease and Improving Quality of Life Among Older Americans*. Atlanta, GA: CDC; 2001.
2. Otis JAD, McGeeney B. Managing pain in the older. *Clin Geriatr* 2001;9:82–88.
3. Ferrell BA, Ferrell BR, Osterweil D. Pain in the nursing home. *J Am Geriatr Soc* 1990;38:409–414.
4. Ferrell BA. Pain management in older people. *J Am Geriatr Soc* 1991;39:64–73.
5. Stein WM, Miech RP. Cancer pain in the older hospice patient. *J Pain Symptom Manage* 1993;8:474–482.
6. Ferrell BA. Pain evaluation and management in the nursing home. *Ann Intern Med* 1995;123:681–687.
7. Mobily P, Herr K. Barriers to managing resident's pain. *Contemp Long Term Care* 1996;19:60A–60B.
8. Gaston-Johansson F, Johansson F, Johansson N. Undertreatment of pain in the older: causes and prevention. *Ann Long-Term Care* 1999;7:190–196.
9. American Geriatrics Society Panel on Chronic Pain in Older Persons. AGS clinical practice guidelines: the management of chronic pain in older persons. *J Am Geriatr Soc* 1998;46:635–651.
10. American Medical Directors Association. *Chronic Pain Management in the Long-Term Care Setting: Clinical Practice Guideline*. Baltimore, MD: American Medical Directors Association; 1999.
11. Schuckit MA. Geriatric alcoholism and drug abuse. *Gerontologist* 1977;17:168–174.
12. Jacox A, Carr DB, Payne R, et al. *Management of Cancer Pain. Clinical Practice Guideline Number 9*. Rockville, MD: Agency for Health Care and Policy Research; US Department of Health and Human Services; 1994: AHCPR Publication No. 94-0592.
13. Fulmer TT, Mion LC, Bottrell MM. Pain management protocol. *Geriatr Nurs* 1996;17:222–227.
14. Verdu E, Ceballos D, Vilches JJ, Navarro X. Influence of aging on peripheral nerve function and regeneration. *J Peripher Nerv Syst* 2000;5(4):191–208.
15. Alder G, Nacimiento AC. Age-dependent changes in short-latency somatosensory evoked potentials in healthy adults. *Appl Neurophysiol* 1988;51:55–59.
16. Prineas JW, Spencer PS. Pathology of the nerve cell body in disorders of the peripheral nervous system. In: *Peripheral Neuropathy*. Edited by Dyck PJ, Thomas PK, Lambert EH. Philadelphia, PA: W B Saunders; 1975: 253–295.
17. Bergman E, Johnson H, Zhang X, Hokfelt T, Ulfhake B. Neuropeptides and neurotrophin receptor mRNAs in primary sensory neurons of aged rats. *J Comp Neurol* 1996;375(2):303–319.
18. Hukkanen M, Platts LA, Corbett SA, Santavirta S, Polak JM, Konttinen YT. Reciprocal age-related changes in GAP-43/B-50, substance P and calcitonin gene-related peptide (CGRP) expression in rat primary sensory neurones and their terminals in the dorsal horn of the spinal cord and subintima of the knee synovium. *Neurosci Res* 2002;42(4):251–260.
19. Ko ML, King MA, Gordon TL, Crisp T. The effects of aging on spinal neurochemistry in the rat. *Brain Res Bull* 1997;42(2):95–98
20. Iwata K, Fukuoka T, Kondo E, Tsuboi Y, Tashiro A, Noguchi K, et al. Plastic changes in nociceptive transmission of the rat spinal cord with advancing age. *J Neurophysiol* 2002;87(2):1086–1093.
21. Chapman CR, Casey KL, Dubner R, Foley KM, Gracely RH, Reading AE. Pain measurement: an overview. *Pain* 1985;22:1–231.
22. Gracely RH, Lota L, Walter DJ, Dubner R. A multiple random staircase method of psychophysical pain assessment. *Pain* 1988;32(1):55–63.

23. Gagliese L, Melzack R. Age differences in nociception and pain behaviours in the rat. *Neurosci Biobehav Rev* 2000;24(8):843–54
24. Cruce WL, Lovell JA, Crisp T, Stuesse SL. Effect of aging on the substance P receptor, NK-1, in the spinal cord of rats with peripheral nerve injury. *Somatosens Mot Res* 2001;18(1):66–75.
25. Herr, KA. Pain assessment in the older adult with verbal communication skills. In *Pain in Older Persons. Progress in Pain Research and Management, Vol 35*. Edited by Gibson SJ, Weiner DK. Seattle, WA: IASP Press;2005:111–133.
26. American Geriatrics Society Panel on Persistent Pain in Older Persons. Clinical practice guidelines: the management of persistent pain in older persons. *J Am Geriatr Soc* 2002;50:S205–S224.
27. Steinhauser KE, Christakis NA, Clipp EC, et al. Preparing for the end of life: preferences of patients, families, physicians and other care providers. *J Pain Symptom Manage* 2001; 22(3):727–737.
28. Morrison RS, Ahronheim JC, Morrison GR, Darling E, Baskin SA, Morris J, Choi C, Meier DE. Pain and discomfort associated with common hospital procedures and experiences. *J Pain Symptom Manage* 1998;15:91–101.
29. Goodlin SJ. Care of the older patient with pain. *Current Pain Headache Reports* 2004; 8:277–280.
30. Gagliese L, Katz J. Age differences in postoperative pain are scale dependent: a comparison of measures of pain intensity and quality in younger and older surgical patients. *Pain* 2003;103:11–20.
31. Gagliese L, Weizblit N, Ellis W, Chan VWS. The measurement of postoperative pain: a comparison of intensity scales in younger and older surgical patients. *Pain* 2005;117:412–420.
32. Harari D, Martin FC, Buttery A, O'neill S, Hopper A. The older persons' assessment and liaison team 'OPAL': evaluation of comprehensive geriatric assessment in acute medical inpatients. Age Aging. 2007 Jul 26.
33. Hadjistavropoulos T. Assessing pain in older persons with severe limitations in ability to communication. In *Pain in Older Persons. Progress in Pain Research and Management, Vol 35*. Edited by Gibson SJ, Weiner DK. Seattle, WA: IASP Press;2005:135–151.
34. Geda YE, Rummans TA. Pain: cause of agitation in elderly individuals with dementia. *Am J Psychiatry* 1999;156(10):1662–1663.
35. Morrison RS. A comparison of pain and its treatment in advanced dementia and cognitively intact patients with hip fracture. *J Pain Symptom Manage* 2000;9:240–248.
36. Hansson RO. Old age: testing the parameters of social psychological assumptions. In *The Social Psychology of Aging*. Edited by Spacapan S, Oskamp S. Newbury, CA: Sage; 1989: 25–52.
37. Lingard EA, Riddle DL. Impact of psychological distress on pain and function following knee arthroplasty. *J Bone Joint Surg Am*. 2007;89(6):1161–9.
38. Simonsick EM. Demography of productive aging. In *Promoting Successful and Productive Aging*. Edited by Bond LA, Cutler SJ, Grams A. Thousand Oaks, CA: Sage; 1995: 69–90.
39. Grams A. Primary prevention in the service of aging. In *Promoting Successful and Productive Aging*. Edited by Bond LA, Cutler SJ, Grams A. Thousand Oaks, CA: Sage; 1995: 5–35.
40. Meeks S. Mental illness in late life: socioeconomic conditions, psychiatric symptoms, and adjustment of long-term sufferers. *Psychol Aging* 1997;12:296–308.
41. Chappell NL. Informal social support. In *Promoting Successful and Productive Aging*. Edited by Bond LA, Cutler SJ, Grams A. Thousand Oaks, CA: Sage; 1995: 171–185.
42. Sorkin BA, Rudy TE, Hanlon RB, Turk DC, Steig RI. Chronic pain in old and young patients: differences appear less important than similarities. *J Gerontol* 1990;45:64–68.
43. Watkins KW, Shifren K, Park DC, Morrell, RW. Age, pain, and coping with rheumatoid arthritis. *Pain* 1999;82:217–228.

44. Parmalee PA. Measuring mood and psychosocial function associated with pain in late life. In *Pain in Older Persons. Progress in Pain Research and Management, Vol 35*. Edited by Gibson SJ, Weiner DK. Seattle, WA: IASP Press; 2005:175–202.
45. Chou KL. Reciprocal relationship between pain and depression in older adults: Evidence from the English Longitudinal Study of Aging. *J Affect Disord* 2007;102(1–3):115–23.
46. Geerlings SW, Twisk JW, Beekman AT, Deeg DJ, van Tilburg W. Longitudinal relationship between pain and depression in older adults: sex, age and physical disability. *Soc Psychiatry Psychiatr Epidemiol* 2002 Jan;37(1):23–30.
47. Richelson E. Pharmacology of antidepressants. *Mayo Clin Proc* 2001, 76:511–527.
48. Lloyd-Williams M, Friedman T, Rudd N. An analysis of the validity of the hospital anxiety and depression scale as a screening tool in patients with advanced metastatic cancer. *J Pain Symptom Manage* 2001;22(6):990–996.
49. von Ammon Cavanaugh S, Furlanetto LM, Creech SD, Powell, LH. Medical illness, past depression, and present depression: a predictive triad for in-hospital mortality. *Am J Psychiatry* 2001; 158:43–48.
50. Bishop KL, Ferraro FR, Borowiak DM. Pain management in older adults: role of fear and avoidance. *Clin Gerontol* 2001;23(1–2):33–42.
51. Wolfe R. Mood disorders in older adults. In *The Practical Handbook of Clinical Gerontology*. Edited by Carstensen LL, Edelstein BA, Dornbrand L. Thousand Oaks, CA: Sage; 1996: 274–303.
52. Waters SJ, Woodward JT, Keefe FJ. Cognitive-behavioral therapy for pain in older adults. In *Pain in Older Persons. Progress in Pain Research and Management, Vol 35*. Edited by Gibson SJ, Weiner DK. Seattle, WA: IASP Press; 2005:239–261.
53. Blazer DG. Depression in late life: review and commentary. *J Gerontol A Biol Sci Med Sci* 2003;58:M249–M265.
54. Gibson MC. Pain in the elderly: psychosocial issues. *Curr Pain Headache Rep* 1998; 2:29–40.
55. Satin DG. The interdisciplinary, integrated approach to professional practice with the aged. In *The Clinical Care of the Aged Person: An Interdisciplinary Perspective*. Edited by Satin DG. New York: Oxford University Press; 1994: 391–403.
56. Pereira J, Bruera E. Depression with psychomotor retardation: diagnostic challenges and the use of psychostimulants. *J Pall Med* 2001;4(1):15–21.
57. Nicassio PM, Moxham EG, Schuman CE, Gevirtz RN. The contribution of pain, reported sleep quality, and depressive symptoms in fibromyalgia. *Pain* 2002;100;271–279.
58. Fishbain DA, Cole B, Cutler RB, Lewis J, Rosomoff HL, Steele-Rosamoff R. Is pain fatiguing? A structured evidence-based review. *Pain Medicine* 2005;4:51–62.
59. Reyes-Gibby CC, Mendoza TR, Wang S, Anderson KO, Cleeland CS. Pain and fatigue in community-dwelling adults. *Pain Medicine* 2003;4231–237.
60. Fishbain DA, Cutler RB, Cole B, Lewis J, Smets E, Rosomoff HL, Steele-Rosamoff R. Are patients with chronic lower back pain or chronic neck pain fatigued? *Pain Medicine* 2004;5:187–195.
61. Fishbain DA, Lewis J, Cole B, Cutler , Smets E, Rosomoff HL, Steele-Rosomoff R. Multidisciplinary pain facility treatment outcome for pain-associated fatigue. *Pain Medicine*. 2005;6:299–304.
62. Dworkin RH, Backonja M, Rowbotham MC, Allen RR, Argoff CR, Bennett GJ, Bushnell MC, Farrar JT, Galer BS, Haythornthwaite JA, Hewitt DJ, Loeser JD, Max MB, Saltarelli M, Schmader KE, Stein C, Thompson D, Turk DC, Wallace MS, Watkins LR, Weinstein SM. Advances in neuropathic pain: diagnosis, mechanisms, and treatment recommendations. *Arch Neurol*. 2003;60(11):1524–1534.
63. Argoff CE, Backonja M-M, Belgrade MJ, Bennett GJ, Clark MR, Cole BE, Fishbain DA, Irving GA, McCarberg BH, McLean MJ, DPNP consensus guidelines: treatment planning and options. *Mayo Clin Proc* (suppl) 2006,81(4):S12–S25.

64. Boswell MV, Trescot AM, Datta S, et al. Interventional techniques: evidence-based practice guidelines in the management of chronic spinal pain. *Pain Physician* 2007; 10;7–111.
65. Harari D, Hopper A, Dhesi J, Babic-Illman G, Lockwood L, Martin F. Proactive care of older people undergoing surgery ('POPS'): designing, embedding,evaluating and funding a comprehensive geriatric assessment service for olderelective surgical patients. *Age Aging* 2007;36(2):190–6.
66. Lewis LD, Miller AA, Rosner GL, Dowell JE, Valdivieso M, Relling MV, Egorin MJ, Bies RR, Hollis DR, Levine EG, Otterson GA, Millard F, Ratain MJ; Cancer and Leukemia Group B. A comparison of the pharmacokinetics and pharmacodynamics of docetaxel between African-American and Caucasian cancer patients: CALGB 9871. *Clin Cancer Res* 2007;13(11):3302–11.
67. Taniguchi A, Urano W, Tanaka E, Furihata S, Kamitsuji S, Inoue E, Yamanaka M, Yamanaka H, Kamatani N. Validation of the associations between single nucleotide polymorphisms or haplotypes and responses to disease-modifying antirheumatic drugs in patients with rheumatoid arthritis: a proposal for prospective pharmacogenomic study in clinical practice. *Pharmacogenet Genomics* 2007;17(6):383–90.
68. Grimaldi MP, Vasto S, Balistreri CR, di Carlo D, Caruso M, Incalcaterra E, Lio D, Caruso C, Candore G. Genetics of inflammation in age-related atherosclerosis: its relevance to pharmacogenomics. *Ann N Y Acad Sci* 2007;1100:123–31.
69. Shah RR. Drug development and use in the elderly: search for the right dose and dosing regimen (Parts I and II). *Br J Clin Pharmacol* 2004;58(5):452–69.
70. Eisenberg DM, Davis RB, Ettner SL, Appel S, Wilkey S, Van Rompay M, et al. Trends in alternative medicine use in the United States, 1990–1997: results of a follow-up national survey. *J Am Med Assoc* 1998;280:1569–1575.
71. Morone NE, Greco CM, Weiner DK. Mindfulness meditation for the treatment of chronic low back pain in older adults: A randomized controlled pilot study. *Pain* 2008;134(3):310–319.
72. Thornberry T, Schaeffer J, Wright PD, Haley MC, Kirsh KL. An exploration of the utility of hypnosis in pain management among rural pain patients. *Palliat Support Care* 2007;5(2):147–52.
73. Brater DC. Effects of nonsteroidal anti-inflammatory drugs on renal function: focus on cyclooxygenase-2-selective inhibition. *Am J Med* 1999;107(suppl 6A):65S–71S.
74. Jasperson D. Drug-induced oseophageal disorders. Pathogenesis, incidence, prevention and management. *Drug Safety* 2000;22:237–249.
75. Shorr RI, Griffin MR, Daugherty JR, Ray WA. Opioid analgesics and the risk of hip fracture in the older: codeine and propoxyphene. *J Gerontol* 1992;47:M111–M115.
76. Weiner D, Hanlon JT, Studenski S. CNS drug-related falls liability in community dwelling older. *Gerontology* 1998;44:217–221.
77. Portenoy RK, Sibirceva U, Smout R, Horn S, Connor S, Blum RH, Spence C, Fine PG. Opioid use and survival at the end of life: a survey of a hospice population. *J Pain Symptom Manage* 2006;32(6):532–40.
78. Moryl N, Kogan M, Comfort C, Obbens E. Methadone in the treatment of pain and terminal delirum in advanced cancer patients. *Palliat Support Care* 2005;3(4):311–7).
79. Peng WL, Wu GJ, Sun WZ, Chen JC, Huang AT. Multidisciplinary management of cancer pain: a longitudinal retrospective study on a cohort of end-stage cancer patients. *J Pain Symptom Manage* 2006;32(5):444–52.
80. Rao JK, Mihaliak K, Kroenke K, Bradley J, Tierney WM, Weinberger M. Use of complementary therapies for arthritis among patients of rheumatologists. *Ann Int Med* 1999;131(6):409–416.
81. Lind BK, Abrams C, Lafferty WE, Diehr PK, Grembowski DE. The effect of complementary and alternative medicine claims on risk adjustment. *Med Care* 2006;44(12):1078–84.
82. Lafferty WE, Tyree PT, Bellas AS, Watts CA, Lind BK, Sherman KJ, Cherkin DC, Grembowski DE. Insurance coverage and subsequent utilization of complementary and alternative medicine providers. *Am J Manag Care* 2006 Jul;12(7):397–404.

83. Bracha Y, Svendsen K, Culliton P. Patient visits to a hospital-based alternative medicine clinic from 1997 through 2002: experience from an integrated healthcare system. *Explore* (NY). 2005;1(1):13–20.

84. Steyer TE, Freed GL, Lantz PM. Medicaid reimbursement for alternative therapies. *Altern Ther Health Med* 2002;8(6):84–8.

85. Astin JA, Pelletier KR, Marie A, Haskell WL. Complementary and alternative medicine use among elderly persons: one-year analysis of a Blue Shield Medicare supplement. *J Gerontol A Biol Sci Med Sci* 2000;55(1):M4–9).

86. Muller JL, Clauson KA. Pharmaceutical considerations of common herbal medicine. *Am J Managed Care* 1997;3:1753–1770.

87. Ernst E. Usage of complementary therapies in rheumatology. A systematic review. *Clin Rheumatology* 1998;17:301–305.

88. Ernst E. Toxic heavy metals and undeclared drugs in Asian herbal medicines. *Trends Pharmacol Sci* 2002;23:136–139.

89. Cappuzzo KA. Herbal product use in a patient with polypharmacy. *Consult Pharm* 2006;21(11):911–5.

90. Wu MT, Hsieh JC, Xiong J, Yang CF, Pan HB, Chen YC, Tsai G, Rosen BR, Kwong KK. Central nervous pathway for acupuncture stimulation: localization of processing with functional MR imaging of the brain-preliminary experience. *Radiology* 1999;212:1133–1141.

91. Han JS. Neurochemical basis of acupuncture. *Annu Rev Pharmacol Toxicol* 1982;22:193–220.

92. Foltz V, St Pierre Y, Rozenberg S, Rossignol M, Bourgeois P, Joseph L, Adam V,Penrod JR, Clarke AE, Fautrel B. Use of complementary and alternative therapies by patients with self-reported chronic back pain: a nationwide survey in Canada. *Joint Bone Spine* 2005;72(6):571–7.

93. Quandt SA, Chen H, Grzywacz JG, Bell RA, Lang W, Arcury TA. Use of complementary and alternative medicine by persons with arthritis: results of the National Health Interview Survey. *Arthritis Rheum* 2005;53(5):748–55.

94. Sharma R, Haas M, Stano M. Patient attitudes, insurance, and other determinants of self-referral to medical and chiropractic physicians. Am J Public Health. 2003;93(12):2111–7.

95. Christensen HW, Vach W, Gichangi A, Manniche C, Haghfelt T, Hoilund-Carlsen PF. Cervicothoracic angina identified by case history and palpation findings in patients with stable angina pectoris. *J Manipulative Physiol Ther* 2005;28(5):303–11.

96. Ea HK, Weber AJ, Yon F, Liote F. Osteoporotic fracture of the dens revealed by cervical manipulation. *Joint Bone Spine* 2004;71(3):246–50.

97. Hawk C, Long CR, Boulanger KT, Morschhauser E, Fuhr AW. Chiropractic care for patients aged 55 years and older: report from a practice-based research program. *J Am Geriatr Soc* 2000;48(5):534–45.

98. *The Cochrane Library* 2005, Issue 4.

99. Ernst E. Chiropractic spinal manipulation for neck pain – a systematic review. Submitted for Publication 2002.

100. Buck T, Baldwin CM, Schwartz GE. Influence of worldview on health care choices among persons with chronic pain. *J Altern Complement Med* 2005;11(3):561–8.

101. Kim S, Hohrmann JL, Clark S, Munoz KN, Braun JE, Doshi A, Radeos MS, Camargo CA Jr. A multicenter study of complementary and alternative medicine usage among ED patients. *Acad Emerg Med* 2005;12(4):377–80.

102. Okmen E, Gurol T, Erdinler I, Sanli A, Cam N. new-onset conduction defects and their relationship with in-hospital major cardiac events in unstable angina pectoris. *Coron Artery Dis* 2003;14(8):521–5.

103. Williamson AT, Fletcher PC, Dawson KA. Complementary and alternative medicine. Use in an older population. *J Gerontol Nurs* 2003;29(5):20–8.

104. Fautrel B, Adam V, St-Pierre Y, Joseph L, Clarke AE, Penrod JR. Use of complementary and alternative therapies by patients self-reporting arthritis or rheumatism: results from a nationwide canadian survey. *J Rheumatol* 2002;29(11):2435–41.

105. Gray CM, Tan AW, Pronk NP, O'Connor PJ. Complementary and alternative medicine use among health plan members. A cross-sectional survey. *Eff Clin Pract* 2002;5(1):17–22).
106. Francoeur RB, Payne R, Raveis VH, Shim H. Palliative care in the inner city. Patient religious affiliation, underinsurance, and symptom attitude. *Cancer* 2007 Jan 15;109(2 Suppl):425–34.
107. Stevenson KM, Dahl JL, Berry PH, Beck SL, Griffie J. Institutionalizing effective pain management practices: practice change programs to improve the quality of pain management in small health care organizations. *Pain Symptom Manage* 2006;31(3):248–61.
108. Alexander BJ, Plank P, Carlson MB, Hanson P, Picken K, Schwebke K. Methods of pain assessment in residents of long-term care facilities: a pilot study. *J Am Med Dir Assoc* 2005;6(2):137–43.
109. Tarzian AJ, Hoffmann DE. Barriers to managing pain in the nursing home: findings from a statewide survey. *J Am Med Dir Assoc* 2005;6(3 Suppl):S13–9.
110. Molony SL, Kobayashi M, Holleran EA, Mezey M. Assessing pain as a fifth vital sign in long-term care facilities: Recommendations from the field. *J Gerontol Nurs* 2005;31(3):16–24.
111. Fox P, Solomon P, Raina P, Jadad A. Barriers and facilitators in pain management in long-term care institutions: a qualitative study. *Can J Aging* 2004;23(3):269–80.
112. Winn PA, Dentino AN. Effective pain management in the long-term care setting. *J Am Med Dir Assoc* 2004;5(5):342–52.
113. Ferrell BA. The management of pain in long-term care. *Clin J Pain* 2004;20(4):240–3.
114. Resnick B, Quinn C, Baxter S. Testing the feasibility of implementation of clinical practice guidelines in long-term care facilities. *J Am Med Dir Assoc* 2004;5(1):1–8.
115. Weissman DE, Griffie J, Muchka S, Matson S. Improving pain management in long-term care facilities. *J Palliat Med* 2001;4(4):567–73.
116. Mrozek JE, Werner JS. Nurses' attitudes toward pain, pain assessment, and pain management practices in long-term care facilities. *Pain Manag Nurs* 2001;2(4):154–62.
117. Ferrell BA.Pain management.Clin Geriatr Med. 2000;16(4):853–74; Pleschberger S. Dignity and the challenge of dying in nursing homes: the residents' view. *Age Aging* 2007;36(2):197–202.
118. Kushel MB, Miaskowski C. End-of-life care for homeless patients: "she says she is there to help me in any situation". *JAMA* 2006;296(24):2959–66.
119. Ouslander J, Osterweil D, Morley J. *Medical Care in the Nursing Home*, 2nd Ed New York, McGraw-Hill; 1997: 1–38.
120. Stein WM. Pain in the nursing home. *Clinics in Geriatric Medicine* 2001;17:575–594.
121. Ferrell BA. Overview of aging and pain. In *Pain in the Elderly*. Edited by Ferrell BA, Ferrell BR. Seattle, WA: IASP Press, 1996: 1–10.
122. Ferrell BA. Pain management. In *Principles of Geriatric Medicine and Gerontology*. Edited by Hazzard WR, Blass JP, Ettinger WH Jr, Halter JB, Ouslander JG. New York, McGraw-Hill, 1999: 413–433.
123. Helm RD, Gibson SJ, Pain in older people. In *Epidemiology of Pain*. Edited by Crombie IK, Croft PR, Linton SJ, LeResche L, Von Korff M. Seattle, WA: IASP Press; 1999: 103–112.
124. Ferrell BA. Pain evaluation and management in the nursing home. *Ann Intern Med* 1995;123:681–687.
125. Ferrell BA. Pain management in older people. *J Am Geriatr Soc* 1991;39:64–73.
126. Otto M, Bach FW, Jensen TS, Sindrup SH. Health-related quality of life and its predictive role for analgesic effect in patients with painful polyneuropathy. *Eur J Pain* 2007;11(5):572–8.
127. Bernabei R, Gambassi G, Lapane K, Landi F, Gatsonis C, Dunlop R, Lipsitz L, Steel K, Mor V. Management of pain in elderly patients with cancer. SAGE Study Group. Systematic Assessment of Geriatric Drug Use via Epidemiology. *JAMA* 1998;279(23):1877–82.
128. Pilotto A, Franceschi M, Vitale D, Zaninelli A, Masotti G, Rengo F; F.I.R.I. (Fondazione Italiana Ricerca Invecchiamento); SOFIA Project Investigators. Drug use by the

elderly in general practice: effects on upper gastrointestinalsymptoms. *Eur J Clin Pharmacol* 2006;62(1):65–73.

129. Boockvar KS, Carlson LaCorte H, Giambanco V, Fridman B, Siu A. Medication reconciliation for reducing drug-discrepancy adverse events. *Am J Geriatr Pharmacother* 2006 Sep;4(3):236–43.

130. Collins RJ, Brokaw DK. A 68-year-old woman with multiple NSAID-induced adverse effects. *Consult Pharm* 2005; 20(8):685–8).

131. Raskin J, Wiltse CG, Siegal A, Sheikh J, Xu J, Dinkel JJ, Rotz BT, Mohs RC. Efficacy of duloxetine on cognition, depression, and pain in elderly patients with major depressive disorder: an 8-week, double-blind, placebo-controlled trial. *Am J Psychiatry* 2007;164(6):900–9.

132. Ouslander JG, Osterweil D, Morley J. *Medical Care in the Nursing Home*, 2nd Ed. New York, McGraw-Hill; 1997: 391–417.

133. Robinson CL. Relieving pain in the elderly. Health Prog. 2007;88(1):48–53, 70.

134. Zyczkowska J, Szczerbinska K, Jantzi MR, Hirdes JP. Pain among the oldest old in community and institutional settings. Pain. 2007;129(1–2):167–76.

135. Vaurio LE, Sands LP, Wang Y, Mullen EA, Leung JM. Postoperative delirium: the importance of pain and pain management. *Anesth Analg* 2006;102(4):1267–73.

136. Rudy TE, Weiner DK, Lieber SJ, Slaboda J, Boston JR. The impact of chronic low back pain on older adults: A comparative study of patients and controls. *Pain* 2007.

137. Fallon WF Jr, Rader E, Zyzanski S, Mancuso C, Martin B, Breedlove L, DeGolia P, Allen K, Campbell J. Geriatric outcomes are improved by a geriatric trauma consultation service. *J Trauma* 2006;61(5):1040–6

138. Zapka JG, Carter R, Carter CL, Hennessy W, Kurent JE, DesHarnais S. Care at the end of life: focus on communication and race. *J Aging Health* 2006;18(6):791–813.

139. Teno JM, Gruneir A, Schwartz Z, Nanda A, Wetle T. Association between advance directives and quality of end-of-life care: a national study. *J Am Geriatr Soc* 2007;55(2):189–94.

140. Trask PC, Teno JM, Nash J. Transitions of care and changes in distressing pain. *J Pain Symptom Manage* 2006;32(2):104–9.

141. Conner TS, Tennen H, Zautra AJ, Affleck G, Armeli S, Fifield J. Coping with rheumatoid arthritis pain in daily life: within-person analysesreveal hidden vulnerability for the formerly depressed. *Pain* 2006;126(1–3):198–209.

142. Morrison LJ, Morrison RS. Palliative care and pain management. *Med Clin North Am* 2006 Sep;90(5):983–1004.

143. Brunier G, Naimark DM, Hladunewich MA. Meeting the guidelines for end-of-life care. *Adv Perit Dial* 2006;22:175–9.

144. Steinhauser KE, Christakis NA, Clipp EC, et al. Preparing for the end of life: preferences of patients, families, physicians and other care providers. *J Pain Symptom Manage* 2001;22(3):727–737.

145. Thornberry T, Schaeffer J, Wright PD, Haley MC, Kirsh KL. An exploration of the utility of hypnosis in pain management among rural pain patients. *Palliat Support Care* 2007;5(2):147–52.

146. Berliner MN, Giesecke T, Bornhovd KD. Impact of transdermal fentanyl on quality of life in rheumatoid arthritis. *Clin J Pain* 2007;23(6):530–4.

147. Larsson A, Wijk H.Patient experiences of pain and pain management at the end of life: a pilot study. *Pain Manag Nurs* 2007;8(1):12–6.

148. Schroepfer TA. Critical events in the dying process: the potential for physical and psychosocial suffering. *J Palliat Med* 2007;10(1):136–47.

149. Miaskowski C, Dodd M, West C, Paul SM, Schumacher K, Tripathy D, Koo P. The use of a responder analysis to identify differences in patient outcomes following a self-care intervention to improve cancer pain management. *Pain* 2007;129(1–2):55–63.

150. Rolnick SJ, Jackson J, Nelson WW, Butani A, Herrinton LJ, Hornbrook M, Neslund-Dudas C, Bachman DJ, Coughlin SS. Pain management in the last six months of life among women who died of ovarian cancer. *J Pain Symptom Manage* 2007;33(1):24–31.

151. Emanuel LL, von Gunten CF, Ferris FD. *The Education for Physicians on End-of-life Care (EPEC) Curriculum.* Chicago, IL: American Medical Association; 1999.
152. Johansson CM, Axelsson B, Danielson E. Living with incurable cancer at the end of life–patients' perceptions on quality of life. Cancer Nurs. 2006;29(5):391–9.
153. Doorenbos AZ, Given CW, Given B, Verbitsky N. Symptom experience in the last year of life among individuals with cancer. J Pain Symptom Manage. 2006;32(5):403–12.
154. Henig RM. Will we ever arrive at the good death? Almost 40 years after the birth of the hospice movement, and despite the rise of living wills and palliative care, the end of life remains anxious and hypermedicalized. Goldie Gold's struggle, and yours, to come to a dignified end. *N Y Times Mag* 2005 Aug 7;26–35, 40, 68.
155. Tsai JS, Wu CH, Chiu TY, Hu WY, Chen CY. Symptom patterns of advanced cancer patients in a palliative care unit. Palliat Med. 2006;20(6):617–22.
156. Rummans TA, Bostwick JM, Clark MM. Maintaining quality of life at the end of life. *Mayo Clin Proc* 2000;75:1305–1310.
157. Fins JJ, Miller FG, Acres CA, et al. End-of-life decision-making in the hospital: current practice and future prospects. *J Pain Symptom Manage* 1999;17(1):6–15.
158. Patrick DL, Engelberg RA, Curtis, JR. Evaluating the quality of dying and death. *J Pain Symptom Manage* 2001;22(3):717–726.
159. Teno JM, Casey VA, Welch LC, Edgman-Levitan S. Patient-focused, family-centered end-of-life medical care: views of the guidelines and bereaved family members. *J Pain and Symptom Management* 2001;22(3):738–751.
160. Kubler-Ross E. *On Death and Dying.* New York: Macmillan; 1969.
161. Yedidia MJ, MacGregor B. Confronting the prospect of dying: reports of terminally ill patients. *J Pain Symptom Manage* 2001;22(4):807–819.
162. Cassem EH. The person confronting death. In *The Harvard Guide to Psychiatry.* 3rd Ed. Edited by AM Nicholi. Cambridge, MA: Belknap Press; 1999:699–731.
163. Prager J, Jacobs M. Evaluation of patients for implantable pain modalities: medical and behavioral assessment. *Clin J of Pain* 2001;17:206–214.
164. Gibson MC, Schroder C. The many faces of pain for older, dying adults. *Am J Hospice & Pall Care* 2001;18(1):19–25.
165. Milch RA. The Dying Patient: pain management at the hospice level. *Curr Rev Pain* 2000;4:215–218.
166. World Health Organization. *Cancer Pain Relief.* Geneva, Switzerland; 1986.
167. Jacox A, Carr DB, Payne R, et al. *Management of Cancer Pain: Clinical Practice Guideline No. 9.* AHCPR Publication No. 94-0592. Rockville, MD. Agency for Health Care Policy and Research, US Department of Health and Human Services, Public Health Service, March 1994.
168. Wrede-Seaman LD. Treatment options to manage pain at the end of life. *Am J Hospice & Pall Care* 2001;18(2):89–101.
169. Beckwith SK, Cole BE. Hospice, cancer pain management and symptom control. In RS Weiner (Ed.) *Pain Management: A Practical Guide for Clinicians.* 5th Ed. Boca Raton, FL: St. Lucie Press; 1998.
170. Mays TA. Antidepressants in the management of cancer pain. *Curr Pain Headache Rep* 2001;5:227–236.
171. Rich BA. A prescription for the pain: the emerging standard of care for pain management. *William Mitchell Law Rev* 2000; 26(1):1–95.
172. Rousseau P. The losses and suffering of terminal illness. *Mayo Clin Proc* 2000;75:197–198.
173. Dickerson, ED. Pain relief pyramid. *Am J Pain Manage* 2002;12(3):99–101.

Healthcare Economic Evaluation of Chronic Pain: Measuring the Economic, Social and Personal Impact of Chronic Pain and its Management

Rebecca L. Robinson and Thomas R. Vetter

Introduction

The aim of this chapter is to provide an overview of the social and personal costs of chronic pain and the role of healthcare economic evaluation methods within the context of chronic pain management, using a standardized and scientific approach. An economic evaluation is essentially the comparative analysis of alternative courses of action in terms of both their costs and consequences (Drummond, Sculpher, Torrance, O'Brien, & Stoddart, 2005). Thus the fundamental tasks of any economic evaluation—including those concerned with heath services—are to identify, measure, value, and compare the costs and consequences of the alternatives being considered (Drummond, Sculpher et al., 2005). The types of healthcare economic evaluations, the categories of cost incorporated in healthcare economic evaluations, the possible perspectives of a healthcare economic evaluation, and a framework for assessing healthcare economic evaluations will first be discussed. The application of such evaluation methods will then be described for two very common, specific chronic pain conditions, namely, chronic low back pain and fibromyalgia. Lastly, the implications and challenges related to the clinical application of healthcare economic evaluations of chronic pain treatment will be discussed.

The Definition and Prevalence of Chronic Pain

Pain is a complex and highly subjective experience (Turk & Okifuji, 2004). Chronic non-cancer pain has been defined by the American Pain Society (2007) as pain that lasts more than 6 months, is ongoing, is due to non-life-threatening causes, has not responded to currently available treatment methods, and may continue for the remainder of the person's life. Chronic pain accompanies a variety of diseases, occurs across the entire life span, and is associated with a number of socioeconomic factors.

R.L. Robinson (✉)
Global Health Outcomes, Eli Lilly and Company, Indianapolis, IN, USA

R.J. Moore (ed.), *Biobehavioral Approaches to Pain*,
DOI 10.1007/978-0-387-78323-9_10, © Springer Science+Business Media, LLC 2009

Pain represents a major clinical, social and economic problem, with estimates of its prevalence ranging from 8% to more than 60%, depending on the patient population (Phillips, 2003). An extensive cross-sectional survey of randomly selected Australian adults revealed a 20% overall prevalence of chronic pain (Blyth et al., 2001). This chronic pain was most often the result of an injury or a co-existing health problem and was frequently associated with substantial disability due to its protracted nature (Blyth, March, Brnabic, & Cousins, 2004). An age-stratified survey of a cohort of Finnish 15–74 year olds revealed an age-standardized 14% prevalence of daily chronic pain (Mäntyselkä et al., 2001). Furthermore, this Finnish study identified the relative frequency and severity of chronic pain to be an independent determinant of the odds ratio of poor self-rated health (Mäntyselkä, Turunen, Ahonen, & Kumpusalo, 2003). Chronic pain is unfortunately also a common pediatric condition, affecting at least one third of adolescents between 12 and 18 years of age (Perquin et al., 2000) (see also Cucchiaro in this Volume).

The Implications of Chronic Pain

Chronic pain is one of the most disabling, burdensome, and costly conditions afflicting patients and thus society. Pain is a leading cause for patients to seek and receive medical care, (Zagari, Mazonson, & Longton, 1996), with pain resulting in an estimated $100 billion in direct medical costs per year in the United States alone (McCarberg & Billington, 2006). Common pain conditions result in an additional estimated $61 billion annual loss in productivity among active US workers (Stewart, Ricci, Chee, Morganstein, & Lipton, 2003). The healthcare costs of patients with chronic diseases, many of which are associated with disabling pain, account for more than 75% of the nation's $1.4 trillion annual healthcare costs (Centers for Disease Control and Prevention, 2005). Given the aging US population and unsustainably increasing percentage of the US gross domestic product (GDP) devoted to healthcare, there is a clear and imminent need for valid healthcare economic evaluation data to establish healthcare funding priorities (Brown, Brown, & Sharma, 2005), including for chronic pain treatment modalities.

The Potential Role of Economic Evaluation in Chronic Pain

Healthcare economic evaluation has matured considerably in the last two decades. However, despite its widespread promotion to this audience, many physicians and researchers remain reluctant to apply economic evaluation methods in their clinical decision-making and clinical trials (Neumann, 2005). Much of this lack of understanding has been attributed to physicians and their innate propensity to think more in terms of clinical effectiveness and advocacy at the individual patient level rather than about cost-effectiveness at the population or policy level (Neumann). This resistance to collecting, analyzing, and incorporating health economic data in the present, well-established era of evidence-based medicine is particularly notable (Neumann).

Numerous conventional biomedical as well as complementary and alternative medicine (CAM) treatment options are available for chronic pain, including a wide range of pharmaceuticals, nutriceuticals, and non-pharmacologic therapies. These various therapies are used singly or in combination. Successful chronic pain treatment requires individualization of therapy based upon not only the etiology and characteristics but also the subjective patient self-reported assessment of pain. However, avoidable costs may be incurred at all stages of care due to inefficiencies in the diagnosis and treatment of patients with chronic pain. Economic evaluations, which balance the expected gain of a specific intervention against its expected cost, can reduce in part such avoidable costs by providing useful information about the relative value of an intervention. The often high cumulative cost and large variability in the management and outcomes of chronic pain naturally lend themselves to health economic evaluation, with the intention that cost savings may eventually be realized.

An Overview of Healthcare Economic Evaluation

The appraisal of a new or existing treatment modality involves three steps (Fig. 1) (Bombardier & Maetzel, 1999; Detsky, 1995; Detsky & Naglie, 1990; Grimes & Schulz, 2002; Kocher & Henley, 2003). Initially, *efficacy* or the treatment achieving its stated clinical goal is demonstrated under "optimal" circumstances in a randomized controlled trial. Subsequently, *effectiveness* or producing greater benefit than harm is assessed under more ordinary or "naturalistic" circumstances, often by way of an analytic cohort study. The *efficiency* or the health status improvement realized for a given amount of resources expended is lastly determined via an economic evaluation. Alternatively, an economic evaluation can provide essential insight into the resources required to deliver the healthcare intervention to a specific population (Kocher & Henley).

Pharmacoeconomics is a sub-discipline of health economics that assess pharmaceutical products specifically. Pharmacoeconomic evaluations are applicable throughout the lifecycle of a pharmaceutical agent (Strom, 1994). Specifically, pharmacoeconomics can be applied by industry to understand the impact of pursuing a new drug for a disease, by national or third-party healthcare payers to maximize the value of their pharmaceutical expenditures, and by healthcare providers and their patients to comprehend the relative benefits of drug therapy choices. New treatments that provide only modest pharmacoeconomic improvements over a less expensive, standard of care may be denied availability by governments or other organizations responsible for maintaining healthcare budgets.

❶ Efficacy

- Achieving its stated clinical goal

- Demonstrated under **optimal** circumstances in a prospective randomized controlled

  trial (RCT) – <u>but</u> the results are limited to the study subjects

❷ Effectiveness

- Producing greater benefit than harm

- Assessed under **ordinary** circumstances in the more general population often by way

  of an observational yet analytic longitudinal cohort study

❸ Efficiency

- Health status improvement for a given amount of resources expended

- Determined via a cost-effectiveness analysis or cost-utility analysis

Fig. 1 The three sequential steps involved in the appraisal of a new or existing healthcare intervention (Bombardier & Eisenberg, 1985; Detsky, 1995; Detsky & Naglie, 1990; Grimes & Schulz, 2002; Kocher & Henley, 2003)

A fundamental characteristic of any economic evaluation is the determination of inputs (costs) *versus* outputs (consequences or outcomes). A full healthcare economic evaluation thus entails identifying, measuring, valuing, and comparing the costs *and* the consequences (both the beneficial and the adverse clinical outcomes) of the alternatives being considered (Drummond, Sculpher et al., 2005). One of these alternative or competing healthcare interventions can legitimately be either the status quo or doing nothing.

The Dimensions of a Healthcare Economic Evaluation

Assessing the relative value of any clinical intervention (e.g., a pharmaceutical) is predicated on three aspects or dimensions of the healthcare economic evaluation (Fig. 2) (Bombardier & Eisenberg, 1985). These three dimensions of a healthcare economic evaluation include: (1) the applied type of analysis, (2) the categories of included costs and consequences (benefits), and (3) the point of view or perspective of the evaluation.

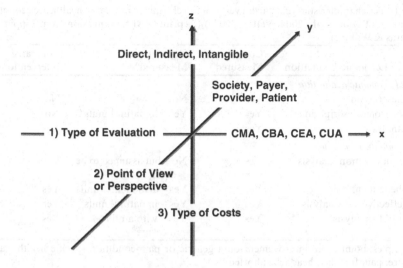

Fig. 2 The three dimensions of healthcare economic evaluations (Bombardier & Eisenberg, 1985). Cost minimization analysis (CMA); cost-benefit analysis (CBA); cost-effectiveness analysis (CEA); cost-utility analysis (CUA)

The Types of Analysis in a Healthcare Economic Evaluation

Full healthcare economic evaluation techniques conventionally include cost-minimization analysis, cost-benefit analysis, cost-effectiveness analysis, and cost-utility analysis (Table 1) (Drummond, Sculpher et al., 2005; Jefferson, Demicheli, & Mugford, 2000; Vetter, 2007a). Of note, the number of healthcare economic evaluations, especially those involving more rigorous analytic methods, is increasing in the chronic pain medicine literature (Fig. 3) (Vetter).

In a *cost-minimization analysis* (CMA), the consequences (clinical outcomes) of the healthcare interventions being evaluated are with statistical rigor assuredly equal. Therefore, the economic analysis can focus exclusively on costs, with the goal of identifying the pain-related intervention or treatment with the lowest possible costs (Jefferson et al., 2000; Robinson, 1993d).

In a *cost-benefit analysis* (CBA) both the costs and the consequences (clinical outcomes) are expressed strictly in monetary terms. This approach proves advantageous when the competing healthcare interventions result in multiple or distinct clinical outcomes that are not readily comparable (Drummond, Sculpher et al., 2005). Cost-benefit analysis, however, requires that a monetary value somehow be placed on health and in some cases a human life (Robinson, 1993a). This monetary value of health can be determined in some settings using a willingness-to-pay approach, in which patients or parents are directly asked how much they would be willing to pay for a specific health outcome (Olsen & Smith, 2001).

In a *cost-effectiveness analysis* (CEA), a single clinical outcome measure is applicable and appropriate. Therefore, the costs of the competing healthcare

Table 1 The characteristics of a partial versus a full chronic pain-related healthcare economic evaluation (Taylor et al., 2004; Vetter, 2007a) (Reprinted with permission from Lippincott Williams & Wilkins)

Type of Economic Evaluation	Costs Measured?	Consequences Measured?	Comparison of Interventions?
Partial economic evaluation			
Cost description	Yes	No	No
Cost-outcome description	Yes	Yes – in natural units[a]	No
Cost analysis	Yes	No	Yes
Full economic evaluation			
Cost-minimization analysis	Yes	No – but assumed to be equal	Yes
Cost-benefit analysis	Yes	Yes – in monetary units	Yes
Cost-effectiveness analysis	Yes	Yes – in natural units[a]	Yes
Cost-utility analysis	Yes	Yes – with a utility measure[b]	Yes

[a] Examples: point score improvement on a generic or pain-condition specific health status measure; pain-free day; headache aborted
[b] Most commonly in the number of quality adjusted life years (QALYs) gained

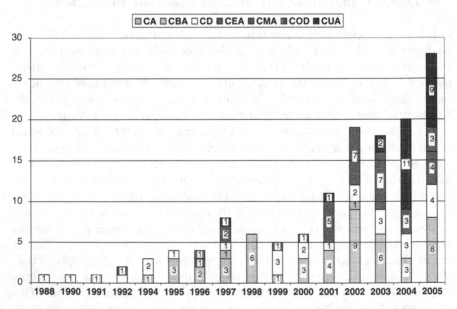

Fig. 3 The chronological distribution of the number and type of chronic-pain related partial and full economic evaluations (y-axis) published between 1988 and 2005. Cost analysis (CA); cost-benefit analysis (CBA); cost-description (CD); cost-effectiveness analysis (CEA); cost-minimization analysis (CMA); cost-outcome description (COD); and cost-utility analysis (CUA) (Vetter, 2007a) (*Reprinted with permission from Lippincott Williams & Wilkins*)

interventions are compared using this single, common clinical outcome measure (Drummond, Sculpher et al., 2005). The marginal (incremental) cost effectiveness is the gain in effectiveness realized for the additional cost between the competing treatments. The result is expressed as the incremental cost effectiveness ratio (ICER). The ICER equals the average difference in costs divided by the average difference in clinical effect for two competing healthcare interventions (Muennig, 2002). The ICER is expressed in natural units of effect, such as cost per life-year gained, cost per migraine headache aborted, or cost per unit reduction in a pain rating scale (e.g., the reduction in visual analogue scale pain score in patients with diabetic neuropathy) (Brown et al., 2005; Robinson, 1993b).

The goal of a CEA is to identify the therapy that has the lowest cost per unit of outcome gained. If drug A is more effective and less costly than drug B, then drug A is an easy choice to make. The more common scenario, especially in the case of new therapies, is that drug A is more effective but also more costly than drug B, making the decision less obvious and requiring a judgment or trade-off be made (O'Brien, Drummond, Labelle, & Willan, 1994). In this latter scenario, more complex inferential statistics and sensitivity analyses, which are beyond the scope of the present discussion, are needed to make a valid cost-effectiveness conclusion (Briggs, 2000, 2001; Briggs & Gray, 1999; Briggs, O'Brien, & Blackhouse, 2002; Briggs, Sculpher, & Buxton, 1994; O'Brien & Briggs, 2002; Obenchain, Robinson, & Swindle, 2005).

As with a cost-effectiveness analysis, in a *cost-utility analysis* (CUA), the costs of competing healthcare interventions are compared using a single, common clinical outcome measure–specifically, the quality-adjusted life year (Robinson, 1993c). In a CUA, the consequences of a healthcare intervention are reflected in its resulting *health-related quality of life* (HRQOL) (Drummond, Sculpher et al., 2005). HRQOL in a CUA, including one that is chronic pain-related, is most commonly measured using an indirect preference-based health status questionnaire, such as the Quality of Well-Being Scale (QWB), the EuroQol-5D (EQ-5D), the Health Utilities Index (HUI2, HUI3), or the Short-Form-6D (SF-6D) (Feeny, 2005; Glick, Doshi, Sonnad, & Polsky, 2007; Tosteson, 2000; Vetter, 2007b).

These patient-elicited health utility scores are in turn used to generate the weighted measure of clinical outcome known as the *quality-adjusted life year* (QALY) (Glick et al., 2007; Jefferson et al., 2000). Quality-adjusted life years (QALYs) are calculated by multiplying the perceived utility or value score for a specific health state (conventionally on a scale from 0.0 equal to death to 1.0 equal to perfect health) by the length of time (in years) spent in that health state (Jefferson et al.). This simple formula converts health-related quality of life, with its various dimensions, into a standard health outcome measure (Nord, 1999). The distinct advantage of the QALY as a measure of healthcare outcome is that it incorporates gains realized from reduced morbidity (health-related *quality* of life gains) as well as reduced mortality (*quantity* of life gains), and integrates the two into a single value (Drummond, Sculpher et al., 2005; Jefferson et al., 2000).

Reading the economic evaluation literature can be confusing given that some authors use the term cost-effectiveness analysis as a general synonym for any full economic evaluation, while others use cost-effectiveness analysis and cost-utility analysis interchangeably (Jefferson et al., 2000; Muennig, 2002). Many authors have historically also used the term cost-benefit analysis when in fact they have only actually performed a simple cost comparison (Zarnke, Levine, & O'Brien, 1997). A distinct nomenclature will be maintained in this review. However, a healthcare intervention shown to be advantageous by way of a cost-utility analysis is referred to as cost-effective rather than cost-utilitarian (Brown et al., 2005).

The Categories of Costs in a Healthcare Economic Evaluations

The identification and computation of all pertinent, healthcare-related costs is a crucial, yet challenging requirement for an economic evaluation (Drummond, Sculpher et al., 2005). The internal and external validity of a CEA or CUA are predicated upon the quality of the collected cost data (Stone, Chapman, Sandberg, Liljas, & Neumann, 2000). There remains a sharp dichotomy, however, between the theory and the practice of cost accounting in healthcare economic evaluation (Brouwer, Rutten, & Koopmanschap, 2001; Brown et al., 2005; Glick et al., 2007; Muennig, 2002). Despite the development of a number of national and international methodological guidelines (Oostenbrink, Koopmanschap, & Rutten, 2002), there continues to be significant variability in the costing methods applied in healthcare cost-effectiveness and cost-utility analyses (Table 2) (Adam, Koopmanschap, & Evans, 2003) including those dealing with chronic pain (Korthals-de Bos, van Tulder, van Dieten, & Bouter, 2004; van der Roer, Boos, & van Tulder, 2006).

Delineating Healthcare Costs

The incremental costs included in a CEA or CUA are commonly divided into *direct costs* and *indirect costs* (Brown et al., 2005; Luce, Manning, Siegel, & Lipscomb, 1996; Oostenbrink et al., 2002; Smith & Brown, 2000). *Direct healthcare costs* include those resulting from laboratory tests and diagnostic studies, medications, supplies, healthcare personnel, and the patient use of inpatient and outpatient healthcare facilities (Brown et al.; Luce et al.). Direct healthcare costs included in economic analyses are more self evident than the other types of cost. *Direct non-healthcare costs*, which are often overlooked, include for instance the cost of transportation to and from a medical facility, the time spent by a family member or volunteer in providing healthcare, and the cost of childcare resulting from treatment (Brown et al.; Luce et al.). The identification and computation of such direct non-healthcare costs is a complex and widely variable process, leading some healthcare economists to conclude

Table 2 Sources of variability in cost-effectiveness analysis costing methods (Adam et al., 2003)

Framework of the analysis
  Perspective: societal versus provider or payer
  Choice of comparative intervention: new versus current or new versus doing nothing

Types of costs included
  Overhead costs
  Shared costs
  Indirect costs (including productivity)
  Healthcare costs associated with unrelated illness during prolonged survival

Data collection methods
  Sources of cost data

Valuation Process
  Bottom-up versus top-down
  Price adjustments, including price distortions and exchange rates
  Valuation of time costs
  Capital costs
  Prices versus charges

Methods of data analysis
  Discounting methods
  Capacity utilization
  Sensitivity analysis of variations in unit costs

Reporting of results
  Ingredient approach and transparency of methods and results

that including direct non-healthcare costs may simply increase methodological disparity and further delay the development of a diverse cost-effectiveness database (Brown et al.).

Indirect productivity costs include those costs resulting from morbidity and mortality and the attendant lost or impaired ability to work (absenteeism or presenteeism, respectively) or to engage in leisure activities as well as the lost economic productivity due to death (Luce et al., 1996). Indirect productivity costing has also been marked by longstanding controversy and methodological uncertainty (Adam et al., 2003). Given a societal perspective (see below), indirect productivity costs can be explicitly measured using either the Human Capital Method (Drummond, Sculpher et al., 2005) or the Friction Cost Method (Koopmanschap, Rutten, van Ineveld, & van Roijen, 1995). If however, the analysis is undertaken from a third-party insurer perspective, indirect productivity costs are presumably accounted for within the QALY (Brown et al., 2005; Luce et al.). Lastly, *intangible costs* include pain, suffering, and grief. These costs are rarely included in healthcare economic analyses, with the exception of willingness to pay analyses, where such intangible costs are more quantifiable.

Additional controversy exists as to whether or not future costs incurred due to the increased longevity conferred by the healthcare intervention (e.g., treatment costs for other eventual acute or chronic illnesses, and the cost of food and shelter) should be included in the economic evaluation (Brouwer et al., 2001;

Drummond, Sculpher et al., 2005). If a third-party insurer perspective is applied, these future costs incurred due to the increased longevity conferred by the healthcare intervention do not need to be included in a CEA or CUA (Brown et al., 2005).

The Point of View or Perspective of a Healthcare Economic Evaluation

A healthcare economic evaluation can be undertaken from the point of view or perspective of the patient, the healthcare provider, the third-party payer (employer or insurer), the government, or society at large (Torrance, Siegel, & Luce, 1996). The perspective of the economic evaluation largely determines what costs are included in the analysis. Applying a societal perspective requires micro-costing, with its attendant comprehensive yet exhaustively detailed identification and measurements of *all* the direct, indirect, and intangible resources consumed by a healthcare intervention as well as its sequelae (Luce et al., 1996). On the other hand, patients and their families are innately concerned only with those direct, indirect, and intangible costs not assumed by others such as insurance companies or employers. In the United States, employees are assuming more healthcare costs and decision making responsibility through employer initiatives such as tiered health insurance premium copayments (i.e., health maintenance organization versus preferred or participating physician organization coverage), tiered prescription medication copayments (i.e., generic versus name brand), and healthcare savings accounts. Third-party payers such as health insurance companies, pharmacy benefit managers, and governmental agencies (e.g., U.S. Centers for Medicaid and Medicare Services and National Health Service in the U.K.) are interested primarily in direct healthcare costs for which they provide reimbursement. Employers focus on not only direct healthcare costs but also direct non-healthcare costs, such as lost worker productivity and disability payments. Lastly, healthcare providers ideally serve as the patient advocate and strive to practice evidence-based medicine yet are facing increasing economic scrutiny through external pay-for-performance initiatives.

In general terms, the all-encompassing societal perspective on costing is not always indicated, especially if some of the costs are not of interest to the primary decision maker or researcher (Russell et al., 1996). The third-party payer perspective is by and large a more practical approach to healthcare costing (Brown et al., 2005), including in chronic pain-related studies. Nevertheless, chronic pain-related societal costs remain noteworthy. For example, in a study of chronic non-malignant pain patients referred to a multidisciplinary pain center in Denmark, healthcare costs were not significantly reduced over nine months, but significant reductions in social transfer payments of sickness benefits, welfare benefits, disability pensions, and retirement pensions were identified (Thomsen, Sorensen, Sjogren, & Eriksen, 2002).

A Framework for Assessing Healthcare Economic Analyses

Seven fundamental questions have been identified that should be answered when assessing a healthcare-related economic analysis (Bombardier & Eisenberg, 1985):

1. What type of analysis was performed?
2. Was the point of view or perspective of the study clearly stated?
3. Were all the important costs and benefits identified?
4. How were the costs measured?
5. Were costs adjusted for differential timings?
6. Were sensitivity analyses performed to determine whether the conclusions change as the assumptions or data are varied?
7. Were the comparisons adequately described?

The dimensions of healthcare economic evaluation as they relate to the seven fundamental questions identified by Bombardier and Eisenberg (1985) are summarized for each of four representative chronic pain studies (Tables 3 and 4).

In the next two sections, chronic low back pain and fibromyalgia will be reviewed with these seven questions in mind. In doing so, each section will discuss the respective pain condition in terms of: (a) its definition and estimated prevalence; (b) the current clinical management of the condition; and (c) examples of economic analyses published on this chronic pain condition.

Chronic Low Back Pain

The Definition and Prevalence of Chronic Low Back Pain

Chronic low back pain (CLBP) is considered to be pain persisting longer than 12 weeks that is located primarily in the lumbosacral region of the spine (Carragee, 2005). While the pathophysiology of CLBP remains somewhat enigmatic, inflammatory mediators as well as mechanical factors appear to play a major role (Biyani & Andersson, 2004). CLBP is most often associated with overuse and muscle strain or repetitive injury sustained over a lengthy period of time, although its often progressive clinical course makes a specific etiology difficult to determine (Hazard, 2007; Rubin, 2007). Pain may also be caused by degenerative conditions such as arthritis or vertebral disc disease, osteoporosis or other bone diseases, infection, irritation of the nerve roots, or congenital abnormalities of the spine (National Institute of Neurological Disorders and Stroke, 2007). Individuals with CLBP frequently experience other comorbid conditions that worsen the clinical prognosis and complicate the economics of their CLBP. These conditions include tension or migraine headaches (Duckro, Schultz, & Chibnall, 1994), cardiovascular disease (Vogt, Nevitt, & Cauley, 1997), psychiatric illness (Atkinson, Slater, Patterson, Grant, &

Garfin, 1991; Polatin, Kinney, Gatchel, Lillo, & Mayer, 1993), and chronic fatigue (Fishbain et al., 2004).

CLBP is the most common and costly of all pain conditions (de Girolamo, 1991; Frymoyer & Cats-Baril, 1991). Summarizing CLBP is mired by methodological inconsistencies across studies, including varying definitions of acute versus chronic back pain (Chou, 2005). For instance, while several studies have documented the high prevalence of generalized back pain (Behrens, Seligman, Cameron, Mathias, & Fine, 1994; Guo et al., 1995; Loney & Stratford, 1999; Patrick et al., 1995); fewer have reported on the prevalence of chronic low back pain (Carey et al., 1995; Newton, Curtis, Witt, & Hobler, 1997; Patrick et al., 1995).

The episodic occurrence of low back pain has been reported to be as high as 70 to 80% in adults during their lifetime (Patrick et al., 1995; Rubin, 2007). The prevalence of CLBP was observed to be 4% in a self-reported telephone survey (Carey et al., 1995), 14% of members in a Health Maintenance Organization where CLBP diagnosis was made by physicians (Newton et al., 1997), and 18% of a national survey of U.S. workers (Guo et al., 1995). In a cohort of chronic pain patients, the prevalence of chronic low back pain was 43% to 48% (Hoffman, Meier, & Council, 2002). Identified risk factors for back pain include increased age, low level of education, job dissatisfaction, poor working conditions, disputed compensation issues, pending litigation, psychological distress, other types of chronic pain, and fear (Carragee, 2005; Phillips, Ch'ien, Norwood, & Smith, 2003).

The Treatment of Chronic Low Back Pain

The clinical management of chronic low back pain varies widely across and within countries (Koes, van Tulder, Ostelo, Burton, & Waddell, 2001). The treatment of CLBP is dependent on its diagnostic classification. For instance, it is recommended that once the pain becomes chronic, both physical and psychological elements be incorporated into the management of CLBP (Grabois, 2005). Treatment options include the use of cold or hot compresses, short term bed rest, exercises both to strengthen back and abdominal muscles and to improve vertebral range of motion, medications, and surgery–and whenever possible, noninvasive or minimally invasive outpatient treatment (National Institute of Neurological Disorders and Stroke, 2007). Frequently, comprehensive management strategies are employed, including multiple, simultaneous therapies and an overall multidisciplinary approach (van Geen, Edelaar, Janssen, & van Eijk, 2007).

However, despite the more recent clinical emphasis on a multidisciplinary approach, CLBP remains a global pain problem. A recent European study of patients presenting with non-specific back pain, showed that approximately 37% still had significant pain and 10% had not improved or worsened after at least two months of treatment (Kovacs et al., 2006). Treatment in this cohort of patients in Spain consisted of medications in 92% of patients and physical therapy or rehabilitation in only 19%, while 10% were referred for surgery (Kovacs et al.). Medications were also found to be prescribed to 80% of back pain patients in the United States (Cherkin, Wheeler, Barlow, & Deyo, 1998), with the most commonly prescribed types of medication being analgesics, non-steroidal anti-inflammatory drugs (NSAIDs), muscle-relaxants, and antidepressants (Cherkin et al., 1998). This observed frequent use of NSAIDs and antidepressants was consistent with a more recent survey of the management of CLBP (Grabois, 2005), which also noted the use of opioids, non-opioid analgesics, corticosteroids, antiepileptic, muscle relaxants, sympathetic nerve blocks, trigger-point injections, epidural steroid injections, and vertebral facet joint injections (Grabois).

Recommended treatments for CLBP include over-the-counter analgesics (aspirin, naproxen, and ibuprofen); other non-narcotic analgesics (tramadol, Cox-2 inhibitors); opioids (codeine, hydrocodone, oxycodone, and morphine); anticonvulsants; antidepressants; muscle relaxants, sleep aids; and injections of local anesthetics, steroids, or narcotics (National Institute of Neurological Disorders and Stroke, 2007). Other non-surgical therapies for CLBP include patient education, physical therapy, exercise, stretching, spinal manipulation, hot/cold packs, ultrasound, massage, transcutaneous electrical nerve stimulation, magnet therapy, acupuncture, biofeedback, traction, relaxation, hypnosis, cognitive behavioral therapy, direct spinal cord neurostimulation, vertebroplasty, and kyphoplasty (Grabois, 2005; National Institute of Neurological Disorders and Stroke).

More invasive treatments, including surgical procedures, are generally pursued when more conservative measures fail or when focal neurological symptoms such as sensory loss and motor weakness are present. Such invasive interventions include discectomy, foraminotomy, intradiscal electrothermal therapy, nucleoplasty, radiofrequency ablation, spinal fusion, spinal laminectomy, and other less common surgical procedures (rhizotomy, cordotomy, dorsal root entry zone operation) (National Institute of Neurological Disorders and Stroke, 2007).

The Burden of Chronic Low Back Pain

The high economic burden of CLBP reported in the literature from 1996 to 2001 was systematically reviewed by Maetzel and Li (2002). Several subsequent publications (Boonen et al., 2005; Ekman, Jonhagen, Hunsche, & Jonsson, 2005; Goetzel, Hawkins, Ozminkowski, & Wang, 2003; Hadler, Tait, & Chibnall, 2007; Kovacs et al., 2006; Luo, Pietrobon, Sun, Liu, & Hey, 2004) support the findings of this earlier review. Collectively, these reports support six conclusions. (1) The cost of CLBP is high and comparable to that from headache, heart disease, and depression. (2) Conclusive cost estimates for CLBP are difficult to obtain given the inconsistencies in the definitions of chronic low back pain versus acute low back pain and in how costs are measured. (3) A small percentage of patients account for a large proportion of CLBP costs. An earlier study found that at least 75% of CLBP costs were attributed to the 5% of patients who become temporarily or permanently disabled (Frymoyer & Cats-Baril, 1991). Another cohort study observed that the top 10% most costly back pain patients were responsible for approximately 100% of the expenditures for inpatient care, 87% for outpatient services, and 90% of the emergency room visits (Luo et al., 2004). (4) The majority of CLBP costs are associated with indirect costs from lost productivity and disability. (5) Some variability in provided services and excessive or inappropriate costs can be documented by country or region. (6) Invasive interventions generally failed to show economic benefit and only provided modest clinical benefit, indicating that more effective or possibly more selective use of such invasive treatments appears needed.

Total annual healthcare costs for back pain in the United States range between $50 billion to $100 billion in 1990 US dollars (Frymoyer & Cats-Baril, 1991) and $91 billion in 1998 US dollars (Luo et al., 2004). The average annual healthcare expenditure for back pain patients is roughly 60% higher than of individuals without back pain ($3,498 vs. $2,178) (Luo et al.). In a Swedish survey of CLBP, 15% of costs were from direct medical care while 85% were indirect costs (Ekman et al., 2005). Higher total healthcare costs have been associated with patients with more severe back pain, more persistent days in pain, a disc disorder/sciatica, and female gender (Ekman et al.; Engel, von Korff, & Katon, 1996). In 1999, low back pain was noted to be the fourth most costly physical health condition among employees in the United States (Goetzel et al., 2003). Payments for mechanical low back disorder were only lower than the chronic maintenance of angina pectoris, essential hypertension, and diabetes mellitus. Total payments (in 1999 U.S. dollars) per eligible employee for mechanical low back disorder were $90.25 for healthcare and productivity management payments (Goetzel et al.).

Direct healthcare costs for back pain are driven primarily by associated inpatient care ($27.9 billion), followed by office-based visits ($23.6 billion) (Luo et al., 2004). Back pain is the third most common reason for surgery, the fifth most common reason for hospitalization, and the fifth most common reason for all physician office visits (Hart, Deyo, & Cherkin, 1995; Turk & Okifuji, 1998). Patients with CLBP average 11 annual medical care visits to a variety of providers, including primary care physicians, orthopedic surgeons, chiropractors, and physical therapists (Carey et al., 1995). While individuals between 25 and 44 years of age, women, African-Americans and Hispanics are more likely to seek back pain-related medical care (Hart et al., 1995), as many as half of those with CLBP do not seek medical care (James Cook University, 2004).

The indirect costs of CLBP, including work disability and absenteeism, are a significant occupational and public health problem. Back pain is a major cause of lost worker productivity (Guo et al., 1995). Workers compensation insurance currently costs employers in the US 2% to 4% of gross earnings (Hadler et al., 2007). Approximately 10% to 15% of individuals with CLBP will become disabled (Indahl, 2004). The total annual compensable cost for all low back pain in the United States has been estimated to be $11.1 billion (Webster & Snook, 1990) The total indirect costs from back pain were $28 billion in 1996 US dollars, with missed work days totaling $18 billion or $4,586 on average per afflicted worker (Rizzo, Abbott, & Berger, 1998).

Economic Evaluation of the Treatment of Chronic Lower Back Pain

An extensive yet diverse array of healthcare economic evaluations of the interventional and the non-interventional treatment of chronic low back pain has been undertaken in the last decade. In a recent review of the economic literature on back pain, van der Roer, Goossens, Evers, & van Tulder (2005) found 17 studies, including five studies of CLBP and four additional studies that combined acute and chronic lower back pain. Most of the studies performed strictly a CEA; however, one study added a CBA, while another study a CUA. Four studies conducted strictly a CUA. One study performed a CMA. A variety of non-interventional therapies were compared, for instance, McKenzie exercises, chiropractic treatment, exercise therapy, multidisciplinary rehabilitation, ergonomic modification, neuroreflexotherapy, bed rest, and worksite visit (van der Roer et al., 2005). The authors concluded that the findings of the published studies could not be synthesized to determine which single therapy was the most cost effective and that more studies were needed in this area (van der Roer et al.).

Another review of healthcare economic evaluations in rheumatology for a single year (2001–2002) identified back pain as the subject of higher quality healthcare economic studies than other areas within rheumatology (Tella, Feinglass, & Chang, 2003). The review included four studies (two CEA; two CBA) that found a dominance of evidence-based medicine over usual care; a dominance of periradicular infiltration with steroids over saline in subgroups with contained herniated vertebral discs but not in subgroups with disc extrusions. However, no conclusions could be drawn regarding multidisciplinary programs as incremental cost-effectiveness ratios were not calculated (Tella et al., 2003).

Included here are specific healthcare economic evaluations in the area of back pain. A CEA has been undertaken of ambulatory care provided by specialists versus general internists to patients with chronic low back pain (Anderson et al., 2002); lumbar spine radiography in primary care patients with low back pain (Miller, Kendrick, Bentley, & Fielding, 2002); long-term intrathecal morphine therapy for failed back surgery syndrome (de Lissovoy, Brown, Halpern, Hassenbusch, & Ross, 1997); lumbar fusion versus nonsurgical treatment for chronic low back pain (Fritzell, Hagg, Jonsson, & Nordwall, 2004); microendoscopic discectomy versus conventional open discectomy in the treatment of lumbar disc

Table 3 The seven fundamental dimensions of a healthcare economic evaluation applied to published studies on chronic low back pain (Bombardier & Eisenberg, 1985)

	Manipulation, exercises, and physician consultation compared to physician consultation alone (Niemisto et al., 2005).	Surgical stabilization of the spine versus intensive rehabilitation (Rivero-Arias et al., 2005).
What type of analysis was performed?	Cost-effectiveness analysis.	Cost-utility analysis.
Was the point of view (perspective) of the study clearly stated?	Yes: Societal perspective.	Yes: Societal perspective.
Were all the important costs and benefits identified?	Yes: Both direct and indirect costs; pain intensity on visual analogue scale, back specific disability on Oswestry Disability Index, HRQOL (15D Quality of Life Instrument).	Yes: Both direct and indirect costs; health utility measured at baseline, six, 12, and 24 months, using patient-completed the EuroQol (EQ-5D) questionnaire.
How were the costs measured?	Patient report of direct healthcare costs, direct non-healthcare costs, and indirect costs.	National average unit approach; patient report of direct (healthcare costs, direct non-healthcare) and indirect costs.
Were costs adjusted for differential timings?	The costs (and effects) were not discounted despite the 2-year timeframe of the study.	Costs (and effects) were effects were discounted at an annual rate of 3.5%.
Was sensitivity analysis performed to check whether the conclusions change as assumptions or data are changed?	Yes: Conclusions remained consistent across the sensitivity analysis of average wage level.	Yes: Uncertainty as to the use of different surgical techniques for spinal stabilization and impact of patients receiving other treatments subsequent to their allocated therapy.
Were the comparison adequately described?	Yes: Combined manipulation/ exercises/ information versus physician consultation alone.	Yes: Full details of the randomized controlled trial were published in parallel with this paper.
Conclusions:	Physician consultation alone was more cost-effective for both healthcare use and work absenteeism, and led to equal improvement in disability and HRQOL.	Spinal fusion surgery as first line therapy for chronic low back pain seems not to be a cost effective use of healthcare resources at two year follow-up.

herniation (Arts, Peul, Brand, Koes, & Thomeer, 2006); neuroreflexotherapy for chronic low back pain in routine general practice (Kovacs et al., 2002); a disability prevention model for back pain management (Loisel et al., 2002); combined manipulation, stabilizing exercises, and physician consultation compared to physician consultation alone for chronic low back pain (Niemisto et al., 2005); intensive group training protocol compared to physiotherapy guideline care for sub-acute and chronic low back pain (van der Roer et al., 2004); self-care interventions to reduce disability associated with back pain (Strong, Von Korff, Saunders, & Moore, 2006); and a multi-stage return to work program for workers on sick-leave due to low back pain (Steenstra et al., 2006).

By the same token, a CUA has been undertaken of early imaging in patients with low back pain (Gilbert et al., 2004); lumbar disectomy for herniated intervertebral disc disease (Malter, Larson, Urban, & Deyo, 1996); epidural steroids for sciatica (Price, Arden, Coglan, & Rogers, 2005); surgical stabilization of the spine versus intensive rehabilitation for chronic low back pain (Rivero-Arias et al., 2005); physiotherapy treatment versus advice in low back pain (Rivero-Arias, Gray, Frost, Lamb, & Stewart-Brown, 2006); spinal cord stimulation for failed back surgery syndrome (Taylor & Taylor, 2005); spinal cord stimulation versus reoperation for failed back surgery syndrome (North, Kidd, Shipley, & Taylor, 2007); acupuncture for chronic low back pain (Ratcliffe, Thomas, Mac-Pherson, & Brazier, 2006; Witt et al., 2006); a brief pain management program compared with physical therapy for low back pain (Whitehurst et al., 2007); physiotherapist-led pain management classes and exercise (Critchley, Ratcliffe, Noonan, Jones, & Hurley, 2007); a brief physiotherapy pain management approach using cognitive-behavioural principles (Solution-Finding Approach) when compared with a commonly used traditional method of physical therapy (McKenzie Approach (Manca et al., 2007)); and manipulation physical treatments for back pain (UK BEAM Trial Team, 2004).

The seven fundamental questions for healthcare economic evaluations identified by Bombardier and Eisenberg (1985) are illustrated here for one CEA and one CUA in chronic lower back pain (Table 3). These two studies were chosen as they were not included in previous reviews (van der Roer et al., 2005; Tella et al., 2003) and they highlight these two diverse treatment options.

Fibromyalgia

The Definition and Prevalence of Fibromyalgia

The1990 American College of Rheumatology (ACR) standardized criteria for the clinical diagnosis of fibromyalgia include a history of chronic pain and significant tenderness to manual palpation at least 11 of 18 specific tendomuscular points (or trigger points) (Wolfe et al., 1990). The condition affects 2% to 4% of the general population, more often females than males (9:1 ratio), and is most commonly diagnosed between the ages of 20–50 years (Raphael, Janal, Nayak, Schwartz, & Gallagher, 2006; Wolfe, Ross, Anderson, Russell, & Hebert, 1995). Fibromyalgia patients experience a wide range of comorbid symptoms, including moderate to severe fatigue, which can wax and wane over time and vary in maximum intensity (Abeles, Pillinger, Solitar, & Abeles, 2007; Chakrabarty & Zoorob, 2007; Staud, 2006; Wolfe et al., 1990).

While there is agreement that there is heightened pain perception in fibromyalgia, the precise underlying mechanisms for this phenomenon are still not clear. The current understanding of fibromyalgia includes several contributing factors, including stress, previous and coexisting medical illness, and a variety of neurotransmitter and neuroendocrine disturbances (Mease, 2005). These disturbances include reduced levels of inhibitory biogenic amines, increased concentrations of excitatory neurotransmitters (including substance P), and dysfunction of the hypothalamic-pituitary-adrenal axis (HPA). One common hypothesis is that fibromyalgia results from global sensitization of the central nervous system (Mease). Other studies note that fibromyalgia arises from peripheral sensitization. And still others analyses indicate that fibromyalgia arises from both peripheral and central sensitization. While various theories exist, one current unifying premise is that there may be multiple factors that contribute to and perpetuate sensitization of the central nervous system and or the peripheral nervous system; therefore, multiple treatment approaches that provide benefit to the fibromyalgia patient may be indicated (Mease).

The Treatment of Fibromyalgia

The goals in the treatment of fibromyalgia are to reduce pain, improve sleep, restore physical function, maintain social interaction, reestablish emotional balance, and reduce the need for expensive healthcare resources (Russell, 2006). The management of fibromyalgia includes non-specific, multimodal, expectant, and symptomatic treatment strategies that incorporate a variety of conventional medical modalities as well as complementary and alternative medical therapies (Bennett, Jones, Turk, Russell, & Matallana, 2007; Goldenberg, 2007; Morris, Bowen, & Morris, 2005; Rooks, 2007; Russell). Medications targeting two or more symptomatic domains, each focusing on unique biochemical, neurophysiologic, and psychological abnormalities, may allow for more successful individualization of treatment (Arnold, 2006; Russell).

Treatment recommendations for fibromyalgia were promulgated by the American Pain Society (APS) in 2004 (Burckhardt, 2006). Goldenberg (2007) has recently updated the initial APS recommendations, incorporating published results with newer medications, including pregabalin, duloxetine hydrochloride, and milnacipran. Other promising new therapies for fibromyalgia may include pramixpexole, ropinirole, dextromethorphan, ketamine, and sodium oxybate (Staud, 2007). The APS currently recommends a multi-tiered approach to the management and treatment of fibromyalgia (Goldenberg). The first step is to confirm the diagnosis, to provide patient education about the condition, and to evaluate and treat any comorbid conditions, particularly mood and sleep disturbances. The second step involves appropriate pharmacological treatment (e.g., a trial of a low-dose of a tricyclic antidepressant) and psychological intervention (Goldenberg). Cognitive behavioral therapy is specifically applicable (Bennett & Nelson, 2006; Garcia, Simon, Duran, Canceller, & Aneiros, 2006; Thieme, Flor, & Turk, 2006; van Koulil et al., 2007). The third step is a subspecialty referral to a rheumatologist, physiatrist, psychiatrist, and/or pain medicine specialist, along with a trial of a selective serotonin reuptake inhibitor (SSRI), a serotonin and norepinephrine reuptake inhibitor (SNRI), tramadol, or an anticonvulsant (Goldenberg). The APS guidelines also include moderate aerobic and muscle strengthening exercises, with consideration given to complementary therapies such as hypnosis and acupuncture (Jones, Adams, Winters-Stone, & Burckhardt, 2006). Multidisciplinary strategies are preferable, particularly in patients who have not responded adequately to previous treatments (Burckhardt). Aside from the weak mu-receptor agonist, tramadol, opioid analgesics should be prescribed with caution and only after all other therapies have been exhausted (Goldenberg; Goldenberg, Burckhardt, & Crofford, 2004). Patients with fibromyalgia may be especially prone to opioid-related side effects and psychological dependency (Furlan, Sandoval, Mailis-Gagnon, & Tunks, 2006).

In 1998, the most widely prescribed types of medications in patients with fibromyalgia have included nonsteroidal anti-inflammatory drugs (NSAIDs) (60%), narcotic analgesics (44%), anti-allergy agents (31%), skeletal muscle relaxants (29%), non-narcotic analgesics (14%), SSRIs (18%), tricyclic antidepressants (12%), and other antidepressants (16%) (Robinson et al., 2003). Based upon two recent retrospective insurance claims studies (Berger, Dukes, Martin, Edelsberg, & Oster, 2007; White et al., 2008), the actual annual rates of use of the current APS recommended medications (Goldenberg, 2007) included tricyclic antidepressants (6% and 11%); SSRIs (19% and 22%), SNRIs (8%), tramadol (8%), and anticonvulsants (10% and 12%). Despite potential dependency issues and an attendant increased risk of depression, the annual rate of opioid use approaches 40% in patients with fibromyalgia (Berger et al., 2007). Concomitant medication use occurs in approximately one-third of fibromyalgia patients, with the most frequent combinations being antidepressants with opioids (23%), antidepressants with anticonvulsants (10%), and opioids with sedative/hypnotic medications (9%) (Berger et al.).

The most effective treatments reported by self-selected respondents to an internet survey were rest, heat, pain medications, antidepressants, and hypnotics (Bennett et al., 2007). The medications perceived by these surveyed patients to be the most effective were hydrocodone preparations, aprazaolam, oxycodone preparations, zolpidem, cyclobenzaprine, and clonazepam (Bennett et al.).

The Burden of Fibromyalgia

The direct and indirect costs of fibromyalgia to both the individual and to society are high. Researchers estimate that fibromyalgia costs in the U.S. range between $12 billion to $14 billion each year and account for a loss of 1% to 2% of the nation's overall productivity (Brandenburg, Mucha, & Silverman, 2007). Numerous studies have addressed the spectrum of costs associated with fibromyalgia, including total healthcare costs, direct healthcare costs, indirect costs, and intangible costs associated with fibromyalgia patients' reduced health-related quality of life and functioning (Berger et al., 2007; Hughes, Martinez, Myon, Taeb, & Wessely, 2006; Martinez, Ferraz, Sato, & Atra, 1995; Penrod et al., 2004; Robinson et al., 2003; Robinson & Jones, 2006).

Total healthcare costs were most recently reported among employees with fibromyalgia, osteoarthritis, and controls without fibromyalgia, who were similar in age, gender, and employment status. Using 2005 US dollars, employees with fibromyalgia generated total healthcare costs of $10,199, which is approximately two times that of matched controls (White et al., 2008). These costs were essentially identical to a 1998 estimate, when adjusted for inflation (Robinson et al., 2003). Both studies found that employee disability, absenteeism, and medical comorbidity associated with fibromyalgia greatly increase its economic burden. The majority of payments were for direct healthcare costs (56% in 1998 and 2005), work loss (26% in 1998 and 29% in 2005), and prescription medication use (18% in 1998 and 16% in 2005) (Robinson et al., 2003; White et al., 2008). Only 6% of the total healthcare costs were attributable to fibromyalgia-specific claims; this equated to one dollar spent on fibromyalgia-specific claims for every $57–$143 spent for additional direct and indirect costs (Robinson et al.).

Although total healthcare costs were similar between fibromyalgia and osteoarthritis patients, some variations were found in the cost components. The fibromyalgia patients had lower direct healthcare costs, including lower inpatient and outpatient costs but greater emergency room visits and no difference in prescription medication use. Fibromyalgia patients also had higher indirect costs and a higher frequency of treatments for conditions commonly coexisting with fibromyalgia, including sleep disturbances, depression, anxiety, and chronic fatigue syndrome (White et al., 2008).

The high cost associated with fibromyalgia has been reported to be even greater when other comorbid conditions are present. For example, in a follow-up study by Robinson et al. (2004), which examined comorbid depression, total healthcare costs for those with fibromyalgia and depressive disorders was $11,899 versus $5,163 (in 1998 U.S. dollars) for fibromyalgia patients without depression. In Wolfe and Michaud's similar study (2004), the medical care of fibromyalgia patients with rheumatoid arthritis was more costly than patients with rheumatoid arthritis alone ($6,447 versus $4,687). Walen and colleagues (2001) similarly found that such fibromyalgia comorbidities were predictive of increased costs among female HMO members.

Other studies have examined just the direct healthcare costs associated with fibromyalgia. A recent report by Berger and colleagues (2007) estimated direct healthcare costs with fibromyalgia to be approximately three times that of patients without fibromyalgia. While Berger's cost estimate differential is somewhat higher than that of White and colleagues (2008), much of this difference is likely due to the lower average age and active employment status in the White et al. sample. In Ontario, Canada, the 1993 direct costs for medical services were $1028 for a representative community sample of patients with fibromyalgia diagnosed by a rheumatologist (White, Speechley, Harth, & Ostbye, 1999c) versus $2274 in 1996 U.S. dollars for medical services and medications (Wolfe et al., 1997a). The major contributors to annual direct healthcare costs in this U.S. study were hospitalization ($882), followed by medications ($731), outpatient visits ($340), and other costs ($320) (Wolfe et al., 1997a). Patients used an average of 2.7 fibromyalgia-related drugs in a six-month study period (Wolfe et al.). Patients averaged almost 10 outpatient medical visits per year, with laboratory and radiology studies being as frequent as medical visits (Wolfe et al.). More recent reports also noted a high use of medications and office visits (Berger et al.; White et al.).

Indirect costs account for about half of the total healthcare costs generated by patient with fibromyalgia (Robinson et al., 2003; White et al., 2008). Indirect costs among employees with fibromyalgia were more than twice those of controls and exceeded such costs among employees with osteoarthritis (White et al.). This equated to approximately 18.1 annual days on disability and an additional 11.6 annual days off work due to medically related absences (White et al.). Although 45% of fibromyalgia patients had filed a disability claim, the majority of the disability claims were not directly related to fibromyalgia but instead to comorbid diseases or other unrelated conditions (Robinson et al.).

Another recent study found that nearly 70% of the costs associated with fibromyalgia were indirect costs (Penrod et al., 2004). Disability is typically measured in terms of disability assistance claims, absenteeism, and productivity loss while at work. Penrod and colleagues extended the scope of indirect costs to include the costs of complementary and alternative medicine services, lost time in the market place and non-market place, and replacement costs for housework and childcare. They estimated the desired labor force participation ratio among female rheumatology patients with fibromyalgia to be 67% (Penrod et al.). This was inferred from 42% of subjects working in the previous 6 months and 25% who were receiving disability assistance or retired because of fibromyalgia. Over half of the women missed some work because of fibromyalgia with an average of four weeks annually (Penrod et al.). Added to this was the loss of work time resulting from women who exited the work force altogether due to fibromyalgia, which increased the average 6-month work losses for the total sample to 12.5 weeks. An additional 80 h of household work were lost over the 6 months because of fibromyalgia-related limitations (Penrod et al.).

Societal costs for individuals with fibromyalgia existing outside of the work-force have not been fully addressed. Estimates of the frequency of patients with fibromyalgia who are not working due to temporary or permanent disability range from 9% to 26% (de Girolamo, 1991; Penrod et al., 2004; Wolfe et al., 1997b) versus only 2% in the general population (Tait, Margolis, Krause, & Liebowitz, 1988) and compared to an approximately 10% disability claim frequency among patients with other chronic pain disorders (White, Speechley, Harth, & Ostbye, 1999b). In Scotland, Al-Allaf (2007) found that 47% of patients with fibromyalgia reported losing their job because of their disease compared to 14% of controls. Additionally, work or school hours were found to be reduced because of health problem in 65% of fibromyalgia patients versus 29% of patients with other chronic, similarly generalized pain syndromes, and 9% of controls, respectively (White et al., 1999b).

Problems that interfere with the employment of patients with fibromyalgia include difficulty in performing repetitive motor tasks, prolonged sitting or standing, loss of mental acuity, performance anxiety, and workplace stressors (Waylonis, Ronan, & Gordon, 1994). One study used computerized worksta-tions to simulate work environments that physically stress the shoulders, spine, wrists, and elbows of fibromyalgia patients, rheumatoid arthritis patients, and healthy controls. Patients with fibromyalgia could only perform 59% of the workload performed by their healthy counterpart, whereas patients with rheumatoid arthritis could perform 62% of the controls' workload (Cathey, Wolfe, & Kleinheksel, 1988). The majority of patients with fibromyalgia have been found to reduce their activities of daily living and spend at least one day in bed during a two-week period because of symptoms (White, Speechley, Harth, & Ostbye, 1999a; White et al., 1999b; Wolfe et al., 1997b).

Other previous research has examined the direct healthcare costs of spouses of patients with fibromyalgia, which were virtually equivalent to controls, as well as the intangible costs stemming from the significant deficits in fibro-myalgia patients' health-related quality of life, loss of social support net-works, and functioning (Affleck, Urrows, Tennen, Higgins, & Abeles, 1996; Bernard, Prince, & Edsall, 2000; Martinez et al., 1995; Reisine, Fifield, Walsh, & Feinn, 2003). Patients with fibromyalgia have also been observed to suffer from medical and social isolation and frank stigma due to its poor prognosis, unclear pathology, and the lack of acceptance of fibromyalgia by the medical community (Asbring & Narvanen, 2002; Cudney, Butler, Weinert, & Sullivan, 2002).

Costs appear be driven by the uncertainties of the etiology and relative lack of objective, more verifiable diagnostic criteria in fibromyalgia. Approximately one-quarter of respondents to an internet survey reported seeing six or more healthcare providers about their symptoms of fibromyalgia before a diagno-sis was made (Bennett et al., 2007). One longitudinal study showed a slight reduction in healthcare resource use at 36 months after diagnosis, although there was a large drop out rate in the study (White et al., 2002). For example, in the U.K., primary care patients with fibromyalgia reported higher rates of illness and healthcare resource use for at least 10 years prior to their diagnosis (Hughes et al., 2006). Some decrease in visits for other comorbidities occurred following diagnosis, with a concomitant decrease in referrals and diagnostic tests (Hughes et al.). However, prescription medication rates initially stabilized after an initial diagnosis but subsequently rose (Hughes et al.).

Costs may be further exacerbated in fibromyalgia patients due to the chronic nature of their pain, the predilection towards polypharmacy, the multidisciplinary treatment strategies commonly employed to manage the complex symptoms and comorbid conditions with this ill-defined syndrome, and the varying standards of care. In this context, economic analyses are more complicated and challenging, albeit ostensibly more necessary. Therefore, interventions associated with changes in concomitant medications, psychosocial issues associated with the clinical course of fibromyalgia, lost work time, disability, and out of pocket costs from complementary and alternative therapies would be especially pertinent for healthcare providers and medical decision makers as they manage patients with fibromyalgia.

Economic Analyses of the Treatment of Fibromyalgia

An extensive review of the literature identified only two published articles that compared the cost effectiveness of interventions for fibromyalgia. Neither study was actually pharmacoeconomic. Instead these analyses focused on non-pharmacological interventions (Goossens et al., 1996; Zijlstra, Braakman-Jansen, Taal, Rasker, & van de Laar, 2007). Multidisciplinary pain management interventions were assessed in the Netherlands to determine if educational programs plus cognitive therapy or educational programs alone (plus group discussion as a placebo) were more clinically efficacious and cost effective (Goossens et al.; Vlaeyen et al., 1996). More recently, the cost-effectiveness of spa treatment for fibromyalgia was examined (Zijlstra et al., 2007). These two studies are summarized using the seven fundamental questions identified by Bombardier and Eisenberg (1985) (Table 4).

This paucity of fibromyalgia economic studies is problematic given the significant economic, social, and personal burdens resulting from the condition. That said, in the absence of pharmacoeconomic evaluations of interventions for fibromyalgia, a number of studies, however, that have addressed the efficacy of interventions for fibromyalgia have also included measures of both cost and patient-reported outcomes (i.e., measures of functioning and HRQOL) (Robinson & Jones, 2006). The most widely applied economic measures were the two work items from the Fibromyalgia Impact Questionnaire. Of the economic outcomes, interference with work was the one measure most likely to improve with treatment (Robinson & Jones).

Table 4 The seven fundamental dimensions of a healthcare economic evaluation applied to published studies on fibromyalgia (Bombardier & Eisenberg, 1985)

	Cognitive educational treatment (Goossens et al., 1996).	Spa treatment (Zijlstra et al., 2007).
What type of analysis was performed?	Cost-utility analysis.	Cost-utility analysis.
Was the point of view (perspective) of the study clearly stated?	Yes: Societal perspective.	Yes: Societal perspective.
Were all the important costs and benefits identified?	Yes: Maastrict Utility Measurement Questionnaire, change in health state using a visual analogue rating scale and standard gamble techniques.	Yes: Total costs and utility measures using the SF-6D (validated utility conversion of the Dutch version of the SF-36 generic HRQOL survey) and a visual analogue scale of general health.
How were the costs measured?	Patient report of direct health care costs, direct non-healthcare costs, and indirect costs.	Patient report of direct healthcare costs, direct non-healthcare costs and indirect costs.
Were costs adjusted for differential timings?	Timings not mentioned, but purchasing power parities were applied between countries.	Costs (and effects) were not discounted as the time horizon of this study was less than 1 year.
Was sensitivity analysis performed to check whether the conclusions change as assumptions or data are changed?	Yes: Conclusions remained consistent across the sensitivity analysis.	Not performed.
Were the comparison adequately described?	Yes: Combined educational/cognitive therapy versus educational therapy alone versus a control group (waiting list).	Yes: Spa treatment (including thalassotherapy, group exercise, patient education, recreational activities, and relaxation) versus usual care.
Conclusions:	Addition of a group discussion component to an educational program was more cost effective than addition of a cognitive component. Neither intervention improved HRQOL.	Spa treatment for fibromyalgia temporarily improves fibromyalgia symptoms and HRQOL. Spa therapy is associated with limited incremental costs per patient.

Implications for the Clinical Application of Healthcare Economic Evaluations of Chronic Pain Management

Can Cost-Effectiveness Analysis Be Performed Simultaneously With an Efficacy Study of Chronic Pain Treatment?

In order to have credibility and hence more likely application among clinicians, healthcare economic evaluations must be focused on practical questions that generate understandable and persuasive findings. To this end, there are two basic approaches to conducting a CEA or CUA (O'Brien, 1996; O'Brien et al., 1994). In deterministic decision analytic modeling, the required cost and clinical outcome data are retrospectively obtained from existing sources and coalesced. Alternatively, in the stochastic "piggy-backed" or trial-based approach, the economic data are prospectively collected alongside a "pragmatic" randomized controlled trial that seeks to mimic real life (Drummond, 2001; O'Brien). It is posited here that the latter approach is innately more credible and hence persuasive to the practicing clinician.

In a general sense, cost-effectiveness analysis seeks to identify the most cost-efficient clinical intervention required to achieve a natural unit of output or clinical outcome. Because of the similarity of questions typically addressed, a CEA and CUA are the healthcare economic evaluation designs most frequently conducted alongside or nested within a randomized clinical trial (RCT). Notionally, an RCT and a CEA/CUA can benefit greatly by their concurrent execution (Jefferson et al., 2000).

However, in addition to being logistically burdensome and more costly to perform, combined clinical and economic trials pose two other overall design concerns (Table 5) (Ramsey, McIntosh, & Sullivan, 2001). The health care

Table 5 Trial design issues when performing a cost-effectiveness analysis or a cost-utility analysis alongside or within a randomized controlled trial (Ramsey et al., 2001)

Clinical care in a randomized controlled trial is not representative of that in routine practice:
  Placebo control group is atypical of standard practice
  Additional protocol-related procedures artificially raise the cost of care
  Screening and selection criteria make clinical trial subjects more homogeneous and more likely compliant
  Sub-specialty care provided by study investigators does not reflect typical practice setting
  Close follow-up increases the probability of diagnosing additional diseases
Clinical trials assess efficacy whereas cost-utility analyses evaluate efficiency and resource allocation:
  Clinical trials focus on benefits/harms in targeted patients; cost-utility analyses take a societal perspective
  Surrogate endpoints are common in clinical trials; cost-utility analyses focus directly on health-related quality of life
  Sample size needed for clinical endpoints may not be sufficient for economic analysis
  Time horizon for a clinical trial is usually shorter than that of a cost-utility analysis

provided in an RCT is very often not representative of that delivered in routine clinical practice. Secondly, as noted above, clinical trial assesses *efficacy* whereas a CEA or CUA evaluates *efficiency* and guides resource allocation (Ramsey et al., 2001).

In an effort to address these issues, the International Society for Pharmacoeconomics and Outcomes Research (ISPOR) has developed guidelines for designing, conducting, and reporting cost-effectiveness analyses conducted as a part of a clinical trial (Ramsey et al., 2005), as well as, guidelines for decision analytic modeling in healthcare economic evaluations (Weinstein et al., 2003).

When Designing an Economic Evaluation to Be Conducted Alongside a Clinical Trial, Upon Which Endpoint Should the Overall Study Sample Size Be Based?

The cost, utility and clinical outcome data collected in a concurrently performed economic evaluation and clinical trial can readily be separately described using generally understood measures of central tendency, dispersion, and correlation, while the observed difference in cost or effect can be subjected to hypothesis testing using conventional confidence intervals and/or an appropriate inferential test statistic (Mullahy & Manning, 1994). Challenges arise, however, when such statistics are performed on the ratio of cost and effect (O'Brien & Briggs, 2002).

An incremental cost-effectiveness ratio (ICER) based upon a single sample is a point estimate and thus innately characterized by uncertainty (Briggs & Gray, 1999; Briggs et al., 1994). The optimal method for addressing the uncertainty of an ICER generated using cost and utility data obtained alongside a prospective clinical trial has been an evolutionary yet mathematically rigorous process (Briggs, 2001; O'Brien & Briggs, 2002; Polsky, Glick, Willke, & Schulman, 1997).

Fundamentally, given the characteristics of a ratio, as the random sample point estimate of the difference in clinical effect in the denominator *decreases* and the difference in costs in the numerator *increases*, the ICER becomes very wide and is not clinically useful (Briggs & Gray, 1999). Furthermore, a simple calculation of the confidence interval for an ICER can be quite problematic, given the non-negligible probability of obtaining a very low value in the denominator (the clinical effect) (Briggs, Mooney, & Wonderling, 1999). This is particularly the case when a CEA or CUA is performed using clinical outcome data from a clinical trial designed and powered to detect very small yet clinically meaningful differences in patient outcome (Mullahy & Manning, 1994).

Healthcare costs generally have greater variance (i.e., standard deviation) than clinical outcomes (Briggs & Gray, 1998). Thus, in the majority of studies, the economic analysis component will require greater patient numbers than the clinical trial to demonstrate a statistical significant difference (Briggs & Gray). Furthermore, when an economic evaluation is conducted alongside a randomized controlled trial, the cost data collected are often positively skewed due to outliers, namely, sample subjects (patients) who utilized a disproportionate amount of healthcare resources (Barber & Thompson, 1998; Thompson & Barber, 2000). This lack of a normal distribution violates one of the basic assumptions for parametric inferential statistical analysis.

Consequently, jointly obtained cost and effect data are more appropriately analyzed using non-parametric methods, including a bootstrapping technique for estimating the ICER and its confidence interval (Briggs et al., 2002; Briggs, Wonderling, & Mooney, 1997; Polsky et al., 1997). Well-described techniques, such as bootstrapping remain challenging for the average clinician. As a consequence, there can be some difficulty in terms of interpreting and applying the published results in his or her practice.

Costs per Country Be Pooled or Remain Separate in Multinational Studies of Chronic Pain?

As the number of multinational clinical trials has increased, so too has the interest among healthcare researchers and policymakers in obtaining concurrent multinational economic data (Pang, 2002; Reed et al., 2005). A primary motivation for conducting an economic evaluation alongside a multinational clinical trial is to further enhance the generalizability (i.e., the external validity) of the results of the study (Drummond & Pang, 2001). To this end, the collection of patient-level data on the quantity of resource use, costs per unit of resource, and where applicable, preference-based health state utility are incorporated into the study protocol (Drummond, Manca, & Sculpher, 2005).

However, in a multinational scenario, confounding study subject variability may not be as adequately controlled for by study group randomization. Geographic and temporal differences in healthcare availability and reimbursement, clinical practice and referral patterns, and relative prices are likewise more problematic and can adversely affect the generalizability or transferability of the aggregate cost-effectiveness or cost-utility results (Drummond, Manca et al., 2005; O'Brien, 1997; Reed et al., 2005; Sculpher et al., 2004). Six basic threats to the transferability of healthcare cost-effectiveness data from one country to another have been elucidated: the demography and epidemiology of disease; clinical practice and conventions; incentives and regulations for healthcare providers; relative price levels; consumer preferences; and opportunity cost of resources (O'Brien).

Once again, an accurate healthcare economic evaluation is predicated upon the soundness of the collected cost data (Halliday & Darba, 2003). Whereas relative differences in patient outcomes can suffice in an RCT that focuses solely on clinical efficacy, estimating a transferable incremental cost-effectiveness ratio (ICER) requires the use of absolute differences in costs and effects (Reed et al., 2005). Not surprisingly, considerable attention has thus been devoted to costing in clinical trial-based multinational economic evaluations (Cook, Drummond, Glick, & Heyse, 2003; Drummond et al., 1992; Koopmanschap, Touw, & Rutten, 2001; Willke, Glick, Polsky, & Schulman, 1998). Nevertheless, definitive guidelines for multinational healthcare economic evaluations have yet to be developed (Pang, 2002), and applied costing methodology has hence varied widely (Halliday & Darba).

Given that pain is a complex and highly subjective experience (Turk & Okifuji, 2004), individual patient and physician preference play an equal and major role in clinical decision making in the treatment of chronic pain (Owens, 1998). Considerable country-level heterogeneity has likewise been observed in the prevalence and symptoms of chronic-pain (Verhaak, Kerssens, Dekker, Sorbi, & Bensing, 1998). In the final analysis, as with other diverse chronic clinical conditions (Drummond et al., 1992), both the collection and transferability of concurrent multinational chronic pain trial clinical and economic data may be simply impractical.

Conclusions

The economic, social and personal impact of chronic pain, its management and treatment are substantial. Just like the healthcare decision making process itself, a legitimate economic evaluation need not be performed only at the macro (societal) level or meta (governmental) level. An economic evaluation can also be performed at the meso level, comparing for instance the costs and consequences of specific treatment guidelines for groups of patients with fibromyalgia or chronic low back pain. The principles can equally be performed at the micro level, involving individual providers and their patients, often as part of a shared decision-making model (Sutherland & Till, 1993; Torrance, 1987, 1997). No matter what the applied perspective of the evaluation, indirect productivity costs and intangible costs, although often less emphasized in the literature, are sizeable in chronic pain conditions like fibromyalgia and chronic low back pain.

While healthcare economic evaluation of chronic pain conditions has matured considerably in the last two decades, it nonetheless remains a work in progress, as health services and clinical researchers strive to refine applicable decision analysis models and the means by which to validly measure costs and outcomes of chronic pain treatments (Goossens, Evers, Vlaeyen, Rutten-van Molken, & van der Linden, 1999; Myriam Hunink et al., 2001). This methodological evolution is exemplified in the body of existing chronic pain-related cost-effectiveness and cost-utility analyses (Vetter, 2007a). The majority of the previous conjoint economic and clinical studies have involved a limited time horizon, which while admittedly a matter of practicality, resulted in a failure to address the protracted costs versus benefits of treating long-term and often episodic or recurrent chronic pain conditions (Vetter).

In their recent review of the literature on fibromyalgia treatment efficacy, Robinson and Jones (2006) found twice as many non-pharmacologic (48) as pharmacologic (23) studies, this despite the widespread use of prescription medications for fibromyalgia. These authors also observed that cost measures were included in less than half of the pharmacologic fibromyalgia treatment studies (10 of 23) versus in a majority of the non-pharmacologic fibromyalgia treatment studies (33 of 48). Less than half of the studies that included cost measures noted significant clinical differences across interventions or in pre- versus post- patient assessments. None of the outcome measures provided consistent results across or within therapies. Inclusion of such patient-reported outcome measures has been a more recent practice, with an emphasis more so on specific functional measures than on general HRQOL. Overall, inconsistent results have been observed regarding the efficacy of many pharmacologic and non-pharmacologic interventions as compared to specific cost reduction (Goldenberg et al., 2004; Robinson & Jones).

Similarly, based upon a review of the published literature, definite conclusions could not be made about the most cost-effective intervention for chronic low back pain due to the heterogeneity of interventions, controls and study populations, as well as a frequently incomplete economic analysis (van der Roer et al., 2005). Thus, it would appear that more studies are needed that conjointly assess the clinical efficacy, pertinent costs, and cost-effectiveness (utility) of interventions for both fibromyalgia and chronic low back pain.

The number and quality of published chronic pain-related, full economic analyses nonetheless appear to be increasing (Fig. 3) (Vetter, 2007a). The trend in pharmacoeconomic evaluations may particularly increase as regulatory agencies approve medications for use in specific chronic pain conditions. Currently only 2 drugs, pregabalin and duloxetine, are approved for fibromyalgia and no medication is approved for chronic lower back pain in the United States. As of 2008 and worldwide, no medication is specifically indicated for chronic lower back pain.

Given the insidious and often refractory nature of both conditions, complementary and alternative medicine (CAM) therapies are widely applied for fibromyalgia and chronic low back pain (Lind, Lafferty, Tyree, Diehr, & Grembowski, 2007; Sherman et al., 2004). At least in the United States, much of the cost for such CAM therapies is borne by patients, many of whom clandestinely seek such care when more conventional medical and surgical interventions prove inadequate (Fleming, Rabago, Mundt, & Fleming, 2007). While capturing these out-of-pocket direct healthcare cost data for CAM therapies is innately more challenging (i.e., requires that patients complete a detailed cost diary rather than simply abstracting an insurance claims database), doing so would appear to be a requisite in order to make future representative and thus valid conclusions about treatment incremental cost-effectiveness.

Despite the attendant methodological challenges, given the present state of affairs, it would appear worthwhile for researchers and clinicians to incorporate healthcare economic evaluations into their treatment and analyses of the costs associated with long term chronic pain (Neumann, 2005; Vetter, 2007a). To do otherwise will likely disenfranchise such strongly invested individuals from the decision-making process already underway in government and among third-party payers, aimed at identifying how to optimally allocate finite resources in the face of a virtually ever increasing demand for health care, including for the now more longitudinal treatment of chronic pain conditions (Neumann, 2005; Vetter, 2007a). Moreover, the seemingly next logical step in the advancement of healthcare policy and point-of-service delivery appears to be the melding of the admittedly presently more well-established principles of evidence-based medicine with both patient-centered outcomes and cost-effectiveness data so as to create the paradigm of value-based medicine (Brown et al., 2005).

References

Abeles, A. M., Pillinger, M. H., Solitar, B. M., & Abeles, M. (2007). Narrative review: The pathophysiology of fibromyalgia. *Annals of Internal Medicine, 146*(10), 726–734.

Adam, T., Koopmanschap, M. A., & Evans, D. B. (2003). Cost-effectiveness analysis: can we reduce variability in costing methods? *International Journal of Technology Assessment in Health Care, 19*(2), 407–420.

Affleck, G., Urrows, S., Tennen, H., Higgins, P., & Abeles, M. (1996). Sequential daily relations of sleep, pain intensity, and attention to pain among women with fibromyalgia. *Pain, 68*(2–3), 363–368.

Al-Allaf, A. W. (2007). Work disability and health system utilization in patients with fibromyalgia syndrome. *Journal of Clinical Rheumatology: Practical Reports On Rheumatic & Musculoskeletal Diseases, 13*(4), 199–201.

American Pain Society. (2007). *APS glossary of pain terminology.* Retrieved November 1, 2007, from http://www.ampainsoc.org/links/pain_glossary.htm

Anderson, J. J., Ruwe, M., Miller, D. R., Kazis, L., Felson, D. T., & Prashker, M. (2002). Relative costs and effectiveness of specialist and general internist ambulatory care for patients with 2 chronic musculoskeletal conditions. *Journal of Rheumatology, 29*(7), 1488–1495.

Arnold, L. M. (2006). Biology and therapy of fibromyalgia. New therapies in fibromyalgia. *Arthritis Research & Therapy, 8*(4), 212.

Arts, M. P., Peul, W. C., Brand, R., Koes, B. W., & Thomeer, R. T. (2006). Cost-effectiveness of microendoscopic discectomy versus conventional open discectomy in the treatment of lumbar disc herniation: A prospective randomised controlled trial. *BMC Musculoskeletal Disorders, 7*, 42.

Asbring, P., & Narvanen, A. L. (2002). Women's experiences of stigma in relation to chronic fatigue syndrome and fibromyalgia. *Qualitative Health Research, 12*(2), 148–160.

Atkinson, J. H., Slater, M. A., Patterson, T. L., Grant, I., & Garfin, S. R. (1991). Prevalence, onset, and risk of psychiatric disorders in men with chronic low back pain: A controlled study. *Pain, 45*(2), 111–121.

Barber, J. A., & Thompson, S. G. (1998). Analysis and interpretation of cost data in randomised controlled trials: review of published studies. *BMJ, 317*(7167), 1195–1200.

Behrens, V., Seligman, P., Cameron, L., Mathias, C. G., & Fine, L. (1994). The prevalence of back pain, hand discomfort, and dermatitis in the US working population. *American Journal of Public Health, 84*(11), 1780–1785.

Bennett, R., & Nelson, D. (2006). Cognitive behavioral therapy for fibromyalgia. *Nature Clinical Practice Rheumatology, 2*(8), 416–424.

Bennett, R. M., Jones, J., Turk, D. C., Russell, I. J., & Matallana, L. (2007). An internet survey of 2,596 people with fibromyalgia. *BMC Musculoskelet Disord, 8*, 27.

Berger, A., Dukes, E., Martin, S., Edelsberg, J., & Oster, G. (2007). Characteristics and healthcare costs of patients with fibromyalgia syndrome. *International Journal of Clinical Practice, 61*(9), 1498–1508.

Bernard, A. L., Prince, A., & Edsall, P. (2000). Quality of life issues for fibromyalgia patients. *Arthritis Care and Research, 13*(1), 42–50.

Biyani, A., & Andersson, G. B. (2004). Low back pain: Pathophysiology and management. *Journal of the American Academy of Orthopaedic Surgeons, 12*(2), 106–115.

Blyth, F. M., March, L. M., Brnabic, A. J., & Cousins, M. J. (2004). Chronic pain and frequent use of health care. *Pain, 111*(1–2), 51–58.

Blyth, F. M., March, L. M., Brnabic, A. J., Jorm, L. R., Williamson, M., & Cousins, M. J. (2001). Chronic pain in Australia: A prevalence study. *Pain, 89*(2–3), 127–134.

Bombardier, C., & Eisenberg, J. (1985). Looking into the crystal ball: Can we estimate the lifetime cost of rheumatoid arthritis? *Journal of Rheumatology, 12*(2), 201–204.

Bombardier, C., & Maetzel, A. (1999). Pharmacoeconomic evaluation of new treatments: Efficacy versus effectiveness studies? *Annals of the Rheumatic Diseases, 58 Suppl 1,* 182–185.

Boonen, A., van den Heuvel, R., van Tubergen, A., Goossens, M., Severens, J. L., & van der Heijde, D. et al. (2005). Large differences in cost of illness and wellbeing between patients with fibromyalgia, chronic low back pain, or ankylosing spondylitis. *Annals of the Rheumatic Diseases, 64*(3), 396–402.

Brandenburg, N., Mucha, L., & Silverman, S. (2007). (939): Impact of fibromyalgia on medical care expenditures and productivity losses. *The Journal of Pain, 8*(4, Supplement 1), S85.

Briggs, A. (2000). Handling uncertainty in cost-effectiveness models. *Pharmacoeconomics, 17*(5), 479–500.

Briggs, A. (2001). Handling uncertainty in economic evaluation and presenting results. In M. Drummond & A. McGuire (Eds.), *Economic evaluation in health care: Merging theory with practice* (pp. 172–214). New York: Oxford University Press.

Briggs, A., & Gray, A. (1998). Power and sample size calculations for stochastic cost-effectiveness analysis. *Medical Decision Making, 18*(2 Suppl), S81–S92.

Briggs, A., & Gray, A. (1999). Handling uncertainty in economic evaluations of healthcare interventions. *BMJ, 319*(7210), 635–638.

Briggs, A., Mooney, C., & Wonderling, D. (1999). Constructing confidence intervals for cost-effectiveness ratios: An evaluation of parametric and non-parametric techniques using Monte Carlo simulation. *Statistics in Medicine, 18*(23), 3245–3262.

Briggs, A., O'Brien, B., & Blackhouse, G. (2002). Thinking outside the box: Recent advances in the analysis and presentation of uncertainty in cost-effectiveness studies. *Annual Review of Public Health, 23*, 377–401.

Briggs, A., Sculpher, M., & Buxton, M. (1994). Uncertainty in the economic evaluation of health care technologies: The role of sensitivity analysis. *Health Economics, 3*(2), 95–104.

Briggs, A., Wonderling, D., & Mooney, C. (1997). Pulling cost-effectiveness analysis up by its bootstraps: A non-parametric approach to confidence interval estimation. *Health Economics, 6*(4), 327–340.

Brouwer, W., Rutten, F., & Koopmanschap, M. A. (2001). Costing in economic evaluation. In M. Drummond & A. McGuire (Eds.), *Economic evaluation in health care: Merging theory with practice* (pp. 68–93). New York: Oxford University Press.

Brown, G. C., Brown, M. M., & Sharma, S. (2005). *Evidence-based to value-based medicine.* Chicago: AMA Press.

Burckhardt, C. S. (2006). Multidisciplinary approaches for management of fibromyalgia. *Current Pharmaceutical Design, 12*(1), 59–66.

Carey, T. S., Evans, A., Hadler, N., Kalsbeek, W., McLaughlin, C., & Fryer, J. (1995). Care-seeking among individuals with chronic low back pain. *Spine, 20*(3), 312–317.

Carragee, E. J. (2005). Clinical practice. Persistent low back pain. *The New England Journal of Medicine, 352*(18), 1891–1898.

Cathey, M. A., Wolfe, F., & Kleinheksel, S. M. (1988). Functional ability and work status in patients with fibromyalgia. *Arthritis Care and Research, 1*(2), 85–98.

Centers for Disease Control and Prevention. (2005). *Chronic disease overview.* Retrieved November 1, 2007, from http://www.cdc.gov/nccdphp/overview.htm

Chakrabarty, S., & Zoorob, R. (2007). Fibromyalgia. *American Family Physician, 76*(2), 247–254.

Cherkin, D. C., Wheeler, K. J., Barlow, W., & Deyo, R. A. (1998). Medication use for low back pain in primary care. *Spine, 23*(5), 607–614.

Chou, R. (2005). Evidence-based medicine and the challenge of low back pain: where are we now? *Pain Practice: The Official Journal of World Institute Of Pain, 5*(3), 153–178.

Cook, J. R., Drummond, M., Glick, H., & Heyse, J. F. (2003). Assessing the appropriateness of combining economic data from multinational clinical trials. *Statistics in Medicine, 22*(12), 1955–1976.

Critchley, D. J., Ratcliffe, J., Noonan, S., Jones, R. H., & Hurley, M. V. (2007). Effectiveness and cost-effectiveness of three types of physiotherapy used to reduce chronic low back pain disability: A pragmatic randomized trial with economic evaluation. *Spine, 32*(14), 1474–1481.

Cudney, S. A., Butler, M. R., Weinert, C., & Sullivan, T. (2002). Ten rural women living with fibromyalgia tell it like it is. *Holistic Nursing Practice, 16*(3), 35–45.

de Girolamo, G. (1991). Epidemiology and social costs of low back pain and fibromyalgia. *The Clinical Journal of Pain, 7* Suppl 1, S1–S7.

de Lissovoy, G., Brown, R. E., Halpern, M., Hassenbusch, S. J., & Ross, E. (1997). Cost-effectiveness of long-term intrathecal morphine therapy for pain associated with failed back surgery syndrome. *Clinical Therapeutics, 19*(1), 96–112.

Detsky, A. S. (1995). Evidence of effectiveness: evaluating its quality. In F. A. Sloan (Ed.), *Valuing health care: costs, benefits, and effectiveness of pharmaceuticals and other medical technologies* (pp. 15–29). Cambridge, UK: Cambridge University Press.

Detsky, A. S., & Naglie, I. G. (1990). A clinician's guide to cost-effectiveness analysis. *Annals of Internal Medicine, 113*(2), 147–154.

Drummond, M. (2001). Introducing economic and quality of life measurements into clinical studies. *Annals of Medicine, 33*(5), 344–349.

Drummond, M., Bloom, B. S., Carrin, G., Hillman, A. L., Hutchings, H. C., & Knill-Jones, et al. (1992). Issues in the cross-national assessment of health technology. *International Journal of Technology Assessment in Health Care, 8*(4), 671–682.

Drummond, M., Manca, A., & Sculpher, M. (2005). Increasing the generalizability of economic evaluations: Recommendations for the design, analysis, and reporting of studies. *International Journal of Technology Assessment in Health Care, 21*(2), 165–171.

Drummond, M., & Pang, F. (2001). Transferability of economic evaluation results In A. McGuire & M. Drummond (Eds.), *Economic evaluation in health care: Merging theory with practice* (pp. 256–276). Oxford: Oxford University Press.

Drummond, M., Sculpher, M. J., Torrance, G. W., O'Brien, B. J., & Stoddart, G. L. (2005). *Methods for economic evaluation of health care programmes* (3rd ed.). New York: Oxford University Press.

Duckro, P. N., Schultz, K. T., & Chibnall, J. T. (1994). Migraine as a sequela to chronic low back pain. *Headache, 34*(5), 279–281.

Ekman, M., Jonhagen, S., Hunsche, E., & Jonsson, L. (2005). Burden of illness of chronic low back pain in Sweden: A cross-sectional, retrospective study in primary care setting. *Spine*, *30*(15), 1777–1785.

Engel, C. C., von Korff, M., & Katon, W. J. (1996). Back pain in primary care: predictors of high health-care costs. *Pain*, *65*(2–3), 197–204.

Feeny, D. H. (2005). Preference-based utility measures: utility and quality-adjusted life years. In P. Fayers & R. Hays (Eds.), *Assessing quality of life in clinical trials* (2nd ed., pp. 406–429). New York: Oxford University Press.

Fishbain, D. A., Cutler, R. B., Cole, B., Lewis, J., Smets, E., & Rosomoff, H. L., et al. (2004). Are patients with chronic low back pain or chronic neck pain fatigued? *Pain Medicine (Malden, Mass.)*, *5*(2), 187–195.

Fleming, S., Rabago, D. P., Mundt, M. P., & Fleming, M. F. (2007). CAM therapies among primary care patients using opioid therapy for chronic pain. *BMC Complementary and Alternative Medicine*, *7*, 15.

Fritzell, P., Hagg, O., Jonsson, D., & Nordwall, A. (2004). Cost-effectiveness of lumbar fusion and nonsurgical treatment for chronic low back pain in the Swedish Lumbar Spine Study: A multicenter, randomized, controlled trial from the Swedish Lumbar Spine Study Group. *Spine*, *29*(4), 421–434.

Frymoyer, J. W., & Cats-Baril, W. L. (1991). An overview of the incidences and costs of low back pain. *Orthopedic Clinics of North America*, *22*(2), 263–271.

Furlan, A. D., Sandoval, J. A., Mailis-Gagnon, A., & Tunks, E. (2006). Opioids for chronic noncancer pain: A meta-analysis of effectiveness and side effects. *CMAJ*, *174*(11), 1589–1594.

Garcia, J., Simon, M. A., Duran, M., Canceller, J., & Aneiros, F. J. (2006). Differential efficacy of a cognitive-behavioral intervention versus pharmacological treatment in the management of fibromyalgic syndrome. *Psychology, Health & Medicine*, *11*(4), 498–506.

Gilbert, F. J., Grant, A. M., Gillan, M. G. C., Vale, L. D., Campbell, M. K., & Scott, N. W., et al. (2004). Low back pain: Influence of early MR imaging or CT on treatment and outcome – Multicenter randomized trial. *Radiology*, *231*(2), 343–351.

Glick, H. A., Doshi, J., Sonnad, S., & Polsky, D. (2007). *Economic evaluation in clinical trials*. New York: Oxford University Press.

Goetzel, R. Z., Hawkins, K., Ozminkowski, R. J., & Wang, S. (2003). The health and productivity cost burden of the "top 10" physical and mental health conditions affecting six large U.S. employers in 1999. *Journal of Occupational and Environmental Medicine*, *45*(1), 5–14.

Goldenberg, D. L. (2007). Pharmacological treatment of fibromyalgia and other chronic musculoskeletal pain. *Best Practice & Research. Clinical Rheumatology*, *21*(3), 499–511.

Goldenberg, D. L., Burckhardt, C., & Crofford, L. (2004). Management of fibromyalgia syndrome. *JAMA*, *292*(19), 2388–2395.

Goossens, M. E., Evers, S. M., Vlaeyen, J. W., Rutten-van Molken, M. P., & van der Linden, S. M. (1999). Principles of economic evaluation for interventions of chronic musculoskeletal pain. *European Journal of Pain*, *3*(4), 343–353.

Goossens, M. E., Rutten-van Molken, M. P., Leidl, R. M., Bos, S. G., Vlaeyen, J. W., & Teeken-Gruben, N. J. (1996). Cognitive-educational treatment of fibromyalgia: A randomized clinical trial. II. Economic evaluation. *Journal of Rheumatology*, *23*(7), 1246–1254.

Grabois, M. (2005). Management of chronic low back pain. *American Journal of Physical Medicine and Rehabilitation*, *84*(3 Suppl), S29–41.

Grimes, D. A., & Schulz, K. F. (2002). An overview of clinical research: The lay of the land. *Lancet*, *359*(9300), 57–61.

Guo, H. R., Tanaka, S., Cameron, L. L., Seligman, P. J., Behrens, V. J., & Ger, J., et al. (1995). Back pain among workers in the United States: National estimates and workers at high risk. *American Journal of Industrial Medicine*, *28*(5), 591–602.

Hadler, N. M., Tait, R. C., & Chibnall, J. T. (2007). Back pain in the workplace. *JAMA*, *297*(14), 1594–1596.

Halliday, R. G., & Darba, J. (2003). Cost data assessment in multinational economic evaluations: some theory and review of published studies. *Applied Health Economics and Health Policy*, *2*(3), 149–155.

Hart, L. G., Deyo, R. A., & Cherkin, D. C. (1995). Physician office visits for low back pain. Frequency, clinical evaluation, and treatment patterns from a U.S. national survey. *Spine*, *20*(1), 11–19.

Hazard, R. G. (2007). Low-back and neck pain diagnosis and treatment. *American Journal of Physical Medicine and Rehabilitation*, *86*(1 Suppl), S59–S68.

Hoffman, P. K., Meier, B. P., & Council, J. R. (2002). A comparison of chronic pain between an urban and rural population. *Journal of Community Health Nursing*, *19*(4), 213–224.

Hughes, G., Martinez, C., Myon, E., Taeb, C., & Wessely, S. (2006). The impact of a diagnosis of fibromyalgia on health care resource use by primary care patients in the UK: An observational study based on clinical practice. *Arthritis and Rheumatism*, *54*(1), 177–183.

Indahl, A. (2004). Low back pain: Diagnosis, treatment, and prognosis. *Scandinavian Journal of Rheumatology*, *33*(4), 199–209.

James Cook University. (2004). Economic burden of back pain tops $9 billion [Electronic Version]. *Outlook*, *16*, 12–13. Retrieved November 6, 2007 from http://www.jcu.edu.au/div1/marketingandpr/Marketing/outlook/outlookoct.pdf.

Jefferson, T., Demicheli, V., & Mugford, M. (2000). *Elementary economic evaluation in health care* (2nd ed.). London: BMJ Publishing Group.

Jones, K. D., Adams, D., Winters-Stone, K., & Burckhardt, C. S. (2006). A comprehensive review of 46 exercise treatment studies in fibromyalgia (1988–2005). *Health and Quality of Life Outcomes*, *4*, 67.

Kocher, M. S., & Henley, M. B. (2003). It is money that matters: Decision analysis and cost-effectiveness analysis. *Clinical Orthopedics and Related Research*(413), 106–116.

Koes, B. W., van Tulder, M. W., Ostelo, R., Burton, A. K., & Waddell, G. (2001). Clinical guidelines for the management of low back pain in primary care: An international comparison. *Spine*, *26*(22), 2504–2513.

Koopmanschap, M. A., Rutten, F. F., van Ineveld, B. M., & van Roijen, L. (1995). The friction cost method for measuring indirect costs of disease. *Journal of Health Economics*, *14*(2), 171–189.

Koopmanschap, M. A., Touw, K. C. R., & Rutten, F. F. H. (2001). Analysis of costs and cost-effectiveness in multinational trials. *Health Policy*, *58*(2), 175–186.

Korthals-de Bos, I., van Tulder, M., van Dieten, H., & Bouter, L. (2004). Economic evaluations and randomized trials in spinal disorders: Principles and methods. *Spine*, *29*(4), 442–448.

Kovacs, F. M., Fernandez, C., Cordero, A., Muriel, A., Gonzalez-Lujan, L., & Gil del Real, M. T. (2006). Non-specific low back pain in primary care in the Spanish National Health Service: A prospective study on clinical outcomes and determinants of management. *BMC Health Services Research*, *6*, 57.

Kovacs, F. M., Llobera, J., Abraira, V., Lazaro, P., Pozo, F., & Kleinbaum, D. (2002). Effectiveness and cost-effectiveness analysis of neuroreflexotherapy for subacute and chronic low back pain in routine general practice: A cluster randomized, controlled trial. *Spine*, *27*(11), 1149–1159.

Lind, B. K., Lafferty, W. E., Tyree, P. T., Diehr, P. K., & Grembowski, D. E. (2007). Use of complementary and alternative medicine providers by fibromyalgia patients under insurance coverage. *Arthritis and Rheumatism*, *57*(1), 71–76.

Loisel, P., Lemaire, J., Poitras, S., Durand, M. J., Champagne, F., & Stock, S., et al. (2002). Cost-benefit and cost-effectiveness analysis of a disability prevention model for back pain management: A six year follow up study. *Occupational and Environmental Medicine*, *59*(12), 807–815.

Loney, P. L., & Stratford, P. W. (1999). The prevalence of low back pain in adults: a methodological review of the literature. *Physical Therapy*, *79*(4), 384–396.

Luce, B. R., Manning, W. G., Siegel, J. E., & Lipscomb, J. (1996). Estimating costs in cost-effectiveness analysis. In M. R. Gold, J. E. Siegel, L. B. Russell, & M. C. Weinstein (Eds.), *Cost-effectiveness in health and medicine* (pp. 176–213). New York: Oxford University Press.

Luo, X., Pietrobon, R., Sun, S. X., Liu, G. G., & Hey, L. (2004). Estimates and patterns of direct health care expenditures among individuals with back pain in the United States. *Spine*, *29*(1), 79–86.

Maetzel, A., & Li, L. (2002). The economic burden of low back pain: A review of studies published between 1996 and 2001. *Best Practice & Research. Clinical Rheumatology*, *16*(1), 23–30.

Malter, A. D., Larson, E. B., Urban, N., & Deyo, R. A. (1996). Cost-effectiveness of lumbar discectomy for the treatment of herniated intervertebral disc. *Spine*, *21*(9), 1048–1054.

Manca, A., Dumville, J. C., Torgerson, D. J., Klaber Moffett, J. A., Mooney, M. P., & Jackson, D. A., et al. (2007). Randomized trial of two physiotherapy interventions for primary care back and neck pain patients: Cost effectiveness analysis. *Rheumatology*, *46*(9), 1495–1501.

Mäntyselkä, P., Kumpusalo, E., Ahonen, R., Kumpusalo, A., Kauhanen, J., & Viinamaki, H. , et al. (2001). Pain as a reason to visit the doctor: A study in Finnish primary health care. *Pain*, *89*(2–3), 175–180.

Mäntyselkä, P., Turunen, J. H., Ahonen, R. S., & Kumpusalo, E. A. (2003). Chronic pain and poor self-rated health. *JAMA*, *290*(18), 2435–2442.

Martinez, J. E., Ferraz, M. B., Sato, E. I., & Atra, E. (1995). Fibromyalgia versus rheumatoid arthritis: A longitudinal comparison of the quality of life. *Journal of Rheumatology*, *22*(2), 270–274.

McCarberg, B. H., & Billington, R. (2006). Consequences of neuropathic pain: quality-of-life issues and associated costs. *American Journal of Managed Care*, *12*(9 Suppl), S263–S268.

Mease, P. (2005). Fibromyalgia syndrome: Review of clinical presentation, pathogenesis, outcome measures, and treatment. *The Journal of Rheumatology. Supplement*, *75*, 6–21.

Miller, P., Kendrick, D., Bentley, E., & Fielding, K. (2002). Cost-effectiveness of lumbar spine radiography in primary care patients with low back pain. *Spine*, *27*(20), 2291–2297.

Morris, C. R., Bowen, L., & Morris, A. J. (2005). Integrative therapy for fibromyalgia: Possible strategies for an individualized treatment program. *Southern Medical Journal*, *98*(2), 177–184.

Muennig, P. (2002). *Designing and conducting cost-effectiveness analyses in medicine and health care*. San Francisco: Jossey-Bass.

Mullahy, J., & Manning, W. (1994). Statistical issues in cost-effectiveness analysis. In F. A. Sloan (Ed.), *Valuing health care* (pp. 149–184). Cambridge, UK: Cambridge University Press.

Myriam Hunink, M. G., Glasziou, P. P., Siegel, J. E., Weeks, J. C., Pliskin, J. S., & Elstein, A. S., et al. (2001). *Decision making in health and medicine: Integrating evidence and values*. Cambridge, UK: Cambridge University Press.

National Institute of Neurological Disorders and Stroke. (2007). *Low back pain fact sheet*. Retrieved November 1, 2007, from http://www.ninds.nih.gov/disorders/backpain/detail_-backpain.htm

Neumann, P. J. (2005). *Using cost-effectiveness analysis to improve health care: Opportunities and barriers*. New York: Oxford University Press.

Newton, W., Curtis, P., Witt, P., & Hobler, K. (1997). Prevalence of subtypes of low back pain in a defined population. *Journal of Family Practice*, *45*(4), 331–335.

Niemisto, L., Rissanen, P., Sarna, S., Lahtinen-Suopanki, T., Lindgren, K. A., & Hurri, H. (2005). Cost-effectiveness of combined manipulation, stabilizing exercises, and physician consultation compared to physician consultation alone for chronic low back pain: A prospective randomized trial with 2-year follow-up. *Spine, 30*(10), 1109–1115.

Nord, E. (1999). *Cost-value in health care: Making sense out of QALYs.* New York: Cambridge University Press.

North, R. B., Kidd, D., Shipley, J., & Taylor, R. S. (2007). Spinal cord stimulation versus reoperation for failed back surgery syndrome: A cost effectiveness and cost utility analysis based on a randomized, controlled trial. *Neurosurgery, 61*(2), 361–368.

O'Brien, B. (1996). Economic evaluation of pharmaceuticals. Frankenstein's monster or vampire of trials? *Medical Care, 34*(12 Suppl), DS99–108.

O'Brien, B. (1997). A tale of two (or more) cities: Geographic transferability of pharmacoeconomic data. *American Journal of Managed Care, 3* Suppl, S33–S39.

O'Brien, B., & Briggs, A. (2002). Analysis of uncertainty in health care cost-effectiveness studies: An introduction to statistical issues and methods. *Statistical Methods in Medical Research, 11*(6), 455–468.

O'Brien, B., Drummond, M. F., Labelle, R. J., & Willan, A. (1994). In search of power and significance: Issues in the design and analysis of stochastic cost-effectiveness studies in health care. *Medical Care, 32*(2), 150–163.

Obenchain, R. L., Robinson, R. L., & Swindle, R. W. (2005). Cost-effectiveness inferences from bootstrap quadrant confidence levels: three degrees of dominance. *Journal of Biopharmaceutical Statistics, 15*(3), 419–436.

Olsen, J. A., & Smith, R. D. (2001). Theory versus practice: a review of 'willingness-to-pay' in health and health care. *Health Economics, 10*(1), 39–52.

Oostenbrink, J. B., Koopmanschap, M. A., & Rutten, F. F. (2002). Standardisation of costs: The Dutch Manual for Costing in economic evaluations. *Pharmacoeconomics, 20*(7), 443–454.

Owens, D. K. (1998). Spine update. Patient preferences and the development of practice guidelines. *Spine, 23*(9), 1073–1079.

Pang, F. (2002). Design, analysis and presentation of mresentation of multinational economic studies – The need for guidance. *Pharmacoeconomics, 20*(2), 75–90.

Patrick, D. L., Deyo, R. A., Atlas, S. J., Singer, D. E., Chapin, A., & Keller, R. B. (1995). Assessing health-related quality of life in patients with sciatica. *Spine, 20*(17), 1899.

Penrod, J. R., Bernatsky, S., Adam, V., Baron, M., Dayan, N., & Dobkin, P. L. (2004). Health services costs and their determinants in women with fibromyalgia. *Journal of Rheumatology, 31*(7), 1391–1398.

Perquin, C. W., Hazebroek-Kampschreur, A. A., Hunfeld, J. A., Bohnen, A. M., van Suijlekom-Smit, L. W., & Passchier, J., et al. (2000). Pain in children and adolescents: A common experience. *Pain, 87*(1), 51–58.

Phillips, C. J. (2003). Pain management: Health economics and quality of life considerations. *Drugs, 63* Spec No 2, 47–50.

Phillips, K., Ch'ien, A. P. Y., Norwood, B. R., & Smith, C. (2003). Chronic low back pain management in primary care. *The Nurse Practitioner, 28*(8), 26–31.

Polatin, P. B., Kinney, R. K., Gatchel, R. J., Lillo, E., & Mayer, T. G. (1993). Psychiatric illness and chronic low-back pain. The mind and the spine–which goes first? *Spine, 18*(1), 66–71.

Polsky, D., Glick, H. A., Willke, R., & Schulman, K. (1997). Confidence intervals for cost-effectiveness ratios: A comparison of four methods. *Health Economics, 6*(3), 243–252.

Price, C., Arden, N., Coglan, L., & Rogers, P. (2005). Cost-effectiveness and safety of epidural steroids in the management of sciatica. *Health Technology Assessment, 9*(33), 1–58.

Ramsey, S., McIntosh, M., & Sullivan, S. (2001). Design issues for conducting cost-effectiveness analyses alongside clinical trials. *Annual Review of Public Health, 22*, 129–141.

Ramsey, S., Willke, R., Briggs, A., Brown, R., Buxton, M., & Chawla, A., et al. (2005). Good research practices for cost-effectiveness analysis alongside clinical trials: the ISPOR RCT-CEA Task Force report. *Value Health, 8*(5), 521–533.

Raphael, K. G., Janal, M. N., Nayak, S., Schwartz, J. E., & Gallagher, R. M. (2006). Psychiatric comorbidities in a community sample of women with fibromyalgia. *Pain, 124*(1–2), 117–125.

Ratcliffe, J., Thomas, K. J., MacPherson, H., & Brazier, J. (2006). A randomised controlled trial of acupuncture care for persistent low back pain: Cost effectiveness analysis. *BMJ, 333*(7569), 626.

Reed, S. D., Anstrom, K. J., Bakhai, A., Briggs, A. H., Califf, R. M., & Cohen, D. J., et al. (2005). Conducting economic evaluations alongside multinational clinical trials: Toward a research consensus. *American Heart Journal, 149*(3), 434–443.

Reisine, S., Fifield, J., Walsh, S. J., & Feinn, R. (2003). Do employment and family work affect the health status of women with fibromyalgia? *Journal of Rheumatology, 30*(9), 2045–2053.

Rivero-Arias, O., Campbell, H., Gray, A., Fairbank, J., Frost, H., & Wilson-MacDonald, J. (2005). Surgical stabilisation of the spine compared with a programme of intensive rehabilitation for the management of patients with chronic low back pain: Cost utility analysis based on a randomised controlled trial. *BMJ, 330*(7502), 1239–1243.

Rivero-Arias, O., Gray, A., Frost, H., Lamb, S. E., & Stewart-Brown, S. (2006). Cost-utility analysis of physiotherapy treatment compared with physiotherapy advice in low back pain. *Spine, 31*(12), 1381–1387.

Rizzo, J. A., Abbott, T. A., 3rd, & Berger, M. L. (1998). The labor productivity effects of chronic backache in the United States. *Medical Care, 36*(10), 1471–1488.

Robinson, R. (1993a). Cost-benefit analysis. *BMJ, 307*(6909), 924–926.

Robinson, R. (1993b). Cost-effectiveness analysis. *BMJ, 307*(6907), 793–795.

Robinson, R. (1993c). Cost-utility analysis. *BMJ, 307*(6908), 859–862.

Robinson, R. (1993d). Costs and cost-minimisation analysis. *BMJ, 307*(6906), 726–728.

Robinson, R. L., Birnbaum, H. G., Morley, M. A., Sisitsky, T., Greenberg, P. E., & Claxton, A. J. (2003). Economic cost and epidemiological characteristics of patients with fibromyalgia claims. *Journal of Rheumatology, 30*(6), 1318–1325.

Robinson, R. L., Birnbaum, H. G., Morley, M. A., Sisitsky, T., Greenberg, P. E., & Wolfe, F. (2004). Depression and fibromyalgia: treatment and cost when diagnosed separately or concurrently. *The Journal Of Rheumatology, 31*(8), 1621–1629.

Robinson, R. L., & Jones, M. L. (2006). In search of pharmacoeconomic evaluations for fibromyalgia treatments: A review. *Expert Opinion on Pharmacotherapy, 7*(8), 1027–1039.

Rooks, D. S. (2007). Fibromyalgia treatment update. *Current Opinion in Rheumatology, 19*(2), 111–117.

Rubin, D. I. (2007). Epidemiology and risk factors for spine pain. *Neurologic Clinics, 25*(2), 353–371.

Russell, I. J. (2006). Fibromyalgia [Electronic Version]. *Essential Science Indicators.* Retrieved November 2, 2007 from http://www.esi-topics.com/fibro/interviews/IJonRussell.html.

Russell, L. B., Siegel, J. E., Daniels, N., Gold, M. R., Luce, B. R., & Mandelblatt, J. S. (1996). Cost-effectiveness analysis as a guide to resource allocation in health: Roles and limitations. In M. R. Gold, J. E. Siegel, L. B. Russell, & M. C. Weinstein (Eds.), *Cost-effectiveness in health and medicine* (pp. 3–24). New York: Oxford University Press.

Sculpher, M. J., Pang, F. S., Manca, A., Drummond, M. F., Golder, S., & Urdahl, H., et al. (2004). Generalisability in economic evaluation studies in healthcare: a review and case studies. *Health Technology Assessment, 8*(49), 1–192.

Sherman, K. J., Cherkin, D. C., Connelly, M. T., Erro, J., Savetsky, J. B., & Davis, R. B., et al. (2004). Complementary and alternative medical therapies for chronic low back pain: What treatments are patients willing to try? *BMC Complementary and Alternative Medicine, 4*, 9.

Smith, A. F., & Brown, G. C. (2000). Understanding cost effectiveness: A detailed review. *British Journal of Ophthalmology, 84*(7), 794–798.

Staud, R. (2006). Biology and therapy of fibromyalgia: Pain in fibromyalgia syndrome. *Arthritis Research & Therapy, 8*(3), 208.

Staud, R. (2007). Treatment of fibromyalgia and its symptoms. *Expert Opinion on Pharmacotherapy, 8*(11), 1629–1642.

Steenstra, I. A., Anema, J. R., van Tulder, M. W., Bongers, P. M., de Vet, H. C., & van Mechelen, W. (2006). Economic evaluation of a multi-stage return to work program for workers on sick-leave due to low back pain. *Journal of Occupational Rehabilitation, 16*(4), 557–578.

Stewart, W. F., Ricci, J. A., Chee, E., Morganstein, D., & Lipton, R. (2003). Lost productive time and cost due to common pain conditions in the US Workforce. *JAMA, 290*(18), 2443–2454.

Stone, P. W., Chapman, R. H., Sandberg, E. A., Liljas, B., & Neumann, P. J. (2000). Measuring costs in cost-utility analyses. Variations in the literature. *International Journal of Technology Assessment in Health Care, 16*(1), 111–124.

Strom, B. L. (1994). *Pharmacoepidemiology* (2nd ed.). New York: John Wiley & Sons.

Strong, L. L., Von Korff, M., Saunders, K., & Moore, J. E. (2006). Cost-effectiveness of two self-care interventions to reduce disability associated with back pain. *Spine, 31*(15), 1639–1645.

Sutherland, H. J., & Till, J. E. (1993). Quality of life assessments and levels of decision making: Differentiating objectives. *Quality of Life Research, 2*(4), 297–303.

Tait, R. C., Margolis, R. B., Krause, S. J., & Liebowitz, E. (1988). Compensation status and symptoms reported by patients with chronic pain. *Archives of Physical Medicine and Rehabilitation, 69*(12), 1027–1029.

Taylor, R. J., & Taylor, R. S. (2005). Spinal cord stimulation for failed back surgery syndrome: a decision-analytic model and cost-effectiveness analysis. *International Journal of Technology Assessment in Health Care, 21*(3), 351–358.

Taylor, R. S., Taylor, R. J., Van Buyten, J. P., Buchser, E., North, R., & Bayliss, S. (2004). The cost effectiveness of spinal cord stimulation in the treatment of pain: A systematic review of the literature. *Journal of Pain and Symptom Management, 27*(4), 370–378.

Tella, M. N., Feinglass, J., & Chang, R. W. (2003). Cost-effectiveness, cost-utility, and cost-benefit studies in rheumatology: A review of the literature, 2001–2002. *Current Opinion in Rheumatology, 15*(2), 127–131.

Thieme, K., Flor, H., & Turk, D. C. (2006). Psychological pain treatment in fibromyalgia syndrome: Efficacy of operant behavioural and cognitive behavioural treatments. *Arthritis Research & Therapy, 8*(4), R121.

Thompson, S. G., & Barber, J. A. (2000). How should cost data in pragmatic randomised trials be analysed? *BMJ, 320*(7243), 1197–1200.

Thomsen, A. B., Sorensen, J., Sjogren, P., & Eriksen, J. (2002). Chronic non-malignant pain patients and health economic consequences. *European Journal of Pain, 6*(5), 341–352.

Torrance, G. W. (1987). Measurement of health utilities for economic appraisals. *Journal of Health Economics, 5*, 1–30.

Torrance, G. W. (1997). Preferences for health outcomes and cost-utility analysis. *American Journal of Managed Care, 3* Suppl, S8–S20.

Torrance, G. W., Siegel, J. E., & Luce, B. R. (1996). Framing and designing the cost-effectiveness study. In M. R. Gold, J. E. Siegel, L. B. Russell, & M. C. Weinstein (Eds.), *Cost-effectiveness in health and medicine* (pp. 54–81). New York: Oxford University Press.

Tosteson, A. N. (2000). Preference-based health outcome measures in low back pain. *Spine, 25*(24), 3161–3166.

Turk, D. C., & Okifuji, A. (1998). Treatment of chronic pain patients: Clinical outcomes, cost-effectiveness, and cost-benefits of multidisciplinary pain centers. *Critical Reviews in Physical and Rehabilitation Medicine, 10*(2), 181–208.

Turk, D. C., & Okifuji, A. (2004). Psychological aspects of pain. In C. A. Warfield & Z. H. Bajwa (Eds.), *Principles and practice of pain medicine* (pp. 139–156). New York: McGraw-Hill.

UK BEAM Trial Team. (2004). United Kingdom back pain exercise and manipulation (UK BEAM) randomised trial: Cost effectiveness of physical treatments for back pain in primary care. *BMJ, 329*(7479), 1381–1385.

van der Roer, N., Boos, N., & van Tulder, M. W. (2006). Economic evaluations: A new avenue of outcome assessment in spinal disorders. *European Spine Journal,* 15 Suppl 1, S109–S117.

van der Roer, N., Goossens, M. E., Evers, S. M., & van Tulder, M. W. (2005). What is the most cost-effective treatment for patients with low back pain? A systematic review. *Best Practice & Research Clinical Rheumatology, 19*(4), 671–684.

van der Roer, N., van Tulder, M. W., Barendse, J. M., van Mechelen, W., Franken, W. K., & Ooms, A. C., et al. (2004). Cost-effectiveness of an intensive group training protocol compared to physiotherapy guideline care for sub-acute and chronic low back pain: Design of a randomised controlled trial with an economic evaluation. *BMC Musculoskeletal Disorders, 5,* 45.

van Geen, J. W., Edelaar, M. J., Janssen, M., & van Eijk, J. T. (2007). The long-term effect of multidisciplinary back training: a systematic review. *Spine, 32*(2), 249–255.

van Koulil, S., Effting, M., Kraaimaat, F. W., van Lankveld, W., van Helmond, T., & Cats, H., et al. (2007). Cognitive-behavioural therapies and exercise programmes for patients with fibromyalgia: State of the art and future directions. *Annals of the Rheumatic Diseases, 66*(5), 571–581.

Verhaak, P. F. M., Kerssens, J. J., Dekker, J., Sorbi, M. J., & Bensing, J. M. (1998). Prevalence of chronic benign pain disorder among adults: a review of the literature. *Pain, 77*(3), 231–239.

Vetter, T. R. (2007a). The application of economic evaluation methods in the chronic pain medicine literature. *Anesthesia and Analgesia, 105*(1), 114–118.

Vetter, T. R. (2007b). A primer on health-related quality of life in chronic pain medicine. *Anesthesia and Analgesia, 104*(3), 703–718.

Vlaeyen, J. W., Teeken-Gruben, N. J., Goossens, M. E., Rutten-van Molken, M. P., Pelt, R. A., & van Eek, H., et al. (1996). Cognitive-educational treatment of fibromyalgia: a randomized clinical trial. I. Clinical effects. *Journal of Rheumatology, 23*(7), 1237–1245.

Vogt, M. T., Nevitt, M. C., & Cauley, J. A. (1997). Back problems and atherosclerosis. The Study of Osteoporotic Fractures. *Spine, 22*(23), 2741–2747.

Walen, H. R., Cronan, P. A., & Bigatti, S. M. (2001). Factors associated with healthcare costs in women with fibromyalgia. *American Journal of Managed Care, 7* Spec No, SP39–S47.

Waylonis, G. W., Ronan, P. G., & Gordon, C. (1994). A profile of fibromyalgia in occupational environments. *American Journal of Physical Medicine and Rehabilitation, 73*(2), 112–115.

Webster, B. S., & Snook, S. H. (1990). The cost of compensable low back pain. *Journal of Occupational Medicine, 32*(1), 13–15.

Weinstein, M. C., O'Brien, B., Hornberger, J., Jackson, J., Johannesson, M., & McCabe, C., et al. (2003). Principles of good practice for decision analytic modeling in health-care evaluation: Report of the ISPOR Task Force on Good Research Practices–Modeling Studies. *Value Health, 6*(1), 9–17.

White, K., Nielson, W. R., Harth, M., Ostbye, T., & Speechley, M. (2002). Does the label "fibromyalgia" alter health status, function, and health service utilization? A prospective, within-group comparison in a community cohort of adults with chronic widespread pain. *Arthritis and Rheumatism, 47*(3), 260–265.

White, K., Speechley, M., Harth, M., & Ostbye, T. (1999a). Comparing self-reported function and work disability in 100 community cases of fibromyalgia syndrome versus controls in London, Ontario: the London Fibromyalgia Epidemiology Study. *Arthritis and Rheumatism, 42*(1), 76–83.

White, K., Speechley, M., Harth, M., & Ostbye, T. (1999b). The London Fibromyalgia Epidemiology Study: Comparing the demographic and clinical characteristics in 100 random community cases of fibromyalgia versus controls. *Journal of Rheumatology, 26*(7), 1577–1585.

White, K., Speechley, M., Harth, M., & Ostbye, T. (1999c). The London Fibromyalgia Epidemiology Study: direct health care costs of fibromyalgia syndrome in London, Canada. *Journal of Rheumatology, 26*(4), 885–889.

White, L. A., Birnbaum, H. G., Kaltenboeck, A., Tang, J., Mallet, D., & Robinson, R. L. (2008). Medical comorbidities, pharmaceutical use and health care costs in patients with fibromyalgia. *Journal of Occupational and Environmental Medicine, 50*, 13–24.

Whitehurst, D. G., Lewis, M., Yao, G. L., Bryan, S., Raftery, J. P., & Mullis, R., et al. (2007). A brief pain management program compared with physical therapy for low back pain: Results from an economic analysis alongside a randomized clinical trial. *Arthritis and Rheumatism, 57*(3), 466–473.

Willke, R. J., Glick, H. A., Polsky, D., & Schulman, K. (1998). Estimating country-specific cost-effectiveness from multinational clinical trials. *Health Economics, 7*(6), 481–493.

Witt, C. M., Jena, S., Selim, D., Brinkhaus, B., Reinhold, T., & Wruck, K., et al. (2006). Pragmatic randomized trial evaluating the clinical and economic effectiveness of acupuncture for chronic low back pain. *American Journal of Epidemiology, 164*(5), 487–496.

Wolfe, F., Anderson, J., Harkness, D., Bennett, R. M., Caro, X. J., & Goldenberg, D. L., et al. (1997a). A prospective, longitudinal, multicenter study of service utilization and costs in fibromyalgia. *Arthritis and Rheumatism, 40*(9), 1560–1570.

Wolfe, F., Anderson, J., Harkness, D., Bennett, R. M., Caro, X. J., & Goldenberg, D. L., et al. (1997b). Work and disability status of persons with fibromyalgia. *Journal of Rheumatology, 24*(6), 1171–1178.

Wolfe, F., & Michaud, K. (2004). Severe rheumatoid arthritis (RA), worse outcomes, comorbid illness, and sociodemographic disadvantage characterize ra patients with fibromyalgia. *Journal of Rheumatology, 31*(4), 695–700.

Wolfe, F., Ross, K., Anderson, J., Russell, I. J., & Hebert, L. (1995). The prevalence and characteristics of fibromyalgia in the general population. *Arthritis and Rheumatism, 38*(1), 19–28.

Wolfe, F., Smythe, H. A., Yunus, M. B., Bennett, R. M., Bombardier, C., & Goldenberg, D. L., et al. (1990). The American College of Rheumatology 1990 Criteria for the Classification of Fibromyalgia. Report of the Multicenter Criteria Committee. *Arthritis and Rheumatism, 33*(2), 160–172.

Zagari, M. J., Mazonson, P. D., & Longton, W. C. (1996). Pharmacoeconomics of chronic nonmalignant pain. *Pharmacoeconomics, 10*(4), 356–377.

Zarnke, K. B., Levine, M. A., & O'Brien, B. J. (1997). Cost-benefit analyses in the health-care literature: don't judge a study by its label. *Journal of Clinical Epidemiology, 50*(7), 813–822.

Zijlstra, T. R., Braakman-Jansen, L. M., Taal, E., Rasker, J. J., & van de Laar, M. A. (2007). Cost-effectiveness of Spa treatment for fibromyalgia: General health improvement is not for free. *Rheumatology, 46*(9), 1454–1459.

Chemotherapy Induced Peripheral Neuropathies (CIPNs): A Biobehavioral Approach

Rhonda J. Moore

"I moan, I try to speak and my soul feels suffocated..."
The 77th Psalm

"The worse pain a person can suffer: to have insight into much and power over nothing."
Herodotus

"Give me life, Give me pain, Give me myself again."
Tori Amos

Abstract Pain is a prevalent symptom in patients with cancer. Chemotherapy Induced Peripheral Neuropathies (CIPNs), as a type of cancer related pain, are an increasingly common neuropathic pain syndrome. In this paper, we offer a biobehavioral approach to understanding the development and perhaps the maintenance of CIPNs. First, CIPNs are defined. This is followed by a description of the epidemiology, symptoms, and barriers associated with CIPNs. Following important research from the fields of pain, behavior and psychoneuroimmunology (PNI), we suggest that injury to peripheral nerves after chemotherapeutic treatments initiates immune to brain communication, which further modulates the biological mechanisms through which life experiences and behavior reinforce and likely perpetuate the experience of CIPN.

Introduction

Pain is a prevalent symptom in patients with cancer [1–28]. Chemotherapy-induced peripheral neuropathies (CIPNs), as a type of cancer pain, are an increasingly common neuropathic pain syndrome in cancer survivors [1–162]. They have been described as the 'end result,' the 'dose limiting' side effect, or as

R.J. Moore (✉)
National Cancer Institute, SRLB/DEA, National Institutes of Health, 6116 Executive Boulevard, Rockville, MD 20852-8329, USA
e-mail: moorerh@mail.nih.gov

R.J. Moore (ed.), *Biobehavioral Approaches to Pain*,
DOI 10.1007/978-0-387-78323-9_11, © Springer Science+Business Media, LLC 2009

the de facto toxic effect which limits the administration of many commonly used anti-neoplastic agents [8–162]. In other words, this specific neuropathic pain syndrome in patients with cancer is caused (at least in part) by injury to nerve structures [8–21]. This damage caused by chemotherapeutic agents can also cause subsequent and long-term functional abnormalities of structural lesions in the peripheral and central nervous system [8–21, 110, 151]. The chemotherapeutic agents most often associated with CIPNs are the platinum-based compounds, taxanes, vinca alkaloids, thalidomide, and bortezomib [8–16, 24–144].

In this paper, we offer a biobehavioral approach to understanding the development and maintenance of CIPNs. CIPNs are defined. This is followed by a description of the epidemiology, symptoms, and barriers associated with CIPNs. Following important research from the fields of pain, neuroscience, behavior and psychoneuroimmunology (PNI), we suggest that injury to peripheral nerves after chemotherapeutic treatments initiates immune to brain communication, which further modulates the biological mechanisms through which life experiences and behavior reinforce and likely perpetuate the experience of CIPN.

Epidemiology

Cancer Pain is a prevalent symptom in cancer patients. It may be present at any time during the course of the illness [8–22, 24–98, 118–136, 148, 152–162]. About 30% to 50% of cancer survivors experience pain while undergoing treatment [118–129, 153–155]. The frequency and intensity of cancer pain also tends to increase with advanced staged disease. Between 75 and 90% of patients with metastatic or advanced stage cancer experience significant cancer-induced pain [1–8, 118–129]. Uncontrolled, under assessed and often under treated, it can also cause significant physical, emotional, and psychological distress and suffering [1–23, 118–129].

CIPNs are as a type of neuropathic pain that develops post-chemotherapeutic treatment in cancer survivors. They are a serious yet understudied consequence of cancer treatment [1–98, 134–136, 152–224]. The sensory and motor symptoms and signs of CIPNs can be disabling, and can have a significant impact on the quality of life (QOL) of cancer patients [8–16]. Even when CIPN is not a dose-limiting side effect, its onset may severely affect QOL and cause chronic discomfort [8–16, 24–98].

The prevalence of CIPNs are not actually known due a lack of adequate standardized assessment, measurement and reporting mechanisms [9, 10]. Incidence may vary and depend on the drugs and schedules used [8–16]. The incidence of severe CIPN has been estimated at 3%–7% in individuals treated with single agents. Risk factors and comorbid conditions have also been associated with worse symptomology. The risk factors include: prior uses of chemotherapies (particularly prior treatments with platinum based therapies), age (older), gender differences (female). There is also recent evidence that the incidence of CIPN is upwards of 38% in those individuals treated with multiple chemotherapeutic agents [8–22, 24–98]. Comorbid conditions that appear to place patients at greater risk for CIPN include diabetes, HIV, alcoholism, pre-existing neuropathies (i.e., diabetic neuropathy), and vitamin B deficiencies [8–15]. Great variability exists in the symptoms associated with CIPNs, and little is known about other risk factors [8–15]. Moreover, even when neurophysiologic methods are used to make a diagnosis, which are associated with an higher incidence, there is still a wide variation in the resultant symptoms [8–16].

In what follows, we briefly describe the symptoms, barriers and risk factors associated with CIPN. This will be followed by a discussion of the etiology of CIPNs.

Symptoms Associated with CIPNs

For an excellent discussion of the symptoms associated with CIPNs, the reader is referred to Paice [13, 15] Wickham [9] Stillman [10] and Manyth [8]. Briefly, the symptoms are described as follows:

- The majority of patients report a gradual onset, although some develop the sensation rapidly [8–15].
- The primary effects are sensory, occurring in a 'stocking-glove distribution' in the toes and fingers [8–15, 17].
- Terms such as "burning," "tingling," "electrical sensation, "painful numbness" have all been used to describe the symptoms associated with CIPNs [13, 15].
- Patients may also report increased pain during walking, with descriptions of sensations such as "walking on shards of glass" or "stepping on razorblades." [13, 15]
- Physical examination may reveal tactile allodynia, cold allodynia, hypersensitivity and loss of deep tendon reflexes [13, 15].
- Patients may also experience a loss of Proprioception. Proprioception is defined as the unconscious perception of movement and spatial orientation arising from stimuli within the body itself. Under normal circumstances, large diameter myelinated A fibers innervating skin, joints and muscles normally conduct non-noxious stimuli including fine touch and vibration as well as proprioceptive information. And under these normal conditions, large sensory neurons do not conduct noxious stimuli. These large myelinated sensory fibers are preferentially injured by chemotherapeutic agents such as the vinca alkaloids, taxanes and platinum-based compounds [13, 15, 17]. Injury or damage to large sensory fibres by chemothereuoutic treatments can also result in the paresthesias, dysesthesias and decreased proprioceptive abilities [8–21]. These stimuli can be detected by nerves within the body itself,

as well as by the semicircular canals of the inner ear. The evaluation for loss of Proprioception includes having the patient close their eyes, move a toe or finger up or down, and state whether the digit is facing upward or downward [8, 13, 15].

- Thes experience can vary and its length cannot be predicted. In other words, it can last from days to a lifetime [8–17].
- Loss of proprioception can also lead to significant safety issues [8, 13, 15]. Patients without proprioceptive sense are at great risk for falls as they also tend to lose all sense of the position of their feet. This raises other concerns regarding their ability to safely drive, particularly when proprioception and sensation are impaired [13, 15]. If patients are unable to feel the brakes or lack the strength to adequately press a pedal, they should not drive [13, 15, 22].

Barriers

Multiple barriers limit optimal pain management in patients with cancer pain and CIPN [8–23, 118–136]. These include Patient, Clinician, Health System and Treatment related factors, racial and ethnic disparities, as well as, wide variation in the phenotypic expression of CIPN symptomology [8–23, 118–136, 152–162].

- *Patient related Factors:*
  Patient related factors include opioid-phobia, under-reporting of cancer related pain due to fears of addiction, fears that the cancer has returned, and beliefs about suffering and poor-clinician patient communication [23, 118–136].
- *Clinician related Factors:*
  Clinician related factors include a lack of knowledge of effective cancer pain management. This also involves a lack adequate knowledge regarding the proper evaluation, assessment, and diagnostic techniques as well as attitudinal barriers by healthcare providers, and poor-clinician patient communication [23, 118–136].
- *Treatment and Health Care System related Factors:*
  Treatments for pain can include physical modalities, exercise, opioids, alternative and complementary medicine, adjuvant medications, and interventional techniques [152–225]. Yet there are also significant barriers to treatments [118–136]. Barriers to treatment may also include side effects, finances, access issues, and attitudes [23, 118–136, 152–224]. In addition, well-intentioned governmental regulations to battle the war on drug abuse often catch pain patients in the crossfire (see also Rich, This Volume). These financial barriers to effective cancer pain management are created by the health care system, and exist in both in the private and public sectors [24, 101–112]. (See also Robinson and Vettner, this Volume)

- **Racial and Ethnic Disparities in Pain:**

  *B*eyond the previously described barriers in cancer pain management, racial and ethnic minorities and other vulnerable populations (e.g. children, women and the elderly) are also at a great risk for inadequate pain management [23, 120–129, 101–112] (See also Cucchiaro, McCarberg and Cole, and Dy, all in this Volume). Individuals from these populations also tend to be under evaluated and treated for pain and related symptoms when compared with non-Hispanic Whites [23, 120–129] Disparities in pain perception, assessment, and treatment have been noted across clinical settings (i.e., postoperative, emergency room) and across all types of pain (i.e., acute, cancer, chronic nonmalignant, and experimental) [23, 120–129]. The sources of pain disparities among racial and ethnic minorities are complex, involving patient (e.g., patient/health care provider communication, attitudes), health care provider (e.g., decision making), and health care system (e.g., access to pain medication) factors [23, 120–129, 24, 101–112].

- **Variation in Symptoms:**

  The clinician cannot simply turn off peripheral nervous system damage post-chemotherapeutic treatments, and the phenomenon of 'coasting,' which is the appearance of neurotoxicity after the discontinuation of chemotherapeutic agents frequently occurs [10]. In addition, it is still quite difficult to predict whether otherwise neurologically normal patients will exhibit susceptibility to the neurotoxic effects of chemotherapy [8–15]. The diagnosis, assessment and management of CIPNs are complicated by therefore existing wide variation in symptoms as well as the lack of a reliable and standardized means to diagnose and monitor patients who are at risk for, or who are symptomatic from, this complication of treatment [8–21, 24–28, 30–98, 130, 148, 152, 155–162]. There are also no well established criteria or guidelines for dose reduction [10].

Heterogeneity in symptoms can range from an almost exclusively sensory or sensory-motor neuropathies, with or without clinical evidence of autonomic impairment [8–22]. For instance, recent, insight from animal and human studies support these findings suggesting that the great heterogeneity in the underlying mechanism(s) of nerve injury caused by individual agents, may partly explain the wide variation in the resultant symptoms [8–22, 137, 149–150].

Chemotherapeutic toxicity is also influenced by multiple genetic factors and nongenetic factors including age, sex and drug-drug interactions [8, 118–137, 154–163]. The manifestations of adverse drug reactions also differ between men and women. For instance, women tend to experience greater toxicity from chemotherapeutic drugs than men [133]. These issues further contribute to the difficulties in predicting which patients from which populations will exhibit long term damage from chemotherapeutic treatments [8–23, 118–37]. Treatments have historically been supportive [8–22, 91, 163–215]. At this time, no medications currently exist that can fully relieve the sensory and motor loss associated with advanced CIPNs. For instance, neuropathic pain management is generally aimed at reducing symptoms, generally by suppressing neuronal activity, and not glial cell activation, which has also been recently associated with the development and maintenance of long-term chronic pain states [8, 29, 99–117].

As a consequence, CIPNs represent a large unmet need for patients due to the absence of adequate assessment and evidence based treatments that could be widely applied across clinical CIPN patient populations and which could potentially prevent or mitigate this increasingly common clinical problem [8–15, 187–224]. Thus, this wide variation in biobehavioral symptomology remains a significant barrier which further contributes to the inadequate pain assessment and management of CIPNs.

A Biobehavioral Approach to Understanding CIPNs

Recent studies over the past decade have begun to explore a biobehavioral approach, one that considers the interactive role of biological, environmental, cultural, emotional and psychosocial processes that directly and indirectly impact the development and course of human illness and disease [31–32]. Pain is also a subjective experience that results from the transduction, transmission or modulation of sensory information. This physiologic input is filtered via an individual's socio-cultural framework, learning and experience, genetic, history, affective or emotional states, as well as, past and current psychological status [8, 31–32].

Biobehavioral research can make an important contribution towards a greater understanding of chronic pain and disability since it focuses on the study of the interactions between biologic factors, behavioral factors and clinical outcomes including disease progression, symptom management and quality of life (QOL) [31–32]. In the context of an evolving understanding of these issues in terms of the development of long term chronic pain states, this shift in emphasis also highlights a growing body of evidence including clinical, animal and experimental data which now clearly shows that immunologic as well as chronic inflammatory factors also significantly contribute to the development and maintenance of long term chronic pain states [8, 31–32, 99–117, 137–147].

Following this important research, in this paper, we suggest that injury to peripheral nerves by cancer and chemotherapeutic treatment activates immune-to-brain communication which also plays a role in the biobehavioral processes underlying the development and perhaps the maintenance of CIPNs [8, 31–32, 99–117, 137–147].

In what follows, we offer some insight as to how these biobehavioral processes and long terms changes in pain states after chemotherapeutic treatment might potentially happen. To begin, we offer a brief overview of healthy peripheral nerves. Then, using Matzinger's Danger theory [149–150]. we briefly explore the environmental context in which peripheral nerve injury post chemotherapeutic treatment(s), as well as, the subsequent biobehavioral processes including activation of the peripheral innate immune system, glial cell activation, immune to brain communication and long term central sensitization occur. We suggest that these biobehavioral processes contribute to the development and maintenance of long term chronic pain states including advanced CIPNs [8, 31–32, 99–117, 137–147].

Healthy Peripheral Nerves

In this paper, we highlight some of the biobehavioral factors and processes associated with the development and perhaps maintenance of CIPNs. As a starting point, we begin with a brief discussion of healthy peripheral nerves. Under normal circumstances, pain serves a highly adaptive normal survival function. In states of health, the majority of ongoing immune surveillance is accomplished by immune cells that reside in the peripheral nerve itself [8, 99, 116]. These cells are "resting" as they provide active surveillance of the nerve's microenvironment. Moreover, they also do not release the proinflammatory mediators as they do upon activation [8, 99, 116].

The Danger Model

The Danger model is a theory proposed by Polly Matzinger at the National Institutes of Health, and it provides an interesting theoretical basis for not only understanding the damage to peripheral nerves post chemotherapeutic treatments [149–150]. It is also an elegant way of explaining the dynamic and constantly-updated response to danger as defined by cellular damage [149–150]. The model suggests that the immune system is more concerned with damage than with foreignness. Immune responses are not initiated by the mere 'foreign-ness' of an antigen but rather by its capacity to create damage [149–150]. Here, the immune response is called into action by 'danger signals' from injured tissues, rather than by the recognition of non-self [149–150]. Thus antigen-presenting cells respond to the 'danger signals' (e.g, from cells undergoing injury, or stress or 'bad cell death', as opposed to apoptosis, controlled cell death). The alarm signals released by these cells let the immune system know that there is a problem requiring an immune response [149–150].

This elegant model is both broad and specific since it readily accounts for both the complexity of the environmental context in terms of the immune response, as in many instances normal as well as pathologic immune responses exist on a continuum [149–150]. Yet, it fails to fully explain why the immune system responds in different ways to different situations [149–150]. Recent evidence supports the possibility that the activation of the peripheral innate immune system, glial cell activations and the brain cytokine system can also be triggered by these 'danger signals,' [8, 31–32, 99–117, 137–147] which include among others heat shock proteins (Hsp) and endogenous nucleic acids that are genomic or mitochondrial in their origin [149–150].

Cancer as a Context

In patients with cancer, the immune response to tumor cells contributes to an already adverse proinflammatory state [8, 19, 146]. Tumoral invasion at central and/or peripheral sites can lead to mechanical damage, proteolysis, and the release of inflammatory pain mediators (including proinflammatory cytokines (i.e. Interleukin 1 (IL-1), Interleukin 6 (Il-6) and Tumor necrosis factor-alpha (TNF-α))which may result in damage to the surrounding tissues [8, 17, 19, 101–105, 146, 149–150]. Cytokines actually function as a motivational signal that tells the brain to change the organism priorities in face of the threat represented by pathogens or 'danger signals.' [138, 141, 149–150] Damaged cells put out 'danger' signals that activate local antigen presenting cells and initiate an immune response [149–150].

Other clinical studies suggest that cytokines, such as tumor necrosis factor (TNF), play a prominent role in the initiation, development and maintenance chronic pain states including neuropathic pain. Members of the TNF super-family also mediate a wide variety of diseases, including cancer, arthritis, bone resorption, and tumor metastases. After injury, TNF- is detected in macro-phages, fibroblasts, neutrophils, and Schwann cells. IL-6, serum levels of IL-6 are increased in patients with neuropathy and other painful conditions. IL-6 is also thought to play an important role in the initiation of painful neuropathies. In neuropathic mice, nerve injury correlates with IL-6 levels and with pain-associated behavior [8, 17, 101–105].

Though the underlying mechanism have yet to be fully elucidated, cancer can be seen as contributing the 'priming of an environmental, psychologic, beha-vioral and physiologic context where peripheral nerve damage could occur, and can accordingly enhance peripheral nerve excitability, exaggerated pain state as well as axonal hyperexcitability, Wallerian degeneration and resultant pain behaviors post chemotherapeutic treatments [8, 17, 19, 101–105, 146, 149–150].

Peripheral Nerve Injury and Peripheral Sensitization

Given the variation in symptoms occurs across various patient populations, it is clear that not all 'damage' is created equal. For example, the 'damage' caused to peripheral nerves by chemotherapeutic treatments depends not only on the anticancer agent(s) used, co-morbidities (i.e. preexisting neuropathies), demographics (age-older; gender-female), the cumulative doses and the delivery method, but also on the capacity of the nerve to cope with the following: the extent of the damage and immune response to these 'danger signals [8, 17, 19, 101–105, 146, 149–150].

Following nerve injury induced by a tumor, tumor-associated cells, or chemotherapeutic agents, many nociceptors alter their response properties and expression of neurotransmitters, receptors and growth factors [8, 17, 19, 101–105, 146]. The injury or functional alterations in nociceptive sensory neurons induced by chemotherapeutic agents may contribute to myalgia, as well as the cold and mechanical allodynia observed in patients receiving chemotherapy [8, 13, 15]. The peripheral, motor, sensory, and autonomic neuronal damage secondary to neurotoxic chemotherapy agents that inactivate the components required to maintain the metabolic needs of the axon [8–21]. In addition, a number of immune cells also release chemokines [101–105, 115]. These proinflammatory chemokines and cytokines, nitric oxide (NO) and reactive oxygen species (ROS) also directly increase nerve excitability, damage myelin, and disrupt the blood–nerve barrier, thus further facilitating the movement of immune products into the damaged nerve [101–103] (ROS) also plays an important pro-inflammatory role, including endothelial cell damage and increased microvascular permeability, release of cytokines, and recruitment of neutrophils at sites of inflammation [101–103, 117].

In addition and, as Watkins (2007) has shown in her important research:

….some activated resident immune cells release degradative enzymes and acids in response to nerve trauma that exposes peripheral nerve proteins (e.g., P0, P2) [01–103]. Nerve proteins such as P0 and P2 are responded to as "non-self" as they are normally buried within the myelin sheath and not detected by immune cells [101–103, 149–150]. Once released, these immune-derived enzymes and acids attack myelin and disrupt the blood–nerve barrier, again allowing increased access of the nerve to bloodborne immune cells… [101–104] …

These activated immune cells and immune-like glial cells can dramatically alter neuronal function and pain states [101–105]. Indeed, the pro-inflammatory cytokines produced by the activation of peripheral innate immune cells and up regulated by glial cell activation are already potentially activated in patients with cancer, and may also play an important role in the peripheral immune response to nerve injury or damage post chemotherapy [8].

Peripheral Nerve Injury and Glial Activation of the Spinal Cord

As we have stated, the recent evidence supports the possibility that the activation of the peripheral innate immune system, glial cell activation and the brain cytokine system can also be triggered by these 'danger' signals [8, 99–117, 138–147, 149–150]. As a consequence of chemotherapy induced damage to sensory neurons, areas of the spinal cord and CNS involved in the processing of somatosensory information also undergo various neurochemical and cellular changes, including glial cell activation

[8, 99–117, 138–147], which facilitate the transmission and conscious awareness of both noxious and non-noxious sensory information [8, 151].

Spinal glia and more recently spinal meninges [120] have also been shown to be activated after injury in response to peripheral immune challenges that activate immune-to-brain communication [8, 99–117, 138–147]. After activation they release chemical modulators that modulate neuronal activity and synaptic strength [102]. Glia (both astrocytes and microglial) in the spinal cord are activated (as inferred from glial activation markers) in response to inflammation, or damage to peripheral tissues, peripheral nerves, spinal nerves, or spinal cord [8, 99–117, 138–147] Activated glia upregulate the release of substance P and other excitatory amino acids from primary afferent neurons in the spinal cord and enhance the excitability of pain transmission neurons. In addition, microglia and astrocytes also release proinflammatory cytokines, such as IL-1, IL-6 and TNF-α. [8, 99–117, 138–147]

Inflammatory cytokines are also induced in the CNS, independent of release of cytokines from the peripheral site of injury. [8, 19, 117] In the CNS, nerve injury also induces structural changes in the dorsal horn, and neuroplasticity. Injured C fiber terminals from the damaged nerve may atrophy and withdraw from lamina I/II and in their place, A-B fibers sprout into the superficial layers of the dorsal horn. In terms of neuroplasticity, the simplest form is that repeated noxious stimulation which may lead to habituation or sensitization [8, 216–218, 223–224]. Prolonged or strong activity of dorsal horn neurons caused by repeated or sustained noxious stimulation may also lead to increased neuronal responsiveness, or central sensitization [8, 216–218, 223–224].

Central sensitization, an activity-dependent increase in the excitability of spinal neurons, is a result of persistent exposure to nociceptive afferent input from the peripheral neurons [8, 216–218, 223–224]. Taken together, these processes (habituation or sensitization contribute to a hypersensitivity state (e.g., spinal wind-up) that is responsible for primary and secondary hyperalgesia and increased pain [8, 216–218, 223–224]. Prolonged central sensitization has the capacity to lead to permanent alterations in the central nervous system, including the death of inhibitory neurons, replacement with new afferent excitatory neurons, axonal sprouting, the establishment of aberrant excitatory synaptic connections and chronic long-term neuropathic pain [8, 216–218, 223–224].

Immune to Brain Communication

Peripheral immune and glial cell activation and signaling to the CNS via proinflammatory cytokine production induces sickness behaviors and sickness responses [8, 99–117, 138–147]. Inflammatory cytokines released during peripheral innate immune response have been implicated in the communication of peripheral inflammatory signals to the brain [8, 99–117, 138–147]. These peripheral cytokines have been shown to communicate with the brain via a fast neural pathway and a slower humoral pathway [117, 142]. The fast neural pathway has been attributed to cytokine activation of vagal afferent nerves, leading to a production of cytokines in the brain [8, 99–117, 138–147]. The importance of the neural pathway in the transmission of the immune message from the periphery to the brain is not the same for all components of sickness behavior [142]. The slower humoral transmission of the cytokine message is represented by the production of molecular intermediates at the level of the blood–brain interface in response to circulating cytokines or micro-organism fragments (e.g., prostaglandins of the E2 series) that propagate into the brain, or by diffusion of cytokines through the blood–brain-barrier. The fast neural pathway and the slow humoral pathway converge in a manner, which remains unknown, to promote the brain expression of IL-1, a predominant mediator of sickness behavior in the brain, because electrical stimulation of the vagus nerve induces the expression of brain IL-1. And it is also possible that the neural immune-to-brain communication pathway recruits various brain areas and sensitizes them to the action of the slowly propagating cytokine message [142].

Sickness Responses and Sickness Behaviors

Animal and human studies highlight the fact that inflammatory cytokines play a central role in mediating sickness-related behaviors by communicating peripheral inflammation to the brain [138–147]. Drawing from animal studies, Dantzer has shown that the expression of sickness behavior is not simply the result of the changes in internal state experienced by sick subjects but the joint function of the changes in their internal state and the environmental constraints or context to which they are exposed [142]. Cytokines actually function as a motivational signal that tells the brain to change the organism priorities in face of the threat represented by pathogens or danger signals. This reorganization of priorities results in changes at the subjective, behavioral and physiological levels [142].

As this Fig. 1 shows, sickness behaviors then may be conceptualized as a normal adaptive reorganization given a threat of the host's homoeostatic and behavioral priorities to facilitate an immune response, rather than simply a detrimental consequence of infection [138–147]. The peripheral immune system also communicates with the central nervous system (CNS) during systemic inflammation, resulting in CNS-mediated effects collectively referred to as sickness responses (e.g., fever, cognitive impairment, reduced social interaction, and pain enhancement) [8, 99–117, 138– 143] This was explained by Watkins (2005) in the following way:

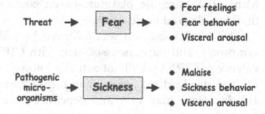

Fig. 1 Motivational Model of Sickness. From Dantzer, R. Cytokine, Sickness Behavior, and Depression. (Neurol Clin. 2006;24(3):441–60)

When you hurt yourself, you become consciously aware of the pain because a chain of neurons carries the pain message from the injury to the spinal cord, and then from the spinal cord up to consciousness in the brain. However, it has been known for more than two decades that neural circuits within the spinal cord (in pathologic pain states) can cause your conscious experience of pain to be amplified-that is, the pain you perceive is out of proportion to the injury that caused it. [104–107]

Put differently, sickness behaviors can become abnormal or pathologic when they occur out of context (ie, in the absence of any inflammatory stimulus), or when over time they are exaggerated in intensity or duration [142].

Dantzer (2005) has also described several conditions which are responsible for these pathologic conditions:

1. Proinflammatory cytokines are produced in higher quantities and for a longer duration than normal.
2. The regulatory molecules that normally down-regulate activation of the molecular and cellular components of the sickness response are faulty or dysregulated. Or,
3. the neuronal circuits that are the targets of inflammatory mediators and organize sickness behavior become sensitized [142].

In pathologic pain states such as CIPNs, sickness behaviors and the sickness responses become abnormal to include exaggerated pain as well as an entire constellation of genetic (e.g.c hanges in gene transcription due to neuroplasticity), biobehavioral, as well as, hormonal changes, which can, over time adversely impact the patient's experience of chronic pain post chemotherapeutic treatment (s) and long term-QOL after cancer [8, 99–117, 138–147].

Conclusions

In this paper, we have described a biobehavioral approach to understanding the development and perhaps the maintenance of Chemotherapy Induced Peripheral Neuropathies (CIPNs). CIPNs are as a type of neuropathic pain that develops post-chemotherapeutic treatment in cancer survivors. They have been described as the *'end result,'* *'dose limiting'* side effect, or the *'de facto'* toxic effect which limits the administration of many commonly used antineoplastic agents [8–162]. The chemotherapeutic agents most often associated with CIPNs are the platinum-based compounds, taxanes, vinca alkaloids, thalidomide, and bortezomib.

This brief discussion was followed by a description of the epidemiology, symptoms, and barriers associated with CIPNs. As we have stated, the prevalence of CIPNs is still not actually known due a lack of adequate and widely utilized standardized assessment, measurement and reporting mechanisms [9, 10]. Incidence may vary and depend on the drugs and schedules used, and incidence has been at between 3%–7% in individuals treated with single agents, and upwards of 38% in those individuals treated with multiple chemotherapeutic agents.

Risk factors and comorbid conditions have also been associated with a adverse phenotype and these include the prior uses of chemotherapies, older age, and being female. Certain comorbid conditions are also risk factors. These include diabetes, HIV, alcoholism, pre-existing neuropathies (i.e., diabetic neuropathy), and vitamin B deficiencies [8–15]. Great variability also exists in the symptoms associated with CIPNs, and little is known about other risk factors [8–15]. Even though there is wide variation in symptoms, the primary effects are sensory, occurring in a 'stocking-glove distribution' in the toes and fingers. These experiences can vary and their length cannot be predicted. In other words, symptoms can last from days to a lifetime. As with other cancer pain syndromes and chronic pain management in general, multiple barriers such as Patient, Clinician, Health System and Treatment related factors, racial and ethnic disparities, as well as wide variation in CIPN symptomology also limit optimal pain management in patients with CIPNs.

Then following important research in the field of pain, behavior, neuroscience and psychoneuroimmunology, we suggest that injury to peripheral nerves after chemotherapeutic treatments initiates immune to brain communication, which further modulates the biological mechanisms through which life experiences and behavior reinforce and likely perpetuate the experience of CIPN. While the underlying biobehavioral processes have not yet been adequately described; we offered some steps in understanding these processes.

First, we briefly described peripheral nerves in states of health, and then used Matzinger's Danger model we emphasized the significance of the proinflammatory environmental context (i.e. cancer) where CIPNs can potentially and perhaps initially develop. Then we proceeded to describe how peripheral nerve injury, peripheral innate immune activation, and proinflammatory cytokines impacts peripheral sensitization. Then we explored how peripheral nerve injury, peripheral innate immune activation, production and circulation of proinflammatory cytokines, and glial (microglial and astrocyte) activation of the spinal cord. Inflammatory cytokines are also induced in the CNS, independent of release of cytokines from the peripheral site of injury. And in the CNS, nerve injury also induces structural changes in the dorsal horn, neuroplasticity, and central sensitization. Then we briefly discussed how peripheral immune and glial cell activation and signaling to the CNS via proinflammatory cytokine production induces sickness behaviors and sickness responses. In pathologic pain states such as CIPNs, sickness behaviors and the sickness responses become abnormal to include exaggerated pain as well as an entire constellation of genetic (e.g. changes in gene transcription due to neuroplasticity), biobehavioral as well as, hormonal changes, which can, over time adversely affect the patient's experience of chronic pain post chemotherapeutic treatment (s) and long term-QOL.

As studies of brain neuroplasticity increasingly show, which can also be applied to our understanding of the development of CIPNs, there is probably a slow but progressive neurochemical and cellular remodelling of both the peripheral and central nervous systems that alters the transmission of somatosensory information from damaged peripheral sensory fibres to the cerebral cortex, which results in a long-term altered, unwanted and perception of noxious and/or non-noxious sensory information [8–15, 17–19, 99–117, 137–146, 216–224]. Prolonged central sensitization has the capacity to lead to permanent alterations in the central nervous system, including the death of inhibitory neurons, replacement with new afferent excitatory neurons, axonal sprouting, the establishment of aberrant excitatory synaptic connections and chronic long-term neuropathic pain [8–15, 99–117, 137–146, 216–224]. Immune and non-immune stressors (e.g. inflammatory) contribute to this scenario and are also involved in the activation of the central sickness-behavioural-system leading to long terms complaints including chronic neuropathic pain syndromes such as CIPNs [8–15, 99–117, 137–146, 216–224].

References

1. Hewitt,M, Greenfield,S, Stovall, E. (Eds). *Cancer Patient to Cancer Survivor: Lost in Transition.* IOM Report, National Academies Press, 2005.
2. Mao JJ, Armstrong K, Bowman MA, Xie SX, Kadakia R, Farrar JT. Symptom burden among cancer survivors: impact of age and comorbidity. *Journal of the American Board of Family Medicine.* 2007;20(5):434–43.
3. von Eschenbach AC. Progress with a purpose: eliminating suffering and death due to cancer. *Oncology* (Williston Park). 2006;20(13):1691–6.
4. Mako C, Galek K, Poppito SR. J Spiritual pain among patients with advanced cancer in palliative care. *Palliative Medicine* 2006 Oct;9(5):1106–13.
5. Shaiova L. Difficult pain syndromes: bone pain, visceral pain, and neuropathic pain. *Cancer Journal* 2006;12(5):330–40.
6. Mystakidou K, Tsilika E, Parpa E, Katsouda E, Galanos A, Vlahos L. Psychological distress of patients with advanced cancer: influence and contribution of pain severity and pain interference. *Cancer Nursing* 2006;29(5):400–5.
7. Trask PC, Teno JM, Nash J. Transitions of care and changes in distressing pain. *Journal of Pain and Symptom Management* 2006;32(2):104–9).
8. Mantyh PW. Cancer pain and its impact on diagnosis, survival and quality of life. *Nature Reviews Neuroscience* 2006;7(10):797–809.
9. Wickham R. Chemotherapy-induced peripheral neuropathy: a review and implications for oncology nursing practice. *Clinical Journal of Oncology Nursing* 2007;11(3):361–76
10. Stillman M, Cata JP. Management of chemotherapy-induced peripheral neuropathy. *Current Pain and Headache Reports* 2006 Aug;10(4):279–87.
11. Cavaletti G, Marmiroli P. Chemotherapy-induced peripheral neurotoxicity. Expert Opin Drug Saf. 2004;3(6):535–46.
12. Dunlap B, Paice JA. Chemotherapy-induced peripheral neuropathy: A need for standardization in measurement. *Journal of Supportive Oncology* 2006 Sep;4(8):398–9.
13. Paice JA. Chemotherapy-Induced Peripheral Neuropathy: A Dangerous but Understudied Syndrome. *Pain Management SIG Newsletter* 2008;17(1). http://onsopcontent.ons.org/Publications/SigNewsletters/pm/pm17.1.html Date accessed: 01/01/2008

14. Kannarkat G, Lasher EE, Schiff D. Neurologic complications of chemotherapy agents. *Current Opinion in Neurology*. 2007 Dec;20(6):719–25.
15. Paice, JA. Peripheral neuropathy: Experimental findings, clinical approaches. *Supportive Oncology* 2007;5(2), 61–63.
16. Hausheer, F.H., Schilsky, R.L., Bain, S., Berghorn, E.J., Lieberman, F. Diagnosis, management, and evaluation of chemotherapy-induced peripheral neuropathy. *Seminars in Oncology* 2006;33, 15–49.
17. Dougherty, P. M., Cata, J. P., Cordella, J. V., Burton, A. Weng, H. R. Taxol-induced sensory disturbance is characterized by preferential impairment of myelinated fiber function in cancer patients. *Pain* 2004;109, 132–142.
18. Postma, T. J. , Vermorken, J. B. , Liefting, A. J. , Pinedo, H. M. Heimans, J. J. Paclitaxel-induced neuropathy. *Annals of Oncology* 1995;6, 489–494.
19. Benoliel R, Epstein J, Eliav E, Jurevic R, Elad S. Orofacial pain in cancer: part I – mechanisms. *Journal of Dental Research* 2007;86(6):491–505.
20. Verstappen, C. C. , Postma, T. J. , Hoekman, K. Heimans, J. J. Peripheral neuropathy due to therapy with paclitaxel, gemcitabine, and cisplatin in patients with advanced ovarian cancer. *Journal of Neurooncology* 2003;63, 201–205.
21. Cavaletti G, Bogliun G, Marzorati L, Zincone A, Piatti M, Colombo N, Franchi D. Early predictors of peripheral neurotoxicity in cisplatin and paclitaxel combination chemotherapy. *Annals of Oncology* 2004;15(9):1439–42.
22. Moore, RJ. Transportation Issues in Patients with Cancer. (in preparation, 2008).
23. Moore RJ, Spiegel D. *Cancer Culture and Communication*. Springer, NY, 2004.
24. England JD, Asbury AK. Peripheral neuropathy. *Lancet* 2004;363(9427):2151–61.
25. Postma TJ, Heimans JJ. Grading of chemotherapy-induced peripheral neuropathy. *Annals of Oncology* 2000 May;11(5):509–13]
26. Postma TJ, Hoekman K, van Riel JM, Heimans JJ, Vermorken JB. Peripheral neuropathy due to biweekly paclitaxel, epirubicin and cisplatin in patients with advanced ovarian cancer. Journals of Neurooncology 1999;45(3):241–6.
27. Postma TJ, Heimans JJ, Luykx SA, van Groeningen CJ, Beenen LF, Hoekstra OS, Taphoorn MJ, Zonnenberg BA, Klein M, Vermorken JB. A phase II study of paclitaxel in chemonaïve patients with recurrent high-grade glioma. *Annals of Oncology* 2000 Apr;11(4):409–13.
28. Asbury AK. Peripheral neuropathy. *Lancet*. 2004;363(9427):2151–61.
29. Scholz J, Woolf CJ. The neuropathic pain triad: neurons, immune cells and glia. *Nature Neuroscience* 2007;10(11):1361–1368.
30. Cavaletti G, Zanna C. Current status and future prospects for the treatment of chemotherapy-induced peripheral neurotoxicity. *European Journal of Cancer* 2002 Sep;38(14):1832–7.
31. Bogduk, M, eds. Classification of Chronic Pain, 2nd Edition, *International Association for the Study of Pain Task Force on Taxonomy*. Seattle, Wash: IASP Press; 1994: 209–214.
32. Gatchel RJ, Peng YB, Peters ML, Fuchs PN, Turk DC. The biopsychosocial approach to chronic pain: scientific advances and future directions. *Psychological Bulletin* 2007;133(4):581–624.
33. Argyriou AA, Polychronopoulos P, Koutras A, Iconomou G, Iconomou A, Kalofonos HP,Chroni E. Peripheral neuropathy induced by administration of cisplatin- andpaclitaxel-based chemotherapy. Could it be predicted? *Support Care in Cancer* 2005 Aug;13(8):647–51.
34. Ziegler D, Nowak H, Kempler P, Vargha P, Low PA. Treatment of symptomatic diabetic polyneuropathy with the antioxidant alpha-lipoic acid: A meta-analysis *Diabetic Medicine* 2004;21:114–121.
35. Almadrones L, McGuire DB, Walczak JR, Florio CM, Tian C. Psychometric evaluation of two scales assessing functional status and peripheral neuropathy associated with

chemotherapy for ovarian cancer: A Gynecologic Oncology Group study. *Oncology Nursing Forum* 2004;31:615–623.

36. Almadrones LA. Neurologic complications. In J.M. Yasko (Ed.), *Nursing management of symptom associated with chemotherapy*. Meniscus Health Care Communications, West Conshohocken, PA. 2001, 5th ed., pp. 215–230.
37. Almadrones LA, Arcot, R. Patient guide to peripheral neuropathy. *Oncology Nursing Forum* 1999;26:1359–1361.
38. Aloe L, Manni L, Porperzi F, De Santis S, Fiore M. Evidence that nerve growth factor promotes the recovery of peripheral neuropathy induced in mice by cisplatin: Behavioral, structural, and biochemical analysis. *Autonomic Neuroscience-Basic and Clinical* 2000;86:84–93.
39. Argoff CE, Katz N, Backonja, M. Treatment of postherpetic neuralgia: A review of therapeutic options. *Journal of Pain and Symptom Management* 2004;28:396–411.
40. Argyriou AA, Chroni E, Koutras A, Ellul J, Papapetropoulos S, Katsoulas G, et al. Vitamin E for prophylaxis against chemotherapy-induced neuropathy. A randomized controlled trial. *Neurology* 2005;64:26–31.
41. Argyriou AA, Polychronopoulos P, Koustra A, Iconomou G, Gourzis P, Assimakopoulos K, et al. Is advanced age associated with increased incidence and severity of chemotherapy-induced peripheral neuropathy? *Supportive Care in Cancer* 2006;14:223–229
42. Armstrong T, Almadrones L, Gilbert MR. Chemotherapy-induced peripheral neuropathy. *Oncology Nursing Forum* 2005;32:305–311.
43. Authier N, Gillet JP, Fialip J, Eschalier A, Coudore F. An animal model of nociceptive peripheral neuropathy following repeated cisplatin injections. *Experimental Neurology* 2003;182:12–20.
44. Backonja MM, Serra J. Pharmacologic management part 1: Better-studied neuropathic pain diseases. *Pain Medicine* 2004;5(Suppl. 1), S28–S47.
45. Beydoun A, Backonja MM. Mechanistic stratification of antineuralgic agents. *Journal of Pain and Symptom Management* 2003;25(5, Suppl.), S18–S30
46. Cassidy J, Bjarnason GA, Hickish T, Topham C, Provencio M, Bodoky G, et al. Randomized double blind placebo controlled phase III study assessing the efficacy of xaliproden in reducing the cumulative peripheral sensory neuropathy induced by the oxaliplatin and 5-FU/LV combination (FOLFOX4) in first line treatment of patients with metastatic colorectal cancer, 2006, [Abstract 229].
47. Cavaletti G, Petruccioli MG, Marmiroli P, Rigolio R, Galbiati S, Zoia C, et al. Circulating nerve growth factor level changes during oxaliplatin treatment-induced neurotoxicity in the rat. *Anticancer Research* 2002;22(6C):4199–4204.
48. Boehmke MM, Dickerson SS. Symptom, symptom experiences, and symptom distress encountered by women with breast cancer undergoing current treatment modalities. *Cancer Nursing* 2005;28:382–389.
49. Cascinu S, Catalano V, Cordella L, Lubianca R, Giordano P, Baldelli AM, et al. Neuroprotective effect of reduced glutathione on oxaliplatin-based chemotherapy in advanced colorectal cancer: A randomized, double-blind, placebo-controlled trial. *Journal of Clinical Oncology* 2002;20:3478–3483
50. Cassidy J, Misset JL. Oxaliplatin-related side effects: Characteristics and management. *Seminars in Oncology* 2002;29(Suppl. 15):11–20.
51. Cersosimo RJ. Oxaliplatin-associated neuropathy: A review. *Annals of Pharmacotherapy* 2005;39:128–135.
52. Chaudhry V, Cornblath DR, Corse A, Freimer M, Simmons-O'Brien E, Vogelsang G. Thalidomide-induced neuropathy. *Neurology* 2002;59:1872–1875.
53. Cianfrocca M, Glatters SJ, Bennett GJ, McNicol E, Relias V, Carr D, et al. Peripheral neuropathy in a woman with breast cancer. *Journal of Pain* 2006;7:2–10.
54. Criscuolo S, Auletta C, Lippi S, Brogi F, Brogi A. Oxcarbazepine (Trileptal®) monotherapy dramatically improves quality of life in two patients with postherpetic neuralgia

refractory to carbamazepine and gabapentin. *Journal of Pain and Symptom Management* 2004;28:535–536.

55. De Santis S, Pace A, Bove L, Cognetti F, Properzi F, Fiore M, et al. Patients treated with antitumor drugs displaying neurological deficits are characterized by a low circulating level of nerve growth factor. *Clinical Cancer Research* 2000;6:90–95.

56. du Bois A, Schlaich M, Lück HJ, Mollenkopf A, Wechsel U, Rauchholz M, et al. Evaluation of neurotoxicity induced by paclitaxel second- line chemotherapy. *Supportive Care in Cancer* 1999;7:354–361.

57. Durand JP, Alexandre J, Guillevin L, Goldwasser F. Clinical activity of venlafaxine and topiramate against oxaliplatin-induced disabling permanent neuropathy. *Anti-Cancer Drugs* 2005;16:587–591.

58. Fine PG, Miaskowski C, Paice JA. Meeting the challenges in cancer pain management. *Journal of Supportive Oncology* 2004;2(Suppl. 4):5–22.

59. Frisk P, Stalberg E, Stromberg B, Jakobson A. Painful peripheral neuropathy after treatment with high-dose ifosfamide. *Medical and Pediatric Oncology* 2001;37:379–382.

60. Gamelin E, Gamelin L, Bossi L, Quasthoff S. Clinical aspects and molecular basis of oxaliplatin neurotoxicity: Current management and development of preventive measures. *Seminars in Oncology* 2002;29(Suppl. 15):21–33.

61. Gamelin L, Boisdron-Celle M, Delva R, Guérin-Meyer V, Ifrah N, Morel A, et al. Prevention of oxaliplatin-related neurotoxicity by calcium and magnesium infusions: A retrospective study of 161 patients receiving oxaliplatin combined with 5-fluorouracil and leucovorin for advanced colorectal cancer. *Clinical Cancer Research* 2004;10:4055–4061. Gornet JM, Savier E, Lokiec F, Cvitkovic E, Misset JL, Goldwasser F. Exacerbation of oxaliplatin neurosensory toxicity following surgery. *Annals of Oncology* 2002;13:1315–1318.

62. Grothey A. Oxaliplatin—Safety profile: Neurotoxicity. *Seminars in Oncology* 2003;30(Suppl. 15):5–13.

63. HughesRA. Peripheral neuropathy. *BMJ* 2002;324:466–469

64. Lehky TJ, Leonard GD, Wilson RH, Grem JL, Floeter MK. Oxaliplatin-induced neurotoxicity: Acute hyperexcitability and chronic neuropathy. *Muscle and Nerve* 2004;29:287–292.

65. Grolleau F, Gamelin L, Boisdron-Celle M, Lapied B, Pelhate M, Gamelin E. A possible explanation for a neurotoxic effect of the anticancer agent oxaliplatin on neuronal voltage-gated sodium channels *Journal of Neurophysiology* 2001;85:2293–2297

66. Lazo G, Kantarjian H, Estey E, Thomas D, O'Brien S, Cortes J. Use of arsenic trioxide (As2O3) in the treatment of patients with acute promyelocytic leukemia. *Cancer* 2003;97:2218–2224.

67. Lenz G, Hacker UT, Kern W, Schalhorn A, Hiddemann W Adverse reactions to oxaliplatin: A retrospective study of 25 patients treated in one institution. *Anti-Cancer Drugs* 2003;14:731–733.

68. Moore DH, Donnelly J, McGuire WP, Almadrones L, Cella DF, Herzog TJ, et al. Limited access trial using amifostine for protection against cisplatin- and three-hour paclitaxel induced neurotoxicity: A phase II study of the Gynecologic Oncology Group. *Journal of Clinical Oncology* 2003;21:4207–4213.

69. Nail LM. Long-term persistence of symptoms. *Seminars in Oncology Nursing* 2001;17:249–254.

70. Hausheer FH, Schilsky RL, Bain S, Berghorn EJ, Lieberman F. Diagnosis, management, and evaluation of chemotherapy-induced peripheral neuropathy. *Seminars in Oncology* 2006;33:15–49.

71. Leonard GD, Wright MA, Quinn MG, Fioravanti S, Harold N, Schuler B, et al. Survey of oxaliplatin-associated neurotoxicity using an interview-based questionnaire in patients with metastatic colorectal cancer. *British Medical Journal of Cancer* 2005;5:116–126.

72. Marrs J, Newton S. Updating your peripheral neuropathy "know-how." *Clinical Journal of Oncology Nursing* 2003;7:299–303.

73. Ocean AJ, Vahdat LT. Chemotherapy-induced peripheral neuropathy: Pathogenesis and emerging therapies. *Supportive Care in Cancer* 2004;12:619–625.

74. Openshaw H, Beamon K, Synold TW, Longmate J, Statkin NE, Doroshow JH, et al. Neurophysiological study of peripheral neuropathy after high-dose paclitaxel: Lace of neuroprotective effect of amifostine. *Clinical Cancer Research* 2004;10: 461–467.

75. Paice JA. Mechanisms and management of neuropathic pain in cancer. *Supportive Oncology* 2003;1:107–112.

76. Polomano RC, Bennett GJ. Chemotherapy-evoked painful peripheral neuropathy. *Pain Medicine* 2001;2:8–14.

77. Polomano RC, Farrar JT. Pain and neuropathy in cancer survivors. *American Journal of Nursing* 2006;106(3, Suppl.): 39–47.

78. Poncelet AN. An algorithm for the evaluation of peripheral neuropathy. *American Family Physician* 1998;57:755–764.

79. Postma TJ, Heimans JJ. Grading of chemotherapy-induced peripheral neuropathy. *Annals of Oncology* 2000;11:509–513.

80. Postma TJ, Heimans JJ, Muller MJ, Ossenkoppele GJ, Vermorken JB, Aaronson NK. Pitfalls in grading severity of chemotherapy-induced peripheral neuropathy. *Annals of Oncology* 1998;9:739–744.

81. Quasthoff S, Hartung HP. Chemotherapy-induced peripheral neuropathy. *Journal of Neurology* 2002;249:9–17.

82. Richardson PG, Barlogie B, Berenson J, Singhal S, Jagannath S, Irwin D, et al. A phase 2 study of bortezomib in relapsed, refractory myeloma. *New England Journal of Medicine* 2003;348:2609–2617.

83. Saif MW. Oral calcium ameliorating oxaliplatin-induced peripheral neuropathy. *Journal of Applied Research* 2004;4:576–582.

84. Smith EL, Whedon MK, Bookbinder M. Quality improvement of painful peripheral neuropathy. *Seminars in Oncology Nursing* 2002;18:36–43.

85. Sorich J, Taubes B, Wagner A, Hochster H. Oxaliplatin: Practical guidelines for administration. *Clinical Journal of Oncology Nursing* 2004;8:251–256.

86. Storstein A, Vedeler CA. Neurological symptoms as the first signs of cancer: Paraneoplastic encephalomyelitis and sensory neuronopathy. *American Journal of Oncology Review* 2005;4:31–34.

87. Susman E. Xaliproden lessens oxaliplatin-mediated neuropathy. *Lancet Oncology* 2006;7:288.

88. Sweeney CW. Understanding peripheral neuropathy in patients with cancer: Background and patient assessment. *Clinical Journal of Oncology Nursing* 2002;6: 163–166.

89. Taieb S, Trillet-Lenoir V, Rambaud L, Descos L, Freyer G. Lhermitte sign and urinary retention: Atypical presentation of oxaliplatin neurotoxicity in four patients. *Cancer* 2002;94:2434–2440.

90. Tournigand C, Cervantes A, Figer A, Lledo G, Flesh M, Buyse M, et al. OPTIMOX1: A randomized study of FOLFOX4 or FOLFOX7 in a stop-and-go fashion in advanced colorectal cancer—A GERCOR study. *Journal of Clinical Oncology* 2006;24:394–400.

91. Verstappen CC, Heimans JJ, Hoekman K, Postma TJ. Neurotoxic complication of chemotherapy in patients with cancer: Clinical signs and optimal management. *Drugs* 2003;63:1549–1563.

92. Verstappen CC, Koeppen S, Heimans JJ, Huijgens PC, Scheulen ME, Strumberg D, et al. Dose-related vincristine-induced peripheral neuropathy with unexpected off-therapy worsening. *Neurology* 2005;64:1076–1077.

93. Visovsky C. Chemotherapy-induced peripheral neuropathy. *Cancer Investigation* 2003;21:439–451.

94. Wampler MA, Hamolsky D, Hamel K, Melisko M, Topp K.S. Case report: Painful peripheral neuropathy following treatment with docetaxel for breast cancer. *Clinical Journal of Oncology Nursing* 2005;9:189–193.
95. Wilkes GM. Therapeutic options in the management of colon cancer: 2005 update. *Clinical Journal of Oncology Nursing* 2005;9:31–44.
96. Willis WD. The nervous system. In R.M. Berne M.N. Levy (Eds.), *Principles of physiology*. Mosby, St. Louis, 2000, pp. 68–94.
97. Wilson RH, Lehky T, Thomas RR, Quinn MG, Floeter MK, Grem JL. Acute oxaliplatin-induced peripheral nerve hyperexcitability. *Journal of Clinical Oncology* 2002;20:1767–1774.
98. Winegarden JD, Mauer AM, Otterson GA, Rudin CM, Villalona-Calero MA, Lanzotti VJ, et al. A phase II study of oxaliplatin and paclitaxel inpatients with advanced non-small-cell lung cancer. *Annals of Oncology* 2004;15:915–920
99. Moalem G, Tracey DJ. Immune and inflammatory mechanisms in neuropathic pain. *Brain Research Reviews* 2006 Aug;51(2):240–64.
100. Watkins LR, Hutchinson MR, Milligan ED, Maier SF. Listening" and "talking" to neurons: implications of immune activation for pain control and increasing the efficacy of opioids. *Brain Research Review* 2007;56(1):148–69.
101. Watkins LR, Hutchinson MR, Ledeboer A, Wieseler-Frank J, Milligan ED, Maier SF. Norman Cousins Lecture. Glia as the "bad guys": implications for improving clinical pain control and the clinical utility of opioids. *Brain, Behavior, and Immunity* 2007;21(2):131–46.
102. Wieseler-Frank J, Jekich BM, Mahoney JH, Bland ST, Maier SF, Watkins LR. A novel immune-to-CNS communication pathway: cells of the meninges surrounding the spinal cord CSF space produce proinflammatory cytokines in response to an inflammatory stimulus. *Brain, Behavior, and Immunity* 2007;21(5):711–8.
103. Banks WA, Watkins LR. Mediation of chronic pain: not by neurons alone. *Pain* 2006 Sep;124(1–2):1–2.
104. Watkins LR, Hutchinson MR, Johnston IN, Maier SF. Glia: novel counter-regulators of opioid analgesia. *Trends in Neuroscience* 2005;28(12):661–9.
105. Wieseler-Frank J, Maier SF, Watkins LR. Central proinflammatory cytokines and pain enhancement. *Neurosignals* 2005;14(4):166–74.
106. Milligan ED, Langer SJ, Sloane EM, He L, Wieseler-Frank J, O'Connor K, Martin D, Forsayeth JR, Maier SF, Johnson K, Chavez RA, Leinwand LA, Watkins LR. Controlling pathological pain by adenovirally driven spinal production of the anti-inflammatory cytokine, interleukin-10. *European Journal of Neuroscience* 2005;21(8):2136–48.
107. Wieseler-Frank J, Maier SF, Watkins LR. Immune-to-brain communication dynamically modulates pain: physiological and pathological consequences. *Brain, Behavior Immunity* 2005;19(2):104–11.
108. Watkins LR, Maier SF. Immune regulation of central nervous system functions: from sickness responses to pathological pain. *Journal of International Medecine* 2005;257(2):139–55.
109. Watkins LR, Maier SF. Glia: a novel drug discovery target for clinical pain. *Nature Reviews Drug Discovery* 2003;2(12):973–85.
110. Dworkin RH, Backonja M, Rowbotham MC, Allen RR, Argoff CR, Bennett GJ,Bushnell MC, Farrar JT, Galer BS, Haythornthwaite JA, Hewitt DJ, Loeser JD, Max MB, Saltarelli M, Schmader KE, Stein C, Thompson D, Turk DC, Wallace MS, Watkins LR, Weinstein SM. Advances in neuropathic pain: diagnosis, mechanisms, and treatment recommendations. *Archives of Neurology* 2003;60(11):1524–34.
111. Watkins LR, Milligan ED, Maier SF. Glial proinflammatory cytokines mediate exaggerated pain states: implications for clinical pain. *Advances in Experimental Medecine and Biology* 2003;521:1–21
112. Maier SF, Watkins LR. Immune-to-central nervous system communication and its role in modulating pain and cognition: Implications for cancer and cancer treatment. *Brain, Behavior, and Immunity* 2003;17 Suppl 1:S125–31.

113. Watkins LR, Maier SF. Beyond neurons: evidence that immune and glial cells contribute to pathological pain states. *Physiological Reviews* 2002;82(4):981–1011.
114. Watkins LR, Milligan ED, Maier SF. Glial activation: a driving force for pathological pain. *Trends in Neuroscience* 2001 Aug;24(8):450–5.
115. White FA, Jung H, Miller RJ. Chemokines and the pathophysiology of neuropathic pain. *Proceedings of the National Academy of the Science of the USA*. 2007 Dec 18;104(51):20151–8. Epub 2007 Dec 14.
116. Watkins, LR. Immune and glial regulation of pain *Brain, Behavior, and Immunity* 2007;21(5):519–521.
117. Brydon L, Harrison NA, Walker C, Steptoe A, Critchley HD. Peripheral Inflammation is Associated with Altered Substantia Nigra Activity and Psychomotor Slowing in Humans. *Biological Psychiatry* 2008;63:1022–1029.
118. Bouchardy C, Rapiti E, Blagojevic S, Vlastos AT, Vlastos G. Older female cancer patients: importance, causes, and consequences of undertreatment. *Journal of Clinical Oncology* 2007 May 10;25(14):1858–69.
119. Meghani SH, Keane A. Preference for analgesic treatment for cancer pain among African Americans. *Journal of Pain and Symptom Management*. 2007 Aug;34(2):136–47.
120. Altilio T. Pain and symptom management clinical, policy, and political perspectives. *Journal of Psychosocial Oncology* 2006;24(1):65–79.
121. Randall-David E, Wright J, Porterfield DS, Lesser G. Barriers to cancer pain management: home-health and hospice nurses and patients. *Supportive Care in Cancer* 2003 Oct;11(10):660–5.
122. Anderson KO, Richman SP, Hurley J, Palos G, Valero V, Mendoza TR, Gning I, Cleeland CS. Cancer pain management among underserved minority outpatients: perceived needs and barriers to optimal control. *Cancer* 2002 ;94(8):2295–304.
123. Maxwell T. Cancer pain management in the elderly. *Geriatr Nursing* 2000 May–Jun;21(3):158–63.
124. Portenoy RK, Lesage P. Management of cancer pain. *Lancet* 1999 May 15;353(9165):1695–700
125. Cleeland CS. Undertreatment of cancer pain in elderly patients. *The Journal of the American Medical Association* 1998 Jun 17;279(23):1914–5.
126. Rich BA. A legacy of silence: bioethics and the culture of pain. *Journal of Medical Humanities* 1997 Winter;18(4):233–59.
127. Grossman SA. Undertreatment of cancer pain: barriers and remedies. *Supportive Care in Cancer* 1993;1(2):74–8.
128. Green C, Todd KH, Lebovits A, Francis M; American Academy of Pain Medicine-Council on Ethics. Disparities in pain: ethical issues. *Pain Medicine* 2006;7(6):530–3.
129. Green CR, Anderson KO, Baker TA, Campbell LC, Decker S, Fillingim RB,Kalauokalani DA, Lasch KE, Myers C, Tait RC, Todd KH, Vallerand AH. The unequal burden of pain: confronting racial and ethnic disparities in pain. *Pain Medicine* 2003;4(3):277–94.
130. Bandrés E, Zárate R, Ramirez N, Abajo A, Bitarte N, Garíia-Foncillas J. Pharmacogenomics in colorectal cancer: the first step for individualized-therapy. *World Journal of Gastroenterology* 2007 Nov 28;13(44):5888–901.
131. Mielke S. Individualized pharmacotherapy with paclitaxel. *Current Opinion Oncology* 2007 Nov;19(6):586–9.
132. Rekhadevi PV, Sailaja N, Chandrasekhar M, Mahboob M, Rahman MF, Grover P. Genotoxicity assessment in oncology nurses handling anti-neoplastic drugs. *Mutagenesis* 2007 Nov;22(6):395–401.
133. Wang J, Huang Y. Pharmacogenomics of sex difference in chemotherapeutic toxicity. *Current Drug Discovery Technology* 2007 Jun;4(1):59–68.
134. Stoehlmacher J. Prediction of efficacy and side effects of chemotherapy in colorectal cancer. *Recent Results in Cancer Research* 2007;176:81–8.

135. Ueno H, Kiyosawa K, Kaniwa N. Pharmacogenomics of gemcitabine: can genetic studies lead to tailor-made therapy? *British Journal of Cancer* 2007 Jul 16;97(2):145–51.

136. Land SR, Kopec JA, Cecchini RS, Ganz PA, Wieand HS, Colangelo LH, Murphy K, Kuebler JP, Seay TE, Needles BM, Bearden JD 3rd, Colman LK, Lanier KS, Pajon ER Jr, Cella D, Smith RE, O'Connell MJ, Costantino JP, Wolmark N. Neurotoxicity from oxaliplatin combined with weekly bolus fluorouracil and leucovorin as surgical adjuvant chemotherapy for stage II and III colon cancer: NSABP C-07. *Journal Clinical Oncology* 2007;25(16):2205–11.

137. Baba H, Doubell TP, Woolf CJ. Peripheral inflammation facilitates Abeta fiber-mediated synaptic input to the substantia gelatinosa of the adult rat spinal cord. *Journal of Neuroscience*;19(2):859–67.

138. Dantzer R, Capuron L, Irwin MR, Miller AH, Ollat H, Hugh Perry V, Rousey S, Yirmiya R. Identification and treatment of symptoms associated with inflammation inmedically ill patients. *Psychoneuroendocrinology*. 2008;33(1):18–29.

139. Dantzer R, O'Connor JC, Freund GG, Johnson RW, Kelley KW.From inflammation to sickness and depression: when the immune system subjugates the brain. *Nature Reviews Neuroscience* 2008;9(1):46–56.

140. Dimsdale JE, Dantzer R. A biological substrate for somatoform disorders: importance of pathophysiology. *Psychosomatic Medicine*. 2007;69(9):850–4.

141. Dantzer R, O'Connor JC, Freund GG, Johnson RW, Kelley KW. From inflammation to sickness and depression: when the immune system subjugates the brain. *Nature Reviews Neuroscience*. 2008;9(1):46–56.

142. Dantzer R. Cytokine, sickness behavior, and depression. *Neurologic Clinics* 2006; 24(3):441–60.

143. Dantzer R, Kelley KW. Twenty years of research on cytokine-induced sickness behavior. *Brain, Behavior, and Immunity* 2007;21(2):153–60.

144. Dantzer R. Cytokine, sickness behavior, and depression. *Neurologic Clinics* 2006;24(3):441–60.

145. Dantzer R. Somatization: a psychoneuroimmune perspective. *Psychoneuroendocrinology* 2005;30(10):947–52

146. Coussens LM, Werb Z. Inflammation and cancer. *Nature* 2002 ;420(6917):860–7.

147. Jan H. Houtveen and Lorenz J.P. van DoornenMedically unexplained symptoms and between-group differences in 24-h ambulatory recording of stress physiology *Biological Psychology, Volume 76, Issue 3*, October 2007, Pages 239–249

148. Mercadante S. Malignant bone pain: pathophysiology and treatment. *Pain*. 1997;69(1–2):1–18.

149. Matzinger P. Friendly and dangerous signals: is the tissue in control? *Nature Immunology* 2007 Jan;8(1):11–3.

150. Matzinger P. The danger model: a renewed sense of self. *Science*. 2002;296(5566):301–5.

151. Melzack R, Wall PD. Pain mechanisms: a new theory. *Science*.1965; 150:971 –9; Reuben SS, Buvanendran A. Preventing the development of chronic pain after orthopaedic surgery with preventive multimodal analgesic techniques. *Journal of Bone and Joint Surgergy American*. 2007;89(6):1343–58

152. Apolone G, et al. Pain in Cancer: An outcome research project to evaluate the epidemiology, the quality and the effects of pain treatment in cancer patients. *Health and Quality of Life Outcomes* 2006;4:7.

153. Ballantyne JC. Chronic Pain Following Treatment for Cancer: The Role of Opioids. *Oncologist* 2003; 8: 567–575.

154. Kulmatycki KM, Jamali F. Drug disease interactions: role of inflammatory mediators in pain and variability in analgesic drug response. *Journal of Pharmacy and Pharmaceutical Sciences* 2007;10(4):554–66.

155. Cleeland CS, Gonin R, Hatfield AK, Edmonson JH, Blum RH, Stewart JA, Pandya KJ. Pain and its treatment in outpatients with metastatic cancer. *The New England Journal of Medicine* 1994 Mar 3;330(9):592–6.

156. Visovsky C, Collins M, Abbott L, Aschenbrenner J, Hart C. Putting evidence into practice: evidence-based interventions for chemotherapy-induced peripheral neuropathy. *Clinical Journal of Oncology Nursing* 2007;11(6):901–13.
157. Cavaletti G, Zanna C. Current status and future prospects for the treatment of chemotherapy-induced peripheral neurotoxicity. *European Journal of Cancer* 2002;38:1832–1837.
158. Cavaletti G, Frigeni B, Lanzani F, Piatti M, Rota S, Briani C, Zara G, Plasmati R, Pastorelli F, Caraceni A, Pace A, Manicone M, Lissoni A, Colombo N, Bianchi G, Zanna C; Italian NETox Group. The Total Neuropathy Score as an assessment tool for grading the course ofchemotherapy-induced peripheral neurotoxicity: comparison with the National Cancer Institute-Common Toxicity Scale. *Journal of Peripheral Nervous System* 2007 Sep;12(3):210–5.
159. Cavaletti G, Bogliun G, Marzorati L, Zincone A, Piatti M, Colombo N, Franchi D, La Presa MT, Lissoni A, Buda A, Fei F, Cundari S, Zanna C. Early predictors of peripheral neurotoxicity in cisplatin and paclitaxelcombination chemotherapy. *Annals of Oncology* 2004 Sep;15(9):1439–42.
160. Cavaletti G, Bogliun G, Marzorati L, Zincone A, Piatti M, Colombo N, Parma G, Lissoni A, Fei F, Cundari S, Zanna C. Grading of chemotherapy-induced peripheral neurotoxicity using the Total Neuropathy Scale. *Neurology* 2003 Nov 11;61(9):1297–300.
161. Cavaletti G, Zanna C. Current status and future prospects for the treatment of chemotherapy-induced peripheral neurotoxicity. *European Journal of Cancer* 2002 Sep;38(14):1832–7
162. Armstrong T, Almadrones L, Gilbert M. Chemotherapyinduced peripheral neuropathy. *Oncology Nursing Forum* 2005;32:305–311.
163. Bianchi G, Vitali G, Caraceni A, Ravaglia S, Capri G, Cundari S, et al. Symptomatic and neurophysiological responses of paclitaxel- or cisplatin-induced neuropathy to oral acetyl-L-carnitine. *European Journal of Cancer* 2005;41:1746–1750.
164. Bove L, Picardo M, Maresca V, Jandolo B, Pace A. A pilot study on the relation between cisplatin neuropathy and vitamin E. *Journal of Experimental and Clinical Cancer Research* 2001;20:277–280.
165. Cascinu S, Cordella L, Del Ferro E, Fronzoni M, Catalano G. Neuroprotective effect of reduced glutathione on cisplatin-based chemotherapy in advanced gastric cancer: A randomized double-blind placebo-controlled trial. *Journal of Clinical Oncology* 1995;13:26–32.
166. Bartolomucci A, Palanza P, Sacerdote P, Panerai AE, Sgoifo A, Openshaw H, Beamon K, Synod TW, Longmate J, Slatkin NE, Doroshaw JH, et al. Neurophysiolgical study of peripheral neuropathy after high-dose paclitaxel: Lack of neuroprotective effect of amifostine. *Clinical Cancer Research* 2004;10:461–467.
167. Wolfe GI, Trivedi JR. Painful peripheral neuropathy and its nonsurgical treatment. *Muscle and Nerve* 2004;30:3–19.
168. Abuaisha BB, Costanzi JB, Boulton AJ. Acupuncture for the treatment of chronic painful peripheral diabetic neuropathy: A long-term study. *Diabetes Research and Clinical Practice* 1998;39:115–121.
169. Almadrones L, Arcot R. Patient guide to peripheral neuropathy. *Oncology Nursing Forum* 1999;26:1359–1360.
170. Argyriou AA, Chroni E, Koutras A, Ellul J, Papapetropoulos S, Katsoulas G, et al. Vitamin E for prophylaxis against chemotherapy-induced neuropathy: A randomized controlled trial. *Neurology* 2005;64:26–31.
171. Armstrong T, Almadrones L, Gilbert M. Chemotherapy-induced peripheral neuropathy. *Oncology Nursing Forum* 2005;32:305–311.
172. Arnall DA, Nelson AG, Lopez L, Sanz N, Iversen L, Sanz I, et al. The restorative effects of pulsed infrared light therapy on significant loss of peripheral protective sensation in patients with long-term type 1 and type 2 diabetes mellitus. *Acta Diabetologica* 2006;43:26–33.
173. Ashton-Miller J, Yeh M, Richardson JK, Galloway T. A cane reduces loss of balance in patients with peripheral neuropathy: Results from a challenging unipedal balance test. *Archives of Physical Medicine and Rehabilitation* 1996;77:446–452.

174. Balducci S, Iacobellis G, Parisi L, Di Biase N, Calandriello E, Leonetti F, et al. Exercise training can modify the natural history of diabetic peripheral neuropathy. *Journal of Diabetes and Its Complications* 2006;20:216–223.
175. Bianchi G, Vitali G, Caraceni A, Ravaglia S, Capri G, Cundari S, et al. Symptomatic and neurophysiological responses of paclitaxel- or cisplatin-induced neuropathy to oral acetyl-L-carnitine. *European Journal of Cancer* 2005;41:1746–1750.
176. Bove L, Picardo M, Maresca V, Jandolo B, Pace A. A pilot study on the relation between cisplatin neuropathy and vitamin E. *Journal of Experimental and Clinical Cancer Research* 2001;20:277–280.
177. Cascinu S, Catalano V, Cordella L, Labianca R, Giordani P, Baldelli AM, et al. Neuroprotective effect of reduced glutathione on oxaliplatin-based chemotherapy in advanced colorectal cancer: A randomized, double-blind, placebo-controlled trial. *Journal of Clinical Oncology* 2002;20:3478–3483.
178. Cascinu S, Cordella L, Del Ferro E, Fronzoni M, Catalano G. Neuroprotective effect of reduced glutathione on cisplatin-based chemotherapy in advanced gastric cancer: A randomized double-blind placebo-controlled trial. *Journal of Clinical Oncology* 1995;13:26–32.
179. Cata JP, Cordella JV, Burton AW, Hassenbusch SJ, Weng HR, Dougherty PM. Spinal cord stimulation relieves chemotherapy-induced pain: A clinical case report. *Journal of Pain and Symptom Management* 2004;27:72–78.
180. Davis ID, Kiers L, MacGregor L, Quinn M, Arezzo J, Green M, et al. A randomized, double-blinded, placebo-controlled phase II trial of recombinant human leukemia inhibitory factor (rhuLIF, emfilermin, AM424) to prevent chemotherapy-induced peripheral neuropathy. *Clinical Cancer Research* 2005;11:1890–1898.
181. Eckel F, Schmelz R, Adelsberger H, Erdmann J, Quasthoff S, Lersch C. [Prevention of oxaliplatin-induced neuropathy by carbamazepine. A pilot study.] *Deutsche Medizinische Wochenschrift* 2002;127:78–82.
182. Hammack J, Michalak J, Loprinzi C, Sloan J, Novotny P, Soori G, et al. Phase III evaluation of nortriptyline for alleviation of symptoms of cisplatinum-induced peripheral neuropathy. *Pain* 2002;98:195–203.
183. Hilpert F, Stahle A, Tome O, Burges A, Rossner D, Spathe K, et al. Neuroprotection with amifostine in the first-line treatment of advanced ovarian cancer with carboplatin/paclitaxel-based chemotherapy. A double blind, placebo-controlled, randomized phase II study from the Arbeitsgemeinschaft Gynakologische Onkologoie (AGO) Ovarian Cancer Study Group. *Supportive Care in Cancer* 2005;13:797–805.
184. Jiang H, Shi K, Li X, Zhou W, Cao Y. Clinical study on the wrist-ankle acupuncture treatment for 30 cases of diabetic peripheral neuritis. *Journal of Traditional Chinese Medicine* 2006;26:8–12.
185. Forst T, Nguyen M, Forst S, Disselhoff B, Pohlmann T, Pfutzner A. Impact of low frequency transcutaneous electrical nerve stimulation on symptomatic diabetic neuropathy using the new Salutaris device. *Diabetes, Nutrition and Metabolism* 2004;17:163–168.
186. Forst T, Pohlmann T, Kunt T, Goitom K, Schulz G, Lobig M, et al. The influence of local capsaicin treatment on small nerve fibre function and neurovascular control in symptomatic diabetic neuropathy. *Acta Diabetologica* 2002;39:1–6.
187. Phillips KD, Skelton WD, Hand GA. Effect of acupuncture administered in a group setting on pain and subjective peripheral neuropathy in persons with human immunodeficiency virus disease. *Journal of Alternative and Complementary Medicine* 2004;10:449–455.
188. Prendergast JJ, Miranda G, Sanchez M. Improvement of sensory impairment in patients with peripheral neuropathy. *Endocrine Practice* 2004;10:24–30.
189. Reichstein L, Labrenz S, Ziegler D, Martin S. Effective treatment of symptomatic diabetic polyneuropathy by high-frequency external muscle stimulation. *Diabetologia* 2005;48:824–828.

190. Gamelin L, Boisdron-Celle M, Delva R, Geurin-Meyer V, Ifrah N, Morel A, et al. Prevention of oxaliplatin-related neurotoxicity by calcium and magnesium infusions: A retrospective study of 161 patients receiving oxaliplatin combined with 5-fluorouracil and leucovorin for advanced colorectal cancer. *Clinical Cancer Research* 2004;10:4055–4061.

191. Leonard DR, Farooqi MH, Myers S. Restoration of sensation, reduced pain, and improved balance in subjects with diabetic peripheral neuropathy: A double-blind, randomized, placebo-controlled study with monochromatic near-infrared treatment. *Diabetes Care* 2004;27:168–172.

192. Lindeman E, Leffers P, Spaans F, Drukker J, Reulen J, Kerckhoffs M, et al. Strength training in patients with myotonic dystrophy and hereditary motor and sensory neuropathy: A randomized clinical trial. *Archives of Physical Medicine and Rehabilitation* 1995;76:612–620.

193. Maestri A, De Pasquale Ceratti A, Cundari S, Zanna C, Cortesi E, Crino L. A pilot study on the effect of acetyl-L-carnitine in paclitaxel- and cisplatin-induced peripheral neuropathy. *Tumori* 2005;91:135–138.

194. Marrs J, Newton S. Updating your peripheral neuropathy "know how." *Clinical Journal of Oncology Nursing* 2003;7:299–303.

195. Moore D, Donnelly J, McGuire WP, Almadrones L, Cella DF, Herzog TJ, et al. Limited access trial using amifostine for protection against cisplatin and three hour paclitaxel-induced neurotoxicity: A phase II study of the Gynecologic Oncology Group. *Journal of Clinical Oncology* 2003;21:4207–4213.

196. Pace A, Savarese A, Picardo M, Maresca V, Pacetti U, Del Monte G, et al. Neuroprotective effect of vitamin E supplementation in patients treated with cisplatin chemotherapy. *Journal of Clinical Oncology* 2003;21:927–931.

197. Richardson JK, Sandman D, Vela S. A focused exercise regimen improves clinical measures of balance in patients with peripheral neuropathy. *Archives of Physical Medicine and Rehabilitation* 2001;82:205–209.

198. Richardson JK, Thies S, DeMott T, Ashton-Miller JA. Interventions improve gait regularity in patients with peripheral neuropathy while walking on an irregular surface under low light. *Journal of the American Geriatrics Society* 2004;52:510–515.

199. Shlay JC, Chaloner K, Max MB, Flaws B, Reichelderfer P, Wentworth D, et al. Acupuncture and amitriptyline for pain due to HIV-related peripheral neuropathy: A randomized controlled trial. *JAMA* 1998;280:1590–1595.

200. Smyth JF, Bowman A, Perren T, Wilkinson P, Prescott RJ, Quinn KJ, et al. Glutathione reduces the toxicity and improves quality of life of women diagnosed with ovarian cancer treated with cisplatin: Results of a double-blind, randomized trial *Annals of Oncology* 1997;8:569–573.

201. Stubblefield MD, Vahdat LT, Balmaceda AB, Troxel AB, Hesdorffer CS, Gooch CL. Glutamine as a neuroprotective agent in high-dose paclitaxel-induced peripheral neuropathy: A clinical and electrophysiologic study. *Clinical Oncology* 2005;17:271–276.

202. Vahdat L, Papadopoulos K, Lange D, Leuin S, Kaufman E, Donovan D, et al. Reduction of paclitaxel-induced peripheral neuropathy with glutamine. *Clinical Cancer Research* 2001;7:1192–1197.

203. Weijl NI, Hopman GD, Wipkink-Bakker A, Lentjes EG, Berger HM, Cleton FJ, et al. Cisplatin combination chemotherapy induces a fall in plasma antioxidants of cancer patients. *Annals of Oncology* 1998;9:1331–1337.

204. White CM, Pritchard J, Turner-Stokes L. Exercise for people with peripheral neuropathy. *Cochrane Database of Systematic Reviews* 2004;4. Art. No.: CD003904. DOI: 10.1002/14651858.CD003904.pub2.

205. Wong R, Sagar S. Acupuncture treatment for chemotherapy-induced peripheral neuropathy—A case series. *Acupuncture in Medicine* 2006;24(2):87–91

206. Pace A, Savarese A, Picardo M, Maresca V, Pacetti U, Del Monte G, et al. Neuroprotective effect of vitamin E supplementation in patients treated with cisplatin chemotherapy. *Journal of Clinical Oncology* 2003;21:927–931.
207. Phillips KD, Skelton WD, Hand GA. Effect of acupuncture administered in a group setting on pain and subjective peripheral neuropathy in persons with human immunodeficiency virus disease. *Journal of Alternative and Complementary Medicine* 2004;10:449–455.
208. Reichstein L, Labrenz S, Ziegler D, Martin S. Effective treatment of symptomatic diabetic polyneuropathy by high-frequency external muscle stimulation. *Diabetologia* 2005;48:824–828.
209. Richardson JK, Sandman D, Vela S. A focused exercise regimen improves clinical measures of balance in patients with peripheral neuropathy. *Archives of Physical Medicine and Rehabilitation* 2001;82:205–209.
210. Richardson JK, Thies S, DeMott T, Ashton-Miller JA. Interventions improve gait regularity in patients with peripheral neuropathy while walking on an irregular surface under low light. *Journal of the American Geriatrics Society* 2004;52:510–515.
211. Shlay JC, Chaloner K, Max MB, Flaws B, Reichelderfer P, Wentworth D, et al. Acupuncture and amitriptyline for pain due to HIV-related peripheral neuropathy: A randomized controlled trial. *JAMA* 1998;280:1590–1595.
212. Smyth JF, Bowman A, Perren T, Wilkinson P, Prescott RJ, Quinn KJ, et al. Glutathione reduces the toxicity and improves quality of life of women diagnosed with ovarian cancer treated with cisplatin: Results of a double-blind, randomized trial. *Annals of Oncology* 1997;8:569–573.
213. Stubblefield MD, Vahdat LT, Balmaceda AB, Troxel AB, Hesdorffer CS, Gooch CL. Glutamine as a neuroprotective agent in high-dose paclitaxel-induced peripheral neuropathy: A clinical and electrophysiologic study. *Clinical Oncology* 2005;17:271–276.
214. Vahdat L, Papadopoulos K, Lange D, Leuin S, Kaufman E, Donovan D, et al. Reduction of paclitaxel-induced peripheral neuropathy with glutamine. *Clinical Cancer Research* 2001;7:1192–1197.
215. Weijl NI, Hopman GD, Wipkink-Bakker A, Lentjes EG, Berger HM, Cleton FJ, et al. Cisplatin combination chemotherapy induces a fall in plasma antioxidants of cancer patients. *Annals of Oncology* 1998;9:1331–1337.
216. Reuben SS, Buvanendran A. Preventing the development of chronic pain after orthopaedic surgery with preventive multimodal analgesic techniques. *Journal of Bone and Joint Surgery America.* 2007;89(6):1343–58.
217. Coderre TJ, Katz J, Vaccarino AL, Melzack R. Contribution of central neuroplasticity to pathological pain: review of clinical and experimental evidence. *Pain*1993; 52:259–85
218. Flor H, Nikolajsen L, Staehelin Jensen T. Phantom limb pain: a case of maladaptive CNS plasticity? *Nature Reviews Neuroscience* 2006 Nov;7(11):873–81.
219. Woolf CJ, Salter MW. Neuronal plasticity: increasing the gain in pain. *Science* 2000; 288:1765–1769.
220. Perkins FM, Kehlet H. Chronic pain as an outcome of surgery. A review of predictive factors. *Anesthesiology* 2000;93:1123–1133.
221. Macrae WM, Davies HTO. Chronic postsurgical pain. In: Crombie IK, Croft PR, Linton SJ, Leresche L, Von Korff, M, editors. Epidemiology of pain: a report on the Task Force on Epidemiology. Seattle: IASP Press; 1999. pp. 125–142.
222. Diatchenko L, Slade GD, Nackley AG, Bhalang K, Sigurdsson A, Belfer I, Goldman D, Xu K, Shabalina SA, Shagin D, Max MB, Makarov SS, Maixner W. Genetc basis for individual variations in pain perception and the development of a chronic pain condition. *Human Molecular Genetics* 2005;14:135–43.
223. Eisenberg E. Post-surgical neuralgia. *Pain* 2004;111:3–7; Melzack R, Wall PD. Pain mechanisms: a new theory. *Science* 1965; 150:971 –

224. Shavit Y, Fridel K, Beilin B. Postoperative pain management and proinflammatory cytokines: animal and human studies. *Journal of Neuroimmune Pharmacology* 2006 Dec;1(4):443–51.
225. Seruga B, Zhang H, Bernstein LJ, Tannock IF. Cytokines and their relationship to the symptoms and outcome of cancer. *Nature Reviews Cancer* 2008 Oct 10. [Epub ahead of print].

Pain and Use of Health Services Among Persons Living with HIV

Aram Dobalian, Jennie C.I. Tsao, and Lonnie K. Zeltzer

Abstract Pain is a significant factor in a person's decision to use health services. Moreover, pain is a particularly important factor in the use of health services among persons living with chronic conditions such as human immunodeficiency virus (HIV)/acquired immunodeficiency syndrome (AIDS). In addition, pain has a far-reaching impact on the health-related quality of life (HRQOL) of persons living with HIV. Nevertheless, the manner in which pain influences an individual to seek out health care remains poorly understood despite the fact that pain is a common experience for both adults and children. This chapter summarizes the role of pain in HIV and begins with a synopsis of epidemiologic studies on the prevalence of pain symptoms with a focus on chronic pain. This is followed by a synthesis of the existing evidence-base of studies of pain and the use of health services using Andersen's Behavioral Model of Health Services Use and includes discussions of both conventional health services and complementary and alternative medicine (CAM) approaches where such studies exist. In this conceptual framework, pain should be considered a perceived need characteristic since a person assesses his or her own pain. Pain is also currently conceptualized as a multidimensional construct that includes social, psychological, and physiological components. Thus, it is not surprising that pain often co-occurs with other health conditions. This chapter also addresses the role of comorbid psychological disorders and substance abuse in the use of health services among persons experiencing pain. Finally, the chapter describes gaps in existing knowledge regarding the role of pain in the use of health services among persons living with HIV, and makes suggestions regarding future directions for this field.

A. Dobalian (✉)
HSR&D Center of Excellence for the Study of Healthcare Provider Behavior, VA Greater Los Angeles Healthcare System; Department of Health Services, UCLA School of Public Health, 10960 Wilshire Blvd., Ste. 1550, Los Angeles, CA 90024, USA
e-mail: aram.dobalian@ucla.edu

R.J. Moore (ed.), *Biobehavioral Approaches to Pain*,
DOI 10.1007/978-0-387-78323-9_12, © Springer Science+Business Media, LLC 2009

Introduction

Research conducted during the past two decades suggests that pain is a significant factor in a person's decision to use health services. Moreover, pain may play a particularly important role in the use of health services among persons living with chronic conditions such as human immunodeficiency virus (HIV)/ acquired immunodeficiency syndrome (AIDS). Furthermore, pain has a far-reaching impact on the health-related quality of life (HRQOL) of populations with chronic diseases. Nevertheless, the manner in which pain influences an individual to seek out health care remains poorly understood despite the fact that pain is a common experience for both adults and children.

This chapter summarizes the role of pain in HIV and begins with a synopsis of epidemiologic studies on the prevalence of pain symptoms with a focus on chronic pain. This is followed by a synthesis of the existing evidence-base on pain and the use of health services using Andersen's Behavioral Model of Health Services Use and includes discussions of complementary and alternative medicine (CAM) approaches where such studies exist. The Behavioral Model of Health Services Use posits that both contextual and individual predisposing, enabling, and need characteristics determine whether an individual ultimately uses health services. In this conceptual framework, an individual's propensity to use different types of health services is influenced by his or her predisposing characteristics, including, for example, age, gender, health status, and race. However, these characteristics are not directly responsible for use. Enabling characteristics such as economic and social resources serve to facilitate or impede the receipt of health care. Finally, need characteristics refer to the presence or severity of illness, as assessed by both a clinician (evaluated need) and by an individual (perceived need). Therefore, pain should be considered a perceived need characteristic since a person assesses his or her own pain (i.e. pain is self-reported).

Pain may also be conceptualized as a multidimensional construct that includes social, behavioral, and physiological components. Thus, it is not surprising that pain often co-occurs with other conditions, and accordingly any consideration of the role of pain in the use of health services should also examine the role of other commonly comorbid need characteristics in the use of health services. Consequently, this chapter also addresses the role of comorbid psychological disorders and substance abuse in the use of health services among persons experiencing pain. Finally, the chapter describes gaps in existing knowledge regarding the role of pain in the use of health services among persons living with HIV. Future directions for research are also proposed.

Prevalence of Pain in the General Population of Adults

To provide a comparison for the importance of pain among persons living with HIV, this section begins with a brief focus on pain in the general population of adults. Estimates of the prevalence of pain vary widely even in the general adult population. Frolund and Frolund (Frolund & Frolund, 1986) reported that the proportion of medical visits for acute and chronic pain was 61% and 39%, respectively. Verhaak, Kerssens, Dekker, Sorbi, & Bensing (1998) reviewed 15 studies on the prevalence of "benign chronic pain" at either the population or primary care level among persons 18 to 75 years old. The authors selected epidemiological studies that examined pain, but which did not exclusively focus on acute pain or on pain as a consequence of a clearly defined disease such as cancer or rheumatoid arthritis. The studies spanned several countries including the United States (U.S.) (4 studies), the United Kingdom (U.K.) (3 studies), Denmark (2 studies), Sweden (2 studies), Canada, Finland, Germany, and New Zealand (1 study each).

Verhaak et al. (Verhaak et al., 1998) reported that the median estimate of the prevalence of chronic pain was 15%, but estimates ranged between 2% (Kohlmann, 1991) and 40%. (Brattberg, Thorslund, & Wikman, 1989) The 15 studies used similar definitions of chronicity (i.e. ranging from less than 1 month to greater than 6 months). The estimates of prevalence were not greatly affected by variations in the time period used to define chronic pain. In some of the studies, chronic pain was assessed using a graded approach that included measures of severity and persistence. Other studies used more basic measures of chronic pain such as whether pain was present or absent. However, both approaches yielded similarly varying estimates. The studies that employed the more complex, graded definition of chronic pain found a median prevalence rate of 13.5%, compared to those that employed simpler definitions, which found a median prevalence rate of 16%. Similarly, the methods used to assess pain varied across each of these studies and included telephone surveys, mailed questionnaires, interviews, and general practitioner assessments. However, Verhaak et al. (Verhaak et al., 1998) found that the differences in prevalence could not be explained by variations in the studies methods. The authors concluded that a conservative estimate for the prevalence of chronic pain in the general population was 10%. Seven of the 15 studies reported that chronic pain was more prevalent among women than men, although two studies found similar prevalence rates between the two genders. Prevalence of pain generally increased with age, although some of the studies reported that prevalence peaked between the ages of 45 and 65 years. In general, lower income groups reported higher prevalence rates. Musculoskeletal pain (back pain, neck pain, shoulder pain) was the most common pain complaint, although headaches and abdominal pain were also frequently mentioned.

Following the review by Verhaak et al. (Verhaak et al., 1998), four additional studies have been published that examined the prevalence of chronic pain in the general adult population. Chrubasik, Junck, Zappe, & Stutzke (1998) mailed a survey to a sample in Germany, and found that 40% reported prolonged pain. These findings are consistent with two prior studies in Sweden (Brattberg et al., 1989) and the U.S. (Von Korff, Dworkin, Le Resche, & Kruger, 1988) that were included in the Verhaak et al. review. Chrubasik et al. (Chrubasik et al., 1998) also found that older respondents and women were more likely to report experiencing pain. A telephone survey conducted by Blyth et al. (Blyth et al., 2001) in Australia reported that the prevalence of chronic pain was 17% in men and 20% in women. The researchers also found that older age, less education, and a lack of private health insurance were significantly associated with having chronic pain. Furthermore, the presence of chronic pain was associated with receiving disability or unemployment benefits, being unemployed for health reasons, having poor self-rated health, and high levels of psychological distress. More recently, Haetzman et al. (Haetzman, Elliott, Smith, Hannaford, & Chambers, 2003) reported that 54% of respondents endorsed having chronic pain in a study that employed mailed surveys in the U.K.

Breivik, Collett, Ventafridda, Cohen, & Gallacher (2006) recently conducted a computer-assisted telephone survey to examine the prevalence, severity, treatment and impact of chronic pain in Israel and 15 countries in Europe. The researchers used screening interviews among 46,394 respondents aged 18 years or older. Pain was assessed using the 10-point Numeric Rating Scale (NRS; 1 = no pain, 10 = worst pain imaginable). About 19% reported chronic pain, with an average pain intensity of 5 during the last episode of pain. The researchers also conducted in-depth interviews with 4,839 respondents who reported chronic pain. Among this sub-sample, 66% reported moderate pain (NRS = 5–7), 34% endorsed severe pain (NRS = 8–10), and 59% reported that they had suffered with pain for two to 15 years. The researchers found that the observed prevalence of chronic pain varied from 12% in Spain and 13% in the UK and Ireland to 26% and 27% in Italy and Poland and 30% in Norway. Breivik et al. (2006) hypothesized that the observed variations may relate to random variation among the samples in each country (about 300 pain sufferers were interviewed in each nation), differences in the ages of the populations, lifestyle differences, and perhaps variations in pain perception and treatment. It should also be noted that telephone surveys tend to exclude the oldest, the sickest, and those with a lower socio-economic status.

Prevalence of Pain Among the General Population of Children

There are few published studies that have examined the epidemiology of pain among children that did not focus on a particular condition. Perquin et al. (Perquin et al., 2000) examined pain among children in the Netherlands. The study included a random sample of 1,300 children aged 0–3 years old and a representative sample of 5,336 children aged 4–18 years. Parents completed the survey for children under 8 years old, while children age 8 and older completed the surveys themselves. About 54% of respondents reported experiencing pain during the prior three months, although only 25% reported chronic pain. Chronic pain, defined as existing recurrently or continuously for more than three months, was most frequently reported by children aged 12–15 years. Chronic pain was reported more often by girls than boys, except among children under age 4.

Campo, Comer, Jansen-Mcwilliams, Gardner, & Kelleher (2002) studied the predictors of recurrent pain in children aged 4 to 15 years using data derived from the Child Behavior Study (CBS). The CBS included 395 clinicians from 204 practices in 44 States, Puerto Rico and 4 Canadian provinces (Campo, Jansen-McWilliams, Comer, & Kelleher, 1999; Kelleher et al., 1997). Parents reported on their children's pain, school attendance/performance, psychological distress, and family functioning. Children were then categorized as complaining "often" or "sometimes/never" about aches and pain. Female gender, age, health status, symptoms of anxiety and/or depression, high rates of health service use, lower levels of parent education, and family support more often predicted membership in the frequent pain group (Campo et al., 2002).

Roth-Isigkeit, Thyen, Raspe, Stoven, & Schmucker (2004) used the survey developed by Perquin and colleagues (Perquin et al., 2000) to examine the prevalence of pain in 715 German children aged 10 to 18 years. Children completed the surveys themselves. Respondents reported that the most common pains were headache, abdominal pain, limb pain and back pain. About 46% reported pain lasting longer than three months, including 35% who reported pain lasting longer than six months. Older children were more likely to report pain, a finding that is consistent with Perquin et al. (Perquin et al., 2000). In addition, girls aged 13 and up were more likely to report pain and this sex difference increased with age.

Prevalence of Pain in Adults and Children Living with HIV

Pain is a common experience for persons with HIV. Pain is the leading source of disability among persons living with HIV. (Gonzalez-Duarte, Cikurel, & Simpson, 2007; Lebovits, Lefkowitz, & McCarthy, 1989; Norval, 2004) HIV-related pain is a source of psychological distress, leads to lower HRQOL, and produces greater functional impairment among persons living with HIV (Douaihy, Stowell, Kohnen, Stoklosa, & Breitbart, 2007a,b).

A nationally representative survey of 2,267 persons living with HIV found that 67% of respondents reported experiencing pain in the prior four-week period. (Dobalian, Tsao, & Duncan, 2004) One earlier study of 438 HIV-positive persons in New York found that more than 60% experienced some pain in the two week period prior to the survey. (Breitbart, McDonald et al., 1996) Estimates of the prevalence of pain among persons living with HIV vary from 25% to 80% depending on the characteristics of the sample, how the respondents were recruited, and the methodology used by the researchers. (McCormack, Li, Zarowny, & Singer, 1993; Schofferman & Brody, 1990; Simmonds, Novy, & Sandoval, 2005; Singer et al., 1993) Thus, the prevalence of chronic pain among persons with HIV is likely significantly greater than in the general adult population. Nevertheless, pain is often underrecognized and undertreated by clinicians providing care to persons with HIV. (Larue, Fontaine, & Colleau, 1997)

One study of pain among persons living with HIV found that women reported more pain than men, and that racial and ethnic minorities reported more pain than whites. (Breitbart, McDonald et al., 1996) No differences in pain between African Americans and Hispanics were reported in the study. In contrast, a more recent nationally representative study reported that African Americans reported less pain than whites. (Dobalian et al., 2004) Differences in the sample characteristics, the measures of pain, and the stage of HIV illness may have led to the disparate findings. Indeed, other socioeconomically disadvantaged populations, including injection drug-using women, the less educated, and the unemployed, reported a higher prevalence of pain in the more recent study. (Dobalian et al., 2004) The researchers speculated that the increased severity of pain in these populations may relate to a greater degree of economic and social stressors in these vulnerable populations, as well as greater barriers to accessing health services.

Few studies have examined the prevalence of pain among children living with HIV. (Gaughan et al., 2002; Lavy, 2007; Lolekha et al., 2004) Gaughan et al. (2002) conducted a prospective cohort study using the General Health Assessment for Children as part of the Pediatric Late Outcomes Study. Pain was assessed for the prior month using 7 questions administered to 985 children living with HIV. The study found that the prevalence of pain in the population remained relatively constant at around 20% over the course of a one-year period. Risk factors for experiencing pain included lower CD4 levels, female gender, and a diagnosis with HIV/AIDS. Pain was associated with an increased risk of mortality.

Lolekha and colleagues (Lolekha et al., 2004) sought to determine the prevalence of pain among children living with HIV in Thailand. The researchers conducted a cross-sectional study in an outpatient facility in Bangkok, and age-matched 61 children aged 4 to 15 years old with HIV to children without chronic illness. They found that 44% of the children living with HIV reported pain compared to 13% of the children in the control group. The prevalence of chronic pain among the children living with HIV was 7%. Children living with HIV most commonly reported that pain occurred in the abdomen, lower limbs or head. The study also found that only 44% of children who experienced pain received analgesia.

Lavy (Lavy, 2007) studied 95 children referred for palliative care in a hospital in Malawi. Seventy-seven percent of the children had HIV and 17% had cancer. The study found that pain was the most common symptom (27%) and that it was significantly more common among children with cancer than those with HIV.

Pain and Health Status

Types of Pain

The majority of studies summarized in this chapter examine the role of chronic pain, rather than acute pain, on the use of health services. Definitions of chronic pain vary. Chronic pain is defined by the International Association for the Study of Pain (IASP) as continuous or recurrent pain that persists for longer than the normal time for healing, generally considered to be approximately three months. (Merskey, Bogduk, & editors., 1994) However, pain that persists for as short a duration as one month may be considered to be chronic pain depending on the health condition underlying the source of that pain. In addition, some pain specialists prefer to classify chronic pain using a prior definition which required pain to persist for longer than six months in order to be considered chronic rather than acute. In contrast to chronic pain, acute pain is usually of brief duration. The intensity of acute pain also tends to decrease after the healing process begins. The causes of pain vary. For example, acute pain may result from disease or injury. Failure to properly treat pain during the acute phase may lead to delayed recovery, and in this manner, acute pain may develop into chronic pain.

Persons living with HIV who endorse pain typically describe two or three simultaneous sources of that pain. (Breitbart & McDonald, 1996) A number of studies note that stage of HIV infection is related to severity of pain. (McCormack et al., 1993; Schofferman & Brody, 1990; Simmonds et al., 2005; Singer et al., 1993) Nevertheless, pain may be significant regardless of disease stage. In addition, pain is associated with current HIV symptoms and the presence of infections related to HIV. (Breitbart, McDonald et al., 1996; Singer et al., 1993) There is also additional evidence to suggest that pain may increase as HIV progresses.

The development and spread of effective antiretroviral therapies beginning in the 1990s has increased the life expectancy of persons living with HIV. These therapies have also led to a need for better understanding and recognition of pain syndromes among this population. (Vogl et al., 1999) Typically pain is divided into two broad categories, nociceptive (caused by tissue damage in the skin, bone, connective tissue, muscle or viscera) and neuropathic (caused by injury or disease in the nerve tissue). (Emanuel & Emmanuel, 2004; Gonzalez-Duarte et al., 2007) This distinction is often important in determining the etiology of pain and directing its effective management. Although pain management has improved in recent years, pain continues to be a significant concern for persons with HIV due in part to the recognition that pain in persons living with HIV may become chronic and multifactorial. (Hewitt et al., 1997; Vogl et al., 1999)

Undertreatment of Pain

A number of studies suggest that pain is undertreated among persons living with HIV. (Breitbart, McDonald et al., 1996; Breitbart, Rosenfeld et al., 1996; Frich & Borgbjerg, 2000) As more fully detailed in section III of this chapter, persons living with HIV who report more pain use more health services than those who do not report pain. In addition, pain appears to be a more important determinant of health services utilization than other symptoms associated with

HIV such as low energy. (Dobalian et al., 2004; Tsao, Dobalian, & Naliboff, 2004) Undertreatment of pain leads to unnecessary suffering and may promote harmful health behaviors such as self-medicating with illicit drugs. (Tsao, Dobalian, Myers, & Zeltzer, 2005a) Self-medication may in turn lead to poorer health status and subsequent worsening of pain.

Barriers to accessing health services may be greater for certain racial and ethnic minority populations such as Native Americans and Asian/Pacific Islanders. These barriers to care may relate to language and culture, resulting in less use of health services relative to non-Hispanic whites. (Dobalian et al., 2004) Women who are HIV-positive and have a history of injection drug-use report more intense pain and are less likely to receive analgesia than are men with a similar history. (Breitbart, McDonald et al., 1996; Breitbart, Rosenfeld et al., 1996; Dobalian et al., 2004) In addition, injection drug-users living with HIV are less likely to receive adequate analgesia than men who have sex with men and other persons living with HIV, even after controlling for age, socioeconomic status, and health insurance. (Dobalian et al., 2004)

Other studies suggest that the undertreatment of pain among injection drug-users may relate to physicians' concerns regarding drug-seeking behavior and fears of criminal prosecution. (Dobalian et al., 2004) Moreover, despite the severity and frequency of pain among hospitalized persons living with HIV, pain reported by these patients may still be underestimated by healthcare providers. This underestimation may also lead to undertreatment. (Aires & Bammann, 2005)

Healthcare providers may create additional barriers to effective pain management among persons living with HIV. Many providers believe that they lack knowledge regarding pain management or have little access to experts who may provide consultations. (Breitbart, Kaim, & Rosenfeld, 1999) Facilities and communities may also lack adequate psychological support and drug treatment services. Furthermore, providers may be concerned about the potential for addiction and substance abuse.

Persons living with HIV may also engage in behaviors that also lead to undertreatment of pain. For example, many individuals report concerns regarding the potential for addiction to pain medications and adverse effects associated with opioid treatment. (Breitbart et al., 1998)

Taken together, the findings from these studies highlight the importance of early detection of patients with risk factors for developing pain. Healthcare providers need additional training in order to recognize the behaviors that may indicate the potential for addiction or misuse of prescription medications. This training should also address providers' own concerns about treatment of pain, particularly in patients with substance abuse histories.

Pain and Functional Impairment

Pain impacts HRQOL indirectly through physical and psychological symptoms that are associated with pain among persons living with HIV. (Lorenz, Shapiro,

Asch, Bozzette, & Hays, 2001) Severity of pain is associated with impaired functional ability. Persons living with HIV who experience pain report significantly decreased HRQOL and declines in functioning. Initial studies of persons living with HIV found that 60% of patients with moderate to severe pain reported impairment in functional ability. (Breitbart, McDonald et al., 1996; Rosenfeld et al., 1996) One survey found that pain typically impaired activities of daily living (a measure of physical functioning) and quality of life, including ability to walk, work, sleep, interact with others, and overall enjoyment. (Breitbart, McDonald et al., 1996) One more recent study that evaluated both pain and fatigue found that pain had a significant impact on both physical functioning and quality of life, while fatigue impacted only physical functioning. (Simmonds et al., 2005) The development of more effective interventions for treating pain in turn may lead to improvements in overall HRQOL.

Psychological Distress and Pain

A number of studies have demonstrated a correlation between psychological distress and chronic pain. For example, in a review of epidemiologic studies on chronic pain, Verhaak et al. (Verhaak et al., 1998) asserted that the presence of chronic pain was associated with a higher prevalence of psychological symptoms (e.g., anxiety, depression) in the studies that investigated such relationships. (Croft, Rigby, Boswell, Schollum, & Silman, 1993; Potter & Jones, 1992; Von Korff et al., 1988) Breivik et al. (2006) conducted in-depth interviews with 4,839 respondents who endorsed chronic pain. Among this group, the researchers found that 21% reported that they had been diagnosed with depression because of their pain. Many of the respondents also indicated that their pain had a significant impact on their employment status: 61% were unable or less able to work outside the home, 19% had lost their job, and 13% had changed jobs because of their pain.

The prevalence of psychological disorders is higher among persons living with HIV than in the general population. For example, the lifetime prevalence of major depressive disorder among persons living with HIV is estimated to be 5% to 45%. (Basu, Chwastiak, & Bruce, 2005) Anxiety disorders, including generalized anxiety disorder, panic disorder, and posttraumatic stress disorder (PTSD) are also prevalent among persons living with HIV with estimated prevalence rates as high as 20%. (Vitiello, Burnam, Bing, Beckman, & Shapiro, 2003)

Tsao et al. (2004) examined the relationship between panic disorder and pain among persons living with HIV. Using data from the HIV Cost and Services Utilization Study (HCSUS), a nationally representative sample of persons receiving medical care for HIV, the researchers found that panic disorder was a stronger predictor of pain than either depression or PTSD. The researchers suggested that the relationship between panic disorder and pain may be related to a tendency of persons with panic disorder to catastro-phize physical symptoms and bodily sensations, leading to increased panic and more intense pain.

Smith, Egert, Winkel, & Jacobson (2002) investigated the interaction between PTSD and pain, and found that PTSD predicted increased pain intensity and greater functional interference in both mood and daily activities. These findings are similar to relationships that have been found in other victims of trauma such as veterans. The researchers suggested that many persons living with HIV encounter traumatic stressors that may lead to PTSD. Typical stres-sors include the initial diagnosis with HIV, sudden declines in CD4 counts, and loss of friends and family to HIV. Many persons living with HIV also have a history of trauma related to physical or sexual abuse, homelessness, and sub-stance abuse. (Liebschutz, Feinman, Sullivan, Stein, & Samet, 2000)

Leserman and colleagues (Leserman et al., 2005) investigated how trauma, severe stressful events, PTSD, and depressive symptoms are related to physical functioning and health utilization in 611 HIV-infected men and women living in rural areas of five Southern states. The researchers found that patients with more lifetime trauma, stressful events, and PTSD symptoms reported more bodily pain, and poorer physical, role, and cognitive functioning than those without such trauma. Both this study and the study by Tsao et al. (2004) found that PTSD and depression were both associated with reports of greater pain even after controlling for HIV disease stage.

Many persons living with HIV also have a history of substance abuse. More than one-third of HIV infections in the U.S. are due to injection drug use, and the rate is higher among women and adolescents. (Centers for Disease Control and Prevention, 2005) Persons living with HIV who use illicit substances report more pain and have a greater burden of illness. (Tsao et al., 2004) Current drug use is more strongly related to experiencing pain than is a history of past substance use. (Tsao, Dobalian, & Stein, 2005b)

Some research indicates that healthcare providers may find it more difficult to manage patients with chronic pain who have a history of substance use. (Rosenblatt & Mekhail, 2005) These persons may be more prone to aberrant drug-taking behaviors. This risk factor may lead some healthcare providers to be more reticent to provide adequate pain management and may make this population more prone to undertreatment. (See also Heit and Lipman, This Volume)

Extant research on the relationship between pain and aberrant use of prescription analgesics in persons living with HIV is more limited than the aforementioned research on illict drug abuse. In a recent study, Tsao, Stein, & Dobalian (2007) investigated the associations among pain, aberrant use of opioids, and problem drug use history in a sample of 2,267 persons from the HCSUS. Using structural equation modeling, the researchers tested a con-ceptual model wherein persons living with HIV who had a history of proble-matic drug use were compared to those without such history. The study found that persons with a history of problematic drug use reported more pain, and were more likely to report aberrant use of prescription analgesics, even after controlling for key demographic and socioeconomic characteristics. In addition, those with a history of problematic drug use reported more use of such medications specifically for pain, compared to patients without such history.

The study also found a trend toward greater stability of aberrant opioid use over time in problem drug users compared with non-problem users. (Tsao et al., 2007) The researchers suggested that these finding indicate a persistent pattern of inappropriate medication use in the former group. Although persons with a history of problematic drug use reported on-going patterns of using prescription analgesics specifically for pain, these patients continued to experience persistently higher levels of pain during the two follow-up surveys, relative to non-problem users.

Various studies have posited many possible causes that may underlie the increased prevalence of psychological disorders among persons living with HIV. (Atkinson et al., 1988; Pugh et al., 1994; Sambamoorthi, Walkup, Olfson, & Crystal, 2000) For example, it has been suggested that stigma plays a role in creating psychological distress among persons living with HIV. (Foster, 2007) Other factors include limited social support, and the overall health burden of being HIV-positive and dealing with its associated health complications. In particular, pain related to HIV has been shown to be associated with a number of symptoms associated with depression, including hopelessness, negativism, anhedonia, difficulty sleeping, and loss of appetite. Pain may also exacerbate existing psychological disorders or other health conditions, or may lead directly to the development of depression and anxiety. For example, increasing severity of pain may worsen the symptoms of depression and lead to declines in HRQOL. (Rosenfeld et al., 1996) Furthermore, pain, stress, and lack of adequate social support are factors that may lead to poor quality sleep among persons living with HIV. (Vosvick et al., 2004) In turn, poor sleep quality among persons living with HIV is associated with a greater likelihood of depression and anxiety. (Robbins, Phillips, Dudgeon, & Hand, 2004)

Consequently, it is important for health care providers to recognize and treat psychological disorders among persons living with HIV, and this may be particularly true for patients with chronic pain. Detection of depression may be challenging among persons living with HIV as there is substantial overlap in symptoms among depression, HIV, and chronic pain. Each may be associated with poor sleep quality and fatigue.

Additional research is needed on the relationship between health beliefs about pain, psychological distress, and the use of health services. In light of the strong evidence-base concerning the correlation between chronic pain and psychological factors, future studies on the role of pain in the decision to seek health care should include validated measures of a range of psychological symptoms, including particularly anxiety, depression, and somatization.

Pain and Access to Health Services

Access to Health Services

Numerous factors influence whether a person chooses to access health care. Various conceptual models have been proposed by researchers seeking to understand why a person uses health care. Most of these models are based on either a psychological (Rosenstock, 1974) or sociological framework. For example, the Health Beliefs Model (Harrison, Mullen, & Green, 1992), a psychologically-based model, hypothesizes that the use of health services is determined by a person's beliefs about disease and the effectiveness of the health care system in preventing or treating disease. In this model, a person's beliefs include perceptions of susceptibility to a disease and its seriousness. Demographic characteristics such as gender, psychological characteristics such as personality, and structural characteristics such as knowledge of the disease and prior experience with it are factors that modify the likelihood of seeking care. Furthermore, a person may experience cues to action such as mass media campaigns that are designed to heighten awareness of a particular disease, and which in turn influence the perceived seriousness of the threat of a particular disease. In this framework, pain may influence the perceived seriousness of a disease. Pain may also impede action if, for example, the treatment is likely to be painful. Criticisms of the Health Beliefs Model have tended to focus on the relative lack of emphasis placed on cultural factors and socioeconomic status.

One commonly used sociological model for understanding utilization of health services is Andersen's Behavioral Model of Health Services Use. (Andersen, 1968, 1995) This conceptual framework is based on a systems perspective, and incorporates both individual and contextual (environmental) characteristics as important factors that influence whether an individual accesses health care. (Phillips, Morrison, Andersen, & Aday, 1998) Within this model, individual characteristics are specific to a particular person, such as, for example, the person's age and the health insurance plan in which the person is enrolled. In contrast, contextual factors include, for example, aspects of the community, its healthcare organizations and healthcare providers, and the environment in which the person resides.

According to the Behavioral Model of Health Services Use, both individual and contextual characteristics are divided into three groups: predisposing, enabling, and need. (Andersen, 1968, 1995) Predisposing characteristics are based on the hypothesis that factors such as age, gender, and race influence an individual's propensity to use different types of health services. Nevertheless, these predisposing characteristics are not directly responsible for a person's use of health care. Contextual predisposing characteristics include, for example, the age and gender makeup of a community since the availability of different types of healthcare organizations and healthcare providers is dependent on the demographic composition of the community. For example, communities with more elderly residents would be more likely to have a greater number of nursing homes and geriatricians. Enabling characteristics include the economic and social resources at both the individual and contextual levels that serve to either facilitate or impede care. These enabling characteristics include, for example, whether an individual has health insurance coverage, and whether an individual has a usual source of health care. Finally, need characteristics refer to the presence or severity of disease or illness, as assessed by both laypersons (perceived need) and healthcare providers (evaluated need). Contextual need characteristics include health-related measures of the environment such as air quality. Under the Behavioral Model of Health Services Use, pain is an individual perceived need characteristic because pain is an aspect of how people think about their health and functional status. It is the perceived need characteristics that are ultimately responsible for whether an individual seeks health care. Prior studies that use this conceptual framework have generally found that the need characteristics have the greatest influence on the use of health services. (Korten et al., 1998; McCallum et al., 1996) This chapter uses the Behavioral Model of Health Services Use to provide the context for a discussion of the role of pain in accessing health care.

HIV and the Healthcare System

HIV is a chronic infection that progressively weakens the body's immune system and leads to opportunistic infections and other diseases. The successful treatment of HIV requires the use of highly active antiretroviral therapy (HAART). The use of HAART has greatly extended the life expectancy of persons living with HIV. (Detels et al., 1998; Palella et al., 1998) However, such treatments are not curative.

The management of HIV requires access to a broad range of health services, including both generalist and specialist medical care, HAART, treatments for HIV-related diseases, social services, mental health services, and treatment for substance abuse. Dental care also plays an important role for persons living with HIV because HIV has a significant impact on oral health. (Parveen et al., 2007; Ramirez-Amador, Ponce-de-Leon, Anaya-Saavedra, Crabtree Ramirez, & Sierra-Madero, 2007) More than one-third of persons living with HIV develop oral lesions (Silverman, Migliorati, Lozada-Nur, Greenspan, & Conant, 1986), and some estimates indicate that more than 90% of persons living with HIV will have at least one oral manifestation. (McCarthy, 1992; Weinert, Grimes, & Lynch, 1996) The consequences of untreated oral disease are significant, including interference with talking, chewing, and swallowing, which may lead to weight loss and malnutrition. (Weinert et al., 1996) Dobalian et al. (2003) conducted a longitudinal study using structural equation modeling and data from the HCSUS to examine use of dental services among persons living with HIV. The authors used the Behavioral Model of Health Services Use and controlled for key predisposing (e.g., gender, drug use, race, education), enabling (e.g., income, insurance, regular source of care), and need characteristics (e.g., mental, physical, and oral health). They found that more education, dental insurance, having a usual source of dental care, and poor oral health predicted a higher probability of having a dental visit. However, African Americans, Hispanics, those exposed to HIV through drug use or heterosexual contact, and those in poor physical health were less likely to have a visited a dentist. In addition, African Americans and persons with poor mental health also had fewer visits. These studies suggest that persons with more HIV-related symptoms and a diagnosis of AIDS have a greater need for dental care than those with fewer symptoms and without AIDS, but that more pressing needs for physical and mental health services may further limit their access to dental services. (Dobalian et al., 2003)

Funding for HIV-Related Services

Persons living with HIV who have health insurance are mostly covered through public insurance programs including Medicaid, Medicare, the Ryan White CARE Act, and state AIDS Drug Assistance Programs (ADAPs). The total costs of care for HIV according to the HCSUS were estimated at $6.7 to $7.8 billion in 1996. (Bozzette et al., 1998; Hellinger & Fleishman, 2000) The current total costs of care for HIV are unknown, but the fiscal year 2007 estimate for federal spending is $23.4 billion.

Despite improvements in care for persons living with HIV, the disease can be disabling and may require individuals to leave the workforce. Individuals without income and access to employer-based health insurance may be eligible for Medicaid, the major financing mechanism in the U.S. for low-income citizens. Medicaid is the largest funding source for HIV care in the U.S. Persons living with HIV may have difficulty meeting eligibility requirements for Medicaid because having HIV does not automatically qualify as a disability even if an individual has low income. (Keefe, 2003) Many low-income people with HIV are ineligible for Medicaid until they become disabled, despite available therapies for HIV that may prevent disability. The HCSUS found that Medicaid covered 44% of persons living with HIV (including 12–13% covered by Medicare). (Bozzette et al., 1998) The HCSUS also found that among persons living with HIV, African Americans and Latinos were more likely to be covered by Medicaid than whites, and women were more likely to be covered by Medicaid than men.

Most persons living with HIV qualify for Medicare because of their disability status rather than because they are age 65 or older. Individuals under age 65 with permanent disability who have adequate work credits and have received Social Security Disability Insurance (SSDI) payments for two years or longer may be eligible for Medicare. The HCSUS found that more than 80% of those covered by Medicare were under the age of 50. (Bozzette et al., 1998) Medicare provides health insurance coverage for 19% of persons living with HIV according to the HCSUS.

The Ryan White CARE Act provides medical care, HIV testing, counseling, and community and psychosocial support services for individuals and families affected by HIV. Funds are provided directly to states, cities, and providers. More than half a million people receive at least one medical, health, or related support service through Ryan White each year, although many individuals receive services from multiple parts of Ryan White. Most Ryan White clients are low-income, male, ages 25 to 44, members of racial and ethnic minority groups, and either uninsured or publicly insured. (Health Resources and Services Administration, 2006)

ADAPs provide FDA-approved HIV-related medications to low-income persons living with HIV who have limited or no health insurance for prescription drugs. Eligibility requirements for ADAPs vary from state to state. ADAPs provide assistance to about one-fourth of all persons living with HIV in the U.S. (Kates, Penner, Crutsinger-Perry, Carbaugh, & Singleton, 2006) Individuals receiving assistance through ADAPs are mostly low-income, uninsured, male, ages 25 to 44, members of racial and ethnic minority groups, and have more advanced HIV disease.

Barriers to Accessing Health Care Among Persons Living with HIV

Approximately one-third to one-half of the HIV infected population is either not diagnosed or not receiving care. (Bozzette et al., 1998) There are multiple barriers to accessing healthcare, including lack of health insurance and under-insurance, the high costs of health care, competing subsistence needs, lack of available transportation, healthcare provider attitudes, lack of continuity of health care, language barriers, and cultural differences. It is important to recognize and reduce these barriers to care because a lack of access or delayed access to needed health care may result in clinical presentation at more advanced stages of HIV disease.

Racial and ethnic minorities with HIV generally have poorer access to health services even after controlling for health insurance status. (Smedley, Stith, & Nelson, 2002) Indeed, despite the widespread availability of effective HIV treatments, disparities in survival persist among persons living with HIV. Some studies in persons living with HIV have found that survival rates are lower among African Americans and persons living in lower socioeconomic status communities. (Blair, Fleming, & Karon, 2002; Cunningham et al., 2005; Jain, Schwarcz, Katz, Gulati, & McFarland, 2006; McFarland, Chen, Hsu, Schwarcz, & Katz, 2003; Morin et al., 2002) Researchers have also found that African Americans, as well as Native Americans and Asian/Pacific Islanders, are less likely to have an infectious disease specialist as a regular source of care than are whites. (Heslin, Andersen, Ettner, & Cunningham, 2005) Heslin et al. also found that physicians of Latino patients living with HIV had higher HIV caseloads than the physicians of white patients. Infectious disease specialists are more likely to properly answer questions concerning the appropriate use of HAART. (Landon et al., 2002)

The HCSUS found that African Americans and Hispanics had poorer access to care than whites based on several measures of access. (Shapiro et al., 1999) This is of particular concern given that the HCSUS sampled persons living with HIV who were receiving medical care, and thus may have underrepresented socio-economically disadvantaged groups who confront even greater barriers to accessing health care. African Americans and Hispanics also received poorer quality of care than whites. These disparities diminished over time, but persisted throughout the duration of the study. The HCSUS further found that African Americans and Hispanics were more likely to postpone needed medical care because they lacked transportation, were too sick to visit a physician, or had other competing needs. (Cunningham et al., 1999) Another study used data from the HCSUS and found that Hispanics were more likely than whites to delay care after receiving a diagnosis of HIV. (Turner et al., 2000) A more recent study by Fleishman and colleagues (Fleishman et al., 2005) using data collected from 11 HIV primary and specialty care sites during 2000–2002 found higher rates of hospitalization among African Americans living with HIV, but no statistically significant differences in outpatient utilization.

Research also suggests that women living with HIV may encounter more barriers to accessing health care and receive poorer quality of care than men. The HCSUS found that women living with HIV were less likely to receive HAART and had poorer access to many other measures of access compared to men. (Shapiro et al., 1999) Women living with HIV were more likely to report that they postponed needed care because they either lacked transportation (26%) or were too sick to go to the doctor (23%) than men (12% and 14%, respectively). (Cunningham et al., 1999) The study by Fleishman and colleagues found that women living with HIV had higher rates of hospitalization and used more outpatient visits compared to men. (Fleishman et al., 2005)

One recent study by Tobias et al. (Tobias et al., 2007) sought to examine differences between those persons who received some care and those who had received no care in the six months prior to the start of the study. Persons receiving "no care" had significantly poorer mental health status, were more likely to be actively using drugs or binge drinking, and had more unmet support service needs compared to those receiving "some care." The "no care" group was also more likely to endorse the health belief of "fatalism" when they reported that they did not seek medical care for HIV because they did not think there was a cure for HIV. Mistrust of the health care system was also more prevalent among the "no care" group. The authors suggested that ensuring case management services to link support services and medical care may improve the likelihood that the "no care" group would seek care.

Within the U.S., the HIV epidemic first emerged among gay men and injection drug users, groups that are socially marginalized. Consequently, negative societal responses to these groups influenced the experiences of persons living with HIV. Many persons living with HIV thus felt stigmatized. Such HIV-related stigma is thought to be one of the major barriers to efforts to address the HIV epidemic both within and outside the U.S. (Sayles, Ryan, Silver, Sarkisian, & Cunningham, 2007; Valdiserri, 2002)

Kinsler, Wong, Sayles, Davis, & Cunningham (2007) recently conducted a study to evaluate the relationship between perceived stigma from a health care provider and access to health care among 223 low income, HIV-infected individuals in Los Angeles County. The researchers found that one-fourth of the sample reported perceived stigma from a health care provider at baseline, and one-fifth continued to report healthcare provider stigma at follow up. In addition, the study found that more than half of the respondents reported difficulty accessing health care at both time-points. The researchers further found that perceived stigma was associated with low access to care, even after controlling for sociodemographic characteristics. The authors suggested that interventions such as educational programs and modeling of non-stigmatizing behavior are needed to reduce perceived stigma.

Pain and the Healthcare System

The role of pain in the use of health services is understudied. Nonetheless, researchers have noted the importance of pain in care-seeking behavior for some time. For example, Von Korff, Wagner, Dworkin, & Saunders (1991) reported that conditions associated with chronic pain are among the most common motives for accessing health care, particularly ambulatory (outpatient) care. (Koch, 1986) Of note, Von Korff et al. (1991) recognized that it does not necessarily follow that persons with chronic pain consume more health services than those without chronic pain. Instead, the higher frequency of health care visits for chronic pain may merely be the result of a higher prevalence of such pain conditions in the general population rather than above average rates of health services utilization by persons with chronic pain. Therefore, researchers subsequently sought to better understand the prevalence and importance of pain in access to health care by conducting epidemiologic studies of pain in the general population.

Chronic Pain and the Use of Conventional Health Services

Despite the recognition that chronic pain is a significant problem in the general adult population, few studies have examined the role of chronic pain and the use of health services and even fewer have focused on persons living with HIV.

Therefore, it is necessary to briefly summarize some of the existing research on the use of health services among the general adult population. Most extant studies have focused on use of conventional medical care including visits to a general practitioner or physical therapist, inpatient hospital stays lasting one or more nights, and visits to the emergency department. A limited number of studies have examined self-care practices and the use of complementary or alternative medicine (CAM) approaches. It should be noted that many of these studies have been conducted in other nations, each with its own healthcare system. Nonetheless, there are some commonalities that cut across national boundaries.

The first study that examined the association between chronic pain and health services utilization was conducted by Von Korff et al. (1991) in a probability sample of 1,016 adult enrollees in a Health Maintenance Organization (HMO) in the U.S. This study sought to determine whether pain and psychological distress predicted the likelihood of care-seeking behavior for a painful symptom, and examined the impact of chronic pain on the use of ambulatory care. The authors assessed pain using a questionnaire which asked about pain problems of the back, head, abdomen, chest and temporomandibular region. Temporomandibular pain was included to allow comparison with 242 patients with temporomandibular disorder (TMJ). The researchers assessed the persistence of the pain over the previous six months, daily duration of pain, typical intensity of pain, pain-related interference with daily activities, and the number of days in the prior six months when the respondent was unable to conduct usual activities due to pain. In addition, the authors asked respondents to indicate whether they had sought care from a doctor, physical therapist, chiropractor, or other health care professional in the previous six months for each reported pain problem. For respondents with temporomandibular disorder pain and headaches, the questionnaire substituted dentists for physical therapists.

The study found that pain severity and pain persistence were the strongest and most consistent predictors of contact with a healthcare provider after controlling for age, sex, recency of pain onset, self-rated health, and psychological distress. (Von Korff et al., 1991) The authors also found that poorer self-reported health status was associated with increased care-seeking for headache and abdominal pain, but that psychological distress was not associated with increased use of health services. Age and gender were not significant predictors of contact with a healthcare provider.

The researchers also showed that a small proportion of respondents with severe persistent pain and disability of 7 or more days in the past six months used more health services relative to the average rates of utilization. (Von Korff et al., 1991) Those with recurrent and non-disabling severe-persistent pain did not differ in their use of health services compared to the general population. In effect, this study suggests that chronic pain is not uniformly associated with higher rates of health services utilization.

Chrubasik et al. (1998) conducted a mailed survey of 1,304 adults in Germany and asked respondents whether they experienced prolonged pain in the previous six months. The survey asked respondents to identify the location, duration, severity and persistence of pain, and requested that they state the number and types of healthcare providers that had been consulted, the extent of self-care, and satisfaction with each treatment. About 47% of the respondents reported prolonged pain, and of those, about 87% indicated that the duration of pain was more than one year. The most common complaint was musculoskeletal pain. Approximately one-third of the respondents with prolonged pain indicated that they sought care from a healthcare provider, most often a general practitioner or specialist in physical medicine. Among those who reported pain, 12% used self-care or consulted non-healthcare providers, 49% consulted one healthcare provider, 24% consulted two healthcare providers, 4% consulted three healthcare providers and 0.7% consulted four or more healthcare providers.

Increased use of health services was also positively associated with age, increased pain intensity, number of pain sites, and pain duration. (Chrubasik et al., 1998) Overall, satisfaction with treatment was rated 75% among those with pain, but only 30% in those with persistent and intolerable pain. Satisfaction was also lower among respondents who were older, and those who had consulted more healthcare providers or who had indicated more pain sites or more intense pain.

Andersson, Ejlertsson, Leden, & Schersten (1999) also used a mailed survey to assess chronic pain and use of health care in the general adult population, although their study was conducted in Sweden. The researchers defined chronic pain as recurrent or persistent pain lasting for more than three months. Use of health services was determined by a count of the number of visits to physicians, physical therapists and CAM practitioners during the past three months. In contrast to the earlier studies by Von Korff et al. (1991) and Chrubasik et al. (Chrubasik et al., 1998), Andersson et al. (1999) did not ask respondents to specify whether they sought care specifically for pain. Respondents with pain most often consulted with their primary care providers. About 40% of the respondents who reported chronic pain visited a primary care provider compared to 26% of those without pain. However, the study found no differences in rates of hospitalization between respondents with and without chronic pain. The authors reported that respondents with shorter pain duration had more visits (59%) than those with pain lasting more than six months (34%).

In addition, the authors separately examined respondents who reported high intensity pain and found that those with depression, insomnia, nervousness, and widespread pain were more likely to visit a primary care provider than those without these characteristics. Andersson et al. (1999) concluded that use of health services among individuals with chronic pain depends primarily on perceptions of pain intensity independent of the location of pain, but that use is also influenced by ethnicity (including immigration status), age, socioeconomic status, and depression.

Haetzman et al. (Haetzman et al., 2003) conducted a mailed survey in the U.K. to assess use of both conventional and alternative therapies by respondents who reported chronic pain. Use of health services was evaluated only among individuals with chronic pain lasting three months or longer. The authors examined how often these respondents visited a general practitioner, a hospital specialist, a physical therapist, or an alternative practitioner in the prior year. Approximately 67% of respondents reported having visited their general practitioner, while 34% visited a hospital specialist, and 26% visited a physical therapist. The likelihood of utilization for each type of healthcare provider was greater among respondents with increased pain severity.

Blyth, March, Brnabic, & Cousins (2004) conducted a telephone survey to examine chronic pain and the use of health services in Australia. The authors used the Behavioral Model of Health Services Use as the conceptual basis to examine chronic pain and the use of three types of health services during the prior year: general practitioner consultations, emergency department visits, and inpatient hospitalizations. In this study, use of health services was not necessarily confined to pain-specific use. Chronic pain was defined as pain that persisted for three months or longer during the six months preceding the survey. The study also assessed pain-related interference in daily activities and found that the mean number of health care visits was higher in respondents with pain, and increased with rising levels of pain-related interference. The authors concluded that there is a need for better interventions to manage pain in order to prevent the development of disability.

Breivik et al. (2006) conducted in-depth interviews with 4,839 individuals from 15 European countries and Israel. They reported that 60% of respondents with chronic pain visited their doctor for their pain two to nine times during the last six months, and 11% had visited a physician 10 or more times during that period. Only 2% of those with chronic pain were currently being treated by an expert in pain management, and 31% were currently not being treated.

Chronic Pain and the Use of Complementary and Alternative Therapies

A high proportion of persons who visit a CAM provider have chronic pain. (Astin, 1998; Stoney and Mansky, This Volume) However, a limited number of studies have investigated the use of CAM in adults with chronic pain. Eisenberg et al. (Eisenberg et al., 1993) interviewed a national sample of U.S. residents and found that the use of CAM therapies was highest for back problems (36%), anxiety (28%), headaches (27%), chronic pain (26%), and cancer (24%). In a follow-up survey conducted six years later, Eisenberg et al. (Eisenberg et al., 1998) reported that the highest condition-specific rates of CAM use were for neck (57%) and back (47.6%) problems. Pain is likely a significant problem for both conditions. Astin (1998) reported that chronic pain was the most frequently cited health problem for which CAM was used in a national sample of U.S. residents (37%). Each of these studies defined CAM use as including both self-care (e.g., high-dose megavitamins) and visits to CAM practitioners.

The aforementioned study on the use of health services by Andersson et al. (1999) also examined visits to acupuncturists, chiropractors, homeopaths, and naturopaths. During the three months prior to the survey, about 6% of respondents with chronic pain visited a CAM provider, most often a chiropractor or acupuncturist. The corresponding rate of CAM use among respondents without chronic pain was 1.2%. By contrast, access to general practitioners in the surveyed areas was good and consultation rates were comparable to other similar studies. Greater intensity of pain was associated with more use of CAM providers, after controlling for age, socioeconomic status, ethnicity, depression, and diagnosis of chronic disease.

Of note, the authors found that use of self-care and CAM was not associated with lower utilization of conventional health services. In particular, respondents who used self-care reported higher use of each type of health services, including CAM. Thus, this study suggests that persons experiencing chronic pain are high-utilizers of self-care, conventional medicine, and CAM and they do not substitute self-care or CAM for conventional health care.

Haetzman et al. also examined the relationship between chronic pain and use of CAM in the general population. (Haetzman et al., 2003) However, the authors did not compare use of CAM by respondents with and without chronic pain. This study found that 18% of respondents with chronic pain consulted alternative therapists and 16% used alternative medicine. These rates of CAM use were much higher than those reported by Anderson et al. (1999), but this earlier study assessed utilization over a three month period rather than during a one-year period.

Haetzman et al. (Haetzman et al., 2003) also found that 67% of respondents who visited an alternative therapist also visited conventional healthcare providers. Similarly, a majority of respondents who reported taking alternative medicines (85.9%) also used conventional medicine. Men and older respondents were less likely to use CAM than women and younger respondents. The authors found that the percentage of those with chronic pain who used both conventional and alternative therapists also increased with increasing severity of pain. Higher socioeconomic status predicted increased use of CAM therapists and greater use of alternative meds but less reliance on prescription medications. Higher socioeconomic status and more education have been shown to be associated with increased use of CAM in other studies. (Astin, 1998; Bausell, Lee, & Berman, 2001; Ni, Simile, & Hardy, 2002)

Breivik et al. (2006) also examined use of some CAM therapies among the 4,839 respondents with whom they conducted in-depth interviews. The most common non-drug treatments for chronic pain included massage (30%), physical therapy (21%), and acupuncture (13%). In comparison, 55% reported taking over-the-counter NSAIDs and 44% were using prescription NSAIDs.

Psychological Distress, Pain, and Use of Health Services

There is little extant research on the role of psychological symptoms on the use of health services related to pain. Few studies have incorporated measures of psychological distress when investigating the relationship between pain and utilization. In their review, Von Korff et al. (1991) suggested that illness behavior theory posits three psychosocial processes that influence the likelihood of care-seeking for pain: (1) symptom perception, (2) symptom appraisal, and (3) situational adaptation to illness. According to illness behavior theory, symptoms perceived to be more persistent and severe should be more likely to prompt a person to seek health care than would transient, more mild symptoms. (Prohaska, Keller, Leventhal, & Leventhal, 1987) It has been suggested that psychological distress may alter an individual's perceptions of a symptom and in turn increase the likelihood of seeking health care. (Barsky, 1986; Bridges & Goldberg, 1985; Katon, Kleinman, & Rosen, 1982a,b)

The second process, symptom appraisal, refers to the meaning a person associates with particular bodily sensations. Mechanic (Mechanic, 1972) theorized that a psychologically distressed person is more likely to attribute such sensations to a disease. It has also been suggested that symptoms are part of an individual's cognitive schema concerning the causes, identity (symptom pattern and diagnostic label), duration and consequences of a bodily sensation such as pain, and that these schemata influence how a persons responds including seeking health services. (Leventhal, 1986)

Finally, the process of situational adaptation indicates that a person seeks health care when he or she is no longer able to suppress, ignore, or otherwise conceal symptoms in a way that allows the person to continue with daily activities and obligations. (Alonzo, 1984, 1985) If pain impairs an individual's adaptive capacity, psychological distress may therefore increase the likelihood that an individual will use health services.

In sum, illness behavior theory asserts that persons who seek health care for a painful symptom should display more distress than those who do not seek health care for such symptoms. Nevertheless, the evidence base supporting this theory in adults is somewhat mixed. Illness behavior theory has primarily been tested in patients with irritable bowel syndrome (IBS). IBS is a syndrome that is characterized by abdominal pain and disrupted defecation. Some of these studies have found greater psychological distress among patients with IBS in comparison to untreated persons with IBS. (Drossman et al., 1988; Whitehead, Bosmajian, Zonderman, Costa, & Schuster, 1988) However, other studies indicate no differences in psychological distress between IBS patients, untreated persons with IBS, and healthy controls. (Welch, Hillman, & Pomare, 1985) Nonetheless, the lack of support for the theory in this latter study should be interpreted with some caution, since somatization (diffuse physical symptoms without medical cause) has been shown to be elevated in IBS patients and nonpatients relative to controls.

A study by Andersson et al. (1999) lent support to illness behavior theory when it found that persons with depression, insomnia, and general nervousness were more likely to use primary health care for pain compared to those that did not endorse these symptoms. In contrast, Von Korff et al. (1991) found that symptoms of depression and anxiety did not increase the likelihood of use of health services, although distressed respondents were more likely to report pain in multiple locations. The divergent findings in these two studies may relate to differences in their measures of psychological distress although both studies used symptom lists to assess psychological distress. In particular, it should be noted that there is substantial empirical support for the psychometric properties of the Symptom Checklist Revised (SCL-90R), the measure used in the Von Korff study. (Derogatis, 1994)

A population-based survey conducted in Belgium (Szpalski, Nordin, Skovron, Melot, & Cukier, 1995) found that health beliefs significantly predicted the likelihood of visiting a health care provider for low-back pain. Persons who believed that low-back pain would be a lifelong problem were more likely to visit a provider. However, this study did not assess psychological distress.

Chronic Pain and the Use of Conventional Health Services and Complementary and Alternative Therapies Among Persons Living with HIV

A limited number of studies have focused on the role of pain in health services utilization among persons living with HIV and AIDS. Based on the studies described above that established the negative impact of pain on HRQOL for persons living with HIV and on the hypothesis that pain may be an important factor in seeking medical care, Dobalian et al. (2004) examined the effect of pain on the use of health services among a nationally representative sample of adults receiving medical care for HIV in the contiguous U.S. This study included 2,267 respondents from the HCSUS, and used Poisson regression to analyze the use of outpatient health services based on respondents' reports of the number of times they visited an outpatient healthcare provider (including an HMO, private physician, community clinic, hospital clinic, other medical clinic, or usual provider) during a six-month period. The conceptual framework for the study was Andersen's Behavioral Model of Health Services Use. Key predisposing characteristics included in the study were gender, race, and ethnicity. Enabling characteristics included income and insurance, and need characteristics included pain, CD4 count, and diagnosis with AIDS (a measure of disease stage).

Pain itself was assessed using the bodily pain subscale of the Short Form-36 Health Survey (SF-36), a widely used and psychometrically validated instrument for measuring the health status of respondents. (Hays & Morales, 2001;

Stewart & Ware, 1992) The pain scale was derived from the following two questions: (1) "During the past four weeks, how much did pain interfere with your normal work (including work outside the house and housework)? Would you say: not at all (1), a little bit (2), moderately (3), quite a bit (4), or extremely (5)?" and 2) "How much bodily pain have you had during the past four weeks? Would you say: none (1), very mild (2), mild (3), moderate (4), severe (5), or very severe (6)?"

The researchers noted that 67% of respondents endorsed experiencing pain during the previous four week period. Self-reported pain was higher among persons with an AIDS diagnosis, women who were exposed to HIV via intravenous (IV) drug use, those without a baccalaureate degree, and the unemployed, but lower among African Americans. The study also found that patients who reported more pain and those developed more pain between the baseline survey and six month follow-up survey used more outpatient health services. In addition, poorer health as assessed by CD4 count (specifically, CD4 counts below 50 cells/mm^3), and less energy (as assessed by the vitality subscale of the SF-36) were also associated with more use of health services.

In addition, Dobalian et al. (2004) also modeled predicted values for the number of annual outpatient visits based on varying levels of pain to demonstrate the size of the effect of pain on outpatient health services use. The authors found that based on their findings, the predicted difference in the number of visits between those without pain and those with the maximum amount of pain at follow-up was approximately 4.1 visits annually. The researchers concluded that pain is an important need characteristic by itself, even when adjusting for objective clinical indicators of health status (i.e. CD4 count and diagnosis with AIDS), and noted that increasing pain over time had a substantial impact on health services utilization even after controlling for health status. Accordingly, the authors suggested that improved pain management for persons with pain and better detection of persons at risk for developing pain might reduce the use of outpatient health services and decrease health-related expenditures.

A few studies have examined the use of CAM among persons living with HIV without examining pain (Josephs, Fleishman, Gaist, & Gebo, 2007; London, Foote-Ardah, Fleishman, & Shapiro, 2003) or examined pain among persons living with HIV without examining use of health services. (Abrams et al., 2007) A more limited number of studies have examined the role of pain in the use of alternative therapies by persons living with HIV and AIDS. However, the generalizability of these studies is limited since they used relatively small convenience samples. For example, Fairfield et al. (Fairfield, Eisenberg, Davis, Libman, & Phillips, 1988) found that pain or neuropathy was the most common reason for visiting a CAM provider among a convenience sample of 180 HIV patients, representing about one-third of respondents. A second study of 256 HIV-positive persons reported that pain was associated with the use of CAM. (Ostrow et al., 1997) In contrast, a third study sampled 70 HIV-positive gay men and found that respondents with little or no pain were more likely to use CAM. (Knippels & Weiss, 2000) The size of the samples in these studies particularly limits the generalizability of the findings with respect to racial and ethnic minority groups.

Tsao et al. (2005a) investigated the relationship of bodily pain to the use of CAM using data from a different wave of the HCUS. In this nationally representative study that included 2,466 adults living with HIV, the researchers also conceptualized pain as a need characteristic using Andersen's Behavioral Model of Health Services Use. This study used the same bodily pain subscale from the SF-36 used in Dobalian et al. (2004) The study used multivariate analyses to examine the association of baseline predisposing, enabling, and need characteristics with the use of CAM about six months later. The researchers included the use of five CAM-specific domains based on groupings outlined by the National Center for Complementary and Alternative Medicine (NCCAM; http://nccam.nih.gov/health/whatiscam/ website viewed 4/9/05) (See also Stoney and Manksy, This Volume). The five domains were: mind-body interventions (i.e., relaxation, spiritual healing, self-help groups, imagery, biofeedback, and hypnosis), biologically-based therapies (i.e., herbal medicine, megavitamin therapy, underground/unlicensed drugs, and lifestyle diets), manipulative/body-based methods (i.e., massage and chiropractic care), alternative medical systems (i.e., homeopathy, acupuncture, and folk remedies), and energy therapies (i.e., energy healing). The study also examined the role that changes in pain had in the use of CAM. The researchers found that pain at baseline predicted subsequent CAM use across four of the five domains, and noted that the lack of an association between pain and the fifth domain, energy healing, may have been due to the small number of patients who used that particular therapy.

In contrast to most prior studies of health services utilization, the Tsao et al. (2005a) study included psychological symptoms (e.g., anxiety, depression) and substance abuse (i.e., drug dependence, heavy alcohol drinker) as additional need characteristics. Anxiety and depressive disorder during the past year were classified based on the short form of the World Health Organization's Composite International Diagnostic Interview (CIDI-SF). Drug dependence was defined by the researchers as use of any of eight classifications of drugs (analgesics, amphetamines, cocaine, hallucinogens, heroin, inhalants, marijuana, sedatives) during the past 12 months, either without a doctor's prescription, in larger amounts than prescribed, or for a longer period than prescribed. The respondent must also have reported using more than intended or having emotional/psychiatric problems related to the use. Heavy alcohol drinkers were classified as persons who drank on at least half of the days in the four weeks prior to the baseline interview and who typically had had three or more drinks on those days. The study found that depression was independently associated with use of CAM, even after controlling for pain. Respondents who screened positive for depression were more likely to report having used at least one CAM therapy and were more likely to use mind-body and biologically-based therapies. In addition, respondents who screened positive for depression were more likely to use a greater number of CAM therapies.

The Tsao et al. (2005a) study demonstrated that pain is an important predictor of use of CAM among persons living with HIV, including both self-care and visits to CAM providers. Furthermore, respondents whose pain declined over the course of the study were less likely to have used biologically-based therapies, specifically underground/unlicensed drugs that have the potential to harm the user (e.g., oral interferon-α, disulfiram, and dinitrochlorobenzene). The authors commented that the study's findings are consistent with the hypothesis that pain that is poorly controlled may lead persons living with HIV to seek out untested drug treatments with the potential for adverse health effects. Accordingly, they suggest that greater efforts at alleviating pain be directed at HIV populations in order to reduce the use of underground or unproven drug therapies.

In sum, there is evidence to suggest that pain predicts use of both conventional health services and CAM, including both self-care and visits to CAM providers, among persons living with HIV. Furthermore, these associations between pain and utilization hold even after controlling for clinical indicators of health status including CD4 count and diagnosis with AIDS. One nationally representative study found that HIV-positive women with a history of IV-drug use may be at heightened risk for pain. (Dobalian et al., 2004) This finding suggests that undertreatment of pain may be of particular concern among persons with a history of substance abuse. (See also Heit and Lipman, This Volume) Nevertheless, additional research is necessary to determine the validity of the self-medication hypothesis, which in this context, proposes that persons in pain may abuse substances in an attempt to mitigate their pain. For example, one study found that symptoms of depression were independently correlated with use of CAM, even after controlling for pain. (Tsao et al., 2005a)

Conclusion

Pain is a common experience for the general adult population, and may be more prevalent among chronically-ill populations such as persons living with HIV. Furthermore, there is ample evidence indicating that pain, particularly chronic pain, has an adverse impact on health-related quality of life (HRQOL) in these populations. HIV-related pain leads to significant psychological distress, worsens HRQOL, and produces considerable functional impairment among persons living with HIV. This chapter has summarized the existing research suggesting that pain may be an important factor in seeking health care among persons living with HIV.

There is a significant need for additional research aimed at improving our understanding of the relationship between pain among persons living with HIV and the use of health services. One significant limitation of the literature on pain and use of health services is the lack of prospective studies. In addition, many studies have failed to include a broad range of factors that may facilitate or impede care-seeking. These factors, including measures of pain-related disability, psychological distress, and substance use, may be of particular importance for persons living with HIV.

To date, healthcare providers have a poor record of recognizing and treating pain caused by a variety of illnesses despite the relatively recent recognition of pain as the "fifth vital sign" and the existence of effective pain therapies for many years. (Marcus, Kerns, Rosenfeld, & Breitbart, 2000) In light of the high prevalence of pain among persons living with HIV and the potentially disabling impact of untreated or undertreated chronic pain, it may be advisable for healthcare providers to assess pain at every visit.

Existing research on the relationship between pain and the use of health services has sought to improve our understanding of the factors associated with pain in the general population as well as persons living with HIV and other sub-populations. Improving our understanding of the risk factors that predict increased use of health services among persons experiencing chronic pain, may allow healthcare providers, policy-makers, patients, and other key stake-holders researchers to develop better systems and processes of care that lead to lower use of health care, lower health care costs, and improved HRQOL for persons experiencing pain.

Future Directions

The current conceptualization of pain is as a multidimensional construct that incorporates social, psychological/behavioral, and physiological aspects. Additional research is needed to better understand how each of these distinct dimensions of pain interacts with other predisposing, enabling, and need characteristics within Andersen's Behavioral Model of Health Services.

In particular, more research is needed that evaluates the relationship between health beliefs about pain, psychological distress, and the use of health services. In light of the strong evidence-base concerning the correlation between chronic pain and psychological factors, future studies on the role of pain in the decision to seek health care should include validated measures of a range of psychological symptoms, including particularly anxiety, depression, and somatization.

There is also a need for research which examines whether alleviating pain symptoms actually leads to reductions in the use of health services. As Kerns et al. (Kerns, Otis, Rosenberg, & Reid, 2003) noted, studies on the efficacy of behavioral rehabilitation programs among persons with chronic pain have demonstrated significant reductions in the use of health services. (Caudill, Schnable, Zuttermeister, Benson, & Friedman, 1991; Simmons, Avant, Demski, & Parisher, 1988) Improved palliative care may lead to decreased health services utilization, reductions in health-related expenditures, and improved HRQOL for persons experiencing pain. Future studies should examine whether effective pain management leads to decreased use of health services and improvements in HRQOL.

A number of studies have identified that pain may be greater among certain vulnerable populations, including women (Blyth et al., 2001; Campo et al., 2002; Chrubasik et al., 1998; Dobalian et al., 2004; Perquin et al., 2000; Verhaak et al., 1998) and persons who abuse substances. (Dobalian et al., 2004; Tsao et al., 2005a) There are many possible causes of these variations in self-reported pain, but undertreatment of pain likely plays an important role for these groups. In turn, undertreatment of pain in these populations may be related to other barriers to accessing health care. In most of the studies summarized in this chapter, these groups did not report higher levels of health services use. There is a need for additional research examining the causes of these disparities. Nevertheless, the causes of many barriers to accessing health care are known. Yet there remains a need for more effective interventions that can decrease this treatment gap and thus improve quality of care for these vulnerable populations.

There are few studies that have examined the prevalence of pain among children living with HIV (Gaughan et al., 2002; Lavy, 2007; Lolekha et al., 2004) and consequently there is a significant need for epidemiologic studies on this vulnerable population. In addition, no studies have examined the role of pain in the use of health services among children living with HIV.

The research linking chronic pain and psychosocial problems with use of health services is somewhat mixed among adults, although the larger population-based studies such as hcsus do provide support for such a link among adults living with hiv. When drawing conclusions from these studies, it is important to recognize that unlike the Von korff et al. (1991) and Chrubasik et al. (chrubasik et al., 1998) studies, the Blyth et al. (2004) and andersson et al. (1999) studies were general studies of the use of health services and were not specifically designed to examine the role of pain. Accordingly, these latter studies should be interpreted with some caution with respect to pain and the use of health services. Thus additional work in this area is also warranted.

Acknowledgments Research by the first and second authors is supported in part by R03 DA017026 (PI: Tsao) awarded by the National Institute on Drug Abuse.

References

Abrams, D. I., Jay, C. A., Shade, S. B., Vizoso, H., Reda, H., Press, S., et al. (2007). Cannabis in painful HIV-associated sensory neuropathy: A randomized placebo-controlled trial. *Neurology, 68*(7), 515–521.

Aires, E. M., & Bammann, R. H. (2005). Pain in hospitalized HIV-positive patients: Clinical and therapeutical issues. *The Brazilian Journal of Infectious Diseases, 9*(3), 201–208.

Alonzo, A. A. (1984). An illness behavior paradigm: A conceptual exploration of a situational-adaptation perspective. *Social and Science Medicine, 19*(5), 499–510.

Alonzo, A. A. (1985). An analytic typology of disclaimers, excuses and justifications surrounding illness: A situational approach to health and illness. *Social and Science Medicine, 21*(2), 153–162.

Andersen, R. M. (1968). *A behavioral model of families' use of health services* (No. Research Series no. 25). Chicago: Center for Administration Studies, University of Chicago.

Andersen, R. M. (1995). Revisiting the behavioral model and access to medical care: Does it matter? *Journal of Health and Social Behavior, 36*(1), 1–10.

Andersson, H. I., Ejlertsson, G., Leden, I., & Schersten, B. (1999). Impact of chronic pain on health care seeking, self care, and medication. Results from a population-based Swedish study. *Journal of Epidemiology and Community Health, 53*(8), 503–509.

Astin, J. A. (1998). Why patients use alternative medicine: Results of a national study. *JAMA, 279,* 1548–1553.

Atkinson, J. H., Jr., Grant, I., Kennedy, C. J., Richman, D. D., Spector, S. A., & McCutchan, J. A. (1988). Prevalence of psychiatric disorders among men infected with human immunodeficiency virus. A controlled study. *Archives of General Psychiatry, 45*(9), 859–864.

Barsky, A. J. (1986). Palliation and symptomatic relief. *Archives of Internal Medicine, 146*(5), 905–909.

Basu, S., Chwastiak, L. A., & Bruce, R. D. (2005). Clinical management of depression and anxiety in HIV-infected adults. *Aids, 19*(18), 2057–2067.

Bausell, R. B., Lee, W., & Berman, B. M. (2001). Demographic and health-related correlates of visits to complementary and alternative medical providers. *Medical Care, 39,* 190–196.

Blair, J. M., Fleming, P. L., & Karon, J. M. (2002). Trends in AIDS incidence and survival among racial/ethnic minority men who have sex with men, United States, 1990–1999. *Journal of Acquired Immune Deficiency Syndromes, 31*(3), 339–347.

Blyth, F. M., March, L. M., Brnabic, A. J., & Cousins, M. J. (2004). Chronic pain and frequent use of health care. *Pain, 111*(1–2), 51–58.

Blyth, F. M., March, L. M., Brnabic, A. J., Jorm, L. R., Williamson, M., & Cousins, M. J. (2001). Chronic pain in Australia: A prevalence study. *Pain, 89*(2–3), 127–134.

Bozzette, S., Berry, S., Duan, N., Frankel, M., Leibowitz, A., Lefkowitz, D., et al. (1998). The care of HIV-infected adults in the United States. HIV Cost and Services Utilization Study Consortium. *The New England Journal of Medicine, 339*(26), 1897–1904.

Brattberg, G., Thorslund, M., & Wikman, A. (1989). The prevalence of pain in a general population. The results of a postal survey in a county of Sweden. *Pain, 37*(2), 215–222.

Breitbart, W., Kaim, M., & Rosenfeld, B. (1999). Clinicans' perceptions of barriers to pain management in AIDS. *Journal of Pain and Symptom Management, 18,* 203–212.

Breitbart, W., & McDonald, M. V. (1996). Pharmacologic pain management in HIV/AIDS. *Journal of International Association of Physicians in AIDS Care, 2*(7), 17–26.

Breitbart, W., McDonald, M. V., Rosenfeld, B., Passik, S. D., Hewitt, D., Thaler, H., et al. (1996). Pain in ambulatory AIDS patients. I: Pain characteristics and medical correlates. *Pain, 68*(2–3), 315–321.

Breitbart, W., Passik, S., McDonald, M., Rosenfeld, B., Smith, M., Kaim, M., et al. (1998). Patient-related barriers to pain management in ambulatory AIDS patients. *Pain, 76,* 9–16.

Breitbart, W., Rosenfeld, B. D., Passik, S. D., McDonald, M. V., Thaler, H., & Portenoy, R. K. (1996). The undertreatment of pain in ambulatory AIDS patients. *Pain, 65*(2–3), 243–249.

Breivik, H., Collett, B., Ventafridda, V., Cohen, R., & Gallacher, D. (2006). Survey of chronic pain in Europe: Prevalence, impact on daily life, and treatment. *European Journal of Pain, 10*(4), 287–333.

Bridges, K. W., & Goldberg, D. P. (1985). Somatic presentation of DSM III psychiatric disorders in primary care. *Journal of Psychosomatic Research, 29*(6), 563–569.

Campo, J. V., Comer, D. M., Jansen-Mcwilliams, L., Gardner, W., & Kelleher, K. J. (2002). Recurrent pain, emotional distress, and health service use in childhood. *Journal of Pediatrics, 141*(1), 76–83.

Campo, J. V., Jansen-McWilliams, L., Comer, D. M., & Kelleher, K. J. (1999). Somatization in pediatric primary care: Association with psychopathology, functional impairment, and use of services. *Journal of American Academy Child and Adolescent Psychiatry, 38*(9), 1093–1101.

Caudill, M., Schnable, R., Zuttermeister, P., Benson, H., & Friedman, R. (1991). Decreased clinic use by chronic pain patients: Response to behavioral medicine intervention. *Clinical Journal of Pain, 7*(4), 305–310.

Centers for Disease Control and Prevention. (2005). *HIV/AIDS Surveillance Report. 16*, 20.

Chrubasik, S., Junck, H., Zappe, H. A., & Stutzke, O. (1998). A survey on pain complaints and health care utilization in a German population sample. *European Journal of Anaesthesiology, 15*(4), 397–408.

Croft, P., Rigby, A. S., Boswell, R., Schollum, J., & Silman, A. (1993). The prevalence of chronic widespread pain in the general population. *Journal of Rheumatology, 20*(4), 710–713.

Cunningham, W. E., Andersen, R. M., Katz, M. H., Stein, M. D., Turner, B. J., Crystal, S., et al. (1999). The impact of competing subsistence needs and barriers on access to medical care for persons with human immunodeficiency virus receiving care in the United States. *Medical Care, 37*(12), 1270–1281.

Cunningham, W. E., Hays, R. D., Duan, N., Andersen, R., Nakazono, T. T., Bozzette, S. A., et al. (2005). The effect of socioeconomic status on the survival of people receiving care for HIV infection in the United States. *Journal of Health Care for the Poor and Underserved, 16*(4), 655–676.

Derogatis, L. R. (1994). *SCL-90-R Symptom Checklist-90-R*. Mineapolis, MN: National Computer Systems, Inc.

Detels, R., Munoz, A., McFarlane, G., Kingsley, L. A., Margolick, J. B., Giorgi, J., et al. (1998). Effectiveness of potent antiretroviral therapy on time to AIDS and death in men with known HIV infection duration. Multicenter AIDS Cohort Study Investigators. *JAMA, 280*(17), 1497–1503.

Dobalian, A., Andersen, R. M., Stein, J. A., Hays, R. D., Cunningham, W. E., & Marcus, M. (2003). The impact of HIV on oral health and subsequent use of dental services. *Journal of Public Health Dentistry, 63*(2), 78–85.

Dobalian, A., Tsao, J. C. I., & Duncan, R. P. (2004). The role of pain in the use of outpatient services among persons with HIV: Results from a nationally representative survey. *Medical Care, 42*, 129–138.

Douaihy, A. B., Stowell, K. R., Kohnen, S., Stoklosa, J. B., & Breitbart, W. S. (2007a). Psychiatric aspects of comorbid HIV/AIDS and pain, Part 1. *AIDS Reader, 17*(6), 310–314.

Douaihy, A. B., Stowell, K. R., Kohnen, S., Stoklosa, J. B., & Breitbart, W. S. (2007b). Psychiatric aspects of comorbid HIV/AIDS and pain, Part 2. *AIDS Reader, 17*(7), 350–352, 357–361.

Drossman, D. A., McKee, D. C., Sandler, R. S., Mitchell, C. M., Cramer, E. M., Lowman, B. C., et al. (1988). Psychosocial factors in the irritable bowel syndrome. A multivariate study of patients and nonpatients with irritable bowel syndrome. *Gastroenterology, 95*(3), 701–708.

Eisenberg, D. M., Davis, R. B., Ettner, S. L., Appel, S., Wilkey, S., Van Rompay, M., et al. (1998). Trends in alternative medicine use in the United States, 1990–1997. *JAMA, 280*, 1569–1575.

Eisenberg, D. M., Kessler, R. C., Foster, C., Norlock, F. E., Calkins, D. R., & Delbanco, T. L. (1993). Unconventional medicine in the United States: Prevalence, costs, and patterns of use. *TheNew England Journal of Medicine, 328*, 246–252.

Emanuel, E. J., & Emmanuel, L. L. (2004). Palliative and end-of-life care. In D. L. Kasper, E. Braunwald, A. S. Fauci, S. L. Hauser, D. L. Longo & J. L. Jameson (Eds.), *Harrison's Principles of Internal Medicine* (16th ed., pp. 53). New York: McGraw-Hill.

Fairfield, K. M., Eisenbeg, D. M., Davis, R. G., Libman, H., & Phillips, R. S. (1988). Patterns of use, expenditures, and perceived efficacy of complementary and alternative therapies in HIV-infected patients. *Archives of Internal Medicine, 158*, 2257–2264.

Fleishman, J. A., Gebo, K. A., Reilly, E. D., Conviser, R., Christopher Mathews, W., Todd Korthuis, P., et al. (2005). Hospital and outpatient health services utilization among HIV-infected adults in care 2000–2002. *Medical Care, 43*(9 Suppl), III40–52.

Foster, P. H. (2007). Use of Stigma, Fear, and Denial in Development of a Framework for Prevention of HIV/AIDS in Rural African American Communities. *Family and Community Health, 30*(4), 318–327.

Frich, L. M., & Borgbjerg, F. M. (2000). Pain and pain treatment in AIDS patients: a Longitudinal study. *Journal of Pain and Symptom Management, 19*(5), 339–347.

Frolund, F., & Frolund, C. (1986). Pain in general practice. Pain as a cause of patient-doctor contact. *Scandinavian Journal of Primary Health Care, 4*(2), 97–100.

Gaughan, D. M., Hughes, M. D., Seage, G. R., 3rd, Selwyn, P. A., Carey, V. J., Gortmaker, S. L., et al. (2002). The prevalence of pain in pediatric human immunodeficiency virus/ acquired immunodeficiency syndrome as reported by participants in the Pediatric Late Outcomes Study (PACTG 219). *Pediatrics, 109*(6), 1144–1152.

Gonzalez-Duarte, A., Cikurel, K., & Simpson, D. M. (2007). Managing HIV Peripheral Neuropathy. *Current HIV/AIDS Reports, 4*(3), 114–118.

Haetzman, M., Elliott, A. M., Smith, B. H., Hannaford, P., & Chambers, W. A. (2003). Chronic pain and the use of conventional and alternative therapy. *Family Practice, 20*(2), 147–154.

Harrison, J. A., Mullen, P. D., & Green, L. W. (1992). A Meta-Analysis of Studies of the Health Belief Model. *Health Education Research, 7*, 107–116.

Hays, R. D., & Morales, L. S. (2001). The RAND-36 measure of health-related quality of life. *Annals of Medicine, 33*(5), 350–357.

Health Resources and Services Administration. (2006). *Ryan White CARE Act Annual Data Summary (for Calendar Year 2004)*. Washington, DC: U.S. Department of Health and Human Services.

Hellinger, F. J., & Fleishman, J. A. (2000). Estimating the national cost of treating people with HIV disease: Patient, payer, and provider data. *Journal of Acquired Immune Deficiency Syndrome, 24*(2), 182–188.

Heslin, K. C., Andersen, R. M., Ettner, S. L., & Cunningham, W. E. (2005). Racial and ethnic disparities in access to physicians with HIV-related expertise. *Journal of Genral Internal Medicine, 20*(3), 283–289.

Hewitt, D. J., McDonald, M., Portenoy, R. K., Rosenfeld, B., Passik, S., & Breitbart, W. (1997). Pain syndromes and etiologies in ambulatory AIDS patients. *Pain, 70*(2–3), 117–123.

Jain, S., Schwarcz, S., Katz, M., Gulati, R., & McFarland, W. (2006). Elevated risk of death for African Americans with AIDS, San Francisco, 1996–2002. *Journal of Health Care for the Poor and Underserved, 17*(3), 493–503.

Josephs, J. S., Fleishman, J. A., Gaist, P., & Gebo, K. A. (2007). Use of complementary and alternative medicines among a multistate, multisite cohort of people living with HIV/ AIDS. *HIV Medicine, 8*(5), 300–305.

Kates, J., Penner, M., Crutsinger-Perry, B., Carbaugh, A. L., & Singleton, N. (2006). *National ADAP Monitoring Project, Annual Report, 2006*. Washington, DC: The National Alliance of State and Territorial AIDS Directors.

Katon, W., Kleinman, A., & Rosen, G. (1982a). Depression and somatization: A review. Part I. *American Journal of Medicine, 72*(1), 127–135.

Katon, W., Kleinman, A., & Rosen, G. (1982b). Depression and somatization: A review. Part II. *American Journal of Medicine, 72*(2), 241–247.

Keefe, R. H. (2003). Containing the cost of care for people living with HIV/AIDS: An examination of the Medicaid managed care approach. *Journal of Health and Social Policy, 17*(3), 41–53.

Kelleher, K. J., Childs, G. E., Wasserman, R. C., McInerny, T. K., Nutting, P. A., & Gardner, W. P. (1997). Insurance status and recognition of psychosocial problems. A report from the Pediatric Research in Office Settings and the Ambulatory Sentinel Practice Networks. *Archives of Pediatrics and Adolescent Medicine, 151*(11), 1109–1115.

Kerns, R. D., Otis, J., Rosenberg, R., & Reid, M. C. (2003). Veterans' reports of pain and associations with ratings of health, health-risk behaviors, affective distress, and use of the healthcare system. *Journal of Rehabilitation Resarch and Development, 40*(5), 371–379.

Kinsler, J. J., Wong, M. D., Sayles, J. N., Davis, C., & Cunningham, W. E. (2007). The Effect of Perceived Stigma from a Health Care Provider on Access to Care Among a Low-Income HIV-Positive Population. *AIDS Patient Care STDS, 21*(8), 584–592.

Knippels, H. M. A., & Weiss, J. J. (2000). Use of alternative medicine in a sample of HIV-positive gay men: An exploratory study of prevalence and user characteristics. *AIDS Care, 12*, 435–446.

Koch, H. (1986). *The management of chronic pain in office-based ambulatory care: National Ambulatory Medical Care Survey. Advance Data for Vital and Health Statistics, no. 123. DHHS publ. no. (PHS) 86–1250.* Hyattsville, MD: Public Health Service.

Kohlmann, T. (1991). Schmerzen in der Lubecker Bevolkerung. Ergebnisse einer bevolker-ungsepidemiologischen studies. *Der Schmerz, 5*, 208–213.

Korten, A. E., Jacomb, P. A., Jiao, Z., Christensen, H., Jorm, A. F., Henderson, A. S., et al. (1998). Predictors of GP service use: A community survey of an elderly Australian sample. *Australian and New Zealand Journal of Public Health, 22*(5), 609–615.

Landon, B. E., Wilson, I. B., Wenger, N. S., Cohn, S. E., Fichtenbaum, C. J., Bozzette, S. A., et al. (2002). Specialty training and specialization among physicians who treat HIV/AIDS in the United States. *Journal of General Internal Medicine, 17*(1), 12–22.

Larue, F., Fontaine, A., & Colleau, S. M. (1997). Underestimation and undertreatment of pain in HIV disease: Multicentre study. *BMJ, 314*(7073), 23–28.

Lavy, V. (2007). Presenting symptoms and signs in children referred for palliative care in Malawi. *Palliative Medicine, 21*(4), 333–339.

Lebovits, A. H., Lefkowitz, M., & McCarthy, D. (1989). The prevalence and mangement of pain in patients with AIDS: A review of 134 cases. *The Clinical Journal of Pain, 5*, 245–248.

Leserman, J., Whetten, K., Lowe, K., Stangl, D., Swartz, M. S., & Thielman, N. M. (2005). How trauma, recent stressful events, and PTSD affect functional health status and health utilization in HIV-infected patients in the south. *Psychosomatic Medicine, 67*(3), 500–507.

Leventhal, H. (1986). Symptom reporting: A focus on process. In S. McHugh & T. M. Vallis (Eds.), *Illness Behavior: A Mulidisciplinary Model.* New York: Plenum Press.

Liebschutz, J. M., Feinman, G., Sullivan, L., Stein, M., & Samet, J. (2000). Physical and sexual abuse in women infected with the human immunodeficiency virus: Increased illness and health care utilization. *Archices of Internal Medicine, 160*(11), 1659–1664.

Lolekha, R., Chanthavanich, P., Limkittikul, K., Luangxay, K., Chotpitayasunodh, T., & Newman, C. J. (2004). Pain: A common symptom in human immunodeficiency virus-infected Thai children. *Acta Paediatrica, 93*(7), 891–898.

London, A. S., Foote-Ardah, C. E., Fleishman, J. A., & Shapiro, M. F. (2003). Use of alternative therapists among people in care for HIV in the United States. *American Journal of Public Health, 93*(6), 980–987.

Lorenz, K. A., Shapiro, M. F., Asch, S. M., Bozzette, S. A., & Hays, R. D. (2001). Associations of symptoms and health-related quality of life: Findings from a national study of persons with HIV infection. *Annals of Internal Medicne, 134*(9 Pt 2), 854–860.

Marcus, K. S., Kerns, R. D., Rosenfeld, B., & Breitbart, W. (2000). HIV/AIDS-related pain as a chronic pain condition: Implications of a biopsychosocial model for comprehensive assessment and effective management. *Pain Medicine, 1*(3), 260–273.

McCallum, J., Simons, L., Simons, J., Wilson, J., Sadler, P., & Owen, A. (1996). Patterns and costs of post-acute care: A longitudinal study of people aged 60 and over in Dubbo. *Australian and New Zealand Journal of Public Health, 20*(1), 19–26.

McCarthy, G. (1992). Host factors associated with HIV-related oral candidiasis. A review. *Oral Surgery, Oral Medicine, and Oral Pathology*, *73*, 181–186.

McCormack, J. P., Li, R., Zarowny, D., & Singer, J. (1993). Inadequate treatment of pain in ambulatory HIV patients. *Clinical Journal of Pain*, *9*(4), 279–283.

McFarland, W., Chen, S., Hsu, L., Schwarcz, S., & Katz, M. (2003). Low socioeconomic status is associated with a higher rate of death in the era of highly active antiretroviral therapy, San Francisco. *Journal of Acquired Immune Deficiency Syndromes*, *33*(1), 96–103.

Mechanic, D. (1972). Social psychologic factors affecting the presentation of bodily complaints. *The New England Journal of Medicine*, *286*(21), 1132–1139.

Merskey, H., Bogduk, N., & editors. (1994). *Classification of chronic pain: Description of chronic pain syndromes and definitions of pain terms*. Seattle: IASP Press.

Morin, S. F., Sengupta, S., Cozen, M., Richards, T. A., Shriver, M. D., Palacio, H., et al. (2002). Responding to racial and ethnic disparities in use of HIV drugs: Analysis of state policies. *Public Health Reports*, *117*(3), 263–272; discussion 231–262.

Ni, H., Simile, C., & Hardy, A. M. (2002). Utilization of complementary and alternative medicine by United States adults: Results from the 1999 national health interview survey. *Medical Care*, *40*, 353–358.

Norval, D. A. (2004). Symptoms and sites of pain experienced by AIDS patients. *S African Medical Journal*, *94*(6), 450–454.

Ostrow, M. J., Cornelisse, P. G., Heath, K. V., Craib, K. J., Schechter, M. T., O'Shaughnessy, M., et al. (1997). Determinants of complementary therapy use in HIV-infected individuals receiving antiretroviral or anti-opportunistic agents. *J Acquir Immune Defic Syndr Hum Retrovirol*, *15*, 115–120.

Palella, F. J., Jr., Delaney, K. M., Moorman, A. C., Loveless, M. O., Fuhrer, J., Satten, G. A., et al. (1998). Declining morbidity and mortality among patients with advanced human immunodeficiency virus infection. HIV Outpatient Study Investigators. *The New England Journal of Medicine*, *338*(13), 853–860.

Parveen, Z., Acheampong, E., Pomerantz, R. J., Jacobson, J. M., Wigdahl, B., & Mukhtar, M. (2007). Effects of highly active antiretroviral therapy on HIV-1-associated oral complications. *Current HIV Research*, *5*(3), 281–292.

Perquin, C. W., Hazebroek-Kampschreur, A. A., Hunfeld, J. A., Bohnen, A. M., van Suijlekom-Smit, L. W., Passchier, J., et al. (2000). Pain in children and adolescents: A common experience. *Pain*, *87*(1), 51–58.

Phillips, K. A., Morrison, K. R., Andersen, R., & Aday, L. A. (1998). Understanding the context of healthcare utilization: Assessing environmental and provider-related variables in the behavioral model of utilization. *Health Service Research*, *33*(3 Pt 1), 571–596.

Potter, R. G., & Jones, J. M. (1992). The evolution of chronic pain among patients with musculoskeletal problems: A pilot study in primary care. *British Journal of Genral Practice*, *42*(364), 462–464.

Prohaska, T. R., Keller, M. L., Leventhal, E. A., & Leventhal, H. (1987). Impact of symptoms and aging attribution on emotions and coping. *Health Psychology*, *6*(6), 495–514.

Pugh, K., Riccio, M., Jadresic, D., Burgess, A. P., Baldeweg, T., Catalan, J., et al. (1994). A longitudinal study of the neuropsychiatric consequences of HIV-1 infection in gay men. II. Psychological and health status at baseline and at 12-month follow-up. *Psychological Medicine*, *24*(4), 897–904.

Ramirez-Amador, V., Ponce-de-Leon, S., Anaya-Saavedra, G., Crabtree Ramirez, B., & Sierra-Madero, J. (2007). Oral lesions as clinical markers of highly active antiretroviral therapy failure: A nested case-control study in Mexico City. *Clinical Infectious Diseases*, *45*(7), 925–932.

Robbins, J. L., Phillips, K. D., Dudgeon, W. D., & Hand, G. A. (2004). Physiological and psychological correlates of sleep in HIV infection. *Clinical Nursing Research*, *13*(1), 33–52.

Rosenblatt, A. B., & Mekhail, N. A. (2005). Management of pain in addicted/illicit and legal substance abusing patients. *Pain Practice*, *5*(1), 2–10.

Rosenfeld, B., Breitbart, W., McDonald, M. V., Passik, S. D., Thaler, H., & Portenoy, R. K. (1996). Pain in ambulatory AIDS patients. II: Impact of pain on psychological functioning and quality of life. *Pain, 68*(2–3), 323–328.

Rosenstock, I. M. (1974). Historical origins of the Health Belief Model. *Health Education Monograph, 2*, 344.

Roth-Isigkeit, A., Thyen, U., Raspe, H. H., Stoven, H., & Schmucker, P. (2004). Reports of pain among German children and adolescents: An epidemiological study. *Acta Paediatrica, 93*(2), 258–263.

Sambamoorthi, U., Walkup, J., Olfson, M., & Crystal, S. (2000). Antidepressant treatment and health services utilization among HIV-infected medicaid patients diagnosed with depression. *Journal of General Internal Medicine, 15*(5), 311–320.

Sayles, J. N., Ryan, G. W., Silver, J. S., Sarkisian, C. A., & Cunningham, W. E. (2007). Experiences of Social Stigma and Implications For Healthcare Among a Diverse Population of HIV Positive Adults. *Journal of Urban Health, 84*(6), 814–818.

Schofferman, J., & Brody, R. (1990). Pain in far advanced AIDS. In R. Chapman & K. Foley (Eds.), *Advances in Pain Research and Therapy* (Vol. 16, pp. 379–386). New York: Raven Press.

Shapiro, M. F., Morton, S. C., McCaffrey, D. F., Senterfitt, J. W., Fleishman, J. A., Perlman, J. F., et al. (1999). Variations in the care of HIV-infected adults in the United States: Results from the HIV Cost and Services Utilization Study. *JAMA, 281*(24), 2305–2315.

Silverman, S. J., Migliorati, C., Lozada-Nur, F., Greenspan, D., & Conant, M. (1986). Oral findings in people with or at high risk for AIDS: A study of 375 homosexual males. *Journal of American Dental Association, 112*(2), 187–192.

Simmonds, M. J., Novy, D., & Sandoval, R. (2005). The differential influence of pain and fatigue on physical performance and health status in ambulatory patients with human immunodeficiency virus. *Clinical Journal of Pain, 21*(3), 200–206.

Simmons, J. W., Avant, W. S., Jr., Demski, J., & Parisher, D. (1988). Determining successful pain clinic treatment through validation of cost effectiveness. *Spine, 13*(3), 342–344.

Singer, E. J., Zorilla, C., Fahy-Chandon, B., Chi, S., Syndulko, K., & Tourtellotte, W. W. (1993). Painful symptoms reported by ambulatory HIV-infected men in a longitudinal study. *Pain, 54*(1), 15–19.

Smedley, B. D., Stith, A. Y., & Nelson, A. R. (Eds.). (2002). *Unequal Treatment: Confronting Racial and Ethnic Disparities in Health Care*. Washington, DC: National Academies Press.

Smith, M. Y., Egert, J., Winkel, G., & Jacobson, J. (2002). The impact of PTSD on pain experience in persons with HIV/AIDS. *Pain, 98*(1–2), 9–17.

Stewart, A. L., & Ware, J. E. (1992). *Measuring functioning and well-being : The medical outcomes study approach*. Durham: Duke University Press.

Szpalski, M., Nordin, M., Skovron, M. L., Melot, C., & Cukier, D. (1995). Health care utilization for low back pain in Belgium. Influence of sociocultural factors and health beliefs. *Spine, 20*(4), 431–442.

Tobias, C. R., Cunningham, W., Cabral, H. D., Cunningham, C. O., Eldred, L., Naar-King, S., et al. (2007). Living with HIV but without medical care: Barriers to engagement. *AIDS Patient Care STDS, 21*(6), 426–434.

Tsao, J. C., Dobalian, A., Myers, C. D., & Zeltzer, L. K. (2005a). Pain and use of complementary and alternative medicine in a national sample of persons living with HIV. *Journal of Pain and Symptom Management, 30*(5), 418–432.

Tsao, J. C., Dobalian, A., & Naliboff, B. D. (2004). Panic disorder and pain in a national sample of persons living with HIV. *Pain, 109*(1–2), 172–180.

Tsao, J. C., Dobalian, A., & Stein, J. A. (2005b). Illness burden mediates the relationship between pain and illicit drug use in persons living with HIV. *Pain, 119*(1–3), 124–132.

Tsao, J. C., Stein, J. A., & Dobalian, A. (2007). Pain, problem drug use history, and aberrant analgesic use behaviors in persons living with HIV. *Pain, 133*(1–3), 128–137.

Turner, B. J., Cunningham, W. E., Duan, N., Andersen, R. M., Shapiro, M. F., Bozzette, S. A., et al. (2000). Delayed medical care after diagnosis in a US national probability sample of persons infected with human immunodeficiency virus. *Archived of Internal Medicine, 160*(17), 2614–2622.

Valdiserri, R. O. (2002). HIV/AIDS stigma: An impediment to public health. *American Journal of Public Health, 92*(3), 341–342.

Verhaak, P. F., Kerssens, J. J., Dekker, J., Sorbi, M. J., & Bensing, J. M. (1998). Prevalence of chronic benign pain disorder among adults: A review of the literature. *Pain, 77*(3), 231–239.

Vitiello, B., Burnam, M. A., Bing, E. G., Beckman, R., & Shapiro, M. F. (2003). Use of psychotropic medications among HIV-infected patients in the United States. *American Journal of Psychiatry, 160*(3), 547–554.

Vogl, D., Rosenfeld, B., Breitbart, W., Thaler, H., Passik, S., McDonald, M., et al. (1999). Symptom prevalence, characteristics, and distress in AIDS outpatients. *Journal of Pain and Symptom Management, 18*(4), 253–262.

Von Korff, M., Dworkin, S. F., Le Resche, L., & Kruger, A. (1988). An epidemiologic comparison of pain complaints. *Pain, 32*(2), 173–183.

Von Korff, M., Wagner, E. H., Dworkin, S. F., & Saunders, K. W. (1991). Chronic pain and use of ambulatory health care. *Psychosomatic Medicine, 53*(1), 61–79.

Vosvick, M., Gore-Felton, C., Ashton, E., Koopman, C., Fluery, T., Israelski, D., et al. (2004). Sleep disturbances among HIV-positive adults: The role of pain, stress, and social support. *Journal of Psychosomatic Research, 57*(5), 459–463.

Weinert, M., Grimes, R., & Lynch, D. (1996). Oral manifestations of HIV infection. *Annals of Internal Medicine, 125*, 485–496.

Welch, G. W., Hillman, L. C., & Pomare, E. W. (1985). Psychoneurotic symptomatology in the irritable bowel syndrome: A study of reporters and non-reporters. *British Medical Journal (Clinical Research Ed), 291*(6506), 1382–1384.

Whitehead, W. E., Bosmajian, L., Zonderman, A. B., Costa, P. T., Jr., & Schuster, M. M. (1988). Symptoms of psychologic distress associated with irritable bowel syndrome. Comparison of community and medical clinic samples. *Gastroenterology, 95*(3), 709–714.

Pain Measurement

Sydney Dy

Introduction

Pain is one of the most common symptoms in clinical medicine. Many types of medications and other interventions to treat pain are supported by strong evidence (Carr et al., 2004) and guideline-based pain treatments can lead to significant reductions in pain severity and pain-related outcomes such as quality of life (Chang, Hwang, & Kasimis 2002). However, the fundamental biobehavioral issues which underlie the development of chronic or intractable pain are not well understood. Pain management is often suboptimal in situations where it is critical, such as in patients with cancer or other advanced disease (Cleeland et al., 1994). Deficits in pain evaluation, management and treatment have been described across clinical settings, including hospitals, outpatient clinics, emergency rooms and nursing homes, and are often more severe in vulnerable populations, such as the elderly, those with dementia, children, and minorities. (Johnson, Teno, Bourbonniere, & Mor, 2005; Mercadante, 2004; Cleeland et al., 1994; Herr, Bjoro, & Decker, 2006; Todd et al., PEMI Study Group, 2007).

In this chapter, we describe methods of pain measurement, including both measurement tools and quality measures. We also discuss methods for improving the management of pain, including population and system-based interventions as well as interventions oriented at health care professionals and at patients. Although pain assessment, measurement and evaluation are central to under-standing the impact of pain in a variety of disease states, in this chapter, we will primarily focus on the assessment and evaluation of pain in the context of palliative care, including management of patients with serious or advanced disease. The chapter also builds on evidence-based systematic reviews and expert panels aiming to standardize and improve the quality of care. We describe tools and interventions aimed at more general populations and for vulnerable popula-tions, where appropriate. Finally, where applicable, we describe differences

S. Dy (✉)
The Johns Hopkins School of Public Health, Room 609, 624 N. Broadway, Baltimore,
MD 21205, USA
e-mail: sdy@jhsph.edu

R.J. Moore (ed.), *Biobehavioral Approaches to Pain*,
DOI 10.1007/978-0-387-78323-9_13, © Springer Science+Business Media, LLC 2009

among populations and how pain management interacts with other physical and psychiatric symptoms and psychosocial issues.

Measuring Pain

Pain can be a difficult symptom to measure. There are many barriers to effective assessment, such as underestimating the impact of pain, fear of consequences of pain management such as addiction, and a lack of knowledge on the part of patients and clinicians. That said, screening to determine who may have pain is a necessary first step both in the effective management and treatment of pain and in the proper conduct of research and quality improvement. (National Comprehensive Cancer Center Network, 2006; Lorenz et al., 2006) Without regular screening, many patients with significant pain do not have pain documented in the medical record and do not receive adequate analgesia. (Rhodes, Koshy, Waterfield, Wu, & Grossman, 2001) Effective measurement begins with patient self-report: without asking the patient, the clinicians' assessments of pain are usually inaccurate. One study found little correlation between physicians' and nurses' assessments of cancer patients' pain and the patients' reports of pain, and correlation was lowest for patients with severe pain. (Grossman, Sheidler, Sweden, Mucenski, & Piantadosi, 1991) Discrepancies between patients and physicians in their perceptions of pain severity are also predictive of inadequate pain management. (Cleeland et al., 1994)

The need for routine assessment of pain is well-accepted and supported by pain clinical practice guidelines. (National Comprehensive Cancer Center Network, 2006) However, quantitative pain measurement alone is insufficient to improve pain outcomes, (Mularski et al., 2006), as more detailed quantitative and qualitative assessment is necessary to determine how best to treat patients. (Lorenz et al., 2006) Assessment may also need to be tailored to the setting, or to the patients' characteristics, including cultural or cognitive factors, which may impact if and how patients report the symptom, the meaning of the pain, and the patient's response. Assessment should also include physical and psychiatric symptoms as well as spiritual, psychosocial, and environmental distress, as these can adversely interact with physical pain or impact the effectiveness of pain treatments. (National Comprehensive Cancer Center Network, 2006)

While the use of standard, well-developed and evaluated assessment tools is key to high-quality pain research and advancing knowledge in the field, they are often not used in clinical care, and are inconsistently used in research. A recent review of tools used in end-of-life interventions found that studies used a wide variety of instruments, with little overlap. (Mularski et al., 2007) In another review of pain measurement methods in clinical trials, 69% of 68 trials used only unidimensional pain rating tools, such as visual analog scales (VAS) which are not adequate for the assessment of pain, rather than questionnaires. While VAS can access the severity of pain at a particular point in time, more detailed questionnaires are also needed to provide an in-depth portrait of the patient's pain experience. This includes the impact of pain on social or physical functioning, psychosocial facets of the pain experience, other distress and related suffering. (Wilson et al., 2007; Graves et al., 2007; Mako, Galek, & Poppito, 2006; Shaiova, 2006).

Assessment Instruments

Pain assessment instruments are tools designed to measure the characteristics of pain in an individual patient. In this section, we describe several systematic reviews that have addressed the variety of tools that have been developed for pain assessment, how they have been used, and recommendations for their use. The focus here is on palliative care and two populations where assessment is often difficult, patients with dementia and children. Recently, a comprehensive, systematic review of instruments potentially applicable to end-of-life care, the Toolkit (Toolkit of Instruments to Measure End-of-Life Care) (Teno 2000) was updated as part of a more recent systematic review of end-of-life care and outcomes. (Mularski et al., 2007) Other recent reviews have addressed the applicability of available pain measurement instruments to palliative care (Hølen et al., 2006) and tools for assessment of pain in nonverbal adults with dementia. (Herr et al., 2006)

Pain assessment tools recommended by the reviews are shown in Table 1. As previously described, although visual analog scales are useful for screening and monitoring the outcomes of pain treatments, they are insufficient for clinical pain assessment or studies requiring information on causality or multidimensionality of pain. Scales that also address other symptoms often closely related to pain, such as fatigue or depression, or that address different measures and qualities of the pain experience are generally preferable for full assessment. However, many of the longer versions may suffer from relatively high rates of incompletion, particularly in ill populations. (Hølen et al., 2006).

The Toolkit (Teno 2000) identified sixty-four pain and physical symptom management instruments that could potentially be useful in end-of-life care; Mularski et al. (2007) identified 10 additional instruments for use in this domain. Hølen et al. (2006) conducted an extensive literature and book search, and described 80 assessment tools including at least one item for pain, forty-eight of which were pain-specific instruments. Thirty-three percent were unidimensional, usually for pain intensity, and an additional 38% addressed only two dimensions. They identified 48 studies of pain assessment in advanced cancer, which included 16 instruments. Sixty-one percent used a visual analog or numerical rating scale, 13% used the Brief Pain Inventory (BPI), and 13% used the McGill Pain Questionnaire (MPQ). Using different pain tools across studies often made comparisons difficult or impossible. (Hølen et al., 2006,Mularski et al., 2007)

Table 1 Recommended pain assessment tools

Tool Pain assessment tools	Description	Recommended by*
Memorial Pain Assessment Card, Visual Analog Scales	Assessment of pain intensity	EAPC, Toolkit
Brief Pain Inventory (BPI)	Measures pain intensity, functionality and impact on life Long and short versions available	EAPC
McGill Pain Questionnaire	Focus on pain quality, especially particular pain syndromes Long and short versions available	EAPC, Toolkit
Wisconsin Brief Pain Questionnaire	Measures pain history, intensity at its worst, usual, and now, relief from medication, and interference.	Toolkit
Multisymptom tools		
ESAS (Edmonton Symptom Assessment System)	Visual analog scales for 9 symptoms	Toolkit
MSAS (Memorial Symptom Assessment Scale)	Prevalence, characteristics, and distress of 32 common symptoms	Toolkit

*EAPC – European Association for Palliative Care Expert Working Group (Caraceni, Brunelli, Martini, Zecca, & De Conno, 2005); Toolkit – Toolkit of Instruments to Measure End-of-Life Care (Teno, 2000)

Extensive descriptions and assessments of these tools are available in these references; most tools are available through the City of Hope Pain & Palliative Care Resource Center Website, www.cityofhope.org/prc.

Since pain tools are often developed for specific syndromes (e.g., low back pain) or populations (chronic pain), they may not adequately assess other types of pain (e.g., neuropathic pain syndromes) or illnesses associated with significant pain (e.g., diabetes, rheumatoid arthritis). Moreover, few have been developed for or tested in palliative care or advanced cancer populations. Hølen et al. (2006) used an expert panel to rate the relative importance of each of 10 dimensions of pain assessment for palliative care. The highest-ranked dimensions, in order of importance, were as follows: intensity, temporal pattern (fluctuation, variations in intensity and occurrence), treatment and exacerbating/relieving factors, location, interference with quality of life, quality, affect (emotional component of pain), duration, beliefs (attitudes and coping strategies), and pain history (including prior pain experiences). They then compared these dimensions to the contents of pain tools. They found that, although the majority of pain tools included in the analysis addressed pain intensity, only 16% addressed the second-most highly-ranked dimension, temporal issues. Another recent review showed that only 2% of cancer pain tools actually addressed this dimension. (Jensen, 2003) Finally, none of the tools which actually addressed all five of the most highly-rated pain dimensions for palliative care were appropriate for palliative care research assessment. (Hølen et al., 2006)

Additional drawbacks of pain assessment instruments include a lack of conceptual research to determine the best timeframe for evaluating pain. (Hølen et al., 2006) Important issues also include how to incorporate different measures, such as worst compared to average pain, and how to incorporate patients' or significant others' goals for pain control. As described by clinical practice guidelines (National Comprehensive Cancer Network, 2006) in clinical care, these instruments are currently best used for initial screening. Clinical assessment of pain requires qualitative assessment of many of the domains described above, which are not adequately addressed by these structured instruments. Since pain is a subjective experience, individual patients experience and rate pain differently, and better tools for adjusting individual ratings are needed before intensity can be used as an comparative measure of pain across individuals or groups. That said, more detailed questionnaires customized to specific illnesses, or changes in pain intensity across time, are currently the best research outcome measures for pain control. (Dionne, Bartoshuk, Mogil, &Witter, 2005)

Assessing Pain in Non-Verbal Populations

Assessing pain in patients with cognitive or communication difficulties can be even more challenging than the assessment of pain in verbal patients. Herr et al. (2006) identified ten behavioral assessment tools for nonverbal dementia patients. These tools are based on indicators of potential pain, including the six types in the American Geriatrics Society (AGS) framework: facial expressions such as grimacing, verbalizations or vocalizations such as moaning, body movements such as rocking, changes in interpersonal interactions such as resisting care, or changes in activity patterns or routines such as refusing food. (AGS Panel on Persistent Pain in Older Persons, 2002) This comprehensive evaluation concluded that all tools were in the early stages of development, and there was no standardized tool to broadly recommend for patient assessment. The only tool with strong evidence for reliability was the Discomfort in Dementia of the Alzheimer's Type scale (DS-DAT), and only two had undergone evaluation in a setting outside the original study. The problems associated with these tools included variability among patients in behaviors potentially related to pain; comprehensiveness in meeting the criteria of the AGS framework; difficulty with demonstrating validity, given the lack of a gold standard; and concerns about the validity of combining ratings of behaviors into a quantitative scale. The review and the AGS guidelines therefore recommend a clinical approach to pain assessment, including observation for potential pain behaviors and a trial of analgesics if pain is suspected, particularly in situations where there are pathological reasons for the patient to have pain. (AGS Panel on Persistent Pain in Older Persons, 2002)

A broader review of instruments for assessment of pain in older persons with cognitive impairment (Stolee et al., 2005) identified 30 instruments, including the behavioral tools described above as well as self-report scales using faces or other graphical representations for pain. This review concluded that none of these instruments had sufficient psychometric testing. Similar issues apply to other types of patients unable to report pain, such as patients in the intensive care unit or with hypoactive delirium at the end of life. (Mularski et al., 2007). None of these reviews identified studies addressing measurement issues in vulnerable populations of underserved ethnic minorities or in those with low health literacy.

Measuring Pain in Children

Some instruments developed for adults may also be appropriate for the measurement of pain in children. For instance, the Memorial Symptom Assessment Scale has undergone validity testing for children between the ages of 7 through 12 years old. (Collins et al., 2002) However, these scales cannot be used for smaller children, except with parental reporting of pain, and developmental factors and differential experience of pain often make specially designed assessment tools preferable (see also Cucchiaro, This Volume). A systematic review of observational (behavioral) measures for children between the ages of 3 and 18 years of age identified 20 behavioral checklists and rating scales. Scales were recommended for acute pain only and for specific settings, and varied in terms of inclusion criteria for physiological or other distress items and reporter status (parent or health care professional for very young children or those with severe cognitive disability, vs the child). Scales judged to have good psychometric properties and clinical applicability included two for procedural pain, two for postoperative pain, one for critical care, and two for pain-related distress. (Baeyer & Spagrud, 2007) A systematic review of single-item self-report intensity measures in children (Stinson, Kavanagh, Yamada, Gill, & Stevens, 2006) identified 34 measures. This review identified six scales, including the Faces Pain Scale-Revised, Wong-Baker FACES Pain Scale, and Oucher numerical rating and VAS scales, with high-quality psychometric evaluation and utility for measuring research outcomes, although there was variation in feasibility and applicability to specific populations. (Stinson et al., 2006).

Other measures include quality of life instruments such as the Child Health and Illness Profile (CHIP), which has undergone reliability and validity testing in child and adolescent editions and has a parental report version as well. (Riley et al., 2004) Finally, a recent systematic review of neonatal pain assessment instruments identified 35 tools, 17 of which were multidimensional. Although no instrument was considered ideal, and many require further psychometric testing, tools are available with a variety of characteristics that may be appropriate for specific populations and research needs. (Duhn & Medves, 2004, See also Cucchiaro, This Volume)

Other Instruments

Other instruments for assessing related constructs may be useful when researching chronic pain. Two recent end-of-life systematic reviews (Teno, 2000) (Mularski et al., 2007) described additional instruments, including questionnaires addressing knowledge about pain (e.g., Patient Pain Questionnaire) and barriers to taking pain medications (Barriers Questionnaire, BQ-II). In chronic pain populations, opioid misuse may be a concern, and instruments such as the Pain Medication Questionnaire can help to assess risk. (Holmes et al., 2006) Many other types of instruments also include measures for the assessment of pain, including many quality of life and needs assessment instruments. Other domains to assess may include those related to pain, such as psychological symptoms or spiritual well-being (including existential issues associated with the experience, management and treatment of pain), particularly since pain is often multidimensional and may not be limited to physical issues, or those that may be affected by pain, such as functional status. (Mularski et al., 2007)

Quality Measures

A quality or performance measure is a descriptive statement related to the quality of medical care and expressed as a measurable standard of care. Two recent reviews have summarized in detail pain quality measures available in measurement sets or used in quality improvement projects for end-of-life care and cancer. (Dy & Lynn 2006, Lorenz et al., 2006) Pain quality measures are critical for overall good-quality medical practice, and have been included in large general measurement sets, such as the RAND Quality Assessment (QA) tools and Assessing Care of Vulnerable Elders (ACOVE). (Dy & Lynn 2006, Lorenz 2006) Categories of quality measures, and some examples, are shown in Table 2. For assessment, these include screening and regular and appropriate measurement; for treatment, addressing high pain scores and appropriate changes in treatment; and for follow-up, whether pain was controlled and satisfaction. (Dy & Lynn 2006, Lorenz 2006)

The quality measures developed to date target only a few areas in the spectrum of quality pain management, have generally not been rigorously developed or evaluated, and are not in wide or regular use. For example, there are no evidence-based best standards for the use of these measures in many settings where pain is common, such as hospitals or outpatient cancer care. Indeed, the measures are often so specific that they cannot be applied

Table 2 Potential pain quality measures (Lorenz et al., 2006, Dy & Lynn, 2006)

Domain Domain	Example	Measurement sets*
Screening	All cancer patients should be screened for pain on every outpatient visit	QA Tools, UHC
Assessment	All hospitalized patients should be assessed using a numeric pain scale within 48 hours	UHC, VHA, ACOVE
Treatment	All cancer patients with uncontrolled pain should be offered a change in treatment within 24 hours	QA tools, Cancer Care Ontario
Management of pain side effects	All patients prescribed opioids should also be prescribed a bowel regimen if not contraindicated	UHC
Outcome	Proportion of patients whose pain was brought down to a comfortable level within 48 hours	NHPCO, VHA
Satisfaction	Patients who responded "yes, completely" when asked if everything was done to control their pain	Cancer Care Ontario

*QA Tools: Quality Assessment Tools; UHC: University Health Consortium; VHA: VHA, Inc; NHPCO: National Hospice and Palliative Care Organization; ACOVE: Assessing Care of Vulnerable Elders

across clinical settings to evaluate a patients' overall pain care, and they fail to adequately address continuity across sites of care. These quality measures also do not generally address the interaction between symptoms, such as the need for assessment of anxiety or depression in patients newly reporting pain symptoms. Additional validity and reliability testing is also needed, as the few measures that are currently being used, such as the Minimum Data Set (MDS, for nursing homes) and National Hospice and Palliative Care Organization (NHPCO) measures, have undergone little rigorous evaluation. (Lorenz et al., 2006) These measures are also often not used as part of quality improvement projects, which complicates the ability to compare results across studies or follow whether improvements in the assessment of pain are actually sustained over time.

Other studies have identified problematic exclusions from pain quality measures. Pain quality measures generally do not address specific treatments or pain syndromes and do not address followup. They also generally exclude those who cannot report their pain, which is problematic in vulnerable populations with a high percentage of nonverbal patients, such as the seriously or terminally ill or nursing home populations. In addition, patients with some degree of cognitive impairment or sedation may also be excluded from pain measures, even though many of these patients are actually able to report their pain. (Ferrell, Ferrell, & Rivera, 1995) Variable exclusion of these patients limits the utility of pain assessment measures for comparisons across populations, between facilities, or over time. There has also been limited measure development in children, although some guidelines are available, such as a position paper on end-of-life pain management for the child with cancer. (Hooke,

Hellsten, Stutzer, & Forte, 2002; See also Cucchiaro, This Volume) Other studies indicate that the measurement of pain outcomes is even more important in vulnerable populations, since cognitively impaired adults receive less pain medication than those who are cognitively intact. Untreated pain may also lead to higher rates of adverse outcomes, such as delirium. (Morrison et al., 2003) The use of surrogates for pain measurement, retrospective pain measurement by patients or family members, and accounting for missing data or different methods of assessment are all important issues in vulnerable populations where pain assessment may be challenging, may vary across patients, or may not be possible for everyone.

Improving Pain Management

Quality Improvement

Quality improvement involves the development and use of interventions to improve the management of pain by addressing barriers to effective care at the health care professional (such as knowledge deficits), individual patient (such as inadequate assessment), or health system level (such as changing or measuring processes of care). Several multicenter pain quality improvement projects based on the use of performance measures have shown significant effects on outcomes. The Veterans Health Administration – Institute for Healthcare Improvement (VHA-IHI) initiative used the IHI rapid change "Breakthrough Series Model". (Cleeland et al., 2003) Seventy-three teams addressed pain management in settings including ambulatory care, rehabilitation, oncology, and long-term care. Measures included screening (pain as the 5th vital sign), care plans for patients with moderate to severe pain, and the provision of educational materials. Improvements were noted in all measures, and the percentage of patients with moderate or severe pain on intervention units decreased from 24% to 17%. In another study, a collaborative with a state Quality Improvement Organization achieved improvements in several pain management process and outcome measures in 21 nursing homes in the US, (Baier et al., 2004) although the project was limited by structural factors, including staff turnover.

A review of comprehensive interventions targeting processes of care within institutions found four interventions that improved processes of pain management; only one evaluated outcomes, and did not show a significant impact. (Allard, Maunsell, Labbe, & Dorval, 2001) A rapid-cycle quality improvement intervention in two surgical intensive care units, targeting pain assessment and treatment and incorporating staff education, improved pain assessment (proportion of nursing of intervals where VAS was used increased from 42 to 94%), treatment, and outcome (percentage of 4-hour intervals with pain >3 decreased from 41 to 6%), without an increase in adverse events (as measured by naloxone administration). (Erdek & Pronovost, 2004) A multimodal pain intervention study, including standardized assessment, education, feedback of pain scores, and decision support, resulted in increased pain assessment and use of opioids, but had no significant effect on pain outcomes. (Morrison et al., 2006) In summary, although pain quality improvement interventions can successfully improve processes of care for pain management, such as increased measurement, the results on patient pain outcomes are more mixed, and more research is needed to better assess and effect systems change.

Interventions Targeting Health Care Professionals

Interventions targeting health care professionals include educational interventions to improve knowledge and attitudes and the implementation of protocols or standard care processes to more closely align clinical care with recommendations from clinical practice guidelines and evidence. Two systematic reviews addressed educational interventions, one on improving knowledge about pain control (Allard et al., 2001) and one on improving knowledge about palliative care and cancer pain (Alvarez & Agra, 2006). Studies used a variety of different educational experiences, including didactics, case discussion, distribution of guidelines, clinical experience, and an internet–based study. The systematic review of educational interventions to improve pain control (Allard et al., 2001) found that the 25 interventions they identified (only 4 of which were RCTs) generally had a significant impact on health care professionals' knowledge, attitudes, and satisfaction, but the evidence for impact on patient outcomes was limited. Seven studies of role model training helped health care professionals become active in cancer pain improvement projects, but the only study that evaluated the impact on patients' pain showed no effect. Five studies for nurses all showed improvement in this group's knowledge and attitudes. (Allard et al., 2001)

In a recent review of educational interventions for cancer pain or palliative care for primary care physicians (which included 5 of the studies described in the above review), (Alvarez & Agra, 2006) fourteen of the 17 studies evaluating palliative care or cancer pain knowledge showed an improvement in this outcome. However, the impact of this intervention on pain assessment and opioid prescribing was mixed in the two studies evaluating these outcomes, and of two studies evaluating pain management as an outcome, neither showed an improvement with the intervention. Six studies described in the above review (Allard et al., 2001) investigated interventions which provided pain assessment and management tools, with mixed results. Two RCTs evaluated the use of cancer pain protocols or guideline implementation. A multicenter RCT of an analgesic protocol for patients with moderate to severe cancer pain showed a significant increase in responders (48% had no or mild pain compared to 15% with usual care, $p = 0.008$). (Cleeland et al., 2005) Another RCT investigating the use of a pain algorithm showed a significantly greater reduction in pain in the intervention as compared to the control group (p<0.02). (Du Pen et al., 1999)

The internet and computerized order entry systems have greatly increased the possibilities for implementing protocols, educational interventions and practice guidelines for pain assessment and management. Indeed, more recent interventions are increasingly using web-based educational materials. One study whose aim was to evaluate teaching of clinical diagnosis skills related to pain found similar examination performance with a web-based compared to a standardized patient educational program. (Turner, Simon, Facemyer, Newhall, & Veach, 2006) Other resources are also now available on the web, such as opioid conversion programs to help with equivalency tables (e.g., Hopkins Opioid Program, www.hopweb.org). Decision support tools that are web-based can also assist in the implementation of evidence-based practice guidelines. Several of these tools have undergone preliminary testing, although more development is needed. (Huang et al., 2003; Im & Chee, 2006) A study of medication prescribing errors in hospitals (Bobb et al., 2004) found that pain medications had the highest percentage of errors that could potentially be prevented with computerized order entry, although no studies have yet addressed whether computerized entry actually does reduce these errors. Electronic toolkits and pain websites may also aid in the dissemination of successful interventions and tools to facilitate quality improvement and educational interventions.

Assessment, Educational, and Psychosocial Interventions Targeting Patients

There is clinical and research evidence to support the use of multidisciplinary interventions to improve pain management in patients. These include interventions to improve assessment, educational interventions about pain to improve patients' adherence to pain regimens, and interventions to address the psychosocial aspects of pain and its management. Two systematic reviews have summarized the evidence on cancer pain interventions including education and/or supportive care directed at psychosocial issues. Allard et al. (2001) included 8 studies of cancer pain educational interventions for patients and caregivers; two were RCTs. These interventions varied from a 15-minute nurse counseling intervention to multivisit and multimodal interventions, which often included educational materials. All six studies evaluating cancer pain knowledge or attitudes noted statistically significant improvement, and three of the four studies included in this analysis of pain outcomes also showed significant improvement. Devine (2003) included 25 controlled studies in meta-analyses of psycho-educational interventions for cancer pain, including interventions such as education, supportive counseling, and cognitive-behavioral therapy, alone or in combination. Overall, the d + (average, unbiased, weighted effect size) was 0.41 (95% CI, 0.29, 0.52) (a d + of 0 is no effect), with similar results when limiting to the 9 highest-quality randomized trials.

Evidence-based guidelines also support other types of interventions for the management of pain. These include complementary and alternative medical approaches such as relaxation and meditation, as well as other cognitive-behavioral interventions and supportive counseling. Another type of intervention which demonstrates potential is narration in the form of expressive writing. A study of breast cancer patients completing treatment randomized patients to expressive writing interventions oriented towards emotional expression or benefit-finding. Patients randomized to expressive writing had fewer physical symptoms at follow-up than those randomized to a fact-writing arm. (Creswell et al., 2007)

Other recent pain interventions for patients have also been translated into e-health methods, particularly electronic versions of the pain diary, a critical component for the careful monitoring of pain. These diaries have been evaluated in various cancer and noncancer populations, including RCTs in children and patients unfamiliar with the use of computers, and have frequently improved compliance and satisfaction, with increased accuracy in some studies. (Palermo, Valenzuela, & Stork, 2004; Gaertner, Elsner, Pollmann-Dahman, Radbruch, & Sabatowski, 2004) Electronic versions have the additional advantage of streamlining data collection, as well as the possibility of real-time monitoring of patients and the response by clinical staff. E-health interventions also afford the assessment of different elements of pain from narrative speech through natural-language processing. (Levin & Levin, 2006) Finally, there are additional e-health interventions undergoing evaluation, including web-based pain educational programs and electronic coaching tools to help patients evaluate their pain management, improve communication skills, to improve their interactions with their physicians and the clinical tream. (www.ehealthinnovation.org)

Conclusion

Appropriate pain assessment and measurement is a necessary prerequisite for adequate pain management and control. Screening is a prerequisite to good clinical pain management and treatment, and standard screening tools are available. Measurement tools useful in clinical practice and research, and applicable to different illnesses and settings, are necessary for adequate identification of pain, assessment of pain characteristics and etiology, and monitoring the effectiveness of interventions. Although a number of tools are available, testing is generally limited and there is little standardization across studies. More development is particularly needed for vulnerable populations, including those patients who are unable to verbally report their pain. Future research which takes a multidisciplinary approach to measure both the physiologic as well as the behavioral manifestations of pain is also needed to further enhance the adequate assessment, measurement and treatment of pain in clinically diverse pain patients.

Quality measures are an important method for monitoring and improving processes of care for pain; although some are currently available, none are in wide use, and further development is ongoing. Finally, there is evidence that population-based pain outcomes can be improved by health care quality improvement interventions. These include interventions targeting patients, including education, assessment methods, and psychosocial interventions; and interventions which target health care professionals, including education and implementation of guidelines through protocols or decision support. E-health as a specific intervention also shows promise for improving the measurement and management of pain through interventions such as web-based education, natural language processing of patients' pain narratives, and decision support.

References

AGS Panel on Persistent Pain in Older Persons. (2002). The management of persistent pain in older persons. *Journal of the American Geriatrics Society*, *50*, S205–S224.

Allard, P., Maunsell, E., Labbe, J., & Dorval, M. (2001). Educational interventions to improve cancer pain control: a systematic review. *Journal of Palliative Medicine*, *4*, 191–203.

Alvarez, M.P., & Agra, Y. (2006) Systematic review of educational interventions in palliative care for primary care physicians. *Palliative Medicine*, *20*, 673–683.

Baeyer, C.L., & Spagrud, L.J. (2007) Systematic review of observational (behavioral) measures of pain for children and adolescents aged 3 to 18 years. *Pain*, *127*, 140–150.

Baier R.R., Gifford D.R., Patry G., Banks S.M., Rochon T., DeSilva D., et al. (2004). Ameliorating pain in nursing homes: a collaborative quality-improvement project. *Journal of the American Geriatrics Society*, *52*, 1988–95.

Bobb, A., Gleason, K., Husch, M., Feinglass, J., Yarnold, P.R., et al. (2004). The epidemiology of prescribing errors: the potential impact of computerized prescriber order entry. *Archives of Internal Medicine*, *164*, 785–92.

Caraceni, A., Brunelli, C., Martini, C., Zecca, E., & De Conno, F. (2005). Cancer pain assessment in clinical trials. A review of the literature (1999–2002). *Journal of Pain and Symptom Management*, *29*, 507–19.

Carr, D.B., Goudas, L.C., Balk, E.M., Bloch, R., Ioannidis, J.P., & Lau, J. (2004). Evidence report on the treatment of pain in cancer patients. *Journal of the National Cancer Institute Monographs*, *32*, 23–31.

Chang, V.T., Hwang S.S., & Kasimis B. (2002). Longitudinal documentation of cancer pain management outcomes: A pilot study at a VA medical center. *Journal of Pain and Symptom Management*, *24*, 494–505.

Cleeland, C.S., Gonin, R., Hatfield, A.K., Edmonson, J.H., Blum, R.H., Stewart, J.A., et al. (1994). Pain and its treatment in outpatients with metastatic cancer. *New England Journal of Medicine*, *330*, 592–596.

Cleeland, C.S., Portenoy, R.K., Rue, M., Mendoza, T.R., Weller, E., Payne, R., et al. (2005). Does an oral analgesic protocol improve pain control for patients with cancer? An intergroup study coordinated by the Eastern Cooperative Oncology Group. *Annals of Oncology*, *16*, 972–80.

Cleeland, C.S., Reyes-Gibby, C.C., Schall, M., Nolan, K., Paice, J., Rosenberg, J.M, et al. (2003). Rapid improvement in pain management: the Veterans Health Administration and the Institute for Healthcare Improvement collaborative. *Clinical Journal of Pain*, *19*, 298–305.

Collins, J.J., Devine, T.D., Dick, G.S., Johnson, E.A., Kilham, H.A., Pinkerton, C.R., et al. (2002). The measurement of symptoms in young children with cancer: the validation of the Memorial Symptom Assessment Scale in children aged 7–12. *Journal of Pain and Symptom Management*, 23, 10–6.

Creswell, J.D., Lam, S., Stanton, A.L., Taylor, S.E., Bower, J.E., & Sherman, D.K. (2007). Does self-affirmation, cognitive processing, or discovery of meaning explain cancer-related health benefits of expressive writing? *Personality and Social Psychology Bulletin*, 33, 238–250.

Duhn, L.J., & Medves, J.M. (2004). A systematic integrative review of infant pain assessment tools. *Advances in Neonatal Care*, 4, 126–40.

Devine, E.C. (2003). Meta-analysis of the effect of psychoeducational interventions on pain in adults with cancer. *Oncology Nursing Forum*, 30, 75–89.

Dionne, R.A., Bartoshuk, L., Mogil, J., & Witter, J. (2005). Individual responder analyses for pain: does one pain scale fit all? *TRENDS in Pharmacological Sciences*, 26, 125–130.

Du Pen, S.L., Du Pen, A.R., Polissar, N., Hansberry, J., Kraybill, B.M., Stillman, M., et al. (1999). Implementing guidelines for cancer pain management: results of a randomized controlled clinical trial. *Journal of Clinical Oncology*, 17, 361–70.

Dy, S.M., & Lynn, J. (2006). Palliative/ end-of-life performance measures, Appendix J. In Committee on Redesigning Health Insurance Performance Measures, Payment, and Performance Improvement Programs, Board on Health Care Services, Institute of Medicine, *Performance Measurement: Accelerating Improvement*. Washington, D.C.: National Academies Press.

Erdek M., Pronovost P. (2004). Improving assessment and treatment of pain in the critically ill. *International Journal of Quality in Health Care*, 16, 59–64.

Ferrell, B.A., Ferrell, B.R., & Rivera, L. (1995). Pain in cognitively impaired nursing home patients. *Journal of Pain and Symptom Management*, 10, 591–598.

Gaertner, J., Elsner, F., Pollmann-Dahmen, K., Radbruch, L., & Sabatowski, R. (2004). Electronic pain diary: a randomized crossover study. *Journal of Pain and Symptom Management*, 28, 259–67.

Graves, K.D., Arnold, S.M., Love, C.L., Kirsh, K.L., Moore, P.G., & Passik, S.D. (2007). Distress screening in a multidisciplinary lung cancer clinic: prevalence and predictors of clinically significant distress. *Lung Cancer 55*, 215–24.

Grossman, S.A., Sheidler, V.R., Swedeen, K., Mucenski, J., & Piantadosi, S. (1991). Correlation of patient and caregiver ratings of cancer pain. *Journal of Pain and Symptom Management*, 6, 53–57.

Herr, K., Bjoro, K., & Decker, S. (2006). Tools for assessment of pain in nonverbal older adults with dementia: A state-of-the-science review. *Journal of Pain and Symptom Management*, 31, 170–192.

Hølen, J.C., Hjermstad, M.J., Loge, J.H., Fayers, P.M., Caraceni, A., De Conno, F., et al. (2006). Pain assessment tools: Is the content appropriate for use in palliative care? *Journal of Pain and Symptom Management*, 32, 567–580.

Holmes, C.P., Gatchel, R.J., Adams, L.L., Stowell, A.W., Hatten, A., Noe, C., et al. (2006). An opioid screening instrument: Long-term evaluation of the utility of the pain medication questionnaire. *Pain Practice*, 6, 74–88.

Hooke, C., Hellsten, M.B., Stutzer, C., & Forte, K. (2002). Pain management for the child with cancer in end-of-life care: APON position paper. *Journal of Pediatric Oncology Nursing*, 19, 43–7.

Huang, H.Y., Wilkie, D.J., Zong, S.P., Berry, D., Hairabedian, D., Judge, M.K., et al. (2003). Developing a computerized data collection and decision support system for cancer pain management. *Computers, Informatics, Nursing*, 21, 206–17.

Im, E.O., & Chee, W. (2006). Evaluation of the decision support computer program for cancer pain management. *Oncology Nursing Forum*, 33, 977–82.

Jensen, M.P. (2003). The validity and reliability of pain measures in adults with cancer. *Journal of Pain*, 4, 2–21.

Johnson, V.M., Teno, J.M., Bourbonniere, M., & Mor, V. (2005). Palliative care needs of cancer patients in U.S. nursing homes. *Journal of Palliative Medicine, 8*, 273–9.

Levin, E., & Levin, A. (2006). Evaluation of spoken dialogue technology for real-time health data collection. *Journal of Medical Internet Research, 8*, e30.

Lorenz, K.A., Lynn, J., Dy, S., Wilkinson, A., Mularski, R.A., Shugarman, L.R., et al. (2006). Quality measures for symptoms and advance care planning in cancer: a systematic review. *Journal of Clinical Oncology, 24*, 4933–8.

Mako, C., Galek, K., Poppito, S.R. (2006). Spiritual pain among patients with advanced cancer in palliative care. *Journal of Palliative Medicine, 9*, 1106–13.

Mercadante, S. (2004). Cancer pain management in children. *Palliative Medicine, 18*, 654–62.

Morrison, R.S., Magaziner, J., Gilbert, M., Koval, K.J., McLaughlin, M.A., Orosz, G., et al. (2003). Relationship between pain and opioid analgesics on the development of delirium following hip fracture. *Journal of Gerontology Series A: Biological Sciences and Medical Sciences, 58*, 76–81.

Morrison, R.S., Meier, D.E., Fischberg, D., Moore, C., Degenholtz H., Litke A., et al. (2006). Improving the management of pain in hospitalized adults. *Archives of Internal Medicine, 2006*, 1033–9.

Mularski, R.A., Dy, S.M., Shugarman, L.R., Wilkinson, A.M., Lynn, J., Shekelle, P.G., et al. (2007). for the Southern California Evidence-Based Practice Center, RAND Health. A systematic review of measures of end-of-life care and its outcomes. *In press, Health Services Research, 42*, 1848–70.

Mularski, R.A., White-Chu, F., Overbay, D., Miller, L., Asch. S.M., & Ganzini, L. (2006). Measuring pain as the 5th vital sign does not improve quality of pain management. *Journal of General Internal Medicine, 21*, 607–12.

National Comprehensive Cancer Network. (2006). Adult Cancer Pain. http://www.nccn.org/professionals/physician_gls/PDF/pain.pdf

Palermo, T.M., Valenzuela, D., & Stork, P.P. (2004). A randomized trial of electronic versus paper pain diaries in children: Impact on compliance, accuracy, and acceptability. *Pain, 107*, 348–56.

Riley, A.W., Forrest, C.B., Rebok, G.W., Starfield, B., Green, B.F., Robertson, J.A., et al. (2004). The Child Report Form of the CHIP-Child Edition: reliability and validity. *Medical Care, 42*, 221–31.

Rhodes, D.J., Koshy, R.C., Waterfield, W.C., Wu, A.W., & Grossman S.A. (2001). Feasibility of quantitative pain assessment in outpatient oncology practice. *Journal of Clinical Oncology, 19*, 501–508.

Shaiova, L. (2006). Difficult pain syndromes: Bone pain, visceral pain, and neuropathic pain. *Cancer Journal, 12*, 330–40.

Stinson, J.N., Kavanagh, T., Yamada, J., Gill, N., & Stevens, B. (2006). Systematic review of the psychometric properties, interpretability and feasibility of self-report pain intensity measures for use in clinical trials in children and adolescents. *Pain, 125*, 143–157.

Stolee, P., Hillier, L.M., Esbaugh, J., Bol, N., McKellar, L., & Gauthier, N. (2005). Instruments for the assessment of pain in older persons with cognitive impairment. *Journal of the American Geriatrics Society, 53*, 319–26.

Teno, J. (2000). Center for Gerontology and Health Care Research, Brown Medical School. Time: Toolkit of Instruments to Measure End-of-life Care. http://www.chcr.brown.edu/pcoc/toolkit.htm.

Todd, K.H., Ducharme, J., Choiniere, M., Crandall, C.S., Fosnocht, D.E, Homel, P., et al. (2007). PEMI Study Group. Pain in the emergency department: Results of the Pain and Emergency Medicine Initiative (PEMI) Multicenter Study. *In press, Journal of Pain, 8*, 460–6.

Turner, M.K., Simon, S.R., Facemyer, K.C., Newhall, L.M., & Veach, T.L. (2006). Web-based learning versus standardized patients for teaching clinical diagnosis: a randomized, controlled, crossover trial. *Teaching and Learning in Medicine, 18*, 208–14.

Wilson, K.G., Chochinov, H.M., McPherson, C.J., LeMay, K., Allard, P., Chary, S., et al. (2007). Suffering with advanced cancer. *Journal of Clinical Oncology, 25*, 1691–7.

Phantom Pain

Jan H.B. Geertzen and Pieter U. Dijkstra

Introduction

Amputation of a limb may be required in the case of critical ischemia, a life-threatening condition of a limb (cancer or diabetes), severe tissue damage due to a trauma, or severe untreatable longstanding infection. Although amputation may be beneficial from a medical point of view, the loss of a limb can have a considerable psychological affect on the patient (e.g. grieving, stress, coping problems) (Geertzen & Rietman, 2008). The process of grief post-amputation is similar to the grieving process after the loss of a spouse, or significant other. Emotions such as shock, fear, depression, denial, guilt, shame and anger may also develop after the amputation (Geertzen & Rietman, 2008). Amputees may also go through a coping process where denial can modulate this process. An amputation may have also an adverse impact on the patient's health related quality of life (Schans van der, Geertzen, Schoppen & Dijkstra, 2002). Other negative sequelae include limitations in walking ability,or walking distance Activities of Daily Living (ADL) problems (e.g., clothing, bathing, house keeping, etc.,), loss of employment, and pain (Geertzen, Bosmans, Schans van der & Dijkstra, 2005).

Phantom Pain, a neuropathic pain syndrome, resulting from functional changes in the peripheral and central pain pathways is challenging to treat. Pain and other sensations felt in the amputated (or absent) limb, so called "phantom pain" and "phantom sensations," are also a frequently described phenomena (Flor, Nikolajsen, & Jensen, 2006). Other recurrent post-amputation pain complaints arise from the stump itself in the form of stump pain (residual limb pain) (Jensen, Krebs, Nielsen & Rasmussen, 1983). Phantom pain must be clinically differentiated from non-painful phantom phenomenon,

J.H.B. Geertzen (✉)
Center for Rehabilitation, Northern Center for Health Care Research, University Medical Center Groningen, University of Groningen, PO Box 30.001, 9700 RB Groningen, The Netherlands
e-mail: j.h.b.geertzen@rev.umcg.nl

R.J. Moore (ed.), *Biobehavioral Approaches to Pain*,
DOI 10.1007/978-0-387-78323-9_14, © Springer Science+Business Media, LLC 2009

residual limb pain, as well as, non-painful residual limb pain (Schmidt, Taka-hashi, & Posso, 2005).

One of the first authors to describe sensations in the absent limb was van de Meij (1995). However, the term "phantom" was actually used for the first time by Silas Weir Mitchell (1871). In this seminal paper "*Phantom limbs,*" Mitchell described the experiences of war victims of the American Civil War. He discussed these symptoms as sensory hallucinations and related them to an inferior intellect. Mitchell also accurately described symptoms such as chorea of the phantom, the strange position of the phantom, its relation to cold, heat and other provoking factors. He wrote:

> "The limb is rarely felt as a whole; nearly always the foot or the hand is the part more distinctly recognized, and, on careful questioning, we learn that the fingers and toes are readily perceived; next to these the thumb; then more rarely the ankle or wrist; and, still less frequently, the elbow and knee." (Mitchell, 1871).

Since these early papers, there has been significant research on the phenomenon of phantom pain and phantom sensations. Yet, despite the various explanations that have been proposed, the underlying mechanisms and the etiology of phantom pain are still not completely understood (Hanley, Jensen, Smith, Ehde, Edwards & Robinson, 2006b; Nikolajsen, Ilkjaer, Kroner, Christensen & Jensen, 1997; Flor et al., 2006).

In this chapter, we take a biopsychosocial approach to understanding phantom limb pain since biological, neurological, psychosocial and environmental factors *all* play a significant role in the experience of phantom limb pain and phantom limb sensations. First, we define and describe phantom limb pain and phantom sensations: Phantom limb pain is defined as any phantom sensation so intense that it is experienced as painful. Stump pain is defined as any painful sensation localized in the stump post-amputation (Merskey & Bogduk, 1994). Indeed, after an amputation, the amputee may continue to have an awareness of the limb and to experience sensations from it. Phantom sensations are defined as all non-painful sensations in the amputated part of the extremity. While phantom pain has also been described in a variety of other clinical conditions including: breast amputation, tooth extraction, tongue amputation, penis amputation, amputation of the ear or nose, and after resection of an organ (e.g. rectum, uterus, bladder, stomach); in this chapter, we will primarily focus on phantom limb pain and phantom sensations in upper and lower extremity amputees (Dijkstra, Rietman & Geertzen, 2007; Sherman, Devor, Jones, Katz & Marbach, 1997). Then, we evaluate the epidemiology and risk factors associated with the development of chronic phantom limb pain and phantom sensations. In the next section, we proceed to discuss the etiology and the theories which have generally been used to try and explain the causes of chronic phantom limb pain. Then, we describe a variety of evidence-based treatments (psychologic, surgical, pharmacologic and supportive) that have been used in the attempt to manage and treat chronic phantom limb pain.

Describing Phantom Limb Pain and Phantom Sensations

One of the most striking features of phantoms is their reality and their vividness to the amputee, particularly directly after post-amputation (Jensen, Krebs, Nielsen & Rasmussen, 1983; Melzack, 1992; Omer, 1981; Flor et al., 2006). There are a wide range of phantom sensations. Frequently described sensations include tingling, coldness, burning, cramping, as"pins and needles,' stabbing, squeezing, shooting, shocking, crushing and heaviness. In certain instances, the absent limb is perceived to be in an unnatural position. The amputee may also experience the amputated limb to still be in the position it was in prior to the amputation (i.e., in a contracted position). Other patients report: that the phantom tends to'move spontaneously,' or 'if to still keep balance.' These words articulate certain aspects of the phantom pain experience. The experience of phantom pain is perhaps best described by Alfred van Loen, a sculptor, painter, illustrator, poet and full-knee amputee in his narrative text titled, *Phantom Pain* (1993). He eloquently states:

> *"Phantom, now that I am walking well, you are redoubling your efforts to floor me. The pain you bring my right foot I now also feel in my left foot. You are a very convincing player, and you make me sit down in my wheelchair to catch my breath. Even my bottom hearts*

In the majority of amputees, phantom sensations and phantom limb pain tend to appear immediately post-amputation. The pain may be continuous, or occasionally present, as it is also usually felt in the distal portions of the limbs (Davis, 1993; Melzack, 1971; Montoya et al., 1997; Omer, 1981; Hunter, Katz, & Davis, 2005). Another remarkable feature of phantom limb pain and phantom sensations is that even some subjects with a congenital limb defects also report having them (Davis, 1993; Fisher & Hanspal, 1998; Kooijman, Dijkstra, Geertzen, Elzinga & van der Schans, 2000; Saadah & Melzack, 1994). For a long time, this phenomenon was not thought to exist since it was assumed that if no amputation was performed, then the nerves could not have been damaged, and no pain could be experienced. More recent evidence suggests that the quality, as well as, the intensity of phantom pain and phantom sensations, are not nearly as strong in subjects with congenital limb defect, as in those following an acquired amputation (Davis, 1993; Fisher & Hanspal, 1998; Kooijman, Dijkstra, Geertzen, Elzinga & van der Schans, 2000; Saadah & Melzack, 1994; Flor et al., 2006).

Another symptom commonly described by the phantom limb amputee is the 'telescoping effect or fade away phenomenon'. Approximately two-thirds of all amputees experience the presence of telescoping (Shukla, Suha, Tripathi, & Gupta, 1982a,b).The effect is best described as occurring when the proximal part of the phantom limb is experienced as fading away (or withdrawing) both in terms of size as well as length of the phantom (over time). These are also typical characteristics of phantom sensations even when the amputee remains aware of the distal parts of the phantom limb. In other instances, amputees state that this experience "feels as if the distal part of the phantom is still directly attached to the stump" (Acker van, 1985; Davis, 1993; Doetsch, 1997; Jensen et al., 1983; Melzack, 1971, 1992; Saadah & Melzack, 1994). While many amputees report experiencing these particular symptoms, there is still no consensus regarding the treatment of the 'telescoping effect or 'the fade away phenomenon' (Krane & Heller, 1995). Moreover, the quality of phantom sensations, frequency, intensity, relation to pre-amputation pain has not been adequately described in a variety of clinical amputee populations such as children (Krane & Heller, 1995; Ingelmo, 2004; Rusy, Troshynski, Weisman, 2001).

Apart from spontaneous phantom sensations, sensations on the missing limb can sometimes be evoked by touching 'trigger zones' on other parts of the body. Indeed, many amputees report having one or several trigger zones. Stimulation of these zones, usually located on the stump, another limb, or on the head (face), may trigger phantom sensations or even phantom limb pain. While the underlying mechanisms have not been fully elucidated, these trigger zones are predominantly ipsilateral to the amputation (Doetsch, 1997; Ramachandran, Rogers-Ramachandran, & Stewart, 1992; Yang, Gallen, Schwartz, Bloom, Ramachandran & Cobb, 1994). Other triggers include defecation, urination, or ejaculation (Melzack, 1971; Sherman, Devor, Jones, Katz & Marbach, 1997).

Epidemiology

Chronic phantom limb pain after surgical amputation affects between 50–80% of patients, and is difficult to treat (Bone, Critchley et al., 2002).The estimated prevalence of phantom pain (for the whole group of amputees: upper and lower limbs) varies between 41% to 83%. (Dijkstra, Geertzen, Stewart & Schans van der, 2002; Jones & Davidson, 1995; Kalauokalani & Loeser, 1999; Kooijman et al., 2000; Montoya et al., 1997; Sherman, Sherman & Parker, 1984; Wilkins, McGrath, Finley & Katz 1998). This wide range in estimated prevalence may be attributed to differences in research techniques such as study design, assessment methodologies, and a failure to adequately distinguish between phantom limb pain, stump pain and phantom sensations. Other factors which could potentially impact reporting include those issues related to selection bias in terms of the specific population included in the study (Kalauokalani & Loeser, 1999). Moreover, the prevalence of phantom pain can also change considerably (7–22%) when different cut off points for phantom pain symptomology are applied (Borsje, Bosmans, Schans van der, Geertzen & Dijkstra, 2004). For instance, the prevalence of phantom pain in lower limb amputees in a total group of 536 amputees (19% upper limb amputee and 81% lower limb amputees) documented that the prevalence of pain in lower limb amputees was approximately 80% (95% CI: 76–83%), and for upper limb amputees it was about 41% (95% CI: 31–51%). In the total group, the overall prevalence was approximately 72% (95% CI: 68–76%) (Dijkstra et al., 2002).

Risk Factors

Potential risk factors for developing phantom sensations and phantom pain include early onset stump pain and phantom pain sensation, pre-existing pain prior to amputation, sex, the reason or cause of the amputation (e.g., a blood clot), prosthetic use, and the time elapsed since the amputation (Kooijman et al, 2000; Jensen et al, 1985; Weich, Preibl, & Birbaumer, 2000; Nikolajsen, Ilkjaer, Kroner, Christensen & Jensen 1997; Lotze, Grodd, Birbaumer, Erb, Huse & Flor, 1999; Sherman et al, 1984; Wartan, Hamann, Wedley & McColl, 1997). Stump pain and phantom sensations have also been shown to be significant risk factors for chronic phantom pain. Different risk factors exist for phantom pain and impediment of phantom pain. However, these risk factors change when different cut off points are applied for phantom pain or impediment (Borsje et al., 2004). There are also a limited number of studies which have evaluated the relationship of blood clot to incident phantom limb pain. There is also some evidence that sudden blood clot as the primary reason for amputation is associated with higher levels of phantom pain as compared to other reasons for amputation (Weiss & Lindell, 1996). The influence of sex differences have not been evaluated in these particular analyses.

There is some evidence that pain prior to an amputation is a risk factor for chronic phantom limb pain or phantom sensations. Yet, the association between phantom sensations, phantom limb pain and pain prior to amputation remains quite controversial. For example, a positive correlation between the existence of pain prior to the amputation and the development of phantom pain, or phantom sensations afterwards has also been shown in certain studies (Hanley et al., 2006b; Jensen et al, 1985; Melzack, 1971; Nikolajsen et al., 1997). This association has not generally been accepted (Flor et al., 1995). In prospective studies, while pre-amputation pain was associated with phantom pain immediately after the amputation, phantom pain persisting for two years after the amputation was less influenced by the existence of the pre-amputation pain (Jensen, Krebs, Nielsen & Rasmussen, 1985; Nikolajsen et al, 1997). One potential reason for this controversy stems from the retrospective character of the majority of these studies and recall bias of the amputees concerning the existence of pre-operative pain which may influence the outcome of these studies. Our clinical experience suggests that there is no relationship between the (severity of) pre-operative pain and the potential (severity) of post-operative phantom pain.

Significant sexual dimorphism in chronic pain has also been observed across a variety of chronic pain conditions (Butkevich, Barr, & Vershinina, 2007; O'Connor, Bragdon, & Baumhauer, 2006; Giles & Walker, 1999). Yet these findings remain controversial since the underlying mechanisms are still not well understood. Moreover, there are significant cultural, linguistic, ethnic and gender differences in activities, awareness, attribution, and willingness to report pain that may modulate the experience of pain, including pain perception and expression (Mailis-Gagnon et al., 2007; Pool, Schwegler, Theodore, & Fuchs, 2007; Garofalo, Lawler, Robinson, Morgan, & Kenworthy-Heinige, 2006). These issues could also potentially influence the interpretation of the outcomes of certain studies (Wilkins, McGrath, Finley, & Katz, 2004). It is therefore not suprising given the observed sexual dimorphism in pain that clinical findings also indicates that while the majority of phantom limb patients are males, women tend to report a higher intensity of phantom pain experienced when compared with men and that a greater percentage of women tend to report their experiencing phantom pain (Gallagher, Allen & McLachlan, 2001; Weiss & Lindell, 1996). Other clinical studies, however, fail to support these previously observed sex differences in the experience and reporting of of phantom limb pain (Jensen et al., 1983, 1985; Sherman et al., 1984).

A lack of prosthetic use has also been associated with an increased risk of chronic phantom pain. Prosthetic use (myoelectrical prostheses) has also been shown to be a potential protective factor against the development of chronic phantom pain in a small group of upper limb amputees (Lotze et al, 1999). Still other studies note that with an increase in time elapsed since the amputation, there is a corresponding decrease in the intensity of the phantom pain, which occurs in approximately half of amputees (Sherman et al, 1984). Yet, there is still some debate regarding the extent to which time is also a "healing" factor. One important study partially supports this finding,since the prevalence of phantom pain did not decline with time, however the duration of the pain attacks diminished significantly over time (Nikolajsen et al., 1997). And still other studies failed to find any correlation between phantom pain and time elapsed since amputation (Flor et al., 1995; Wartan et al., 1997).

Etiology

Current concepts regarding the cause of chronic phantom limb pain and phantom sensations have focused primarily on the role of the peripheral and central nervous system in the development of chronic phantom limb pain and phantom limb sensations (Flor et al., 2006). Still, the underlying mechanisms regarding the causes of phantom pain are not completely understood. As a consequence, however, there is still no general consensus regarding the etiology of phantom pain. Here we describe four general theories that have been used to try to explain the cause of phantom limb pain and phantom sensations.

Phantom Pain as a Psychiatric Problem

Historically, attempts to explain phantom pain and phantom sensations have been made on a psychiatric basis since amputees complained about pain in a non existent limb. As a consequence of such complaints, however, the amputee was often presumed to have a psychiatric disorder. Other explanations used to support the psychiatric theory suggest that the phantom limb pain and phantom sensations are just an overly emotional responses to the loss of a limb. These explanations are now considered to be rather out of date, though it is clear that similar to other chronic pain syndromes, psychosocial and emotional factors do contribute to the quality, duration, and intensity of the phantom pain and phantom sensations.

Neuromata

Another proposed explanation regarding the cause of phantom pain and phantom pain sensations is the neuromata (Geraghty & Jones, 1996) After an amputation, the remaining nerves at the end of the stump may grow into neuromata, or a benign swelling of nerve tissue. The neuromata continues to generate pulses, which reach the somatosensory areas of the cortex via the spinal cord and the thalamus. These impulses have previously been interpreted as if coming from the amputated limb. However, more recent data show that since the removal of the neuromata is often not a successful cure for phantom pain and phantom sensations, this theory fails to fully account for all symptoms (Ramachandran, 1993). Higher central nervous centers must also be involved.

Neurons of the Spinal Cord

Another theory proposes that neurons of the spinal cord are the primary cause of phantom pain and phantom sensations. According to this theory, neurons of the spinal cord, due to injury, lose their normal inhibition through sensory input, and begin to fire spontaneously. This information is then transmitted to the cortex and subsequently processed as if it comes from the the amputated limb. Yet, clinical observations of patients with a complete lesion of the spinal cord prove that this hypothesis is flawed as italso fails to fully explain all symptoms. Patients with a spinal cord lesion may sometimes feel severe pain in the legs and groin while the spinal neurons which carry the information from those areas to the brain originate below the level of the lesion. Put differently, if the impulses started in those neurons, they would never reach the cortex since they could not traverse the lesion (Sherman et al., 1996).

Reorganization (Remapping)

As we have stated, the underlying mechanisms regarding the causes of phantom pain are still not completely understood. A more recent theory suggests that phantoms arise in the brain due to changes, 'remapping,' or the 'reorganization' of peripheral and central mechanisms (Flor et al., 2006).

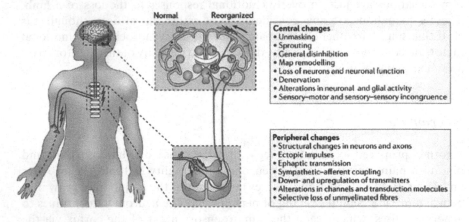

Flor et al. Nature Reviews Neuroscience 7, 873–881 (November 2006) | doi:10.1038/nrn1991

(Permissions from Nature reviews Neuroscience granted 5/21/2007/2007)

As highlighted by this visual, functional and morphological changes in peripheral, spinal, subcortical and cortical structures are responsible for decreased thresholds and increased responsivity at all levels of pain perception (Woolf, 1999; Weich et al., 2000; Flor et al., 2006). Moreover long-term changes like axonal sprouting and formation of new cell assemblies may also contribute to a permanently altered reorganization (Merzenich, 1998). Other studies support these findings. Recent human studies note that reorganisation of the somatosensory and motor system may occur post-amputation (Chen, Cohen, & Hallet, 2002). Moreover, pathological neuronal activity in the residual limb or the dorsal root ganglion, which can be enhanced by sympathetic activation, could be one of the more important factors in the etiology and development of chronic phantom limb pain (Flor et al., 2006). Sensations in the phantom limb can be elicited by somatosensory stimulation of the face and upper body (Chen, Cohen, & Hallet, 2002). The cortical area, originally corresponding to the amputated limb, is taken over by adjacent areas and it is this shift in the cortical representation which has been associated with the presence of phantom sensations and pain (Flor et al., 1995; Weich, et al, 2000; Knecht et al., 1996). For instance, the cortical area corresponding to the hand is taken over by the face. If this remapping process interferes with the "proprioceptive" maps, a stimulus of the face may induce the sensation of a phantom hand. The face acts as a trigger-zone for phantom pain and phantom sensations in the hand. Yet, the extent of the shift in cortical representation is correlated with the amount of the phantom (Flor et al., 1995; Kew et al, 1994; Chen, Cohen, & Hallet, 2002).

The (topographical) phenomenon of remapping, or reorganisation is also supported by magnetoencephalograhy (MEG) studies which reveal medial displacement of the face area toward hand representation in the somatosensory cortex (Elbert et al., 1994; Flor et al., 1995; Chen, Cohen, & Hallet, 2002). Cortical reorganization has also been shown in Positron Emission Tomography (PET) studies on pain, where regional cerebral blood flow is increased in the contralateral cortex with movement of the amputated side compared to the normal side in amputees with a congenital reduction defect and in traumatic upper limb amputees (Kew et al., 1994; Willoch et al., 2000).

In other studies the site of motor reorganization following amputation has been investigated by stimulating the central nervous system at different levels with various techniques, including transcranial magnetic stimulation (TMS). Supraspinal changes seem to be important and might have a special focus in the cortex, where maladaptive map reorganization has been found to be closely associated with the magnitude of the phantom pain experienced (Flor et al., 2006). What these studies suggest is that while excitability of the motor system to TMS is increased on the amputated side, the excitability of subcortical and spinal structures also remains unchanged and motor reorganization following amputation occurs predominantly in the cortex (Chen, Cohen & Hallett, 2002). So once again, this theory fails to fully explain the reasons for all aspects of phantom limb and phantom sensations, as highlighted by the experience of phantom limbs in patients with congenital reduction defects (Flor et al., 1995, Ramachandran et al., 1992, 1993; Yang et al., 1994).

To summarise, the phenomenon commonly described as phantom limb and phantom limb sensations are probably caused by a combination of these proposed theories. The development of phantom limbs (i.e. phantom pain and phantom sensations) might initially begin with the injury and changes in central mechanism as well as peripheral mechanisms and alterations in the spinal cord and brain (Sherman et al., 1996). An example will perhaps make this point clearer: Because of the more intense use of the dominant arm, the cortical area corresponding to that limb receives more stimuli as compared to the non-dominant side. As a result, this part of the cortex is more developed. Understandably post- amputation, the loss of stimuli and inhibition coming from the amputated limb side is more severe following an amputating of this dominant arm. Therefore, one can test the hypothesis that a more intense use of the arm in the past (dominant side), is one potential risk factor for the development of phantom pain and phantom sensations (Shukla et al., 1982b). And while it is still uncertain if the experience of phantom pain or phantom sensations is influenced by the use of a prosthesis; there are two different hypotheses that might potentially explain a possible relationship between prosthetic use and phantom pain. According to the first hypothesis, the use of a prosthesis, while experiencing phantom pain or phantom sensations is uncomfortable. One could, imagine the strange situation where the amputee experiences the phantom limb to be of another shape or length or position other than that of the prosthesis. One would expect an inverse relationship between these variables. In other words: if phantom pain or phantom sensations are present and persistent, then the use of the prosthesis decreases (Lotze et al., 1999; Weiss, Miltner, Adler, Bruckner & Taub, 1999).

Another example to clarify this point: It might be possible that the presence of a prosthesis makes the experience of phantom pain or a phantom limb less bothersome or strange. One might then expect a positive relation between these variables. In other words: If phantom pain or phantom sensations are present, prosthetic use increases. However, another study found that there was no relationship at all between these variables (Jones & Davidson, 1995). Other studies found no significant differences between subjects reporting phantom pain, and those without phantom pain concerning the use of a prosthesis. Only 8% of amputees experienced more phantom limb pain while using a prosthesis (Jones & Davidson, 1995; Wartan et al., 1997), or only one case (1/32) when prosthetic use ceased due to an increase in phantom limb pain (Geraghty & Jones, 1996).

That said, under conditions of prosthetic use or non-use; the physiologic impact of the experience of phantom pain and phantom sensations cannot be divorced from psychosocial and emotional variables including stress, fear, catastrophising and related coping problems which also contribute to the experience and meaning of chronic phantom pain.

Treatments

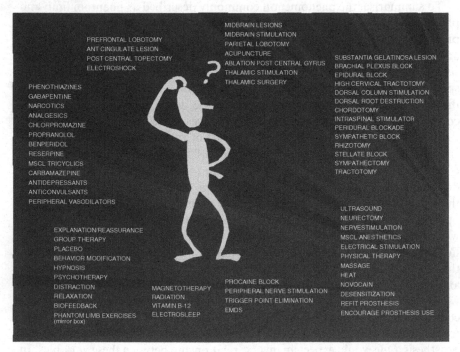

Phantom limb pain has been characterized by changes in cortical processing and organization, negative psychosocial sequelae, perceptual disturbances, and a poor response to conventional treatments (Flor et al., 2006). Despite the pre-valence of pain in this patient population; the literature describing the effective management and treatment of phantom limb pain or stump pain is in its infancy. While numerous treatments have been described, there is little clinical evidence supporting drug therapy, psychological therapy, interventional techniques or surgery since there is no single evidence-based treatment that is superior for the treatment of phantom limb pain. Moreover, given the variety of psychosocial and physiologic symptoms, the optimal management of patients with chronic phantom pain requires a multidisciplinary approach. Yet, multiple therapies have been used with mixed success, and unfortunately, there are no protocols that can adequately predict which therapy is likely to benefit a particular amputee. In this section, we will not cover all treatments used for phantom limb pain. Instead, we will highlight the efficacy and limitations of existing psycho-social, pharma-cologic, surgical, supportive and self management approaches to theh treatment of chronic phantom limb pain. (Flor et al., 2006).

In 1980, an important survey was published where sixty-eight methods for treating chronic phantom pain were identified. The study found that only a very few treatments produced adequate pain control and that placebo responses were very common (Sherman, Sherman & Gall, 1980). These treatments ranged from psychosurgeries including lobotomies to "phantom" exercises where the amputee had to reflect, control, or just attempt to ignore the phantom pain. The majority of the studies included in this survey were clinical, single group studies with follow-ups of less than 6 months. Other studies by the same authors (Sherman & Sherman, 1983, 1985, Sherman ct al., 1984) of more than 11,700 amputees, noted that only 1% of the respondents reported benefits from the host of available treatments (e.g., 0.7 % had a major reduction in pain and 0.4% was cured). A more recent systematic evidence based review evaluated the management of acute and chronic phantom pain (Halbert, Crotty & Cameron, 2002). The existing literature from 1966 till 1999 was reviewed. Significant limitations in pain management, such as poor quality research and contra-dictory results, were identified. Other recent randomized and controlled trials have also failed to any provide evidence to support any treatment for phantom pain in either the acute phase or in the chronic phase. At this time, for the early/ acute phases in the development of chronic phantom pain, there are no more effective treatments than administration of opioid analgesics, in doses with an acceptable level of risk of adverse effects.

That said, a variety of different treatments do exists. These different treat-ments should be divided into three treatment modalities; surgical (including neurosurgical), pharmacological, psychological, and supportive. Finally, there is one treatment modality of which very little is known: patient-self-management (Hanley, Ehde, Campbell, Osborn & Smith, 2006a; Mortimer, Steedman, McMillan, Martin & Ravey, 2002). With respect to all the previously mentioned treatments, aggressive treatment for chronic phantom pain is not always required. There is some evidence that only approximately 28% of the amputees report experiencing phantom pain at least every day, and only 23% of those amputees who had phantom pain experience it as a sever impediment to their normal activities of daily living (Borsje et al., 2004).

Surgical treatments

Surgical procedures, including the exploration of the stump or re-amputation, are often unsuccessful in the long term. This is probably because operative procedures produce an initial afferent barrage of pain signals and generate a secondary inflammatory response, both of which contribute substantially to postoperative pain (Reuben & Buvanendran, 2007). These signals have the capacity to initiate prolonged changes in both the peripheral and the central nervous system which lead to the amplification and prolongation of postoperative pain. Peripheral sensitization, a reduction in the threshold of nociceptor afferent peripheral terminals, is a result of inflammation at the site of surgical trauma (Melzack & Wall, 1965; Reuben & Buvanendran, 2007). Central sensitization, an activity-dependent increase in the excitability of spinal neurons, is a result of persistent exposure to nociceptive afferent input from the peripheral neurons (Melzack &Wall, 1965). Taken together, these two processes contribute to a postoperative hypersensitivity state (a so-called spinal wind-up) that is responsible for primary and secondary hyperalgesia (Reuben & Buvanendran, 2007). Prolonged central sensitization has the capacity to lead to permanent alterations in the central nervous system, including the death of inhibitory neurons, replacement with new afferent excitatory neurons, axonal sprouting, and the establishment of aberrant excitatory synaptic connections (Coderre, Katz, Vaccarino, & Melzack, 1993; Reuben & Buvanendran, 2007; Flor et al., 2006). These alterations can also lead to a prolonged state of sensitization, resulting in intractable postoperative pain that remains unresponsive to many traditional analgesics (Woolf & Salter, 2000; Reuben & Buvanendran, 2007; Perkins & Kehlet, 2000; Macrae & Davies, 1999; Diatchenko et al., 2005; Eisenberg, 2004; Melzack & Wall, 1965; Coderre, Katz, Vaccarino, & Melzack, 1993; Woolf & Salter, 2000; Moiniche, Kehlet, & Dahl, 2002).

Some examples to clarify the point: The excision of neuromata has proved to be quite successful in the reduction of stump pain. Yet, it generally fails to substantially decrease the intensity of phantom pain (Geraghty & Jones, 1996). Neuroablative procedures, including a variety of destructive procedures to the central nervous system such as chordotomies, and rhizotomies have also rarely offered substantial relief, and may under certain conditions, cause more widespread pain and morbidity (Omer, 1981; Davis, 1993; Loeser, 2006). Moreover, other, less dramatic procedures such as sympathectomies have also been tried, all without much success (Sherman et al., 1996)., These poor results in sensory pathway abalation also suggest that structures other than the spinothalamic tract and somatosensory relay nuclei of the thalamus are involved in the pathogenesis of chronic phantom pain (Loeser, 2006).

Pharmacological treatments

Before an amputee can be considered for an ablative procedure, nonsurgical therapies including pharmacologic therapies must be attempted and fully evaluated for therapeutic failure (Loeser, 2006). Pharmacological treatments can be divided in the pre-operative, intra-operative, early post-operative and late post-operative management (Halbert et al., 2002). Epidural analgesia before limb amputation is a commonly used pharmacological intervention to reduce post-amputation acute pain in the immediate post-operative phase but also for the relief and management of phantom pain. A recent study evaluating the effects of epidural, spinal, and general anesthesia on pain after lower-limb amputation noted that patients who received epidural anesthesia and those who received spinal anesthesia recalled better analgesia in the first week after their amputation than did patients who received general anesthesia. Anesthetic technique had no effect on stump pain, phantom limb sensation, or phantom limb pain at 14 months after lower-limb amputation (Ong, Arneja, & Ong, 2006; Cohen, Christo, & Moroz, 2004).

Many combinations of analgesics have been used in the attempt to provide effective relief for phantom limb pain and phantom sensations. These include opioids, paracetamol, acetylsalicylic acids, regional nerve blocks (perineural and epineural bupivacaine blocks), morphine, ketamine, oral dextromethophan, gabapentin, calctonin, amitryptiline and peri-operative epidural blocks. For instance, while there is certainly conflicting evidence regarding the efficacy of peri-operative epidural blocks; some studies do suggest that peri-operative epidural blocks, started 24 hours before amputation, are more effective than an infusion of local anesthetics via a perineural catheter in the prevention of phantom pain (Lambert et al., 2001). Another study showed that in 11 patients after a preoperative lumbar epidural block the incidence of phantom pain (compared to 14 patients receiving no preoperative lumbar epidural blockade) was reduced during the first 12 months post amputation (Bach, Noreng & Tjellden, 1988). Other studies using epidural anesthesia failed to provide sufficient evidence to support its routine use (Halbert et al., 2002).

All studies with respect to regional nerve blocks (perineural and epineural bupivacaine blocks) showed no difference in stump pain and/or phantom pain between the intervention and control groups during the post-acute period (Elizaga, Smith, Sharar, Edward & Hansen, 1994; Fisher & Meller, 1991; Nikolajsen, Ilkjaer, & Jensen, 1998; Pinzur, Garla, Pluth & Vrbos, 1996).

Salmon Calcitonin

Salmon calcitonin (s-CT) has been shown to be a valuable analgesic in phantom limb pain in several case reports (Braga et al, 1994; Kessell 1987; Jaeger 1992). Calcitonin is a thirty-two amino acid polypeptide hormone that is produced in

350   J.H.B. Geertzen and P.U. Dijkstra

humans primarily by the Parafollicular (also known as C) cells of the thyroid. The hormone participates in calcium (Ca^{2+}) and phosphorus metabolism. It is also presumed that the principal mechanism is its action on the movement of ionic calcium in neuronal membranes and particularly in the brain (small intracerebral doses of calcium ions increase the permeability and reverse (Mannarini, Fincato, Galimberti, Maderna, & Greco, 1994). The analgesic effect of calcitonin has been initially attributed to its ability to block bone re-absorbtion, but pain relief occurs very early, likely before any antiosteoclastic activity. Other explanations have therefore been proposed. Calcitonin, with its high-molecular weight peptide, should not play a direct effect on the cortex, except if a blood barrier transport mechanism by special carrier proteins is present (Appelboom, 2002; Kessel & Worz, 1987). Salmon calcitonin induces the release of propiomelanocortin, a β endorphin precursor, and increases the activity in the nucleus raphe magnus, consequently activating the serotoninergic descending pathway and inhibiting substance P release. Moreover, intrathecal administration in animals and now in humans confirms that salmon calcitonin exerts a direct central analgesic effect that is not reversible by naloxone, or on selective κ and μ antagonists of opiate receptors (Braga, 1994). Intravenous administration of calcitonin (200 IU) compared to a placebo showed a reduction in phantom pain in the early post-operative period. That said, phantom pain in the longer term follow-up was not adequately controlled and the study group was small (n = 21) (Jaeger & Maier, 1992).

Oral Dextromethorphan

Dextromethorphan (DM) is a noncompetitive N-methyl-d-aspartate (NMDA) receptor antagonist, which is widely used as an antitussive agent. DM not only prevents neuronal damage and modulates pain sensation via noncompetitive antagonism of excitatory amino acids, it has also been found to be useful in the treatment of cancer pain, in the treatment of methotrexate-induced periopheral neurotoxicity, and for phantom limb pain (Siu & Drachtman, 2007; Abraham, Marouani & Weinbroum, 2003). Oral dextromethorpan (120–270 mg/day) has been shown to be effective in a three-period double-blind crossover placebo-controlled trial in reducing phantom pain by > 50% with no side effects (Abraham, Marouani & Weinbroum, 2003). In another small study of the same authors (n = 3) this effect was also noted, however in one patient, one month after the treatment, DM was stopped as the pain recurred (Abraham, Marouani, Kollender, Meller & Weinboum, 2002).

Gabapentin

Gabapentin is an anticonvulsant that has antinociceptive and antihyperalgesic properties (Rose & Kam, 2002). It has a well-established role in the treatment of chronic pain (Wiffen et al., 2005) with particular efficacy in the treatment of neuropathic pain syndromes including (Bennett & Simpson, 2004) diabetic neuropathy (Backonja et al., 1998), postherpetic neuralgia (Rowbotham et al., 1998), and complex regional pain syndrome (van de Vusse et al., 2004). It works by binding the α-2-δ subunits of voltage-dependent calcium ion channels and blocks the development of hyperalgesia and central sensitization (Ho, Gam, & Habib, 2006). Used in the treatment of phantom limb pain; Gabapentin (after 6 weeks) and intravenous morphine (within an hour) seems to have a pain reducing effect on the development of chronic phantom limb pain (Bone, Critchley & Buggy, 2002; Wu et al., 2002). However, another study showed that gabapentine administered in the first 30 days postoperative after amputation failed to reduce the incidence, intensity of phantom pain as well as that of the post-amputation pain (Nikolajsen et al., 2006). The side-effects of gabapentin include sedation, drowsiness and dizziness.

Amitryptiline

Pain after amputation is common but difficult to treat. Yet few controlled treatment studies exist. Amitryptiline, a tricyclic antidepressant drug, inhibits serotonin and noradrenaline reuptake almost equally. In randomized controlled clinical trials (RCT's) to evaluate whether amitryptiline was more effective for treatment of phantom pain that placebo, amitryptiline was as effective as placebo in the improvement of symptoms associated with chronic phantom pain. Based on the findings, it was not recommended as a front-line standard treatment for chronic phantom limb pain (Robinson et al., 2004). Yet, more recent studies have validated the efficacy of amitryptiline in the treatment of phantom limb pain. For example, one study, characterized responses to treatment with tramadol, amitryptiline and placebo. Ninety-four treatment-naive posttraumatic limb amputees with phantom pain (intensity: mean visual analog scale score [0–100], 40 [95% confidence interval, 38–41]) were randomly assigned to receive individually titrated doses of tramadol, placebo (double-blind comparison), or amitriptyline (open comparison) for one month. In treatment-naive patients, both amitriptyline and tramadol, provided excellent and stable phantom limb and stump pain control with no major adverse events. Moreover, both drugs demonstrated consistent and large antinociceptive effects on both the stump and the intact limbs (Wilder-Smith, Hill, & Laurent, 2005).

Ketamine

Persistent phantom limb pain has been reported in up to 80% of patients post-amputation. The mechanisms are not fully understood, but nerve injury during amputation is important, with evidence for the crucial involvement of the spinal

N-methyl d-aspartate (NMDA) receptor in central changes (Wilson, Nimmo, Fleetwood-Walker, & Colvin, 2007). Ketamine is also a NMDA antagonist which has been shown to have an some efficacy in the treatment of post-amputation pain and sensory processing. A recent study showed that there was a decrease in the incidence of stump pain and phantom pain in a group of patients treated with perioperative ketamine infusion. However, the sample size is too small (n = 45) to draw any definitive conclusions in terms of broad efficacy of these findings. These results must be validated in a larger sample size of phantom pain patients (Hayes et al., 2004). Another more recent analysis of 53 patients undergoing lower limb amputation who received a combined intrathecal/epidural anaesthetic for surgery followed by a randomised epidural infusion (Group K received racemic ketamine and bupivacaine; Group S received saline and bupivacaine). The improved short-term analgesia and reduced mechanical sensitivity in Group K may also reflect the acute effects of ketamine on central sensitization (Wilson et al., 2007)

Psychological treatments

If the patient experiences phantom pain and no treatments have shown results above the placebo level, then a psychological treatment must also be considered as part of the clinical treatment plan. Treatment modalities include hypnosis, phantom limb exercises, meditation, psychotherapy, biofeedback, relaxation therapy, mirror therapy, cognitive behavioral therapy, and EMDR (Eye Movement Desensibilisation and Reprocessing, a treatment sometimes used for Post Traumatic Stress Disorders) (Hogberg et al., 2007; Meditation Practices for Health: State of the Research. AHRQ, 2007).

There is a qualitative literature which has explored the psychologic and psycho-social impact of phantom pain, distress, depression and anxiety as these can adversely affect the quality of life of the patient with chronic phantom pain (Bosmans et al., 2007). In the not so recent past, phantom limb pain was thought to be primarily a psychological problem that reflected: the patient's grief over the loss of the limb, denial or their desire to believe that the limb was still present (as a healthy or unhealthy response to the loss of a limb). Indeed, while psychological factors do not appear to be the primary cause of phantom pain; early studies on phantom pain do support the thesis that this pain was primarily psychological in origin. For instance, phantom limb pain has also been deemed to be characteristic of certain personality factors, such as compulsive self-reliance' and 'rigidity', all of which served to perpetuate the condition (Whyte & Niver, 2001). Such thinking is not part of the dark ages since a survey of 2700 amputees, 69% stated that their physicians thought that the phantom pain was in their head (Sherman & Sherman, 1983).

In addition, evidence-based best practices for the psychologic treatment of phantom limb pain and phantom sensations is also lacking given the dearth of randomized controlled clinical trials (RCTs) which have been completed (Brodie, Whyte, & Niven, 2007; Halbert, Crotty, & Cameron, 2002; Meditation Practices for Health: State of the Research. AHRQ, 2007). Some case reports provide anecdotal evidence which could support the use of these modalities as part of the overall treatment plan in patients with phantom pain (Muruoka, Komiyama, Hosoi, Mine & Kubo, 1996; Oakley, Whitman, & Halligan, 2002). Additionally, despite the relative dearth in the literature regarding the efficacy of these modalities, it is clear that every effort must be made to understand and prevent the transition from acute phantom pain to long-term chronic phantom pain, as is the case in every pain syndrome.

Supportive treatments

Prosthetic Management

Prosthetic management is usually the first treatment in the supportive treatment regimen. A bad fit may be one of the main reasons that the patient initially reports phantom limb pain or stump pain. Swelling of the stump, decreased blood flow or too high pressure on the soft tissues (and the nerves) caused by the improper fit may initiate or maintain phantom pain. Logs (or daily diaries) of amputees show that in 63% of lower limb amputees there is a relationship between phantom pain and physical activity (Sherman & Arena, 1992).

While a variety of supportive treatments exist; we limit our discussion in this paper to Transcutaneous Electrical Nerve Stimulation (TENS), Farabloc and Mirror Treatment Therapy. Clinically, a summary of treatments that could potentially assist in the treatment of phantom limb pain and phantom sensations should be provided to the clinician because some combination of treatments may provide individual patients with some relief for their pain.

Transcutaneous Electrical Nerve Stimulation (TENS)

The use of low frequency transcutaneous electrical nerve stimulation (TENS) applied at the outer ear has produced modest short-term reductions in the intensity of phantom pain and non-painful phantom upper and lower limb paresthesias (Katz & Melzack, 1991). A study of amputees with phantom pain, treated with TENS applied at the stump (30 minutes, twice a day during two weeks postoperative following amputation), showed that the incidence of phantom pain decreased significantly at 4-week follow-up compared with a control group. However, this effect was not permanent as it did not persist one year later (Finsen et al., 1988; Cohen, Christo, & Moroz, 2004).

Farabloc

Another form of supportive therapy for the treatment of chronic phantom pain is Farabloc. Farabloc is a liner (socket), made of a series of ultra thin steel threads, woven into a linen fabric which can be sewn into a garment. It is worn over the stump as soon as the phantom pain is felt by the patient. The principle is similar to "Farady's Cage" (a mechanism by using for instance an iron cage, to block external magnetic influences), which blocks external magnetic influences. It claims to shield the nerve endings from electrical and magnetic fields. In a double-blind , cross-over design, 34 amputees reported their pain level during a pretreatment period, Farabloc or placebo treatment period, a no-treatment or washout period for the control of any carry-over effect, and an alteration of treatment period. The results were statistically significant in favor for the Farabloc period; yet it was unclear whether this difference is clinically relevant (Conine et al., 1993), as a more recent trial showed only a modest short term reduction of phantom limb pain (Halbert, Crotty, & Cameron, 2002).

Mirror Treatments

Experiments in chronic phantom pain patients highlight the fact that neural connections in adult humans are much more malleable than previously assumed (Ramachandran, 2005; Brodie, Whyte, & Niven, 2007). Such plasticity is further illuminated by the use of mirror treatment, yet another promising therapy for reducing phantom pain (Ramachandran & Rogers-Ramachandran, 1990; MacLachlan, McDonald & Waloch, 2004). It works by inducing vivid sensations of movement originating from the muscles and joints of amputees' phantom limbs (Murray, Patchick, Pettifer, Caillette, & Howard, 2006). For example, the amputee place their intact arm or leg into a box, with a mirror down the mid-line, so that when the amputee views from slightly off-centre, the reflection of their arm or leg, it gives the impression of having two intact arms or legs. By using a series of movement exercises certain patients have reported a considerable reduction in phantom pain and phantom sensations (Ramachandran & Rogers-Ramachandran, 1990; MacLachlan, McDonald & Waloch, 2004; Brodie, Whyte, & Niven, 2007). While this form of treatment has been shown to have some efficacy, the underlying mechanisms are still unclear. (Moseley, 2006; Oakley, Whitman, & Halligan, 2002). A recent study found that though the mirror condition elicited a significantly greater number of phantom limb movements than the control condition, it did not attenuate phantom limb pain and sensations any more than the control condition. That said, the potential benefit of a 'virtual' limb as a treatment for phantom limb pain was discussed in terms of its ability to halt and/or reverse the cortical re-organisation of motor and somatosensory cortex following an acquired limb loss (Brodie, Whyte, & Niven, 2007).

Self Management

Many amputees with phantom pain have found few of these treatments to be useful in the long term management of chronic phantom pain. In addition, the majority of the previously considered supportive treatments have been tried by the amputees as part of their individual self management programs. The use of self management modalities has been well documented in the fields of alcohol, naturopathic care and marijuana (Hanley et al., 2006a; Lundeberg, 1985).

Research studies specific to the amputee population are few and also too small to draw any definitive conclusions (Lundeberg, 1985; Hanley et al., 2006b).

Conclusion

Phantom limb pain refers to pain in a body part that has been amputated, and for many patients, the phantom pain persists despite the blockage of peripheral input by local anesthesics, or surgery. In the past, phantom limb pain and phantom sensations have been described in the clinical context as a psychiatric problem, or as a form of mental disturbance or disorder, or has been assumed to stem from pathological alterations in the amputation stump. And though the etiology is unclear; it is clear that the adult central nervous system is an adaptive and responsive system.

There is no one theory that can explain phantom pain. Rather, it is more a compilation of different theories. What we do know is that phantom limb pain is not a static experience as it varies within and between individuals. Moreover, phantom pain as a phenomenon is not homogeneous; each patient presents with a unique combination of spontaneous or evokes sensations, pain and awareness (Hunter et al., 2005). And while it is clear that amputation can be beneficial from a medical perspective; the underlying mechanisms regarding the transition from the acute phase to chronic phantom pain are still unclear. What is clear is that phantom pain still occurs in approximately 50–80% of all amputees. Moreover, the experience and long term physiologic and psychosocial impact of chronic phantom pain on the patient and their psycho-social world can be very distressing for the amputee (e.g. mourning, stress, coping problems). Indeed, recent evidence suggests that phantom pain might be a phenomenon of the central nervous system that is related to plastic changes at several levels of the neuraxis and especially the cortex (Flor et al., 2006).

Early treatment of phantom limb pain in the acute stage could potentially reduce or prevent the morbidity associated with chronic pain in amputees from 60–80% to 10–20%. (Astra Chemicals Sweden. Ripovacain Product Information. Astra Sweden, 1996). That said, chronic phantom pain persists in the amputee population, in part because it is difficult to treat due to a complex interplay of psychosocial , physiologic, emotional and environmental factors which also work in concert to maintain the pain behaviors associated with chronic phantom pain. Moreover, once the phantom pain becomes a chronic condition, it rarely fades so aggressive evaluation, management and treatment must be a priority.

Many practices with the goal of alleviating the pain and suffering of the patient with phantom pain exist. However, while there is a clear need for early assessment, management and treatment; more evidence based research and practice guidelines and treatment trials are required to adequately guide the clinician towards to the effective prevention, management and treatment of the chronic phantom pain syndromes, Given the continued need for effective treatments; the gap between research, theory and practice in the area of phantom pain continues to persist.

References

Abraham, R. B., Marouani, N., Kollender, Y., Meller, I. & Weinbroum, A. A. (2002). Dextromethorphan for phantom pain attenuation in cancer amputees: A double-blind crossover trial involving three amputees. *Clinical Journal of Pain*, *18*(5), 282–285.

Abraham, R. B., Marouani, N., & Weinbroum, A. A. (2003). Dextromethorphan mitigates phantom pain in cancer amputees. *Annals of Surgical Oncology*, *10*(3), 268–274.

Acker van, R. E. H. (1985). *Fantoompijn* (Dutch) PhD thesis. University of Amsterdam. Koedijk drukkers.

Appelboom, T. (2002). Calcitonin in reflex sympathetic dystrophy syndrome and other painful conditions. *Bone*, *30*(5 Suppl), 84S–86S.

Bach, S., Noreng, M. F., & Tjellden, N. U. (1988). Phantom limb pain in amputees during the first 12 months following limb amputation, after preoperative lumbar epidural blockade. *Pain*, *33*, 297–301.

Bone, M., Critchley, P., & Buggy, D. J. (2002). Gabapentin in postamputation phantom limb pain: A randomized, double-blind, placebo-controlled, cross-over study. *Regional Anesthesia and Pain Medicine*, *27*(5), 486.

Borsje, S., Bosmans, J. C., Schans van der, C. P., Geertzen, J. H. B., & Dijkstra, P. U. (2004). Phantom pain: A sensitivity analysis. *Disability and Rehabilitation*, *26*(14/15), 905–910.

Bosmans, J. C., Suurmeijer, T. P., Hulsink, M., van der Schans, C. P., Geertzen, J. H., & Dijkstra, P. U. (2007). Amputation, phantom pain and subjective well-being: a qualitative study. *International Journal of Rehabilitation Research*, *30*(1), 1–8.

Brodie, E. E., Whyte, A., & Niven, C. A. (2007). Analgesia through the looking-glass? A randomized controlled trial investigating the effect of viewing a 'virtual' limb upon phantom limb pain, sensation and movement. *European Journal of Pain*, *11*(4), 428–436.

Butkevich, I. P., Barr, G. A., & Vershinina, E. A. (2007). Sex differences in formalin-induced pain in prenatally stressed infant rats. *European Journal of Pain*.

Chen, R., Cohen, L. G., & Hallett, M. (2002). Nervous system reorganization following injury. *Neuroscience*, *111*(4), 761–773.

Coderre, T. J., Katz, J., Vaccarino, A. L., & Melzack, R. (1993). Contribution of central neuroplasticity to pathological pain: Review of clinical and experimental evidence. *Pain*, *52*, 259–285.

Cohen, S. P., Christo, P. J., & Moroz, L. (2004). Pain management in trauma patients. *Am J Phys Med Rehabil*, *83*, 142–161.

Conine, T. A., Hershler, C., Alexander, S. T., & Crisp, R. H. (1993). The efficacy of Farabloc in the treatment of phantom limb pain. *Canadian Journal of Rehabilitation, 6,* 155–161.

Davis, R. W. (1993). Phantom sensation, phantom pain and stump pain. *Archives of Physical and Medical Rehabilitation, 74,* 79–90.

Diatchenko, L., Slade, G. D., Nackley, A. G., Bhalang, K., Sigurdsson, A., Belfer, I., Goldman, D., et al. (2005). Genetc basis for individual variations in pain perception and the development of a chronic pain condition. *Human Molecular Genetics, 14,* 135–143.

Dijkstra, P. U., Geertzen, J. H. B., Stewart, R., & Schans van der, C. P. (2002). Phantom pain and risk factors: A multivariate analysis. *Journal of Pain and Symptom Management, 24*(6), 578–585.

Dijkstra, P. U., Rietman, J. S., & Geertzen, J. H. B. (2007). Phantom breast sensations and phantom breast pain: A 2-year prospective study and a methodological analysis of literature. *European Journal of Pain, 11,* 99–108.

Doetsch, G. S. (1997). Progressive changes in cutaneous trigger zones for sensation referred to a phantom hand: A case report and review with implications for cortical reorganisation. *Somatosensory and Motor Research, 14*(1), 6–16.

Eisenberg, E. (2004). Post-surgical neuralgia. *Pain, 111,* 3–7.

Elbert, F., Flor, H., Birbaumer, N., Knecht, S., Hampson, S., Larbig, W., et al. (1994). Extensive reorganization of the somatosensory cortex in adult humans after nervous system injury. *NeuroReport, 5,* 2593–2597.

Elizaga, A. M., Smith, D. G., Sharar, S. R., Edward, W. T., & Hansen, S. T.Jr. (1994). Continuous regional analgesia by intraneural block: Effect on postoperative opioid requirements and phantom limb pain following amputation. *Journal of Rehabilitation Research and Development, 31,* 179–187.

Finsen, V., Persen, L., Lovlien, M., Veslegaard, E. K., Simensen, M., Gsvann, A. K., et al. (1988). Transcutaneous electrical nerve stimulation after major amputation. *Journal of Bone and Joint Surgery (B), 70,* 109–112.

Fisher, A & Meller, Y.(1991). Continuous postoperative regional analgesia by nerve sheath block for amputation surgery: A pilot study. *Anaesthesia and analgesia, 72,*300–303.

Fisher, K. & Hanspal, R. S. (1998). Phantom pain, anxiety, depression and their relation in consecutive patients with amputated limbs: Case reports. *British Medical Journal, 316,* 903–904.

Flor, H., Elbert, T., Knecht, S., Wienbruch, C., Pantev, C., Birbaumer, N., et al. (1995). Phantom-limb pain as a perceptual correlate of cortical reorganization following arm amputation. *Nature, 375,* 482–484.

Flor. H., Nikolajsen, L., & Jensen T. S. (2006). Phantom limb pain: A case of maladaptive CNS plasticity? *Nature Reviews Neuroscience, 7*(11), 873–881.

Garofalo J. P., Lawler C., Robinson R., Morgan M., & Kenworthy-Heinige T. (2006). The role of mood states underlying sex differences in the perception and tolerance of pain. *Pain Practice, 6*(3), 186–196.

Geertzen, J. H. B., & Rietman, J. S. (2008). *Amputation and Prosthetics of the lower extremity* (in Dutch). Lemma BV, Utrecht, The Netherlands.

Geertzen, J. H. B., Bosmans, J. C., Schans van der, C. P., & Dijkstra, P. U. (2005). Claimed walking distance of lower limb amputees. *Disability and Rehabilitation, 27*(3), 101–104.

Geraghty, T. J., & Jones, L.J (1996). Painful neuromata following upper limb amputation. *Prosthetics and Orthotics International, 20,* 176–181.

Giles, B. E., & Walker, J. S. (1999). Gender differences in pain. *Current Opinion in Anaesthesiology, 12*(5), 591–595.

Halbert, J., Crotty, A., & Cameron, I. D. (2002). Evidence for the optimal management of acute and chronic phantom pain: A systematic review. *The Clinical Journal of Pain, 18*(2), 84–92.

Hanley, M. A., Ehde, D. M., Campbell, K. M., Osborn, B., & Smith, D. G. (2006a). Self-reported treatments used for lower-limb phantom pain: Descriptive findings. *Archives of Physical Medicine and Rehabilitation, 87,* 270–277.

Hanley, M. A., Jensen, M. P., Smith, D. G., Ehde, D. M., Edwards, W. T., & Robinson, L. R. (2006 Aug). Preamputation pain and acute pain predict chronic pain after lower extremity amputation. *The Journal of Pain, 8*(2), 102–109.

Hayes, C., Armstrong-Brown, A., & Burstal, R. (2004). Perioperative intravenous ketamine infusion for the prevention of persistent post-amputation pain: A randomized, controlled trial. *Anaesthesia and Intensive Care, 32*(3), 330–338.

Ho, K. Y., Gam, T. J., & Habib, A. S. (2006). Gabapentin and postoperative pain – a systematic review of randomized controlled trials. *Pain, 126*(1–3), 91–101.

Hogberg, G., Pagani, M., Sundin, O., Soares, J., Aberg-Wistedt, A., Tarnell, B., et al. (2007). On treatment with eye movement desensitization and reprocessing of chronic post-traumatic stress disorder in public transportation workers – A randomized controlled trial. *Nordic Journal of Psychiatry, 61*(1), 54–61.

Hunter J. P., Katz J., & Davis K. D. (2005). Dissociation of Phantom Limb Pain from Stump Tactile spatial acuity and sensory thresholds. *Brain 128*(2), 308–320.

Ingelmo P. M., & Fumagalli R. (2004). Neuropathic pain in children. *Minerva Anestesiology, 70*(5), 393–398.

Jaeger, H., & Maier, C. (1992). Calcitonin in phantom limb pain: A double blind study. *Pain, 48*, 21–27.

Jensen, T. S., Krebs, B., Nielsen, J., & Rasmussen, P. (1983). Phantom limb, phantom pain and stump pain in amputees during the first 6 months following limb amputation. *Pain, 17*, 243–256.

Jensen, T. S., Krebs, B., Nielsen, J., & Rasmussen, P. (1985). Immediate and long-term phantom limb pain in amputees: Incidence, clinical characteristics and relationship to pre-term limb pain. *Pain, 21*, 267–278.

Jones, L. E., & Davidson, J. H. (1995). The long-term outcome of upper limb amputees treated at a rehabilitation centre in Sydney. *Disability and Rehabilitation, 17*(8), 437–442.

Kalauokalani, D. A. K., & Loeser, J. D. (1999). Phantom limb pain. In: I. K. Crombie (Ed), *Epidemiology of pain* (pp. 143–153). Seattle: IASP Press.

Katz, J., & Melzack, R. (1991). Auricular transcutaneous electrical nerve stimulation reduces phantom limb pain. *Journal of Pain and Symptom Management, 6*, 73–83.

Kessel, C., & Worz, R. (1987). Immediate response of phantom limb pain to calcitonin. *Pain, 30*, 79–87.

Kew, J. J. M., Ridding, M. C., Rothwell, J. C., Passingham, R. E., Leigh, P. N., Sooriakumaran, S., et al. (1994). Reorganization of cortical blood flow and transcranial magnetic stimulation maps in human subjects after upper limb amputation. *Journal of Neurophysiology, 72*, 2517–2524.

Knecht, S., Henningsen, H., Elbert, T., Flor, H., Hohling, C., Pantev, C., et al. (1996). Reorganization and perceptional changes after amputation. *Brain, 119*, 1213–1219.

Kooijman, C. M., Dijkstra, P. U., Geertzen, J. H. B., Elzinga, A., & van der Schans, C. P. (2000). Phantom pain and phantom sensations in upper limb amputees: An epidemiological study. *Pain, 87*, 33–41.

Krane, E. J., & Heller, L. B. (1995). The prevalence of phantom sensations and pain in paediatric amputees. *Journal of Pain and Symptom Management, 10*, 21–29.

Lambert, A. W., Dashfield, A. K., Cosgrove, C., Wilkins, D. C., Walker A. J., & Ashley, S. (2001). Randomized prospective study comparing preoperative epidural and intraoperative perineural analgesia for the prevention of postoperative stump and phantom limb pain following major amputation. *Regional Anesthesia and Pain Medicine, 26*(4), 316–321.

Loen, van A. (1993). *Phantom pain. Story and drawings.* Brookville, N. Y.: Long Island University.

Loeser, J. D. Other surgical interventions. *Pain Practice, 6*(1), 58–62.

Lotze, M., Grodd, W., Birbaumer, N., Erb, M., Huse, E., & Flor, H. (1999). Does use of a myoelectric prosthesis prevent cortical reorganization and phantom limb pain? *Nature Neuroscience, 2*, 501-502.

Lundeberg, T. (1985). Relief of pain from a phantom limb by peripheral stimulation. *Journal Neurology*, *232*(2), 79–82.

MacLachlan, M., McDonald, D., & Waloch, J. (2004). Mirror treatment of lower limb phantom pain: A case study. *Disability and Rehabilitation*, *14/15*, 901–904.

Macrae, W. M., & Davies, H. T. O. (1999). Chronic postsurgical pain. In: Crombie IK, Croft PR, Linton SJ, Leresche L, & Von Korff, M, (Ed.). *Epidemiology of pain: A report on the Task Force on Epidemiology*. (pp. 125–142). Seattle, WA: IASP Press.

Mailis-Gagnon A., Yegneswaran B., Nicholson K., Lakha S. F., Papagapiou M., Steiman A. J., et al. (2007). Ethnocultural and sex characteristics of patients attending a tertiary care pain clinic in Toronto, Ontario. *Pain Research & Management*, *12*(2), 100–106.

Mannarini, M., Fincato, G., Galimberti, S., Maderna, M., & Greco, F. (1994). Analgesic effect of salmon calcitonin suppositories in patients with bone pain. *Current Therapeutics Research, Clinical and Experimental*, *55*, 1079–1083.

Meditation Practices for Health: State of the Research. AHRQ, (2007 June). www.ahrq.gov/downloads/pub/evidence/pdf/meditation/medit.pdf. Date accessed, July 2, 2007.

Meij van der, W. K. N. (1995). No leg to stand on. Historical relation between amputation surgery and prostheseology. Thesis, Rijksuniversite it Groningen (NL). Turnout (B), Proost Int Book Production.

Melzack, R., & Wall, P. D. (1965). Pain mechanisms: A new theory. *Science*, *150*, 971–979.

Melzack, R. (1971). Phantom limb pain, implications for treatment of pathologic pain. *Anesthesiology*, *35*(4), 409–418.

Melzack, R. (1992). Phantom limbs. *Scientific American*, *226*(4), 120–126.

Merskey, H., & Bogduk, N. (1994). *Classification of chronic pain*. Seattle: IASP Press.

Merzenich, M. (1998). Long Term Change of Mind. *Science*, *282*, 1062–1063.

Mitchel, S. W. (1871). Phantom limbs. *Lippincott's Mag Popular Literature and Science*, *8*, 563–569.

Moiniche, S., Kehlet H. &, Dahl, J. B. (2002) . A qualitative and quantitative systematic review of preemptive analgesia for postoperative pain relief: the role of timing of analgesia. *Anesthesiology*, *96*, 725–41.

Montoya, P., Larbig, W., Grulke, N., Flor, H., Taub. R., & Birbaumer, N. (1997). The relationship of phantom limb pain to other phantom limb phenomena in upper extremity amputees. *Pain*, *72*, 87–93.

Mortimer, C. M., Steedman, W. M., McMillan, I. R., Martin, D. J. & Ravey, J. (2002). Patient information on phantom limb pain: A focus group study of patient experiences, perceptions and opinions. *Health Education Research*, *17*(3), 291–304.

Moseley, G. L. (2006). Graded motor imagery for pathologic pain: a randomized controlled trial. *Neurology*, *67*(12), 2129–2134.

Muraoka, M., Komiyama, H., Hosoi, M., Mine, K., & Kubo, K. (1996). Psychosomatic treatment of phantom limb pain with post–traumatic stress disorder: A case report. *Pain*, *66*(2–3), 385–388.

Murray, C. D.,Patchick, E., Pettifer, S., Caillette, F., & Howard, T. (2006 Apr). Immersive virtual reality as a rehabilitative technology for phantom limb experience: A protocol. *Cyberpsychology Behavior*, *9*(2):167–170.

Nikolajsen, L., Hansen, C. L., Nielsen, J., Keller, J., Arendt-Nielsen, L., & Jensen, T. S. (1996). The effect of ketamine on phantom pain: A central neuropathic disorder maintained by peripheral input. *Pain*, *67*, 69–77.

Nikolajsen, L., Ilkjaer, S., Kroner, K., Christensen, J. H., & Jensen, T. S. (1997). The influence of preamputation pain on postamputation stump and phantom pain. *Pain*, *72*, 393–405.

Nikolajsen, L., Ilkjaer, S., & Jensen, T. S. (1998). Effect of preoperative extradural bupivacaine and morphine on stump sensation in lower limb amputees. *British Journal of Anaesthesia*, *81*, 348–354.

Nikolajsen, L., Finnerup, N. B., Kramp, S., Vimtrup, A. S., Keller, J. & Jensen, T. S. (2006). A randomized study of the effects of gabapentin on postamputation pain. *Anesthesiology*, *105*(5), 1008–1015.

Oakley, D. A., Whitman, L. G., & Halligan, P. W. (2002). Hypnotic imaging as a treatment for phantom limb pain: Two case reports and a review. *Clinical Rehabilitation*, *16*(4), 368–377.

O'Connor, K., Bragdon, G., Baumhauer, & J. F. (2006). Sexual dimorphism of the foot and ankle. *Orthopedic Clinics of North America*, *37*(4), 569–574.

Omer, Jr., G. E. (1981). Nerve, neuroma, and pain problems related to upper limb amputations. *Orthopedic Clinics of North America*, *12*(4), 751–762.

Ong, B. Y., Arneja, A., & Ong, E. W. (2006). Effects of anesthesia on pain after lower-limb amputation. *Journal of Clinical Anesthesia*, *18*(8), 600–604.

Perkins, F. M., & Kehlet, H. (2000). Chronic pain as an outcome of surgery. A review of predictive factors. *Anesthesiology*, *93*, 1123–1133.

Pinzur, M., Garla, P. G., Pluth, T., & Vrbos, L. (1996). Continuous postoperative infusion of a regional anaesthetic after an amputation of the lower extremity. *Journal of Bone and Joint Surgery*, *79*, 1752–1753.

Pool G. J., Schwegler A. F., Theodore B. R., & Fuchs P. N. (2007). Role of gender norms and group identification on hypothetical and experimental pain tolerance. *Pain*, *129*(1–2), 122–129.

Ramachandran, V. S. (1993). Behavioral and magnetoencephalographic correlates of plasticity in the adult human brain. *Proceedings National Academic Sciences USA*, *30*, 10413–10420.

Ramachandran, V. S. (2005). Plasticity and Functional Recovers in Neurology. *Clinical Medecine*, *5*(4), 368–373.

Ramachandran, V. S., Rogers-Ramachandran, D., & Stewart, M. (1992). Perceptual correlates of massive cortical reorganisation. *Science*, *258*, 1159–1160.

Ramachandran, V. S., & Rogers-Ramachandran, D. (1996). Synaesthesia in phantom limbs induced with mirrors. *Proceedings of the Royal Society of London*, *263*, 377–386.

Reuben, S. S., & Buvanendran, A. (2007). Preventing the development of chronic pain after orthopaedic surgery with preventive multimodal analgesic techniques. *Journal of Bone and Joint Surgery of American*, *89*(6), 1343–58.

Robinson, L. R., Czerniecki, J. M., Ehde, D. M., Edwards, W. T., Judish, D. A., Goldberg, M. L., et al. (2004). Trial of amitriptyline for relief of pain in amputees: Results of a randomized controlled study. *Archives of Physical and Medical Rehabilitation*, *85*, 1–6.

Rusy L. M., Troshynski T. J., & Weisman S. J. (2001). Gabapentin in phantom limb pain management in children and young adults: Report of seven cases. *Journal of Pain and Symptom Management*, *21*(1), 78–82.

Saadah, E. S. M., & Melzack, R. (1994). Phantom limb experiences in congenital limb-deficient adults. *Cortex*, *30*, 479–485.

Schans van der, C. P., Geertzen, J. H. B., Schoppen, T., & Dijkstra, P. U. (2002). Phantom pain and health-related quality of life in lower limb amputees. *Journal of Pain and Symptom Management*, *24*(4), 429–436.

Schmidt, A., Takahashi, M. E., Posso, I. P. (2005). Phantom Limb Pain induced by spinal anesthesia. *Clinics*, *60*(3), 263–264.

Sherman, R., Sherman, C., & Gall, N. (1980). A survey of phantom limb pain treated in the United States. *Pain*, *8*, 85–99.

Sherman, R., & Sherman, C. (1983). Prevalence and characteristics of chronic phantom limb pain among American veterans. Results of a trial survey. *American Journal of Physical Medicine*, *62*, 227–238.

Sherman, R. A., Sherman, C. J., & Parker, L. (1984). Chronic phantom and stump pain among American veterans: Results of a survey. *Pain*, *18*(1), 83–95.

Sherman, R., & Sherman, C. (1985). A comparison of phantom sensations among amputees whose amputations were of civilian and military origins. *Pain*, *2*, 91–97.

Sherman, R. A., & Arena, J. G. (1992). Phantom limb pain: Mechanisms, incidence, and treatment. *Critical Reviews in Physical and Rehabilitation Medicine, 4*, 1–26.

Sherman, R. A., Devor, M., Jones, D. E. C., Katz, J., & Marbach, J. J. (1997). *Phantom pain.* New York and London, Plenum Press.

Shukla, G. D., Sahu, S. C., Tripathi, R. D., & Gupta, D. K. (1982a). A psychiatric study of amputees. *British Journal of Psychiatry, 141*, 50–53.

Shukla, G. D., Sahu, S. C., Tripathi, R. D., & Gupta, D. K. (1982b). Phantom limb: A phenomenological study. *British Journal of Psychiatry, 141*, 54–58.

Siu, A., & Drachtman, R. (2007). Dextromethorphan: A Review of N-methyl-d-aspartate Receptor Antagonist in the Management of Pain. *CNS Drug Reviews, 13*(1), 96–106.

Wartan, S. W., Hamann, W., Wedley, J. R., & McColl, J. (1997). Phantom pain and sensations among British veteran amputees. *British Journal of Anaesthesia, 78*, 652–659.

Weich K., Preibl H., & Birbaumer N. (2000). Neuroimaging of chronic pain: Phantom Pain and Musculoskeletal Pain. *Scandinavian Journal of Rheumatology,113*, 13–8.

Weiss, S. A., & Lindell, B. (1996). Phantom limb pain and etiology of amputation in unilateral lower extremity amputees. *Journal of Pain and Symptom Management, 11*(1), 3–17.

Weiss, T., Miltner, W. H., Adler, T., Bruckner, L., & Taub, E. (1999). Decrease in phantom limb pain associated with prosthesis-induced increased use of an amputation stump in humans. *Neurosciences letters, 10*, 272(2), 131–134.

Whyte, A. S., & Niver, R. G. N. (2001). Psychological Distress in Amputees with Phantom Limb Pain. *Journal of Pain and Symptom Management, 22*(5), 938–946.

Wilder-Smith, C. H., Hill, L. T., & Laurent, S. (2005). Postamputation pain and sensory changes in treatment-naive patients: characteristics and responses to treatment with tramadol, amitriptyline, and placebo. *Anesthesiology, 103*(3), 619–628.

Wilkins, K. L., McGrath, P. J., Finley, G. A., & Katz, J. (1998). Phantom limb sensations and phantom limb pain in child and adolescent amputees. *Pain, 78*(1), 7–12.

Wilkins, K. L., McGrath, P. J., Finley, G. A.,& Katz, J. (2004). Prospective diary study of nonpainful and painful phantom sensations in a preselected sample of child and adolescent amputees reporting phantom limbs. *Clinical Journal of Pain, 20*(5), 293–301.

Willoch, F., Rosen, G., Tolle, T. R., Oye, I., Wester, H. J., Berner, N., et al. (2000). Phantom limb pain in the human brain: Unraveling neural circuitries of phantom limb sensations using positron emission tomography. *Annals of Neurology, 48*(6), 842–849.

Wilson, J. A., Nimmo, A. F., Fleetwood-Walker, S. M., Colvin, L. A. (2008). A randomised double blind trial of the effect of pre-emptive epidural ketamine on persistent pain after lower limb amputation. *Pain, 135*, 108–110.

Woolf, C. J. (1999). Neuropathic Pain. *Lancet, 353*, 1959–1964.

Woolf, C. J., & Salter, M. W. (2000). Neuronal plasticity: Increasing the gain in pain. *Science, 288*, 1765–1769.

Wu, C. L., Tella, P., Staats, P. S., Vaslav, R., Kazim, D. A., Wesselman, U., et al. (2002). Analgesic effects of intravenous lidocaine and morphine on postamputation pain. *Anesthesiology, 96*, 841–848.

Yang, T. T., Gallen, C., Schwartz, B., Bloom, F. E., Ramachandran, V. S., & Cobb, S. (1994). Sensory maps in the human brain. *Nature, 368*, 592–593.

Pain: Substance Abuse Issues in the Treatment of Pain

Howard A. Heit and Arthur G. Lipman

About 50 million Americans suffer from chronic pain [1]. As our population continues to age, this number is likely to grow, yet unfortunately, pain continues to be undertreated and poorly treated. Forty to 60% of people with severe pain in the context of life-limiting illnesses have difficulty getting their pain adequately treated [2–4]. Lost productive time and cost due to common pain conditions in the United States affects 13% of the total workforce and costs the nation $61.2 billion per year [5].

Millions of persons with pain from chronic diseases such as arthritis, diabetes, headaches, and muscle disorders suffer and have difficulty finding and paying for qualified professionals willing to help them gain access to the medicines, physical and psychological therapies and surgical/anesthetic interventions that can help them lead higher quality and more productive lives.

Chronic pain serves no useful purpose [6] once the underlying cause has been identified. It is no longer a useful clinical monitoring parameter, and it should be treated as effectively as possible. Unfortunately, pain has been and continues to be undertreated. One reason is "opiophobia," which was first described in 1985. The author of that classic paper in which this term was defined wrote, "American physicians markedly undertreat severe pain based on an irrational and undocumented fear that appropriate use will lead patients to become addicts." [7] Moreover, some members of minorities who present to a healthcare professional with pain are inadequately treated due to clinicians' concerns about concurrent addictive disorders or prejudice arising from racism, homophobia, and/or opiophobia [8]. Such undertreatment of pain violates the Hippocratic Oath.

Pain is the most common reason that patients enter the healthcare system, commonly through visits to physicians' offices, presentation at emergency departments, or by visiting community pharmacies [9]. Opioids remain the most effective analgesics that we have for most moderate to severe pain disorders, but these important medications do carry a risk of addiction. Opioids are not

H.A. Heit (✉)
Assistant Clinical Professor of Medicine, Georgetown University School of Medicine, Washington DC
email: howard204@aol.com

R.J. Moore (ed.), *Biobehavioral Approaches to Pain*,
DOI 10.1007/978-0-387-78323-9_15, © Springer Science+Business Media, LLC 2009

contraindicated in patients with the brain disease of addiction, [10] but such use should be under the supervision of appropriately trained specialists with clearly defined boundaries [11,12]. Additionally, patients who have the disease of addiction and who are not currently abusing substances may still be at higher risk for relapse if opioids are used in their clinical care. It is important for clinicians treating pain patients who also have the disease of addiction to be able to understand and weigh the risks and benefits of these important medications in such settings.

Pain does not protect against a concurrent substance use disorder. Patients enrolled in methadone maintenance and treatment programs for opioid addiction often list severe chronic pain as a major problem [13]. The prevalence of addiction has been estimated as 3–16%, most commonly cited as 10% [14]. It seems improbable that the rate of substance use disorders in the chronic pain population would be lower. This rate may underestimate the prevalence of addiction in pain patients [15]. No one specific marker reliably identifies at-risk pain patients. Therefore careful boundary setting for all patients is in order.

Not all aberrant behavior reflects drug misuse or addiction. Some individuals who do not meet the diagnostic criteria for addiction may also use medications and other drugs problematically. The latter are sometimes referred to as "chemical copers." [16] They lack coping skills commonly acquired during childhood and adolescence and tend to turn to external sources for support in dealing with life's problems. For example, stress increases pain [17]. A pain patient who takes inappropriate additional doses of his or her opioid medication after stressful situations to treat anxiety must be educated that this is not the correct response to the situation. Open and honest dialogue with the patient is an appropriate biopsychosocial approach to the problem.

The pain patient who is in recovery from the disease of addiction faces multiple barriers to appropriate pharmacologic pain management. The barriers may be insurmountable if the addictive disease is both active and dominant. The reasons are multifactorial: inadequate education in pain and addiction medicine; [9,18] misunderstanding of common definitions used in pain and addiction medicine; [19] fear of misuse/addiction and diversion secondary to prescribing a controlled substance such an opioid, and/or concerns of sanctions from the regulatory agencies for prescribing a controlled substance. The healthcare professional must know and understand federal regulations for prescribing a controlled substance to a pain patient with or without a history of addiction [19].

The goal of this chapter is to give healthcare providers information they will need to treat pain patients who also have a history of addiction.

A Brief History of Drug Regulation in the United States

Until the twentieth century, American policy toward drug control was essentially libertarian. The Pure Food and Drug Act of 1906 was the first federal drug law; it required proof of safety in marketed drugs but few other controls. The Harrison Narcotics Act of 1914 placed control of narcotics within the medical profession through a taxation scheme that was needed due to international treaty obligations. For the first time American doctors faced restrictions in their prescription of narcotics, and physicians were prohibited from providing these drugs to patients who were already addicted. Similar marijuana legislation enacted in 1937 rapidly evolved into a full prohibition. More comprehensive drug control resulted from the Food Drug and Cosmetic Act of 1938 and several subsequent amendments. A series of political and legal changes in the late 1960s and early 1970s dramatically altered drug control policy.

The Harrison Act remained the cornerstone of American narcotics regulation until the second half of the twentieth century when federal registration was mandated for clinicians to have authority to prescribe many abusable drugs. The Bureau of Narcotics and Dangerous Drugs (BNDD) regulated opioids in the 1960s as an agency of the (then) Department of Health Education and Welfare (DHEW). The BNDD was replaced just a few years later when the Comprehensive Drug Abuse Prevention and Control Act of 1970 (Controlled Substance Act) established the federal Drug Enforcement Administration (DEA) and established five controlled substance schedules that placed varying levels of restriction on prescription and use of drugs and other substances deemed to have high abuse potential. The DEA was established as an agency of the Department of Justice (DOJ), not the Department of Health and Human Services (which was then the federal department responsible for the health-related roles of the former DHEW). Reassigning these responsibilities to DOJ clearly signaled the governmental perspective that control of abusable substances was more a law enforcement than health concern.

The term opioid originally meant opium and its derivatives. The current extensive use of the word in both federal and state legislation to describe a broad range of abusable substances has removed its utility to describe that specific class of drugs. Narcotic is now a value-laden word with strong negative connotations that mediate against its use by clinicians. The term opiate was commonly used in the recent past to describe exogenous derivatives of opium, and opioid to describe endogenous substances that bind at the same receptors as opium derivatives in the human body. Recognizing the similarity of endogenous and exogenous substances, opioid is now the preferred term for the strong analgesics derived from or analogous to opium and its derivatives [20].

All states, territories, and the District of Columbia also have controlled substance acts, most of which simply mirror the federal law. But some place more stringent restrictions on some controlled substances than the CSA. In such cases, the more stringent law prevails.

Risk versus Benefit

An essential philosophical construct for all health care interventions is the need to have a favorable risk to benefit ratio (R:B). The R:B must be determined individually; i.e., it applies to the use of a specific intervention for a specific problem at a specific time. Opioid use can have an unfavorable R:B. When used properly, the R:B is usually highly favorable.

A Continuum of Pain and Opioid Addiction

Opioids used to treat the chronic pain patient may be identified as either "the problem," "the solution" or a mix of both depending upon the frame of reference used [21,22]. This would be especially true with the patient who has moderate to severe pain and a history of heroin addiction or opioid prescription abuse. It is also possible for pain and addiction to exist as comorbid conditions, such as alcohol dependence with peripheral neuropathic pain. While pain and addiction can be comorbid, they may also be considered as a dynamic continuum, with pain at one end and addiction the other [21]. When seeing patients with ongoing inappropriate substance use, e.g. alcohol or cocaine abuse, clinicians should consider co-morbid pain and substance use disorder. But when the drug in question may be a clinically appropriate intervention for the underlying problem, a continuum model may apply, as in the use of opioids for the treatment of chronic pain. Figure 1 illustrates this relationship.

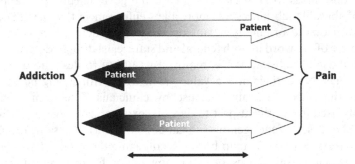

Fig. 1 Pain and addiction continuum. Failure to treat both conditions, when present, will undoubtedly lead to frustration and poor outcomes in both domains [22]

Definitions

Definitions relating to substance misuse were formulated in 1988 by representatives of an international group of professional societies to help achieve greater clarity and uniformity in terminology associated with alcohol and other drug-related problems. The interdisciplinary group of experts produced a list of substance-abuse terms deemed important, along with the most agreed-upon definition for each term. Addiction was defined as "the compulsive use of a substance resulting in physical, psychological, or social harm to the user *and* continued use despite that harm." [23,24]

Nearly two decades later and armed with much greater knowledge about the biological and genetic aspects of addiction, a Liaison Committee on Pain and Addiction (LCPA) of the American Academy of Pain Medicine, the American Pain Society, and the American Society of Addiction Medicine defined addiction, physical dependence, and tolerance. The consensus definitions were approved by the Board of Directors of the three societies and published in 2001 [23,24]. Those definitions are as follows:

- **Addiction** is a primary, chronic, neurobiologic disease, with genetic, psychosocial, and environmental factors influencing its development and manifestations. It is characterized by behaviors that include one or more of the following: impaired control over drug use, compulsive use, continued use despite harm and craving.
- **Physical dependence** is a state of adaptation that is manifested by a drug-class-specific withdrawal syndrome that can be produced by abrupt cessation, rapid dose reduction, decreasing blood level of the drug and/or administration of an antagonist.
- **Tolerance** is a state of adaptation in which exposure to a drug induces changes that result in a diminution of one or more of the drugs effects over time.

Pseudoaddiction

Aberrant drug seeking behavior that appears much like that demonstrated by opioid addicts may result from inadequate pain management. Pseudoaddiction was defined in 1989, [25] as a syndrome that causes patients to seek additional medications appropriately or inappropriately due to inadequate pharmacotherapy being prescribed. Typically when the pain is treated appropriately, the inappropriate behavior ceases.

Pseudotolerance

Pseudotolerance describes the need to increase medication such as opioids for pain when factors other than tolerance to analgesia *per se* are present such as disease progression, new disease, increased physical activity, change in medication, drug interaction, lack of compliance, addiction and/or deviant behavior such as diversion. Most patient requests for increased opioid doses after pain relief has been established and maintained for a period of time are due to one of these factors, not tolerance to the analgesic effect of the drug [26]. Most requests for more pain medication are valid, but some are not. Therefore evaluation of the patient at appropriate intervals is necessary for optimal decisions in prescribing controlled substances.

Multiple Types of Tolerance

Tolerance is a multidimensional phenomenon. Tolerance to analgesia is relatively uncommon and is often confused with pseudotolerance. Tolerance to respiratory depression, pruritus, nausea or vomiting or sedation usually resolves after approximately a week of regularly scheduled opioid therapy [27]. Tolerance to opioid-induced constipation normally does not occur [28].

Iatrogenic Addiction

Iatrogenic is not clearly defined in the literature [15]. In the authors' opinion, iatrogenic addiction occurs when a patient, with a negative personal or family history for alcohol or drug addiction or abuse, is appropriately prescribed a controlled substance and subsequently in the therapeutic course shows signs of abuse or addiction to that substance. The true incidence of iatrogenic addiction to opioids is not known. [15] It is therefore important to set boundaries with all patients before writing the first prescription [22].

It is only by aggressive evaluation and rational pharmacotherapeutic management of the pain that diagnoses such as addiction, pseudoaddiction or iatrogenic addiction can be confirmed. While a diagnosis of addiction is made prospectively, over time, a diagnosis of pseudoaddiction is made retrospectively [22]. When reasonable limits and boundaries are placed on a patient, and yet the patient continues to exceed these limits, addiction and pseudoaddiction should be considered.

When a patient explains aberrant behavior in terms of inadequate analgesia, it is reasonable to consider a careful review of the treatment plan and, where appropriate, to adjust the prescribed medications upward to achieve the desired functional goals. This increase in medication dose should be tied to a tightening of the dispensing interval/boundaries in order to safely test the possibilities of drug misuse, pseudoaddiction or addiction. For example, a patient who continually runs out of medication before the next prescription is due should have the prescribing interval reduced when the decision to increase the dose is made. If the patient continues to run out of medication early, despite the dose being increased, the diagnosis of pseudoaddiction becomes less plausible.

The new consensus definitions should help health professionals better understand addiction, physical dependence and tolerance, and assist in differentiating these from pseudotolerance and pseudoaddiction. This will enable clinicians to more effectively evaluate and treat chronic pain patients with, or without the disease of addiction.

Understanding of addiction, dependence and tolerance is confounded by a second set of definitions found in the Diagnostic and Statistical Manual of Mental Disorders, currently in the fourth-text revised edition (DSM IV-TR) [29]. Under the section "Criteria for Substance Dependence," DSM-IV defines

Table 1 Criteria for a Diagnosis of Substance Dependence

Substance Dependence

A maladaptive pattern of substance use, leading to clinically significant impairment or distress, as manifested by the occurrence of three (or more) of the following during the same 12-month period:

(1) Tolerance, as defined by either of the following: (a) a need for markedly increased amounts of a substance to achieve intoxication or a desired effect, (b) markedly diminished effect with continued use of the same amount of a substance

(2) Withdrawal, as manifested by either of the following: (a) symptoms characteristic of withdrawal from a substance, (b) the ability to take a substance or one closely related to it, to relieve or avoid withdrawal symptoms

(3) A need to take a substance in larger amounts or over a longer period than intended.

(4) A persistent desire or unsuccessful efforts to cut down or control substance use

(5) A great deal of time spent in activities necessary to obtain a substance (e.g., visits to multiple doctors or driving long distances), to use a substance (e.g., chain-smoking), or to recover from its effects.

(6) Abandonment of or absence from important social, occupational, or recreational activities because of substance use.

(7) Continued substance use despite knowledge of having a persistent or recurrent physical or psychological problem that is likely to have been caused or exacerbated by the substance (e.g., continued cocaine use despite recognition of cocaine-induced depression, or continued drinking despite recognition that an ulcer is made worse by alcohol consumption).

substance dependence as "a maladaptive pattern of substance use, leading to clinically significant impairment or distress, as manifested by three (or more) of the following during the same 12-month period." It then lists seven criteria for determining if this disorder exists (Table 1). Without differentiating between physical dependence and addiction, five of the seven criteria for substance use disorder could apply either to a person with the disease of addiction or to a chronic pain patient on opioids. (Table 2)

A heroin addict could be both physically dependent and addicted as per the definitions. Consequently, a pain patient receiving opioids may be misdiagnosed with the disease of addiction when he or she is only physically dependent, a normal physiological consequence of using opioids.

Table 2 Five out of seven of the DSM-IV criteria for substance misuse could be for a pain patient appropriately on opioids or patient with the disease of addiction

1. Tolerance does not equal addiction
2. Withdrawal does not equal addiction
3. Length of use of opioids does not equal addiction
4. Desire to cut down the use of opioids does not equal addiction
5. Time and activity to obtain opioid does always equal addiction

Adapted from Heit HA. Addiction, Physical Dependence, and Tolerance: Precise Definitions to Help Clinicians Evaluate and Treat the Patient with Chronic Pain. J Pain Palliat Care Pharmacotherap. 2003;17(1):15–29.

Until the Liaison Committee on Pain and Addiction (LCPA) definitions are incorporated into a future Substance Use Disorder section of DSM-V, clinicians should understand and apply definitions that reflect accurate and current knowledge in basic science and clinical medicine.

Universal Precautions in Pain Medicine

No single behavior is pathognomonic of addiction [22]. Therefore, it is important for clinicians to obtain drug and alcohol use histories in all patients. Alcoholism, for example, is a disease that intrudes into many aspects of the care of affected patients seeking medical treatment. Unresponsive hypertension, intractable mood disorders, difficult interpersonal conflict and impaired sleep all may adversely impact an untreated alcoholic. Appropriate use of potent medications such as opioids is likely to be more complicated in alcoholic than in nonalcoholic patients. Undiagnosed substance use disorders can make even routine healthcare difficult.

Some clinicians resist taking a drug and alcohol history in all patients. Even asking about drug and alcohol misuse may be seen as minimizing or dismissing the patients' complaints of pain. In no other area of medicine would such an attitude exist. Alcohol and drug addiction are independent of socioeconomic status, race, age or sexual orientation. It is unwise to limit one's inquiry into substance use based on classical societal stereotypes.

Because no one can determine *a priori* which patient may be abusing substances, clinicians should uniformly and respectfully assess all patients. For patients at increased risk for substance use disorders, this basic level of inquiry can be expanded. The term "Universal Precautions" originated from the field of infectious disease (See also CDC: www.cdc.gov/ncidod/dhqp/bp_universal_precautions.html, date accessed: 06/26/2007). In the context of pain management, it is a careful 10-point assessment of all persistent pain patients within the biopsychosocial model. Appropriate "boundary setting" is determined based on the initial evaluation of the patient using a non-judgmental approach before writing the first prescription. By using this approach to the pain patient, stigma can be reduced, patient care improved and overall risk of pain management reduced [22]. The 10 Principles of Universal Precautions are listed in Table 3.

While the treatment of the majority of pain patients who present to primary care providers is unlikely to be complicated by substance use disorders, it may be useful to triage these patients into three groups, according to risk and recommended management strategies [22].

Group I - Primary Care Management Patients

These are patients with no past or current history of substance use disorders. They have a noncontributory family history with respect to substance use

Table 3 The Ten Principles of "Universal Precautions

1. Diagnosis with appropriate differential
2. Psychological assessment including risk of addictive disorders
3. Informed consent (verbal vs written/signed)
4. Treatment agreement (verbal vs written/signed)
5. Pre/post intervention assessment of pain level and function
6. Appropriate trial of opioid therapy +/− adjunctive medication
7. Reassessment of pain score and level of function
8. Regularly assess the "Four A's" of pain medicine *Analgesia, Activity, Adverse reactions, & Aberrant behavior* [32]
9. Periodically review pain and comorbidity diagnoses, including addictive disorders
10. Documentation

disorders and lack major or untreated psychopathology. This group clearly represents the majority of patients who will present to the primary care practitioner.

Group II – Primary Care Patients with Specialist Support

In this group, there may be a past history of a treated substance use disorder or a significant family history of problematic drug use. They may also have a past or concurrent psychiatric disorder. These patients, however, are not actively addicted but do represent increased risk that may be managed in consultation with appropriate specialist support. This consultation may be formal and ongoing (co-managed) or simply with the option for referral back for reassessment should the need arise.

Group III – Specialty Pain Management

This group of patients represents the most complex cases to manage because they have an active substance use disorder or major, untreated psychopathology. These patients are actively addicted and pose significant risk to both themselves and to the practitioners, who often lack the resources or experience to manage them.

It is important to remember that Groups II and III can be dynamic; patients in Group II can move into Group III with relapse to active addiction, while Group III patients can move to Group II with appropriate treatment. In some cases, as more information becomes available to the practitioner, the patient who was originally thought to be low risk (Group I) may become Group II or even Group III. Thus, it is important to continually reassess risk over time.

The purpose of effective pain management for all patients including those with substance use disorders is to reduce pain and improve function while monitoring for unacceptable side effects of the prescribed medication. When a drug does more *to* the patient than *for* the patient, and yet continues to be used, an active addictive disorder must be considered. Failure to identify such a comorbid state will render even the most ardent efforts at pain management ineffective and frustrating. Thus the Universal Precautions approach in pain management helps clinicians to set appropriate boundaries based on mutual trust and honesty with the patient before writing the first prescription [23].

Urine Drug Testing in Pain or Addiction Medicine

Urine drug testing (UDT) is a useful diagnostic tool in pain and addiction management that provides valuable information to assist in diagnostic and therapeutic decisions [30]. To assess compliance, the clinician may look for the presence of prescribed medications as evidence of their use. Not finding the prescribed drug or finding unprescribed or illicit drugs in the urine merits further discussion with the patient while recognizing that laboratory error and test insensitivity can cause a false-negative report. Bingeing by the patient can result in unexpected negative urine reports if the patient runs out of medication prior to sample collection. Therefore, these results by themselves cannot be relied upon to prove drug diversion and may be consistent with addiction, pseudoaddiction or the use of an opioid for non-pain purposes – so called chemical copings [16]. The purpose of UDT should be explained to the patient at the initial evaluation. UDT should be used, like all other diagnostic tests, to improve patient care. UDT can also enhance the relationship between clinicians and patients by providing documentation of adherence to mutually agreed-upon treatment plans [30,31].

Reports of unprescribed or illicit substances in the urine aid in the assessment and diagnosis of drug misuse or addiction. UDT results can be used to encourage change to more functional behaviors, while supporting the positive changes previously made. Thus, the appropriate use of a UDT result requires documentation in the medical record and an understanding on the part of both the patient and the clinician of how these results are to be used [32].

In the pain management setting, the presence of an illicit or unprescribed drug does not necessarily negate the legitimacy of the patient's pain complaints, but it may suggest a concurrent disorder such as drug abuse or addiction. While acute pain can be treated in a patient with an active addictive disorder, it is improbable that one can successfully treat chronic pain in a patient with untreated addiction. The patient must be willing to accept assessment and treatment of both disorders to receive adequate and successful pain management [22] Thus, the diagnosis of a concurrent addictive disorder, when it exists, is vital to the successful treatment of chronic pain.

Specimen Choice

Urine has been the preferred biologic specimen for determining the presence or absence of most drugs since the 1970s [33]. This is in part due to the increased window of detection of one to three days for most drugs or their metabolites [34]. When compared to serum samples, the relatively non-invasive nature of sample collection, ease of storage and low cost of testing favor urine as the specimen of choice.

Whom to Test

The question of whom to test is made easier by having a uniform practice policy. This reduces any stigma while ensuring that patients with pain and substance use disorders may receive optimal treatment. Careful explanation of the purpose of testing normally allays patient concerns [30].

Testing Strategies

The clinician must know the drugs for which to test, appropriate methods and the expected use of the results. If the purpose of testing is to find unprescribed or illicit drug use, Gas Chromatography/Mass Spectroscopy (GC/MS) and High Performance Liquid Chromatography (HPLC) are the most specific for identifying individual drugs or their metabolites [35]. Caution must be exercised when interpreting UDT results in a pain practice. True negative urine results for prescribed medication may indicate a pattern of bingeing rather than drug diversion. Time of last use of the drug(s) can be helpful in the interpretation of UDT results.

A basic routine UDT panel should screen for the following drugs/drug classes:

- cocaine
- amphetamines / methamphetamine
- opioids
- methadone
- marijuana
- benzodiazepines

Urinary creatinine, pH, and temperature should be recorded to assist with interpretation and to increase specimen reliability. The temperature of a urine sample within four minutes of voiding should be between 90 and 100°F [36]. Urinary pH undergoes physiologic fluctuations throughout the day, but should remain within the range of 4.5 to 8.0 [36]. Urinary creatinine varies with daily water intake and hydration; normal human urine has a creatinine concentration greater than 20 mg/dL. Values lower than 20 mg/dL indicate dilution and findings lower than 5 mg/dL are inconsistent with human urine [27]. Test results outside of these ranges should be discussed with the patient and/or the laboratory, as necessary [30].

The detection time of most drugs or their metabolites in urine is usually one to three days, which is influenced by several factors including but not limited to dose, route of administration, metabolism, urine concentration and pH [35,37]. Chronic use of a lipid-soluble drug such as marijuana may extend the window of detection to a week or more [36,38]. Benzodiazepines and their metabolites differ widely in their elimination half-lives, which affect their clinical effect, excretion and detection [39]. The window of detection for commonly tested drugs is presented in Table 4.

The method chosen to detect a particular drug will depend on the reason for undertaking the test. Immunoassay drug tests are most commonly used. They are designed to classify substances as either present or absent and are generally highly sensitive. In pain management, specific drug identification using more sophisticated confirmatory tests is needed. Combined techniques such as GC/MS make accurate identification of a specific drug and/or its metabolites possible. When the patient is being prescribed drugs from several different classes of compounds, such as the case with many pain patients, specific identification is recommended. When properly used, these tests can help reduce cost, ensure accuracy and improve efficiency.

Immunoassay drug tests for natural opioids are very responsive to morphine and codeine, but do not distinguish between the two. UDT by immunoassay also shows a low sensitivity for semisynthetic/synthetic opioids such as

Table 4 Detection Time of Drugs in Urine

Drug	Approximate Retention Time
Amphetamines	48 hours
Barbiturates	Short acting (eg, secobarbital) 24 hours Long acting (eg, phenobarbital) 2–3 weeks
Benzodiazepines	3 days if therapeutic dose ingested Up to 4–6 weeks after extended dosage (ie, 1 or more years)
Cocaine (metab)	2–4 days
Ethanol	2–4 hours
Methadone	Approximately 3 days
Opiates	2 days
Propoxyphene	6–48 hours
Cannabinoids	Moderate smoker (4 times per week) 5 days Heavy smoker (smoking daily) 10 days Retention time for chronic smokers may be 20–28 days
Methaqualone	2 weeks
Phencyclidine	Approximately 8 days Up to 30 days in chronic users (mean value = 14 days)

Note: Interpretation of retention time must take into account variability of urine specimens, drug metabolism and half-life, patient's physical condition, fluid intake, and method and frequency of ingestion. These are general guidelines only.
Adapted from Vandevenne M, et al. Acta Clinica Belgica. 2000;55:323–33.

oxycodone and fentanyl [39,40]. A negative result does not exclude their use. Even though an immunoassay may be negative for consumed oxycodone, it should be positive on HPLC or GC/MS if the drug was used within the window of detection. The clinical importance of this fact with urine drug testing can not be overstated, since compliant patients may have been dismissed from pain management practices secondary to false-negative immunoassay test when looking specifically for prescribed oxycodone.

The synthetic opioid methadone will not be detected on a routine screening immunoassay drug panel unless specifically ordered [31]. The previous detection of a semisynthetic or synthetic drug does not ensure future detection, even when dose and dosing interval have not changed [30].

The presence of a prescribed drug in the urine sample makes monitoring of that class of drugs impossible by immunoassay technique alone. Specific drug identification by chromatographic testing (HPLC or GC/MS) is also necessary to identify which member of the detected class is responsible for the positive screen [30].

The clinician also must know the basic metabolism of opioids so he or she will be able to explain a urine drug test result that is positive for the prescribed opioid and/or its metabolite. For example, codeine is a prodrug that has no intrinsic analgesic activity but is metabolized to morphine for its analgesic properties Fig. 2.

The amount of drug and/or metabolite(s) (i.e., ng/dL) should not be used to extrapolate backward and make specific determinations regarding compliance

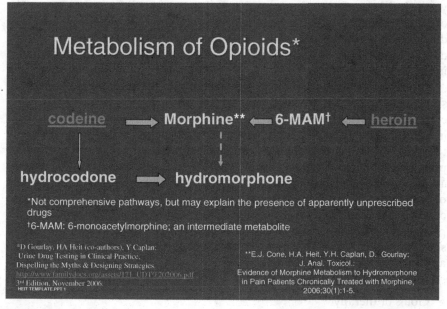

Fig. 2

of ingestion of the prescribed controlled substance. Software and laboratory products have not been fully scientifcally validated in the peer review literature to give this information at this time. Interpreting UDT beyond the current scientific knowledge may possibly put clinicians and patients at medical and/or legal risk [41].

Clinical urine drug testing, like any other medical test, must be used to improve quality of care [42]. Inappropriate interpretation of results may adversely affect clinical decisions; for example, discharge of patients from care when prescribed drugs are not detected (compliance testing) and over- or under diagnosis of addiction/misuse. Healthcare professionals should use UDT results in conjunction with other clinical information when deciding to continue with or adjust the established boundaries of the treatment plan.

A relationship of mutual honesty and trust between the clinician and patient is important when using urine drug testing. Well-thought-out testing strategies and accurate interpretation of results serve the interests of both patient and practitioners. Urine drug testing should be consensual; it should improve patient care and assist clinicians to advocate for their patients [30].

Opioid Agreements

Written opioid agreements facilitate informed consent, patient education and compliance in the management of chronic, noncancer pain [43]. A well-written agreement establishes the responsibilities of clinician to the patient and vice versa. It delineates the treatment plan and documents informed consent. The opioid agreement establishes boundaries and consequences for opioid misuse or diversion. Non-compliance with the agreement can aid in the diagnoses of the disease of addiction or substance-abuse relapse, which would require a change in the treatment plan.

Opioid agreements have the potential to improve the therapeutic relationship [43,44]. The agreement must be part of an environment of care that emphasizes truthful, open dialogue, and in which the process of agreement is fully individualized [44]. It often is easiest and entirely appropriate to simply tell patients that signed medication management agreements are practice policy for all patients taking chronic opioids. The agreement must be reasonable, readable and flexible [45]. In the past, such agreements often were called opioid contracts. Such agreements are not legal contracts, and it is better to call them medication management agreements than opioid contracts. Both the patient and clinicians should sign two copies of the agreement, and the patient should receive a copy. Effective agreements clearly define both the clinician's and the patient's responsibilities.

In general, well-written agreements contain the following elements: [43,44]

- Goals of therapy
- Single prescriber if possible

- Informed consent on all opioid risks
- Definition of addiction, tolerance and physical dependence
- Need for patient disclosure of substance abuse history; psychiatric history including history of sexual, physical or verbal abuse, and medications currently prescribed
- Need for complete, honest self-report of pain relief, side effects and function at each medical visit
- Establishment of regular medical visits
- Requirement for prescription renewal only during regular office hours
- Conditions of noncompliance (For example; evidence of drug hoarding or use of any illegal drug *may* cause termination of the clinician-patient relationship.)
- Use of the word *may* instead of *will* in the agreement, so clinical judgment can be used in each situation
- Patient consent to random urine drug tests and pill counts
- Permission for the practice to contact appropriate sources to obtain or provide information about the patient's care or actions
- Recovery program for substance abusers (Patients with a history of substance abuse must agree to start or continue recovery programs such as Alcoholics Anonymous or Narcotics Anonymous.)

Reality and Responsibility: The Treatment of Pain and Suffering in Our Society

There is a debate over whether opioids are "good" or "bad" and whether or not they should be available. The answer is that opioids are "good" when used appropriately and "bad" when they are abused. Of course they should be made available to the people who need them, but opioids should not be given to all pain patients in exactly the same fashion [45]. The chronic pain population is incredibly heterogeneous and varies tremendously in terms of vulnerability to addiction and abuse. The most effective and safest way to provide pain management is to make it available in a tailored and thoughtful way to reduce pain and suffering in an individualized fashion [45]. The best way to accomplish the goal of keeping opioids available to those who need them is for all of the stakeholders involved in legitimate opioid therapy to openly address the complexity of the issue and to do so in a collaborative way [45].

Major stakeholders in achieving an appropriate balance in the treatment of pain and the prevention of drug abuse and diversion are health professionals, patients, third-party payers, regulatory bodies, law enforcement, industry and the media. If these groups reconcile themselves to the need for thoughtful and unemotional dialogue, opioid treatment can remain available while efforts are made to stem the tide of prescription drug misuse and addiction. Everyone has a stake in this health, economic and social issue. We are all aging and many of us will have pain. Societal solutions are needed now so that we can all enjoy the comfort of knowing that safe and effective pain treatment will be there for us if we need it. It is the responsibility of all to make this a reality [45].

References

1. Verhaak PFM, Kerssens JJ, Dekker J, Sorbi MJ, Bensing JM. Prevalence of chronic benign pain disorder among adults: A review of the literature. Pain, 1998, 77:231–239.
2. Glajchen M, Fitzmartin RD, Blum D, et al. Psychosocial barriers to cancer pain relief. Cancer Practice, 1995, 3(2):76–82.
3. Ramer L, Richardson JL, Cohen MZ, et al. Multimeasure pain assessment in an ethnically diverse group of patients with cancer. Journal of Transcultural Nursing, 1999, 10(2):94–101.
4. Ward SE, Goldberg N, Miller-McCoulry V, et al. Patient-related barriers to management of cancer pain. Pain, 1993, 52:319–324.
5. Stewart WF, Ricci JA, Chee E, Morganstein D, Lipton R Lost Productive Time and Cost Due to Common Pain Conditions in the US Workforce. JAMA, 2003, 290:2443–2454.41.
6. Oaklander, A., The pathology of pain. Neuroscientist, 1999, 5(5):302–310.
7. Morgan JP. American opiophobia: customary underutilization of opioid analgesics. Advances in Alcohol & Substance Abuse, 1985, 5:163–73.
8. Pohl M. Pain. In Special Populations. 3rd ed. Principles of Addiction Medicine, Graham A et al, editors,Chevy Chase MD, American Society of Addiction Medicine, 2003.
9. Glajchen, M, Chronic pain: treatment barriers and strategies for clinical practice. Journal of American Board of Family Practice, 2001, 14(3):211–8.
10. Wise, R.A., Addiction becomes a brain disease. Neuron, 2000, 26(1): p. 27–33.
11. Acute Pain Management Guideline Panel. Acute Pain Management: Operative or Medical Procedures and Trauma; Clinical Practice Guideline. AHCPR Publication Number 92-0032, Rockville MD, Agency for Health Care Policy and Research, U.S. Department of Health and Human Services, Public Health Service, 1992.
12. Jacox A, Carr DB, Payne R, et al. Management of Cancer Pain. Clinical Practice Guideline. AHCPR Publication Number 94-0592, Rockville MD. Agency for Health Care Policy and Research, U.S. Department of Health and Human Services, Public Health Service, 1994.
13. Rosenblum A, Joseph H, Fong C, et al. Prevalence and characteristics of chronic pain among chemicallydependent patients in methadone maintenance and residential treatment facilities. JAMA, 2003, 289(18):2370–8.
14. Savage SR. Long-term opioid therapy: assessment of consequences and risks. Journal of Pain and Symptom Management, 1996, 11(5):274–86.
15. Wassan AD, Correll DJ, Kissin I, O'Shea S, Jamison RN. Iatrogengenic addiction inpatients treated for acute or subacute pain. Journal of Opioid Management, 2006, 2(1): Jan./Feb.:16–21
16. Passik SD, Weinreb HJ. Managing chronic nonmalignant pain: overcoming obstacles to the use of opioids. Advances in Therapy, 2000, 17(2):70–83.
17. Compton, P. and G. Gebhart, The Neurophysiology of Pain and Interfaces with Addiction, in Principles of Addiction Medicine, A. Graham, et al., Editors. 2003, American Society of Addiction Medicine: Chevy Chase, MD. pp. 1385–1404.
18. Hoffman NG, Chang AJ, Lewis DC. Medical student attitudes toward drug addiction policy. Journal of Addictive Diseases, 2000, 19(3):1–12.

19. Heit HA. Addiction, physical dependence, and tolerance: precise definitions to help clinicians evaluate and treat chronic pain patients. Journal of Pain & Palliative Care Pharmacotherapy, 2003, 17(1):15–29.
20. Battin MP, Luna E, Lipman AG et al. Drugs and Justice: Seeking a Consistent, Coherent, Comprehensive View. NY, Oxford University Press, 2007.
21. Heit HA, Gourlay D. Chronic Pain and Addiction. In Chronic Abdominal and Visceral Pain: Theory and Practice. Pasricha PJ, Willis WD, Gebhart GF, editors, NY. Taylor and Francis, 2006.
22. Gourlay D, Heit HA, Almahrezi A. Universal precautions in pain medicine: a rational approach to the treatment of chronic pain. Pain Medicine, 2005, 6(2):107–12.
23. American Academy of Pain Medicine, American Pain Society, and American Society of Addiction Medicine. Definitions Related to the Use of Opioids for the Treatment of Pain, Glenview, IL, American Academy of Pain Medicine, 2001.
24. SR Savage, DE Joranson, EC Covington, SH Schnoll, HA Heit, AM Gilson. Definitions Related to the Medical Use of Opioids: Evolution Towards Universal Agreement. Journal of Pain and Symptom Management, 2003, 26(1):655–67.
25. Weissman DE, Haddox JD. Opioid pseudoaddiction – an iatrogenic syndrome. Pain, 1989, 36(3):363–6.
26. Pappagallo M., The concept of pseudotolerance to opioids. Journal of Pharmaceutical Care in Pain and Symptom Control, 1998, 6:95–8.
27. Lipman AG, Jackson KC. Opioids. In Warfield C, Bajwa Z, editors, Principles and Practice of Pain Management, 2nd edition, New York, McGraw Hill, 2003.
28. Fakata KL, Lipman AG. Opioid Bowel Dysfunction in Acute and Chronic Non-malignant Pain. In Yuan S-H, editor, Opioid Bowel Dysfunction, Binghamton NY, Haworth Medical Press, 2004.
29. Diagnostic and Statistical Manual of Mental Disorders – Text Revised, 4th edition, Washington DC, American Psychiatric Association, 2000.
30. Heit HA, Gourlay D. Urine drug testing in pain medicine. Journal of Pain and Symptom Management, 2004, 27(3):260–7.
31. Gourlay D, Heit HA, Caplan YH. Urine Drug Testing in Primary Care: Dispelling the Myths & Designing Strategies. San Francisco, California Academy of Family Physicians, 2006.
32. Passik SD, Schreiber J, Kirsh KL, Portenoy RK. A chart review of the ordering and documentation of urine toxicology screens in a cancer center: do they influence patient management? Journal of Pain and Symptom Management, 2000, 19:40–4.
33. Caplan YH, Goldberger BA. Alternative specimens for workplace drug testing. Journal of Analytical Toxicology, 2001, 25:396–399.
34. Conigliaro C, Reyes CR, Schultz JS. Principles of screening and early intervention. In: Graham AW, Schultz TK, Mayo-Smith M, Ries RK, Wilford BB, eds. Principles of addiction medicine, third edition. Chevy Chase, MD: American Society of Addiction Medicine, 2003, 323–1
35. Vandevenne M, Vandenbussche H, Verstraete A. Detection time of drugs of abuse in urine. Acta Clinica Belgica, 2000, 55:323–333.
36. Cook JD, Caplan YH, LoDico CP, Bush DM. The characterization of human urine for specimen validity determination in workplace drug testing: a review. Journal of Analytical Toxicology, 2000, 24:579–588.
37. Casavant MJ. Urine drug screening in adolescents. Pediatric Clinics of North America, 2002, 49:317–327.
38. Huestis MA, Mitchell JM, Cone EJ. Detection times of marijuana metabolites in urine by immunoassay and GC–MS. Journal of Analytical Toxicology, 1995, 19:443–44.
39. Simpson D, Braithwaite RA, Jarvie DR, et al. Screening for drugs of abuse (II): cannabinoids, lysergic acid diethylamide, buprenorphine, methadone, barbiturates, benzodiazepines and other drugs. Annals of Clinical Biochemistry, 1997, 34:460–510.
40. Shults TF, St. Clair, S. The Medical Review Officer Handbook. 7th ed. Research Triangle Park NC. Quadrangle Research, 1999.

41. MROALERT November 6 Vol. XVII; No. 9(1–4)
42. American Academy of Pain Management, American Pain Society. The use of opioids for the treatment of chronic pain. Consensus Statement, 1996. www.ampainsoc.org.
43. Fishman SM, Bandman TB, Edwards A, et al. The opioid contract in the management of chronic pain. Journal of Pain and Symptom Management, 1999, 18:27–37.
44. Heit HA. Creating and Implementing Opioid Agreements. Disease Management Digest, 2003, 7(1):2–3, in: Care Management, 2003, 9
45. Passik SD, Heit HA, Kirsh KL. Reality and Responsibility: A Commentary on the Treatment of Pain and Suffering in a Drug-Using Society. Journa of Opioid Management, 2006, 2(3):1–5.

The Use of Complementary and Alternative Medicine for Pain

Catherine M. Stoney, Dawn Wallerstedt, Jamie M. Stagl, and Patrick Mansky

Complementary and Alternative Medicine (CAM) refers to those medical and health care practices, modalities, products, and treatments which are not integrated into conventional medicine in the United States. CAM practices and modalities which are used in conjunction with conventional medical care are considered to be complementary, while those practices and modalities used in place of conventional medicine are considered to be alternative. In both cases, data regarding safety and efficacy are generally not fully available.

Among the 27 institutes and centers at the National Institutes of Health (NIH) is the National Center for Complementary and Alternative Medicine (NCCAM). NCCAM is responsible for sponsoring intramural and extramural research on various CAM modalities for a variety of conditions and populations.

NCCAM defines CAM as those practices falling into four discrete domains or areas of interest.

Biologically active products and practices refer to the use of herbs, foods, and vitamins for health purposes. Examples include the use of dietary supplements, herbal products, and probiotics to promote health and treat various diseases.

Energy Therapies use energy fields in the treatment of disease. CAM energy therapies include biofield therapies, such as Reiki, as well as electromagnetic therapies, such as the use of magnetic fields.

Mind Body Medicine refers to those practices which enhance the ability of the mind and psychological processes to affect the body. Some mind-body medicine practices include the many varieties of meditation, yoga, Tai Chi, hypnosis, and some forms of art and music therapy.

Manipulative and Body-based Practices include practices and procedures which manipulate one or more parts of the body. Chiropractic care, osteopathic manipulation, and massage are all example of manipulative and body-based practices.

C.M. Stoney (✉)
National Center for Complementary and Alternative Medicine, National Institutes of Health, 6707 Democracy Blvd, Suite 401, Bethesda, MD 20892, USA
e-mail: Stoneyc@mail.nih.gov

R.J. Moore (ed.), *Biobehavioral Approaches to Pain*,
DOI 10.1007/978-0-387-78323-9_16, © Springer Science+Business Media, LLC 2009

In addition, NCCAM also considers studies of whole medical systems which have developed from discrete theoretical frameworks, and which can incorporate a variety of different CAM modalities, as CAM. These systems include Traditional Chinese Medicine (TCM), Ayurveda, anthroposophical medicine, naturopathic, and homeopathic medicine. Some practices within these whole medical systems, when conducted in isolation, might fall into one of the four categories above. For example, acupuncture, one technique used frequently in the practice of Traditional Chinese Medicine, is thought to operate by releasing Qi, or the vital energy of the body. Thus, acupuncture might be considered to be a type of energy therapy.

Practices and modalities that are considered CAM do and will change over time as more data become available regarding safety and efficacy of these practices, and as those practices identified as safe and effective become more fully integrated into conventional medical care. Once integrated into conventional care, these practices are generally no longer considered to be CAM.

Individuals who are living with chronic and debilitating conditions, particularly those which are resistant to conventional treatments, are increasingly turning toward CAM modalities for symptomatic relief. Data from the 2002 National Health Interview Survey (NHIS), which included specific questions regarding CAM usage, provides health information of a representative sampling of the US adult civilian population. The 2002 survey data, sampling 36,161 households consisting of 93,386 individuals, indicated that the most frequent conditions for which CAM practices of a variety of types are used in the United States are back pain, colds, neck pain, joint pain, mood disorders, and anxiety. In fact, 33% of all health reasons cited for CAM use were for pain-related conditions, including back, neck and joint pain, migraine, and other forms of recurring pain (Barnes, Powell-Griner, McFann & Nahin, 2004). Among chronic pain patients using long-term opioid therapy, CAM use was reported by 44% of patients, and all therapies were reported to be beneficial in relieving pain by well over half of the patients using them (Fleming, Rabago, Mundt, & Fleming, 2007). Other sources have surveyed use of CAM practices among pediatric pain patients, but the estimates of CAM use in children and adolescents show considerable variation from one survey to another (Davis & Darden, 2003; Hodgson, Nakamura, & Walker, 2007; Tsao & Zeltzer, 2005). Nonetheless, it is clear that the use of CAM practices for pain conditions in both adults and children in the United States is relatively common. Despite the relatively wide-spread use of CAM practices for the alleviation of pain, research investigating the efficacy and the mechanisms of action of CAM therapies in pain management is not equally extensive and results are generally not definitive.

Not all CAM domains, as identified and conceptualized by the National Center for Complementary and Alternative Medicine (NCCAM) at the National Institutes of Health (NIH), have been tested with regard to their potential pain-relieving qualities. Indeed, the domains most frequently tested are manipulative and body-based therapies, some of the variety of mind-body medicine therapies, and energy medicine therapies. Even among these broad categories of CAM domains, not all specific techniques have been explored in the context of pain. For example, while studies of hypnosis and relaxation, two mind-body medicine approaches, have frequently been employed in studies testing efficacy for pain, relatively few investigations of other mind-body medicine techniques, such as meditation, have been systematically tested for their pain relieving qualities.

This chapter will focus on those CAM modalities for which the most investigations have been employed, such as massage, acupuncture, Reiki, hypnosis, yoga, and Tai Chi. Other CAM domains, such as the use of biologically-based products, including herbal products, supplements and vitamins, have some available data, but not sufficient data to be meaningful in a review such as this. Investigations of chiropractic for the relief of pain will not be reviewed here because there are extensive reviews of this modality which already exist (Hawk, Khorsan, Lisi, Ferrance, & Evans, 2007).

Manipulative and Body-Based CAM Therapies for Pain

Massage

Massage therapy is a form of manual therapy which is applied by the hands of a massage therapist to either a single or multiple areas of the body. There are many massage practices, including Swedish massage, Rolfing, Reflexology, and others. In the United States and elsewhere, massage, particularly Swedish massage, is in widespread clinical use for the management and alleviation of both chronic and acute pain, particularly low back and neck pain. Most investigations of massage for pain focus on patient populations with discrete or single pain conditions, such as low back pain, neck pain, or fibromyalgia (Ezzo et al., 2007). The analgesic effects of massage therapy for complex or multiple pain conditions is less well studied and these conditions are generally more difficult to effectively treat. The exception is the increasingly widespread use of massage therapy in clinical practice for decreasing pain and improving quality of life among cancer patients (Calenda, 2006).

Recent reviews have indicated significant evidence for the positive benefits of massage therapy for the relief of chronic low back pain (Furlan, Brosseau, Imamura, & Irvin, 2002), while evidence for the effectiveness of massage therapy for other pain conditions, including headache, shoulder and neck pain, carpal tunnel syndrome, cancer-related pain, and pain due to fibromyalgia, is less compelling (Moyer, Rounds, & Hannum, 2004; Tsao, 2007). A systematic review of investigations of massage for neck pain concluded that the heterogeneity of treatments and poor overall methodological quality of the research in this area precluded conclusions being drawn (Ezzo et al., 2007), and specifically recommended the need for high-quality studies of the optimal frequency and duration of massage for neck pain. A recent meta-analysis (Moyer, Rounds, & Hannum, 2004) echoes this suggestion with the observation that several sessions of massage therapy can have significant effects on a variety of discrete pain conditions over a period of time, but the beneficial effects are not apparent immediately and only emerge after time and multiple massage treatments. The overall conclusions from these reviews suggest that the dose (number of sessions as well as the duration and frequency of sessions) of massage may be an important factor to consider when evaluating the potential for pain relief. Unfortunately, the literature in this area has not systematically evaluated optimal dosing in relation to massage therapy.

In the case of low back pain, massage in combination with conventional therapeutic exercise may be more effective than either therapy alone. This suggestion illustrates the need for the systematic investigation of CAM therapies used in conjunction with established, albeit only partially effective, conventional treatment (that is, therapies used to *complement* conventional treatment). Although CAM therapies are frequently used in such a complementary fashion, they are less frequently researched in this manner, despite the fact that these combined treatments may be the most effective strategy to enhance our ability to clinically treat and manage pain.

Although the mechanisms that operate during massage therapy for the relief of pain are not completely understood, there are data showing that massage can stimulate the endogenous opiate system, as well as stimulate the release of oxytocin (Furlan et al., 2002). As with other therapies, understanding the biological and psychological mechanisms of action that operate to alleviate pain with massage therapy is a crucial step towards optimizing the massage intervention, and basic science studies in this area are needed.

Mind-Body Medicine CAM Therapies for Pain

CAM practices considered to fall into the category of mind-body medicine includes various forms of meditation, such as mindfulness-based meditation, Tai Chi, yoga, mantra meditation, and Transcendental Meditation[TM]; hypnosis and guided imagery; and certain forms of art, music, and dance therapies. Among the most commonly used mind-body medicine CAM therapies for pain include hypnosis and guided imagery, and various meditative techniques, such as yoga, meditation and Tai Chi.

Hypnosis and Imagery

Hypnosis has been used frequently as an alternative type of intervention for pain relief, in addition to being used in a complementary fashion, in conjunction with conventional (primarily pharmacological) pain treatments. Hypnosis consists of an hypnotic induction induced by a trained therapist, followed by suggestions for the relief of pain, and then guidance of the patient out of the hypnotic state. Hypnotic inductions can be self-induced among individuals with adequate hypnotic ability after they are given sufficient guided training. When used for discrete pain, it is sometimes termed focused hypnotic analgesia because the hypnotic focus is targeted toward a specific area of the body (Sharav & Tal, 2006). Although there is substantial disagreement within the field regarding the psychological, physiological, cognitive, and neural changes that occur during hypnosis, the practice is used widely and with significant success for the alleviation of pain. One theory of hypnosis posits that an altered state of consciousness occurs during hypnosis, while other theories suggest that attentional and cognitive changes explain the hypnotic state (Raz, 2005). In the later case, hypnosis may operate by reallocating attention elsewhere or by distraction. Increasingly, research has focused on the neural underpinnings of the hypnotic state. For instance, recent studies suggest that hypnosis may involve brain activation via dopaminergic pathways (Lichtenberg, Bachner-Melman, Gritsenko, & Ebstein, 2000; Montgomery et al., 2007; Raz, 2005; Spiegel, 2007).

A significant body of research has tested the analgesic effects of hypnosis for both chronic and acute pain conditions, with the majority of the available literature suggesting that hypnosis can be efficacious for pain, and many studies suggesting that the analgesic effects can be sustained for several months to a year (Jensen & Patterson, 2006). With regard to acute pain, hypnosis has been quite effectively used for the control of pain associated with labor (Brown & Hammond, 2007; Smith, Collins, Cyna, & Crowther, 2006), medical procedural pain (Lang et al., 2006; Montgomery et al, 2007; Spiegel, 2007), and dental pain. However, the literature in this area is incomplete, the studies are small, and there are significant questions that remain regarding the efficacy and specificity of hypnosis for acute pain relief. For example, the extent to which hypnosis is superior to distraction strategies for acute pain is still unclear.

For chronic pain conditions, somewhat more and better-controlled studies are available demonstrating that hypnosis can diminish pain that results from a variety of chronic pain conditions, such as fibromyalgia (Haanen et al., 1991), cancer pain (Elkins, Cheung, Marcus, Palamara, & Rajab, 2004), and chronic low back pain (Spinhoven & Linssen, 1989). However, in some investigations of hypnosis for chronic pain, hypnosis is found to be equivalent and not superior to comparison conditions such as health education or physical therapy (Elkins, Jensen, & Patterson, 2007), raising questions regarding the specificity of the effects of hypnosis.

Significant individual differences in response to hypnosis are typically apparent and thus hypnosis is not appropriate for all individuals with pain (Benham, Woody, Wilson, & Nash, 2006). These individual differences are most likely due to how effectively some people can be hypnotized and how vividly images can be imagined. In addition, although most investigations of a variety of pain conditions have demonstrated hypnosis to be superior to wait-list or attention control, the data are more mixed when comparing hypnosis to relaxation techniques for pain relief (Gay, Philippot, Luminet, 2002; Patterson & Jensen, 2003). For example, when comparing hypnotically-induced imaginative suggestions with nonhypnotic imaginative suggestions for pain relief, there were no differences in the amount of pain relief reported by those experiencing experimentally-induced acute pain (Milling, Kirsch, Allen, & Reutenauer, 2005). Thus, it is likely that at least part of the analgesic effect of hypnosis for acute pain may be due to expectancy for relief, suggesting that control groups for studies of hypnosis must be carefully considered. Finally, as noted above, the neural mechanisms by which hypnosis operates to modify pain are still not well understood. Taken together, the research to date clearly indicates that hypnosis can be considered an effective treatment for many types of pain for those individuals who are able to be hypnotized. The mechanisms by which hypnosis exerts its effects on pain are not well-studied, but the fact that pain relief is similar between hypnosis and relaxation and imagery suggests that at least some of the pain relieving properties of hypnosis are a function of the relaxation component of hypnosis, the allocation of attention, and/or the expectation for relief.

Guided imagery is a procedure that combines relaxation, focusing of attention, breathing, and visualization of an image. The nature of the image can vary according to the characteristics of the patient and complaint, from a relaxing and pleasant "picture", to a focused image related to a disease or body part. Guided imagery is often conducted with a trained therapist or other individual, but, once learned, can also be practiced individually with the use of audiotapes. Imagery is often used in conjunction with hypnosis and relaxation therapies, in part to enhance the pain-relieving abilities of those therapies. Because relaxation is an important step in initiating a guided imagery session, a specific relaxation technique is commonly practiced at the beginning of each session, such as progressive muscle relaxation.

Guided imagery has been studied as a pain-relieving therapy in a number of conditions and patient populations. In particular, guided imagery has produced promising results when tested among children (Russell & Smart, 2007) and older adults (Morone & Greco, 2007) with procedural and chronic pain. For example, guided imagery among older women with osteoarthritis pain resulted in increased quality of life (with presumably decreased pain; Baird & Sands, 2006). However, many of the same issues outlined above regarding studies examining hypnosis for the relief of pain are also considerations for the study of guided imagery. Thus, well-designed and well-controlled studies are needed to identify the specific elements of and mechanisms by which guided imagery produces its effects on pain.

Yoga

Many forms of yoga are practiced for a variety of physical and mental health conditions, as well as to enhance overall well-being. Yoga typically includes specific breathing exercises, as well as specific physical activity movements or postures, and also can (although not always) include a meditation component. While yoga has traditionally been practiced to relax and rejuvenate, it is now being used for a wide variety of medical conditions, including pain. Despite the fairly wide-spread use of yoga for many pain conditions, only minimal research has investigated the efficacy of yoga to reduce pain, and improve strength and mobility. Data regarding the analgesic mechanisms by which yoga confers these effects is almost non-existent.

There have been a few studies examining the effects of yoga specifically for chronic low back pain (Galantino et al., 2004; Jacobs et al., 2004; Sherman, Cherkin, Erro, Miglioretti, & Deyo, 2005; Williams et al., 2005), and most have reported some positive benefits of yoga. However, the design of the majority of these studies has limited the conclusions that can be drawn regarding the mechanisms by which yoga may be operating to reduce pain; for example, it is not clear how much of the benefit of yoga is derived solely from the exercise component of this therapy. Since physical exercise is generally considered a standard treatment for chronic low back pain, a better understanding of how yoga may improve low back pain above and beyond what is already known to be effective would require the inclusion of a standard exercise group. This is exactly what was tested in a recent study of yoga for chronic back pain (Sherman et al., 2005). As with previous investigations, this study demonstrated that yoga was more effective than was a self-care book for individuals with chronic back pain, and that the beneficial effects persisted for 14 weeks post completion of the intervention (Sherman, et al., 2005). Interestingly, this study also included a third arm, consisting of standard therapeutic exercises for back pain. Although the yoga group showed somewhat more improvement in Roland Disability Scale scores during and following treatment relative to the standard exercise group, these differences were not clinically or statistically significant. While yoga is apparently safe and effective for chronic low back pain, it may not confer any demonstrable benefit over and above standard therapeutic exercises already known to be effective for chronic low back pain. However, as patients with chronic low back pain are particularly interested in exploring CAM treatment modalities (Sherman et al., 2004), there may be individuals who prefer yoga over conventional therapeutic exercises (Jacobs et al., 2004). It is important to point out that the various styles of yoga have not been adequately studied in the context of chronic low back pain. Given the evidence for pain relief demonstrated in the above noted studies, it may be beneficial to conduct more systematic and rigorous investigations testing the efficacy and mechanisms of various forms of yoga for chronic back pain.

Yoga has also been tested, albeit less frequently, among patients with other pain conditions. For example, yoga for osteoarthritis of the knee (Kolasinski et al., 2005) and hands (Garfinkel, Schumacher, Husain, Levy, & Reshetar, 1994) was found to be moderately effective in reducing perceived pain, functional capacity and/or local tenderness. However, an understanding of the optimal dose, the mechanism of effects, and the duration of the effects of yoga on pain await future investigation.

Meditation

Meditation practices vary widely with regard to the specific features of the techniques, but share the common feature of allocating or training attention and level of awareness, often using various breathing or other anchoring strategies, such as repetition of a word or mantra (Meditation Practices for Health: State of the Research, 2007). Meditation has been studied as a means of enhancing quality of life, promoting well-being, and for addressing health concerns including hypertension, substance abuse, and mental health disorders (Arias, Steinberg, Banga, & Trestman, 2006; Grossman, Niemann, Schmidt & Walach, 2004). Clinically, meditation is also sometimes used for pain management, although the literature studying the efficacy and mechanisms of meditation for pain is not extensive. In the context of pain management, meditation is thought to operate by refocusing awareness of pain and responses to pain, by inducing a relaxed and peaceful state, and/or by promoting physiological changes such as alterations in inflammatory processes which may, in turn, lead to diminished pain.

Several early investigations of mindfulness-based stress reduction (MBSR) identified this type of meditation as effective for chronic and remitting pain patients (Kabat-Zinn, Lipworth, & Burney, 1985; Kabat-Zinn, Lipworth, Burney, & Sellers, 1986). In addition, studies employing a combined intervention of a mindfulness-type of meditation, along with other mind-body and psychoeducational components, reported significant reductions in pain ratings among chronic back pain patients (Berman & Singh, 1997). However, more recent investigations have failed to demonstrate a specific and superior analgesic effect of various forms of meditation for low back pain (Mehling, Hamel, Acree, Byl & Hecht, 2005), pain due to fibromyalgia (Astin et al., 2003), and gastrointestinal pain (Keefer & Blanchard, 2001), relative to educational, active, and/or support control groups. Some of these reports, however, did demonstrate pain reductions among the meditation group that were of a similar magnitude to the other, conventional treatments (Mehling et al., 2005). One reported positive effects of meditation on other symptoms, but not pain (Keefer & Blanchard, 2001). Taken together, there is only limited evidence that meditative practices can provide specific analgesic effects among chronic pain patients. However, meditative practices vary dramatically in terms of the specific elements of the practice and none have been systematically investigated with regard to potential pain-relieving qualities.

Tai-Chi and Qi Gong

Beginning as a martial art form in China during the 12 century, Tai Chi (also referred to as Tai Chi Chuan or Taiji) is a form of physical exercise combined with a meditative component and specific breathing exercises. Tai Chi encompasses a series of movements and postures which can be practiced in group settings or individually. Traditional Chinese Medicine identifies pain and illness as the result of an imbalance, blockage, or interruption of "Qi ," the Chinese term for vital energy (Mansky et al., 2006). Tai Chi is proposed to reestablish the flow of Qi to maximize health and provide pain relief. Traditional Chinese Medicine promotes Tai Chi's harmonious effect on two opposing life forces, yin (water) and yang (fire), for optimal (well-being) and physical functioning. The pain-relieving qualities of Tai Chi have been studied among patients with a number of chronic pain conditions such as chronic back pain and pain due to arthritis (Klein & Adams, 2004).

Several investigations have examined the effects of Tai Chi on arthritic pain. For example, a randomized clinical study (Adler, Good, Roberts, & Snyder, 2000) of the effect of Tai Chi on joint pain in a small group of adults with chronic arthritic conditions found those that participants who were randomized to the Tai Chi group and practiced Tai Chi once a week over a ten week study period had a significant decrease in reported joint pain intensity, relative to those who were asked to maintain their normal daily activities. A similar investigation of a small group of elderly patients with pain due to osteoarthritis of the knee also found regular Tai Chi practice over the course of several months demonstrated significant and long-lasting pain relief, relative to a health education control group (Brismee et. al., 2007). Finally, in a study comparing Tai Chi with a group who received phone contact for pain due to osteoarthritis (Song, Lee, Lam & Bae, 2003), 72 women 55 years and older were randomized into one of the two groups and participated in a 12 week study. Joint pain and stiffness were improved with Tai Chi practice compared to the telephone contact control group.

While these studies provide some initial evidence for the pain-relieving effects of Tai Chi for arthritis pain, the studies are generally small and the effects of Tai Chi are compared with a wait list or no-treatment control group. In a more stringent study design, the potential superiority of Tai Chi over an active treatment was examined (Fransen, Nairn, Winstanley, Lam, & Edmonds, 2007). One hundred and fifty-two older persons with painful hip or knee osteoarthritis were randomly assigned to one of three study arms, including Tai Chi, hydrotherapy, and a wait list control group. Participants assigned to the two active arms practiced twice weekly. After a twelve week study period both the Tai Chi and hydrotherapy groups reported improvements in physical function and reductions in pain, although the magnitude of the pain reduction was only significant for the hydrotherapy group. Thus, Tai Chi was less efficacious for pain reduction among these older arthritic patients than was hydrotherapy, but equally effective for improving physical function.

Despite the fact that the bulk of research on Tai Chi has compared those receiving Tai Chi to only wait list or no treatment control groups, there is a promising suggestion that Tai Chi may be an effective strategy to manage chronic pain and improve physical functioning. Considering the low stress, meditative nature of the practice, Tai Chi may be particularly beneficial for pain management and treatment among those who may be candidates for physical therapy but who cannot tolerate high impact physical exercise.

Qi Gong (Qi-gong) is a traditional Chinese practice which has become increasingly recognized in the United States and other westernized countries as contributing to the enhancement of well-being and decreasing stress. Qi Gong involves concentration and relaxation exercises with special breathing techniques to promote Qi (vital energy force) circulation in the body. It is similar to Tai Chi in that they both involve a proscribed set of gentle exercises, with a focus on meditation and relaxation, but Qi Gong also incorporates specific breathing techniques. Recently, there is the new term, medical Qi Gong, which refers to the application of Qi Gong specifically to health. External Qi Gong refers to a Qi Gong master exerting personal Qi to heal a disease, and internal Qi Gong refers to the practitioner using Qi Gong for self-healing or maintaining health. Among elderly patients with significant chronic pain conditions, external Qi Gong was reported to significantly improve reports of pain compared to usual care (Yang, Kim, & Lee, 2005). However, studies of Qi Gong require comparison groups that allow appropriate control for any effects that may be due to interaction with a practitioner, which in some cases may be significant and may in itself have clinically important effects on reports of pain. Although Qi Gong and Tai Chi have many common features, there are many fewer studies of Qi Gong for the alleviation of pain.

Energy Medicine

Reiki

Reiki is an energy healing practice which originated 2,500 years ago from Buddhism. The Japanese term "Reiki" stems from "rei," which means "universal spirit," and "ki," meaning "life energy." Reiki aims to heal and maximize well-being by establishing a mind and body balance and restoring energy flow. According to Reiki's concepts, physical and mental pain are the results of energy deficiency which can be relieved by channeling energy to areas of pain. Practitioners can guide energy by directly touching a clothed patient or by positioning their hands at a 1–2 inch distance from the skin for several minutes. Individuals receiving Reiki may feel a warm, tingling, relaxing sensation while practitioners feel heat in their hands.

There is limited but promising evidence that Reiki may be effective for pain management in acute, post-operative pain. For example, one recent quasi-experimental study measured the effect of Reiki on pain in 22 women undergoing abdominal hysterectomies (Vitale & O'Connor, 2006). The women were randomly assigned to either standard nursing care or standard care complimented by Reiki; those in the Reiki group initially reported a more significant decline in pain than did those in the control group. However, the group differences disappeared within a few days. Thus, although the data suggest that Reiki plus nursing care is more effective than nursing care alone initially, the longer-term benefit of Reiki on surgery-related analgesia is questionable. A study of Reiki for post-operative dental pain examined the effect of Reiki in combination with LeShan healing on postoperative pain (Wirth, Brenlan, Levine, & Rodriguez, 1993). Twenty-one volunteers underwent two surgeries, two weeks apart, for removal of impacted third molar teeth. All participants were given pharmacologic analgesia; the experimental group received Reiki and LeShan healing in addition. In this crossover study design, volunteers became their own controls in the second surgery. Reiki and LeShan healers alternated treating the volunteer beginning at 3 hours post surgery. Postoperative pain intensity was more substantially reduced in the Reiki/LeShan healing group, relative to the pharmacologic control group, suggesting that Reiki (at least in conjunction with LeShan healing) is effective for decreasing acute, postoperative dental pain.

Reiki has also been examined in relation to chronic pain conditions. For example, among HIV patients with disease-related pain, Reiki practice resulted in a significant drop in pain intensity (Miles, 2003). Among cancer patients with pain, Reiki therapy plus pharmacotherapy for pain (opioids) compared with pharmacotherapy alone resulted in a statistically greater decline in pain (Olson, Hanson, & Michaud, 2003). Finally, a randomized, placebo controlled study evaluated Reiki healing in 207 Type II diabetic subjects with painful neuropathy. Subjects were randomized into either the Reiki group, the sham Reiki group, or the usual care control group. This twelve week study period consisted of 2 treatments in the first week, and weekly treatments thereafter. Pain was measured according to the McGill Pain Questionnaire, which found a statistically significant decrease in pain for both the Reiki and sham Reiki groups, and not the control group. Because there were no significant differences found between real Reiki and mimic Reiki compared to the control (Gillespie, Gillespie, & Stevens, 2007), the mechanisms by which Reiki has pain relieving qualities are probably due to attentional or social support factors.

There is limited preliminary evidence that Reiki may provide analgesia for both acute and chronic pain conditions. However, as with many other CAM modalities for pain, large, well-designed studies are lacking and several significant design limitations exist in the studies which are available. Problems with substantial and/or differential attrition rates are particularly problematic in Reiki investigations, and the lack of information regarding mechanisms of action, optimal dosing, timing, and frequency of Reiki to treat pain significantly limit conclusions that can be drawn.

Acupuncture

Acupuncture, a component of Traditional Chinese Medicine (TCM), involves the insertion of thin needles into set anatomical points (acupuncture points) in the body in order to balance Qi or the vital energy of the body. These acupuncture points are located on meridians, along which Qi is thought to circulate throughout the body. After insertion, needles are typically manually stimulated (referred to as "needling"). In addition to needling, acupuncture points can also be stimulated with heat, mild electrical currents, pressure, herbs and herbal extracts, which can be injected or burned at the end of the needle (moxibustion), and laser light (Ernst, 2006; Lao, 1996).

Relief of musculoskeletal pain is one of the most common reasons that Americans seek treatment by acupuncture practitioners (Burke, Upchurch, Dye & Chyu, 2006). An often-cited 1997 NIH Consensus statement concluded that acupuncture has potential benefits in the alleviation of post-operative dental pain, headache, tennis elbow, fibromyalgia, myofascial pain, osteoarthritis, low back pain, and carpal tunnel syndrome (NIH Consensus Panel – Acupuncture, 1997), but the data are inconsistent. Since the time of the Consensus panel, numerous randomized controlled trials (RCTs) have subsequently been conducted in populations with chronic musculoskeletal pain, including low back, elbow, neck, knee, and shoulder pain. Systematic reviews and meta-analyses of these clinical studies of acupuncture for analgesia have concluded that there is mixed evidence for the efficacy of acupuncture. For example, a review of 51 studies of acupuncture for the treatment of chronic pain indicated that slightly fewer than half demonstrated evidence for efficacy, while the remaining were either neutral or reported ambiguous findings (Ezzo et al., 2000). This review suggests that the effects of acupuncture for pain are not uniform across patient population, dose, and pain condition, and the studies in this area vary widely with regard to methodological quality. While the overall conclusions across all pain conditions examined in this review are that there is only limited evidence that acupuncture is more effective than no treatment, placebo, sham acupuncture (e.g., superficial needling at non-acupuncture sites or needle insertion with no needling), and standard care, it is perhaps most informative to review the evidence for acupuncture separately by pain condition.

Low back pain. A review of several investigations of acupuncture for the treatment of low back pain suggests that acupuncture may be more effective than either no treatment or sham acupuncture (Furlan et al., 2005) for chronic back pain, but insufficient studies are available to draw conclusions regarding acute back pain. In addition, although the effects were significant among chronic back pain patients, they dissipated rather rapidly after treatment. An additional review of 10 randomized controlled trials that compared acupuncture, massage therapy, and spinal manipulation for the treatment of chronic back pain concluded that acupuncture was more effective than no intervention or sham treatment, but less effective than massage (Cherkin, Sherman, Deyo, & Shekelle, 2003). Thus, there is no compelling evidence that acupuncture is more effective than other treatments (both conventional and CAM) for the alleviation of chronic low back pain, and modest evidence that acupuncture may be more effective for this condition relative to no treatment.

Elbow pain. Lateral epicondoyle pain, commonly known as 'tennis elbow', has been the subject of several clinical research studies of acupuncture. An initial review of the literature suggested that acupuncture may result in short-term (e.g., less than 24 hours) pain reduction for lateral epicondoyle pain, but at that time there are only a very few small studies available (Green, Buchbinder, & Hetrick, 2005). In a more recent review, 53 studies of acupuncture for epicondoyle pain were identified, although only a small subset were considered to be of sufficient quality to merit inclusion in the review. Nonetheless, this review concluded that acupuncture treatment was more effective than either the control condition or sham acupuncture in the majority of the studies examined (Trinh, Phillips, Ho & Damsma, 2004).

Neck pain. In a recent Cochrane systematic review of 10 RCTs in which acupuncture was used as a treatment intervention in adult populations with chronic neck pain, Trinh et al. found evidence of acupuncture's effectiveness. For chronic mechanical neck disorders, including whiplash-associated disorders, myofascial neck pain, and degenerative changes, this review found moderate evidence of acupuncture's effectiveness in the following three areas: when compared to needling at sham points immediately after treatment; when compared to inactive, sham treatments immediately after treatment and at short-term follow-up; and when compared to a wait-list control at short-term follow-up (Trinh et al., 2006).

Knee pain. A systematic review and meta-analysis of 13 RCTs in which acupuncture was used as an intervention in reducing pain and improving function in patients with chronic knee pain reported that acupuncture was significantly superior to sham acupuncture in both short- and long-term pain reduction and improved function (White, Foster, Cummings, & Barlas, 2007). This effect persisted even when one strongly positive study and when one lower quality study were excluded from the analysis. Although this review provides promising evidence for the efficacy of acupuncture for knee pain, as with many other studies of CAM modalities for pain, more carefully designed and controlled trials are necessary before clinical recommendations can be suggested. However, because the evidence for efficacy among conventional treatments for chronic knee pain is weak, this is one population for whom acupuncture for pain relief may be particularly effective (White, Foster, Cummings, & Barlas, 2007).

Headache. Acupuncture is frequently used clinically for the treatment of patients with tension-type headache, in part to decrease the frequent and long-term use of analgesic medications. The available trials have been somewhat mixed with regard to outcome, however. The majority (Melchart et al., 2005; Karst et al., 2001; Tavola, Gala, Conte, & Invernizzi, 1992) have reported no effects of true acupuncture over sham acupuncture, while 2 (Hansen & Hansen, 1985; Xue et al., 2004) have reported superior pain relief with acupuncture compared to sham acupuncture. However, even the studies reporting null effects provide important conclusions regarding how acupuncture may be operating. For example, a randomized, well-controlled, multi-center trial of 279 patients with tension-type headache examined the efficacy of acupuncture for both episodic and chronic tension headache pain (Melchart et al.,

2005). When acupuncture, sham acupuncture (termed minimal acupuncture, and defined in this study as superficial needling at non-acupuncture points), and a wait list control were compared, after 12 sessions over 8 weeks, the number of days with headache decreased by 7.2 days in the acupuncture group, 6.6 days in the sham acupuncture group, and 1.5 days in wait list group. Thus, acupuncture was found to be more effective than a wait list control, but not significantly more effective than sham acupuncture. The value of the study is its large size and rigorous design. The fact that both the true and sham acupuncture groups, compared to the waitlist group, had significant and clinically important improvements in symptoms that lasted for several months following the completion of treatment suggests that the expectation of relief with an active treatment might have been responsible for part or all of the effects noted (see placebo section, below). Thus, the choice of control group when testing the effects of acupuncture on tension-type headache is particularly important.

A systematic review of acupuncture for the treatment of a variety of other types of idiopathic headache pain, including migraine, tension-type, and cluster headaches (Melchart et al., 2001) indicated that the majority of the 26 studies evaluated were of poor methodological quality, particularly with regard to insufficient reporting of methods and results. Nonetheless, acupuncture was more effective than sham treatment in half of the studies of migraine and tension-type headache patients. However, there was insufficient evidence to determine whether acupuncture was as effective as other headache treatments. Thus, while there is some encouraging evidence regarding the efficacy of acupuncture for the treatment of idiopathic headache, the quality of the study designs is generally not optimal.

Cancer-related pain. Pain is a predominant physical and psychological symptom in persons with cancer and can often present with a neuropathic component. Although several dozen investigations testing the efficacy of acupuncture for the relief of cancer-related pain have been conducted, few of these are randomized, controlled trials, and most are of very small sample sizes (Lee, Schmidt, & Ernst, 2005). One high quality randomized controlled trial of auricular (ear) acupuncture reported statistically significant pain relief among cancer patients, compared to a placebo intervention (Alimi et al., 2003). This particular study is distinguished by its careful study design; however, there is generally inadequate evidence to support the analgesic effect of acupuncture in persons with cancer. Because of the increasingly wide-spread use of the complementary and alternative practice for pain relief in cancer patients, more carefully designed investigations are warranted (Lee, Schmidt, & Ernst, 2005).

Obstetric-gynecologic applications. Acupuncture has been studied in only a limited way as a therapy to diminish pain during labor and delivery, as well as the pain associated with oocyte retrieval during *in vitro* fertilization procedures. A systematic review of acupuncture as a pain management adjunct during labor yielded 3 clinical trials of good methodological quality (Lee & Ernst, 2004).

Each of these provided evidence that acupuncture is superior to either standard labor and delivery care or sham acupuncture for pain management, resulting in lower reports of pain and reduced reliance on pharmacologic analgesic agents during labor. While these results suggest that acupuncture alleviates labor pain and is associated with a reduction in the use of pharmacologic analgesics during labor, the results of this review should be interpreted cautiously due to the small number of evaluated studies.

Two systematic reviews have been performed in evaluating the effects of eletroacupuncture on pain reduction during oocyte retrieval for *in vitro* fertilization (Kwan, Bhattacharya, Knox, & McNeil, 2005; Stener-Victorin, 2005). Although only a small number of studies are available, electroacupuncture is generally not superior to, and is sometimes inferior to, standard pharmacologic analgesia during this procedure. Other forms of acupuncture have not been systematically investigated for the management of pain during oocyte retrieval. In general, electroacupuncture does not appear to be a promising analgesic for this patient population.

Methodological Issues

Researchers face a number of challenges attempting to scientifically validate many CAM therapies as acceptable treatments for pain relief. Numerous case studies and anecdotal evidence, rather than well-controlled, masked investigations, have been published, leading to inconsistent reports and inaccurate estimates of effects. The nature of many CAM therapies require creative thought in creating double-blind, controlled clinical studies in order to determine safety and estimates of efficacy (Phase I and II studies). Late-phase effectiveness trials (Phase III and IV trials) require careful consideration of external validity, feasibility of implementing interventions in community-based settings, and other challenges associated with translating effects of well-controlled interventions to applied settings. However, prior to initiating such Phase III and IV trials, it is essential to have data from rigorous Phase I and II safety and efficacy studies available, and it is these early phase studies that are most relevant to the investigation of many CAM interventions. Some of the design issues related to such early phase studies are outlined below.

Control Groups

One question which frequently arises among investigations of many CAM therapies, particularly mind-body medicine and energy medicine practices, is how to create an appropriate control group. Because many such practices involve significant interaction with participants, there can be substantial effects on some outcomes as a result of this interaction and personal attention, rather than as a function of the other active properties of the intervention. The correct control group should be determined based on the specific questions posed, the hypotheses being tested, the nature and specifics of the intervention, and the outcomes of interest. However, in all cases it is possible and preferable to provide some level of control for the non-specific effects of the intervention being studied. These unintended effects can both enhance and diminish pain relieving qualities of the active treatment, and can include effects due to social interaction for interventions provided in a group setting; attention from a practitioner for interventions with significant practitioner interaction; patient expectations for relief; and effects due to patient burden of participating in particularly intensive or noxious interventions.

Mind-body medicine researchers have dealt with this control group issue in a variety of ways, most effectively by carefully considering the specific questions being tested and outcomes of interest. For example, studies investigating the efficacy of hypnotic induction might construct a control group which provides suggestions for pain relief in the absence of hypnotic induction or design a control group which consists of one or more relaxation interventions without a hypnosis element. Studies of meditation might employ cognitive-behavior therapy as the control condition, or a standard psychoeducational control group that would didactically focus on a variety of general health-promoting behaviors. Importantly, these control conditions should be equivalent to the active intervention in terms of time spent in the intervention, homework required, overall burden and risk, expectations for relief, and whether the intervention is provided in a group or individual setting. Ensuring equivalent expectations for relief requires careful orientation to the groups, a credible control condition, and that practitioner allegiance to the active intervention is minimized (or at least that the practitioner allegiance is equal for both conditions). Thus, differences between the control and active condition can more clearly be ascribed to the "active" ingredients in the active condition. While wait-list groups have the benefit of low cost and provide a control for the passage of time, pain patients can exhibit significant responses to placebo conditions. Thus, control conditions that are equivalent with regard to expectations for relief are particularly important when assessing interventions for pain.

Mechanisms of Action & Placebo

Almost without exception, the psychophysiological mechanisms of action by which the CAM modalities outlined above might have analgesic effects are not well investigated. In addition to providing insight with regard to the expected efficacy of CAM therapies with similar components, understanding the biological underpinnings of how a particular therapy operates to produce the desired effects can assist researchers and clinicians in designing optimally effective treatments for pain. In addition, psychological mechanisms of action also may play a role in mediating part of the analgesic effects of CAM therapies, and these factors, including understanding the impact of expectancy, may also assist in optimizing the ability of any therapy to provide relief of pain. For example, an investigation of irritable bowel syndrome (IBS) patients who were verbally provided with placebo along with the strong suggestion of pain relief during evoked rectal distention reported the same level of analgesia as when they received an application of rectal lidocaine and the same expectation of pain relief (Vase, Robinson, Verne, & Price, 2003). Moreover, patients reporting the highest expectations and desire for relief subsequently reported the most relief. This study underscores the potential clinical utility of maximizing expectations for relief when providing therapies for pain, and additionally suggests that understanding how expectations influence physiological mechanisms of pain relief may be a fruitful area of investigation (See also Pollo A, Benedetti F, This Volume). Toward this end, the neural substrates of placebo analgesia have been identified in an elegant study using PET scans that demonstrated that the endorphin system was activated in pain-related areas of the brain when patients were expecting to receive a pain-relieving medication but in fact received placebo (Zubieta et al., 2005; See also Matre & Tuan, This Volume).

The role of expectations is further underscored by a recent study which directly compared the pain-relieving effects of hypnosis with that of a non-hypnotic suggestion of pain relief and placebo cream, thus providing an estimate of the effects of pain relief due to the expectation for relief (Milling et al., 2005). Those receiving a suggestion of pain relief, either during a hypnotic induction or alone in the absence of hypnotic induction, reported stronger analgesia to an experimental pain, relative to those receiving a placebo cream. These findings suggest that a hypnotic induction prior to providing an imagery-based suggestion of analgesia may not provide significant additional pain relief. Further identification of the psychological processes, as well as the central and peripheral physiological systems, that are activated during placebo analgesia, will advance our understanding of the most efficacious interventions for pain relief.

Another psychological pathway by which some CAM therapies, particularly mind-body therapies, may operate is by reducing stress and increasing the ability to cope with pain. Stress is a particular concern for chronic pain patients who may have experienced years of poorly treated pain, misdiagnoses including psychiatric diagnoses and labels, and significant decrements in functional ability and quality of life. For some pain conditions, both chronic and acute stress can often exacerbate the experience of pain and/or flares, particularly when there is significant anxiety related to the pain condition (Weisenberg, Aviram, Wolf, & Raphaeli, 1984). For example, exposure to chronic stress can decrease thresholds and tolerance for pain and increase sensitivity to pain stimuli in animals (Geerse et al., 2006; Imbe et al., 2006). Human studies have found that intermittent stressors, even when minor, increase reports of pain and other symptoms (Walker et al., 1991). This phenomenon occurs in humans even in the context of experimental pain; children exposed to laboratory stressors before an experimental pain condition exhibited reduced pain thresholds relative to those who did not receive the stressors (Dufton et al., 2007). Thus, stress can occur as part of the experience of pain, particularly chronic pain, but can also affect thresholds for detecting pain.

The physiological underpinnings of this latter phenomenon are not completely understood. Autonomic nervous system stimulation that occurs as part of the stress response can modify the activation of endogenous pain modulation circuits (Mayer, 2000). This may explain, in part, the complex relationship between physiological stress responding and subsequent pain sensitivity. Greater cardiac reactivity to acute stressors is associated with lower pain thresholds in some cases (Caceres & Burns, 1997), but higher blood pressure and lower cortisol reactivity are related to reduce pain sensitivity in others (France & Stewart, 1995).

The ability of mind-body techniques to alter physiological stress responding might provide a mechanism for the beneficial health effects of these therapies, including pain relief. Indeed, after 4 months of Transcendental Meditation (TM) practice, healthy males exhibited lower basal cortisol levels (MacLean et al., 1997). Long-term meditation practice reduces baseline cortisol, blood pressure, and heart rate (Sudsuang, Chentanez, & Veluvan, 1991; Walton et al., 1995; Wallace, Silver, Mills, Dillbeck, & Wagoner, 1983; Vyas & Dikshit, 2002; Solberg et al., 2004) and improves mood states (Walton et al., 1995). Older women completing a TM program have lower levels and slower rises in cortisol responses to a metabolic stressor (glucose challenge) (Walton et al., 2004). In addition, after an 8-week mindfulness-based stress reduction (MBSR) program, women with heart disease have shown a trend in reduced resting levels of cortisol, and breast/prostate cancer patients have reported improvements in quality of life, which were associated with decreases in cortisol levels. However, cortisol plays a complex role in mediating the physiological and psychological effects of stress; it serves as an analgesic during inflammatory pain conditions (Lariviere & Melzack, 2000) and the impact of certain mind-body therapies which reduce circulating cortisol levels might have a smaller effect on reducing pain because of the analgesic benefits associated with cortisol.

Although most studies examining the effects of mind-body programs on immunity have focused on the improvement of NK and T cell number and function (Davidson et al., 1999; Taylor, 1995) and greater antibody responses to a viral vaccine (e.g., influenza) (Davidson et al., 2003), few studies have examined the effects of such interventions on inflammation and/or cytokine responses. One notable exception is a study reporting that breast and prostate cancer patients exhibited a reduction in TH1 (pro-inflammatory) cytokine profiles and enhancement of TH2 (anti-inflammatory) cytokine profiles after participating in an MBSR program (Carlson et al., 2003), reversing the cytokine profile that is often observed in individuals under chronic stress.

It is seldom the case that studies are designed to specifically address the extent to which mind-body CAM therapies operate on psychosocial and physiological processes to have beneficial effects. However, a better understanding of the psychological, in addition to physiological mechanisms operating to reduce perceived pain with CAM therapies is also essential.

Significant strides have been made with regard to understanding mechanisms of action of acupuncture, and several potential pathways have been proposed and tested for acupuncture's effects. These include neurochemical mechanisms, segmental ("gate theory") pathways, autonomic regulation, local effects, and effects on brain function (Rabinstein & Shulman, 2003; Moffet, 2006). Recent neuroimaging data demonstrate that acupuncture modulates brain responses in cortical, limbic and brainstem centers, including regions involved in both sensory and affective pain perception (Dhond, Kettner, & Napadow, 2007). The subsequent release of neurotransmitters and hormones may cause analgesia. Additionally, local effects of peripheral vasodilation and anti-inflammatory responses may be an additional mechanism of action (Berman, 2007). Despite these findings, the exact mechanism of acupuncture's actions in pain management has not been clearly defined, and it is quite possible that multiple mechanisms may be operating under different pain conditions.

Finally, many investigations of CAM therapies for pain conditions are commonly used as complementary treatments, accompanying surgery or pharmacologic therapy for optimal healing and pain relief. Although this strategy likely optimizes the opportunity for pain relief in clinical settings, when used in this way for research purposes, conclusions regarding the mechanisms of action of the CAM therapy cannot be established.

Masking & Dose-Ranging

While both participants and experimenters can typically be masked to the specific intervention they receive during some types of CAM interventions (e.g., herbal products, vitamins), this is not the case for practitioner-administered interventions such as mind-body medicine practices, energy medicine, and acupuncture. Practitioners inevitably know if they are administering verum or "sham" therapies, and participants are aware in at least a general sense of the intervention they are receiving. In order to decrease potential sources of intentional and unintentional bias, several steps can be taken to remedy this latter situation. For example, all research personnel who randomize participants, and who collect, enter and analyze data should be masked to condition. Additionally, practitioners (if they are not the experimenters) and participants can be masked to the specific hypotheses being tested, and control conditions should plausibly have positive benefits. Interventions can be renamed ("movement exercises" can be used in place of, for example, yoga) to diminish preconceived notions of participants. Such steps can significantly diminish the possibility of bias altering the outcomes of the study.

Throughout this review, the lack of information regarding the safest and optimal dose for each of the intervention strategies outlined is a recurring theme. Dose-ranging studies for pharmacologic interventions are a necessary step towards approval of those agents. Dose-ranging studies of this type employ escalating doses to determine the safety profile, as well as the optimal dose for the desired effect. Such dose-escalating studies might also be employed for the CAM therapies outlined above. In addition to establishing safety, dose-ranging studies prevent the premature dismissal of a CAM pain therapy tested at only one dose as being ineffective. Although dose-ranging studies can be particularly complex to conduct with pain conditions that are remitting, failure to identify the correct frequency, timing, and amount of an intervention for the optimal relief of pain will prevent the field from moving forward.

Effects of Age

The specific investigation of age effects on efficacy of CAM modalities for the treatment of pain has not been undertaken. However, several studies have examined the use and ability of CAM interventions to reduce pain among children and adolescents. The conditions studied have included headache and migraine pain, irritable bowel syndrome, and acute pain due to medical interventions and procedures; the children have included very young to adolescent patients. Acupuncture, biofeedback, herbal medications, hypnosis, massage, and music and art therapy have all been studied for their ability to reduce pain among children and adolescents, although the investigations have typically been small and focused on only a few pain conditions. In general, CAM interventions that have been successful for adult populations have shown some efficacy for children and adolescents. For example, hypnosis, guided imagery and biofeedback have all been studied in a variety of pediatric pain conditions (Hermann & Blanchard, 2002; Uman, Chambers, McGrath, & Kisely, 2006; Wild & Espie, 2004), and all have shown some level of efficacy and safety, as well as general willingness of children and their families to try these strategies (Tsao & Zeltzer, 2005). Other techniques, such as acupuncture and meditation, have much less frequently been examined in pediatric pain populations, perhaps in part because it is less likely that children and their families would either accept (acupuncture) or be able to effectively engage (meditation) in these intervention strategies. Certainly, the use of these interventions in clinical practice is also more limited among children, despite some preliminary evidence that they can be tolerated and accepted, particularly by adolescents (Kemper et al., 2000). An exception is a small but well-designed study of acupuncture for pediatric migraine, which demonstrated significant benefit on migraine pain with acupuncture relative to a sham acupuncture group (Pintov, Lahat, Alstein, Vogel, & Barg, 1997). This randomized study is particularly informative because the children, their parents and the researchers maintaining pain ratings were all masked to condition, thus eliminating an important potential source of treatment bias, and because the investigators simultaneously examined evidence for activity of the opioid system during acupuncture, as a way of testing a potential mechanism by which acupuncture may be operating to reduce pain. Although the data did not clearly show group differences in opioid activity at the end of treatment, the acupuncture group did show significantly greater increases from baseline (due to initial baseline differences between the groups). These results reinforce the importance of adequate randomization procedures to ensure baseline equivalence between the groups. In most cases, the optimal way to do this is to employ larger, homogeneous groups with clearly defined inclusionary and exclusionary criteria which remain consistent throughout the recruitment phases of the study.

Standardized Treatments

Because relatively few CAM treatments are completely standardized, there can be tremendous variability in the specific elements and procedures related to how a specific CAM treatment is provided in a clinical setting. Frequently, that variability is echoed in research investigations testing the efficacy of CAM treatments for pain (and other) conditions, often resulting in inconsistent and variable findings (Bardia, Barton, Prokop, Bauer, & Moynihan, 2006). One solution to that problem is to manualize treatment modalities for particular conditions, which might, for example, outline the specific elements of a particular modality, how those elements might be incorporated into treatment, and the frequency of treatments. Toward this end, a taxonomy of massage therapies for the treatment of musculoskeletal pain has recently been described (Sherman, Dixon, Thompson, & Cherkin, 2006). While the ultimate goal of medicine is increasingly to individualize and tailor therapies (both CAM and conventional) to the specific needs of the patient and expertise of the practitioner for optimal treatment effects, early stages of research in all areas of medicine mandate optimal control to evaluate initial proof of concept. The explication of classification schemes across a variety of CAM therapies and modalities can be a valuable step forward in improving the quality of research in CAM treatments for pain.

Limitations and Directions

Although the bulk of the literature reviewed above indicates modest evidence for pain-relieving qualities of selected CAM energy therapies, mind-body medicine therapies, and body-based therapies, the literature in this area is methodologically limited. For example, most of the available studies investigating various CAM therapies for the relief of pain are poorly controlled or uncontrolled, not randomized, and tested in only limited patient populations with only limited types of pain conditions. Whether a particular CAM modality that

C.M. Stoney et al.

has been shown to be effective in treating a specific pain condition will generalize to other pain conditions and populations is not well understood.

Future investigations of CAM therapies for pain should focus on those therapies with the most evidence for pain-relieving ability, such as Qi Gong, hypnosis, and massage. However, the inconsistent findings that have been reported in the literature to date mandate that future studies focus on three specific goals. First, small, tightly-controlled and well-designed efficacy (e.g., early phase II) studies will more definitively demonstrate the extent to which these CAM treatments are able to result in consistent pain relief. Second, identification of the physiological and biological mechanisms by which specific CAM therapies provide pain relief is an essential step in order to design maximally effective interventions, and to predict the potential effectiveness of other CAM (and perhaps conventional) therapies for pain relief. Third, the potential generalizability of specific modalities across patient populations and pain conditions should be investigated, particularly in reference to widely experienced pain conditions. However, the particular CAM treatment for specific pain conditions should be chosen on the basis of a conceptual understanding of the mechanisms by which the intervention operates or is presumed to operate, and the physiology of the pain condition.

While we have attempted to consolidate and summarize a broad literature, in reality there are numerous variations used clinically of each of the therapies mentioned above, and potential differences in therapeutic efficacy with different variations of modalities have not been systematically examined. Thus, although we provide a global understanding of specific CAM therapies for pain conditions, in fact the large variety of each of these therapies in use would assume differences in efficacy. Thus, this chapter should best be understood as providing a framework for future investigations.

References

Adler P., Good M., Roberts B., & Snyder S. (2000). The effects of Tai Chi on older adults with chronic arthritis pain. *Journal of Nursing Scholarship, 32*, 377.

Alimi D., Rubino C., Pichard-Leandri E., Fermand-Brule S., Dubreuil-Lemaire M. L., & Hill C. (2003). Analgesic effect of auricular acupuncture for cancer pain: A randomized, blinded, controlled trial. *Journal of Clinical Oncology, 21*, 4120–4126.

Arias A.J., Steinberg K., Banga A., & Trestman R.L. (2006). Systematic review of the efficacy of meditation techniques as treatments for medical illness. *Journal of Alternative and Complementary Medicine, 12*, 817–832.

Astin J. A., Berman B. M., Bausell B., Lee W-L., Hochberg M., & Forys K. L. (2003). The efficacy of mindfulness meditation plus Qigong movement therapy in the treatment of FM: A randomized controlled trial. *The Journal of Rheumatology, 30*, 2257–2262.

Baird C. L., & Sands L. P. (2006). Effect of guided imagery with relaxation on health-related quality of life in older women with osteoarthritis. *Research in Nursing and Health, 29*, 442–451.

Bardia A., Barton D. L., Prokop L. J., Bauer B. A., & Moynihan T. J. (2006). Efficacy of complementary and alternative medicine therapies in relieving cancer pain: a systematic review. *Journal of Clinical Oncology, 24,* 5457–64.

Barnes P. M., Powell-Griner E., McFann K., & Nahin R. L. (2004). Complementary and alternative medicine use among adults: United States, 2002. *Advance data from vital and health statistics; no 343.* Hyattsville, Maryland: National Center for Health Statistics.

Benham G., Woody E. Z., Wilson K. S., & Nash M. R. (2006). Expect the unexpected: Ability, attitude, and responsiveness to hypnosis. *Journal of Personality and Social Psychology, 91,* 342–350.

Berman B. (2007). A 60-year-old woman considering acupuncture for knee pain. *Journal of the American Medical Association, 297,* 1697–707.

Berman B. M., & Singh B. B. (1997). Chronic low back pain: An outcome analysis of a mind-body intervention. *Complementary Therapies in Medicine, 5,* 29–35.

Brismee J. M., Paige R. L., Chyu M. C., Boatright J. D., Hagar J. M., McCaleb J. A., et al. (2007). Group and home-based Tai Chi in elderly subjects with knee osteoarthritis: A randomized controlled trial. *Clinical Rehabilitation, 21,* 99–111.

Brown D. C., & Hammond D. C. (2007). Evidence-based clinical hypnosis for obstetrics, labor and delivery, and preterm labor. *International Journal of Clinical and Experimental Hypnosis, 55,* 355–371.

Burke A., Upchurch D. M., Dye C., & Chyu L. (2006). Acupuncture use in the United States: findings from the National Health Interview Survey. *Journal of Alternative and Complementary Medicine, 12,* 639–648.

Caceres C., & Burns J. W. (1997). Cardiovascular reactivity to psychological stress may enhance subsequent pain sensitivity. *Pain, 69,* 237–244.

Calenda E. (2006). Massage therapy for cancer pain. *Current Pain and Headache Reports, 10,* 270–274.

Carlson L. E., Speca M., Patel K. D., & Goodey E. (2003). Mindfulness-based stress reduction in relation to quality of life, mood, symptoms of stress and immune parameters in breast and prostate cancer outpatients. *Psychosomatic Medicine, 65,* 571–581.

Cherkin D. C., Sherman K. J., Deyo R. A., & Shekelle P. G. (2003). A review of the evidence for the effectiveness, safety, and cost of acupuncture, massage therapy, and spinal manipulation for back pain. *Annals of Internal Medicine, 138,* 898–906.

Davidson R. J., Coe C. C., Dolski I., & Donzella B. (1999). Individual differences in prefrontal activation asymmetry predict natural killer cell activity at rest and in response to challenge. *Brain, Behavior, and Immunology, 13,* 93–108.

Davidson R. J., Kabat-Zinn J., Schumacher J., Rosenkranz M., Muller D., Santorelli S. F., et al. (2003). Alterations in brain and immune function produced by mindfulness meditation. *Psychosomatic Medicine, 65,* 564–570.

Davis M. P., & Darden P. M. (2003). Use of complementary and alternative medicine by children in the United States. *Archives of Pediatrics and Adolescent Medicine, 157,* 393–6.

Dhond, R. P., Kettner N., & Napadow V. (2007). Do the neural correlates of acupuncture and placebo effects differ? *Pain, 128,* 8–12.

Dufton LM, Konik B, Colletti R, Stanger C, Boyer M, Morrow S et al. (2007). Effects of stress on pain threshold and tolerance in children with recurrent abdominal pain. *Pain, 136*(1–2), 38–43.

Elkins G. R., Cheung A., Marcus J, Palamara L., & Rajab, H. (2004). Hypnosis to reduce pain in cancer survivors with advanced disease: A prospective study. *Journal of Cancer Integrative Medicine, 2,* 167–172.

Elkins G. R., Jensen M. P., & Patterson D. R. (2007). Hypnotherapy for the management of chronic pain. *International Journal of Clinical and Experimental Hypnosis, 55,* 275–287.

Ernst, E. (2006). Acupuncture – A critical analysis. *Journal of Internal Medicine, 259,* 125–37.

Ezzo, J., Berman B., Hadhazy V. A., Jadad A. R., Lao L., & Singh B. B. (2000). Is acupuncture effective for the treatment of chronic pain? A systematic review. *Pain, 86,* 217–25.

Ezzo J., Haraldsson B. G., Gross A. R., Myers C. D., Morien A., Goldsmith C. H., et al. (2007). Massage for mechanical neck disorders: A systematic review. *Spine, 32*, 353–362.

Fleming S., Rabago D. P., Mundt M. P., & Fleming, M. F. (2007). CAM therapies among primary care patients using opioid therapy for chronic pain. *BMC Complementary and Alternative Medicine, 7*, 15–21.

Fransen M., Nairn L., Winstanley J., Lam P., & Edmonds J. (2007). Physical activity for osteoarthritis management: a randomized controlled clinical trial evaluating hydrotherapy or Tai Chi classes. *Arthritis and Rheumatism, 57*, 407–414.

France C. R., & Stewart K. M. (1995). Parental history of hypertension and enhanced cardiovascular reactivity are associated with decreased pain ratings. *Psychophysiology, 52*, 571–578.

Furlan A. D., Brosseau L., Imamura M., & Irvin E. (2002). Massage for low back pain. *Cochrane Database Systematic Review, 2*, CD001929.

Furlan A. D., van Tulder M. W., Cherkin D., Tsukayama H., Lao L., Koes B., et al. (2005). Acupuncture and dry-needling for low back pain: An updated systematic review within the framework of the Cochrane collaboration. *Spine, 30*, 944–963.

Galantino M.L., Bzdewka T.M., Eissler-Russo J.L., Holbrook M.L., Mogck E.P., Geigle P., et al. (2004). The impact of modified Hatha yoga on chronic low back pain: a pilot study. *Alternative Therapies in Health and Medicine, 10*, 56–59.

Garfinkel M.S., Schumacher H. R. Jr, Husain A., Levy M., & Reshetar R.A. (1994). Evaluation of a yoga based regimen for treatment of osteoarthritis of the hands. *Journal of Rheumatology, 21*, 2341–2343.

Gay M. C., Philippot P., & Luminet O. (2002). Differential effectiveness of psychological interventions for reducing osteoarthritis pain: A comparison of Erikson. *European Journal of Pain, 6*, 1–16.

Geerse G.J., van Gurp L.C., Wiegant V.M., & Stam R. (2006). Individual reactivity to the open-field predicts the expression of cardiovascular and behavioural sensitisation to novel stress. *Behavior and Brain Research, 175*, 9–17.

Gillespie, E. A., Gillespie B. W., & Stevens M. J. (2007). Painful diabetic neuropathy: impact of an alternative approach. *Diabetes Care 30*, 999–1001.

Green S., Buchbinder R., & Hetrick S. (2005). Acupuncture for shoulder pain. *Cochrane Database Systematic Review, 8*(2), CD005319.

Grossman P, Niemann L., Schmidt S., & Walach H. (2004). Mindfulness-based stress reduction and health benefits: A meta-analysis *Journal of Psychosomatic Research, 57*, 35–43.

Haanen, H. C., Hoenderdos, H. T., van Romunde, L. K., Hop, W. C., Mallee, C., Terwiel, J. P., et al. (1991). Controlled trial of hypnotherapy in the treatment of refractory fibromyalgia. *Journal of Rheumatology, 18*, 72–75.

Hansen P. E., & Hansen J. H. (1985). Acupuncture treatment of chronic tension headache – a controlled cross-over trial. *Cephalalgia, 5*, 137–142.

Hawk C., Khorsan R., Lisi A. J., Ferrance R. J., & Evans M. W. (2007). Chiropractic care for nonmusculoskeletal conditions: a systematic review with implications for whole systems research *Journal of Alternative and Complementary Medicine, 13*, 491–512.

Hermann C., & Blanchard E. B. (2002). Biofeedback in the treatment of headache and other childhood pain. *Applied Psychophysiology and Biofeedback, 27*, 143–162.

Hodgson D. M., Nakamura T., & Walker A. K. (2007). Prophylactic role for complementary and alternative medicine in perinatal programming of adult health. *Forsch Komplementarmed, 14*, 92–101.

Imbe H., Iwai-Liao Y., & Senba E. (2006). Stress-induced hyperalgesia: animal models and putative mechanisms. *Front Biosci, 11*, 2179–2192.

Jacobs B.P., Mehling W., Avins A.L., Goldberg H.A., Acree M., Lasater J.H., et al. (2004). Feasibility of conducting a clinical trial on Hatha yoga for chronic low back pain: methodological lessons. *Alternative Therapies in Health and Medicine, 10*, 80–83.

Jensen M., & Patterson D. R. (2006). Hypnotic treatment of chronic pain. *Journal of Behavioral Medicine, 29*, 95–124.

Kabat-Zinn J., Lipworth L., & Burney R. (1985). The clinical use of mindfulness meditation for the self-regulation of chronic pain. *Journal of Behavioral Medicine, 8,* 163–190.

Kabat-Zinn J., Lipworth L., Burney R., & Sellers W. (1986). Four-year follow-up of a meditation-based program for the self-regulation of chronic pain: Treatment outcomes and compliances. *Clinical Journal of Pain, 2,* 159–173.

Karst M., Reinhard M., Thum P., Wiese B., Rollnik J., & Fink M. (2001). Needle acupuncture in tension-type headache: a randomized, placebo-controlled study. *Cephalalgia, 21,* 637–642.

Keefer L., & Blanchard E. B. (2001). The effects of relaxation response meditation on the symptoms of irritable bowel syndrome: results of a controlled treatment study. *Behaviour Research and Therapy, 39,* 801–811.

Kemper K. J., Sarah R., Silver-Highfield E., Xiarhos E., Barnes L., & Berde C. (2000). On Pins and Needles? Pediatric Pain Patients' Experience With Acupuncture. *Pediatrics, 105,* 941–947.

Klein P. J., & Adams W. D. (2004). Comprehensive therapeutic benefits of Taiji: a critical review. *American Journal of Physical Medicine and Rehabilitation, 83,* 735–45.

Kolasinski S. L., Garfinkel M., Tsai A. G., Matz W., Van Dyke A., & Schumacher H. R. (2005). Iyengar yoga for treating symptoms of osteoarthritis of the knees: A pilot study. *Journal of Alternative and Complementary Medicine, 11,* 689–693.

Kwan I., Bhattacharya S., Knox F., & McNeil A. (2005). Conscious sedation and analgesia for oocyte retrieval during in vitro fertilisation procedures. *Cochrane Database Systematic Reviews,* CD004829.

Lang E. B., Berbaum K. S., Faintuch S., Hatsiopoulou O., Halsey N., Li X., et al. (2006). Adjunctive self-hypnotic relaxation for outpatient medical procedures: a prospective randomized trial with women undergoing large core breast biopsy. *Pain, 126,* 155–164.

Lao L. (1996). Acupuncture techniques and devices. *Journal of Alternative and Complementary Medicine, 2,* 23–25.

Lariviere W. R., & Melzack R. (2000). The bee venom test: comparisons with the formalin test with injection of different venoms. *Pain, 84,* 111–112.

Lee H., & Ernst E. (2004). Acupuncture for labor pain management: A systematic review. *American Journal of Obstetrics and Gynecology, 191,* 1573–9.

Lee H., Schmidt K., & Ernst E. (2005). Acupuncture for the relief of cancer-related pain – a systematic review. *European Journal of Pain 9,* 437–44.

Lichtenberg P., Bachner-Melman R., Gritsenko I., & Ebstein R. P. (2000). Exploratory association study between catechol-O-methyltransferase (COMT) high/low enzyme activity polymorphism and hypnotizability. *American Journal of Medical Genetics, 96,* 771–774.

MacLean C. R., Walton K. G., Wenneberg S. R., Levitsky D. K., Mandarino J. P., Waziri R., et al. (1997). Effects of the Transcendental Meditation program on adaptive mechanisms: changes in hormone levels and responses to stress after 4 months of practice. *Psychoneuroendocrinology, 22,* 277–295.

Mansky P., Sannes T., Wallerstedt D., Ge A., Ryan M., Johnson L. L., et al. (2006). Tai Chi Chuan: Mind body practice or exercise intervention? Studying the benefit for cancer survivors. *Integrative Cancer Therapies, 5,* 192–201.

Mayer E. A. (2000). The neurobiology of stress and gastrointestinal disease. *Gut, 47,* 861–869.

Meditation Practices for Health: State of the Research, Structured Abstract. Publication No. 07-E010, June 2007. Agency for Healthcare Research and Quality, Rockville, MD. http://www.ahrq.gov/clinic/tp/medittp.htm.

Mehling W. E., Hamel K. A., Acree M., Byl N., & Hecht F. M. (2005). Randomized, controlled trial of breath therapy for patients with chronic low-back pain. *Alternative Therapies in Health and Medicine, 11,* 44–52.

Melchart D., Streng A., Hoppe A., Brinkhaus B., Witt C., Wagenpfeil S., et al. (2005). Acupuncture in patients with tension-type headache: randomized controlled trial. *British Medical Journal, 331,* 376–382.

Melchart D., Linde K., Fischer P., Berman B., White A., Vickers A., et al. (2001). Acupuncture for idiopathic headache. *Cochrane Database Systematic Reviews, 1,* CD001218.

Miles P. (2003). Preliminary report on the use of Reiki for HIV-related pain and anxiety. *Alternative Therapies in Health and Medicine, 9,* 36.

Milling L. S., Kirsch I., Allen G. J., & Reutenauer E. L. (2005). The effects of hypnotic and nonhypnotic imaginative suggestion on pain. *Annals of Behavioral Medicine, 29,* 116–127.

Moffet H. H. (2006). How might acupuncture work? A systematic review of physiologic rationales from clinical trials. *BMC Complementary and Alternative Medicine, 6,* 25.

Montgomery G. H., Bovbjerg D. H., Schnur J. B., David D., Goldfarb A., Weltz C. R., et al. (2007). A randomized clinical trial of a brief hypnosis intervention to control side effects in Breast surgery patients. *Journal of the National Cancer Institute, 99,* 1304–1312.

Morone N. E., & Greco C. M. (2007). Mind-body interventions for chronic pain in older adults: a structured review. *Pain Medicine, 8,* 359–75.

Moyer C. A., Rounds J., & Hannum J. W. (2004). A meta-analysis of massage therapy research. *Psychological Bulletin, 130,* 3–18.

National Institutes of Health Consensus Statement. (1997). Acupuncture. 15,1–34.

Olson K., Hanson J., & Michaud M. (2003). A phase II trial of Reiki for the management of pain in advanced cancer patients. *Journal of Pain and Symptom Management, 26,* 990–997.

Patterson D. R., & Jensen M. P. (2003). Hypnosis and clinical pain. *Psychological Bulletin, 129,* 495–521.

Pintov S., Lahat E., Alstein M., Vogel A., & Barg J. (1997). Acupuncture and the opioid system: Implications in management of migraine. *Pediatric Neurology, 17,* 129–133.

Rabinstein A. A., & Shulman L. M. (2003). Acupuncture in clinical neurology. *Neurologist, 9,* 137–48.

Raz A. (2005). Attention and hypnosis: neural substrates and genetic associations of two converging processes. *International Journal of Clinical and Experimental Hypnosis, 53,* 237–58.

Russell C., & Smart S. (2007). Guided imagery and distraction therapy in paediatric hospice care. *Paediatric Nursing, 19,* 24–25.

Sharav Y., & Tal M. (2006). Focused hypnotic analgesia: Local and remote effects. *Pain, 124,* 280–286.

Sherman K. J., Cherkin D. C., Erro J., Miglioretti D. L., & Deyo R. A. (2005). Comparing yoga, exercise, and a self-care book for chronic low back pain. *Annals of Internal Medicine, 143,* 849–856.

Sherman K. J., Cherkin D. C., Connelly M. T., Erro J., Savetsky J. B., Davis R. B., et al. (2004). Complementary and alternative medical therapies for chronic low back pain: What treatments are patients willing to try? *BMC Complementary and Alternative Medicine, 4,* 9.

Sherman K. J., Dixon M. W., Thompson D., & Cherkin D. C. (2006). Development of a taxonomy to describe massage treatments for musculoskeletal pain. *BMC Complementary and Alternative Medicine, 6,* 24.

Smith C. A., Collins C. T., Cyna A. M., & Crowther C. A. (2006). Complementary and alternative therapies for pain management in labour. *Cochrane Database Systematic Review, 4,* CD003521.

Solberg E. E., Ekeberg O., Holen A., Ingjer F., Sandvik L., & Standal P. A., (2004). Hemodynamic changes during long meditation. *Applied Psychophysiology and Biofeedback, 29,* 213–221.

Song R., Lee E. O., Lam P., & Bae S. C. (2003). Effects of Tai Chi exercise on pain, balance, muscle strength, and perceived difficulties in physical functioning in older women with osteoarthritis: a randomized clinical trial. *Journal of Rheumatology, 30,* 2039–44.

Spiegel D. (2007). The mind prepared: Hypnosis in surgery. *Journal of the National Cancer Institute, 99,* 1280–1281.

Spinhoven P., & Linssen A. C. (1989). Education and self-hypnosis in the management of low back pain: A component analysis. *British Journal of Clinical Psychology, 28,* 145–153.

Stener-Victorin E. (2005). The pain-relieving effect of electro-acupuncture and conventional medical analgesic methods during oocyte retrieval: a systematic review of randomized controlled trials. *Human Reproduction, 20*, 339–49.

Sudsuang R., Chentanez V., & Veluvan K. (1991). Effect of Buddhist meditation on serum cortisol and total protein levels, blood pressure, pulse rate, lung volume and reaction time. *Physiology and Behavior, 50*, 543–548.

Tavola T., Gala C., Conte G., & Invernizzi G. (1992). Traditional Chinese acupuncture in tension-type headache: A controlled study. *Pain, 48*, 325–329.

Taylor D. N. (1995). Effects of a behavioral stress-management program on anxiety, mood, self-esteem, and T-cell count in HIV positive men. *Psychological Reports, 76*, 451–457.

Trinh K. V., Graham N., Gross A. R., Goldsmith C. H., Wang E., Cameron I. D., et al. (2006). Acupuncture for neck disorders. *Cochrane Database Systematic Review, 3*, CD004870.

Trinh K. V., Phillips S. D., Ho E., & Damsma K. (2004). Acupuncture for the alleviation of lateral epicondyle pain: a systematic review. *Rheumatology (Oxford), 43*, 1085–90.

Tsao J. C., & Zeltzer L. K. (2005). Complementary and Alternative Medicine Approaches for Pediatric Pain: A Review of the State-of-the-science. *Evidence-Based Complementary and Alternative Medicine, 2*, 149–159.

Tsao J. C. I. (2007). Effectiveness of massage therapy for chronic, non-malignant pain: A review. *Evidence-Based Complementary and Alternative Medicine, 4*, 165–179.

Uman L. S., Chambers C. T., McGrath P. J., & Kisely S. (2006). Psychological interventions for needle-related procedural pain and distress in children and adolescents. *Cochrane Database of Systematic Reviews, 4*, CD005179.

Vase L., Robinson M. E., Verne G. N., & Price D. D. (2003). The contributions of suggestion, desire, and expectation to placebo effects in irritable bowel syndrome patients: An empirical investigation. *Pain, 105*, 17–25.

Vitale A. T., & O'Connor P. C. (2006). The effect of Reiki on pain and anxiety in women with abdominal hysterectomies: a quasi-experimental pilot study. *Holistic Nursing Practice, 20*, 263–272.

Vyas R., & Dikshit N. (2002). Effect of meditation on respiratory system, cardiovascular system and lipid profile. *Indian Journal of Physiology and Pharmacology, 46*, 487–491.

Walker L. S., & Greene J. W. (1991). Negative life events and symptom resolution in pediatric abdominal pain patients. *J. Pediatric Psychology, 16*(3), 341–360.

Wallace R. K., Silver J., Mills P. J., Dillbeck M. C., & Wagoner D. E. (1983). Systolic blood pressure and long-term practice of the Transcendental Meditation and TM-Sidhi program: effects of TM on systolic blood pressure. *Psychosomatic Medicine, 45*, 41–46.

Walton K. G., Fields J. Z., Levitsky D. K., Harris D. A., Pugh N. D., & Schneider R. H. (2004). Lowering cortisol and CVD risk in postmenopausal women: a pilot study using the Transcendental Meditation program. *Annals of the New York Academy of Sciences, 1032*, 211–215.

Walton K. G., Pugh N. D., Gelderloos P., & Macrae P. (1995). Stress reduction and preventing hypertension: preliminary support for a psychoneuroendocrine mechanism. *Journal of Alternative and Complementary Medicine, 1*, 263–283.

Weisenberg M., Aviram O., Wolf Y., & Raphaeli N. (1984) Relevant and irrelevant anxiety in the reaction to pain. *Pain, 20*, 371–383

White A., Foster, N. E., Cummings M., & Barlas P. (2007). Acupuncture treatment for chronic knee pain: a systematic review. *Rheumatology (Oxford), 46*, 384–90.

Wild M. R., & Espie C. A. (2004). The efficacy of hypnosis in the reduction of procedural pain and distress in pediatric oncology: A systematic review. *Journal of Developmental and Behavioral Pediatrics, 25*, 207–213.

Williams K. A., Petronis J., Smith D., Goodrich D., Wu J., Ravi N., et al. (2005). Effect of Iyengar yoga therapy for chronic low back pain. *Pain, 115*, 107–117.

Wirth D. P., Brenlan D. R., Levine R. J., & Rodriguez C. M. (1993). The effect of complementary healing therapy on postoperative pain after surgical removal of impacted third
   molar teeth. *Complementary Therapies in Medicine 1*, 133–138.
Xue C. C., Dong L., Polus B., English R. A., Zheng Z., DaCosta C., et al. (2004). Electroacupuncture for tension-type headache on distal acupoints only: a randomized, controlled,
   crossover trial. *Headache, 44*, 333–341.
Yang K. H., Kim Y. H., & Lee M. S. (2005). Efficacy of Qi -therapy (external Qi gong) for
   elderly people with chronic pain. *International Journal of Neuroscience, 115*, 949–963.
Zubieta J-K., Bueller J. A., Jackson L. R., Scott D. J., Xu Y., Koeppe R. A., et al. (2005).
   Placebo effects mediated by endogenous opioid activity on opioid receptors. *The Journal
   of Neuroscience, 25*, 7754–7762.

Imaging Modalities for Pain

Dagfin Matre and Tuan Diep Tran

Introduction

Information transfer in the brain takes place by electrical conduction along axons and chemical interaction between neurons. Functional brain imaging is a general term for techniques measuring correlates of neuronal activity. The techniques used most often are functional magnetic resonance imaging (fMRI), positron emission tomography (PET), single photon emission computed tomography (SPECT), electroencephalography (EEG), magnetoencephalography (MEG) and MR spectroscopy (Apkarian et al., 2005). The outputs measured are cerebral blood flow (fMRI/PET), electrophysiology (EEG/MEG), neurochemistry (PET/SPECT) and relative chemical concentrations (MR spectroscopy) (Apkarian et al., 2005). In the context of pain research, fMRI is the most commonly used today; not only for activation studies, but for identifying interactions and connectivities between brain regions during the modulation of pain. PET is decreasing in use for pain activation studies, but is becoming increasingly popular for detecting the neurochemistry of neuronal communication. EEG and MEG are popular mainly for detecting temporal sequences. Although there are a variety of important imaging techniques; in this chapter we will focus on three of the main functional imaging methods used to study pain: MEG, fMRI, and PET.

Background/Historical Overview

The ultimate aim of pain research is prevention and treatment of pain. During the past few decades it has become widely accepted that the field of pain deserves its own research and attention. This is partly because of the enormous socio-economic costs of pain and partly because pain is recognized as a unique experience unlike other sensory modalities. Pain demands attention and always

D. Matre (✉)
National Institute of Occupational Health Oslo, Norway

R.J. Moore (ed.), *Biobehavioral Approaches to Pain*,
DOI 10.1007/978-0-387-78323-9_17, © Springer Science+Business Media, LLC 2009

has an affective component (Eccleston & Crombez, 1999). The most disturbing part of the experience we call pain is probably not the intensity, duration and localization of the pain sensation, but the unpleasantness and meaning that is part of the experience of pain (Price & Bushnell, 2004). Thus, a dedicated focus is needed if the neurobiology of pain is to be revealed.

Almost 40 years ago, Melzack and Casey (1968) pointed to the importance of the sensory, affective, and cognitive aspects of pain. However it is with pain imaging it has become possible to understand the functional neuroanatomy of pain in a more comprehensive manner. The major challenges within functional imaging of pain probably lie in interpreting the vast amount of captured data, and render it useful to guide research and clinical practice.

To better understand the neurobiology of pain it is necessary to compare animal studies with studies in patients and in pain-free individuals. In a given group of patients, large variation can be expected in the emotional and affective aspects of their pain experience, including their neuronal correlates of pain, although their pain experience may be similar. To minimize the variance of these mentioned factors, it is therefore often necessary to recruit pain-free subjects to represent a more homogenous group. On the other hand, if the aim is to study the affective and emotional components of pain, ethical issues may present certain limitations on the use of healthy volunteers. It is clearly not possible to investigate the emotional consequences of, say a (false) cancer diagnosis, in a healthy normal volunteer.

When studying pain it is often necessary to apply an external stimulus to create the experience of pain. This is always the case when using healthy subjects, but may also be necessary when studying patients with pain. Advantages with inducing pain are full control of applied intensity, duration and location, making it possible to do repeated measurements within and across subjects. Yet, several considerations must be made when choosing an external pain stimulus, which is usually given to activate a certain peripheral receptor or fiber type, or to mimic a particular clinical pain syndrome/complaint. In the latter situation the psychophysical properties of the experimental pain are compared with a clinical pain condition to establish the relevance of that particular experimental stimulus under evaluation. Examples are injection of hypertonic saline into the back muscles of healthy individuals to mimic low back pain (Arendt-Nielsen et al., 1996) and into the temporomandibular muscle or joint to mimic temporomandibular disorders (Svensson, 2007). Although muscle pain by far is a larger clinical problem than cutaneous pain, methods to induce cutaneous pain dominate. Experimental stimulus modalities includes heat, cold, ischemia, mechanical pressure, electrical and chemical stimuli. For an overview of methods to induce pain in humans, see Gracely (2005).

The present chapter is divided into three parts. First, the reader is introduced to the basic technical aspects of MEG, PET and fMRI. The second part describes the so-called pain matrix, and how functional imaging has contributed to the understanding of the psychology as well as the neurobiology of pain in normal (pain free) subjects, including how pain is modulated. The third part describes imaging of selected clinical conditions with abnormal pain processing and how the results of basic science studies are translated into useful clinical applications.

Imaging Methodology

Functional brain imaging includes a range of techniques that capture the neural correlates of brain activity. Below the principles for MEG, PET and fMRI are outlined. For a review of other imaging modalities, see for example Apkarian et al. (2005), or Kupers and Kehlet (2006).

Magnetoencephalography (MEG)

The Principles of MEG

If there is an electric current, there is a magnetic field in the neighbor region of the current. When information is being processed in a brain, small currents flow in the neural system and simultaneously producing a weak magnetic field. If an electrical activity in the brain can be measured by electroencephalography (EEG), it is natural to ask if a magnetic filed in the brain can also be measured. Magnetoencephalography (MEG) is a noninvasive measurement of magnetic fields generated by electrical activity in the brain. These fields, however, are very weak. Magnetic field signals from the brain are typically in the range of 50 to 500 fT (femtoTesla; $1 fT = 10^{-15}$ T), which is about a billion times weaker than the earth's magnetic fields. In order to make these weak signals visible, the biomagnetometer employs a low-noise amplifier called a SQUID (superconducting quantum interference device), a sensitive detector of magnetic field, introduced in the late 1960s by James Zimmerman (Zimmerman et al., 1970). The SQUID converts the magnetic signal into an ordinary electrical signal that can be amplified, filtered, and displayed or recorded for subsequent analysis. Current state-of-the-art MEG systems consist of 100-300 channels that allow magnetic signals to be simultaneously recorded throughout the scalp. In short, a MEG system consists of (1) the SQUID sensor unit, (2) a magnetic shielded room, (3) a data acquisition processor and (4) a master analysis processor.

Both MEG and EEG primarily measure intracellular current flow of post-synaptic currents, which are generated by synchronized neuronal activity. The signal generators in the brain are described as current dipoles. While EEG senses both radial and tangential current dipoles, MEG is sensitive only to the tangential component (Cohen, 1972). This means that MEG suits well for studies of fissure cortex. When a source is located in a deep area, the magnetic signals decrease relatively more rapidly in amplitude than the electric potentials. A source in the center of the sphere does not cause any external magnetic field at all, whereas electric potentials can still be recorded on the surface. Therefore, MEG is considered a tool to mainly study cortical activity.

EEG measures the difference in voltage, or potential, between two electrodes. In contrast, MEG measures the absolute magnitude of the magnetic field and does not require a reference. Both EEG and MEG measure brain activity from the surface; from the scalp and outside the skull, respectively. To localize brain activity from the recorded electric and magnetic fields, the so-called inverse problem must be solved. That is, to make a reasonable guess about current sources and their locations based on measurements from the surface. Unfortunately, theory shows that there is no unique solution to this problem. In additon, EEG is affected by the conductivities of the skull and scalp much more than MEG. Therefore, interpretation of EEG signals, in particular for source localization, will require more precise knowledge of the thickness and conductivities of the tissues in the head. Consequently, MEG has a better spatial resolution (Fig. 1). Under favorable conditions the source location can be determined with a precision of a few millimeters (Hari, 1988).

MEG is completely noninvasive and can record physiological signals in the order of milliseconds. Thus, it is possible to follow the rapid neuronal changes in the brain. MEG also provides direct measure of neuronal activity, whereas other functional brain imaging techniques, i.e. single-photon-emission computed tomography (SPECT), positron-emission tomography (PET), and functional magnetic resonance imaging (fMRI), measure hemodynamic response, and so, provide an indirect measure of neuronal activity. The time resolution, therefore, is much better in MEG than in those methods (Fig. 1).

The first measurement of magnetic field in human brain was carried out at the Massachusetts Institute of Technology by David Cohen (1972). He measured the spontaneous activity of a healthy subject and the abnormal brain

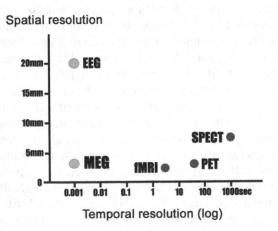

Fig. 1 Temporal and spatial resolution of brain imaging techniques
EEG   Electroencephalography; MEG   Magnetoencephalography; SPECT   Single-photon-emission computed tomography; PET   Positron-emission tomography; fMRI   Functional magnetic resonance imaging

activity of an epileptic patient. Evoked responses were first recorded a few years later (Brenner et al., 1975; Teyler et al., 1975). The first study of pain evoked magnetic fields was conducted in the 1980s (Hari et al., 1983).

Temporal and Spatial Resolution

The excellent temporal resolution of MEG allows us to follow sequential brain activations in response to painful stimulus. For example, the latencies of the peak main evoked magnetic fields following cutaneous A-delta and C fiber activations were approximately 150–200 ms and 750–1000 ms, respectively. Source analyses have also revealed that the earliest pain-induced cortical activities nearly simultaneously originate in S1 and S2, cortical areas responsible for the sensory-discriminative aspect of pain (Ploner et al., 1999; Tran et al., 2002). The activations in S1 and S2 are followed approximately 50–100 ms later by the activation in the anterior cingulate gyrus, which is believed to play a role in cognitive-evaluative aspect of pain processing (Druschky et al., 2000; Kitamura et al., 1997; Maihofner et al., 2002; Ninomiya et al., 2001).

With a precision ranging from 5–10 mm in spatial resolution, some MEG studies have provided information about somatotopic organization of pain in the S1 cortex (Huttunen et al., 1986; Kitamura et al., 1995, 1997).

Positron Emission Tomography (PET)

The Principles of PET

Positron emission tomography was the first technique that could measure brain function in three dimensions and provided a new and exciting tool to investigate human brain activity. In PET, as in fMRI, imaging is based on an assumption of a general coupling of neuronal activity and regional cerebral blood flow (rCBF). There is strong evidence supporting this assumption of neurovascular coupling (Logothetis et al., 2001; Sheth et al., 2004). In PET, cerebral blood flow is measured using diffusible radioactive agents (radiotracers) (Willoch, 2001). Radiotracers are positron-emitting isotopes that are produced and incorporated into molecules of a compound of interest. These labeled compounds are used to 'trace' biological processes. The tracer is injected intravenously into the blood stream and will distribute in the body according to its characteristics. Some of the atoms that are attached to the biological tracer molecules will decay, emitting a positron. The positron collides with electrons in the tissue and annihilates with one of these. This event produces energy which is released in form of two gamma rays that can be detected by external detector systems. The need for radioactive agents to be injected into the blood stream is a disadvantage of PET compared to fMRI. However, unlike fMRI, PET allows determination of the baseline (resting) rCBF in different brain structures. This information can be used for comparison with the activation (stimulus) condition and is essential when investigating the activation of brains with abnormal resting activity (Raichle et al., 2001).

A PET scanner consists of circumferential arrays of scintillation detectors which detect gamma rays. By detecting two simultaneous gamma rays resulting from the same energy emission, the location of the positron emission (in the tissue) can be determined. Finally, using conventional mathematical algorithms, data can be reconstructed into cross-sectional and 3D images of the brain tissue (Bailey, 1992; Shepp & Logan, 1974). In 3D mode acquisition time is reduced, thus reducing the radiation burden for subjects (Bruckbauer et al., 2000).

Radiotracers and Receptor Binding

The first PET study in 1981 used ^{18}F-fluorodiprenorphine (FDG) to show increasing metabolic rates in the human visual cortex in response to visual stimulation (Phelps et al., 1981). The long half-life of ^{18}F, however, does not allow repeated scanning of the same subject within a short time interval. The most used radiotracers are carbon (^{11}C), nitrogen (^{13}N) and oxygen (^{15}O), which all are essential components of the body. These isotopes have half-lives in the range of minutes to hours which makes them ideal for medical purposes (Willoch, 2001).

PET has also been useful in understanding the experience of pain. The endogenous opioid system plays a major role in reducing pain experience. It is activated by analgesic opiate drugs (Jones et al., 1994) and by endogenous opioids, such as during placebo analgesia (Petrovic et al., 2002). With PET it is possible to determine where opiate receptors are localized in the human brain using the receptor binding technique. It is also possible to determine the release of endogenous opioids. The basic principle is that a radioactive drug (ligand), which has a high affinity and a high degree of selectivity for the receptor under study, is injected intravenously. When the radioactive drug binds to the receptor a binding potential is measured as a parameter for the regional cerebral opioid receptor availability (Baumgartner et al., 2006).

Experimental Design and Statistical Analysis

Acquisition of each image for a ^{15}O-water activation study takes approximately 1 minute, which explains the relatively low temporal resolution of PET (Minoshima et al., 2000) (Fig. 1). Radiation exposure to subjects also poses some limitations on the design of PET experiments. As subjects should receive a limited amount of radiation per year, this may imply the use of between-subject designs rather than within-subject designs when comparing two experimental conditions (Sprenger et al., 2006).

Statistical analysis of PET images follows basically the same steps as for fMRI (see next section) with co-registration, movement correction, standardization and statistical modeling. Moreover, to determine the anatomical localization of PET activation, a structural MR image is performed on each subject.

Functional Magnetic Resonance Imaging (fMRI)

The BOLD Response

With increased synaptic activity there is greater local demand for delivery of energy (oxygen). To meet increased metabolic demand, neuronal activation is accompanied by increased local blood flow that overcompensates for the oxygen requirement (Ogawa et al., 1993). This is the theoretical basis for blood oxygen level-dependent (BOLD) imaging. In BOLD imaging a higher signal arises because oxyhaemoglobin does not disturb magnetic resonance signals as much as deoxyhaemoglobin, generating a contrast between activated and inactivated structures such as local draining venules and veins (Ogawa et al., 1993). There is evidence to support the critical assumption in fMRI studies of pain that the BOLD signal is a known and reliable function of the neuronal activity generated by a nociceptive (or pain-producing) signal (Buxton et al., 2004; Sheth et al., 2004). This relationship, however, may depend on how "neuronal activity" is measured. The time course of the BOLD response in a volume element (voxel) is complex and is to a large degree based on studies of the primary sensory cortex (Ernst & Hennig, 1994). A brief stimulus results in a BOLD response lasting about 10 s.

Rather than reflecting activity in single neurons, BOLD reflects activity in a particular region of the brain (Logothetis et al., 2001). Care must be taken during the interpretation of BOLD data, however, since cortical regions presumed to be involved in pain contain a mixed population of pain-signaling and non-pain-signaling neurons (Davis, 2003).

Data Acquisition

fMRI technology has received great interest over the past few years. It owes its popularity to its relatively low cost per examination, the lack of risks to repeated testing of the same individuals, as well as, its fine temporal and spatial resolution (Fig. 1). fMRI scanners are measured in terms of their magnetic field strength. In principle, the higher the field strength the weaker signals can be detected. Depending on the spatial resolution, the whole brain can be scanned in about 2 seconds (Bandettini, 2001).

Stimulus devices in fMRI must be of nonferromagnetic materials such as wood, aluminium or plastic to be compatible with the MRI environment. Most manufacturers of experimental pain devices offer fMRI compatible units today. Magnetic objects will not only interfere with imaging, but also pose a great risk to the subject.

This chapter will focus mainly on BOLD fMRI. Other techniques, such as arterial spin labeling (ASL) (Petersen et al., 2006) has been used less widely in the clinical context of pain, and are not covered in this chapter.

Experimental Design

fMRI designs can broadly be divided into two categories: block designs and event-related designs. In block design the stimulus is usually divided into one or several stimulus blocks (ON) and one or several resting blocks (OFF). Each block lasts relatively long (e.g. 30 sec). Under otherwise similar conditions between ON and OFF blocks, the idea is that only the specific process of interest show up when the resting image(s) are subtracted from the stimulus image(s). The time-course of an individual response is lost within a block. This is not a problem for event-related (single-trial) design. In event-related design the stimulus is on for a relatively short time (e.g. 1–1000 millisec) and activation data are acquired after discrete events. The time course of the BOLD response can then be defined and averaged across several events. Lasers and electrical stimulators are particularly relevant for event-related designs since the pulse is relatively short. Mechanical stimulation and contact-heat stimulation usually have some "ramp up" time until they reach the desired intensity, but may still be used in event-related designs.

Statistical Analysis

The aim of the statistical analysis in the context of pain imaging is to detect those regions of the brain that show increased intensity at the points in time that stimulation was applied (Tracey, 2005). This is performed at each volume element (voxel). Several pre-processing steps are completed before the statistical analysis. These will not be described here, but can be found elsewhere (Hu et al., 2005; Worsley, 2001). The most popular statistical approach is probably the general linear model (GLM). In GLM, a model of explanatory variables is set up and is fitted to the data in each voxel over time. The model provides a general pattern which you expect to see in the data. An example could be a square wave block design (ON/OFF-paradigm) with 30 s of stimulation followed by 30 s rest. To get the best possible fit of the model to the data, the sharp ON/OFF waveform is convolved with the haemodynamic response function (HRF). The convolution mimics the effect that the brain's neurophysiology has on the input function (Smith, 2001).

A simple example of a model with one explanatory variable is as follows:

$$y(t) = \beta * x(t) + c + e(t),$$

where $y(t)$ is the data, $x(t)$ is the model (square wave), c is a constant (rest intensity) and $e(t)$ is the error in the model fitting. β is the parameter estimate for $x(t)$ and represents the peak of the BOLD response. To convert β into a useful statistic, its value is compared with the uncertainty in its estimation (*standard error* (β); determined following multiple stimuli providing a population sample of β). This results in a T value for each voxel, where $T = \beta / standard\ error\ (\beta)$. In this example 'stimulation' is compared to 'rest.' It is also possible to compare two conditions (e.g. two different intensities of heat) by subtracting one β from the other, calculating the standard error for this difference and generating a new T image. Voxels showing statistically higher signals (higher T value) during ON-conditions are considered as "activation," coded with colors and overlaid on a high-resolution referenced anatomical image.

fMRI is extremely sensitive to motion of the head or brain (i.e. movement, respiration or cardiac cycles). All images (whole brain scans) are therefore co-registered to the first image to remove artifacts. To compare or average activation across multiple experiments on different subjects, functional and anatomical images are transformed into a standard stereotaxic space. Spatial and temporal filtering is then typically applied before the statistical analysis is done. More details on statistical modeling of functional imaging data can be found elsewhere (Beckmann et al., 2005; Bullmore et al., 2003; Fair et al., 2006; Flandin & Penny, 2007; Friston, 2005; Kiebel & Friston, 2004; Mitiche & Sekkati, 2006; Parker et al., 2006; Woolrich & Behrens, 2006; Worsley 2001).

Functional Connectivity

Studies of neuroimaging are largely correlative; behavior or symptoms are related to changes in brain activity within specialized regions (Tracey 2005). The consequence is that causality is poorly understood. Functional connectivity, defined as the temporal correlation between spatially remote neurophysiological events (Friston, 1994), is one approach to understand causality. The principle of functional connectivity comes from the concept that function is dependent on the flow of information between brain areas. Pain perception is a complex experience depending on the flow and integration of information between several brain regions and therefore lends itself to connectivity analyses (Tracey 2005). Functional connectivity analyses may be data-driven, making no assumptions about the underlying biology, or hypothesis-driven, based on knowledge of connections between brain regions. One disadvantage of the latter method is that a priori knowledge is required for modeling. Although connectivity analysis indicates causality, it may not give the full answer.

Pharmacological fMRI

fMRI is making a significant contribution to our understanding of drug-effects on brain systems (Wise & Tracey, 2006). When developing new therapeutic drugs, pharmaceutical companies rely to a great deal on so-called biomarkers. Biomarkers are measures of biologically relevant responses to the drug intervention. By applying existing agents to neuroanatomically dissect brain function in the normal and pathological brain, an imaging assay of drug effects on relevant brain function (biomarker) may be characterized. Although there are no current published examples of fMRI applied to novel compounds, fMRI may eventually contribute substantially to decision-making in drug development by demonstrating a proof-of-concept of drug action in a small human cohort, reducing the costs of drug development (Wise & Tracey, 2006).

Imaging Pain

The Pain Matrix

There has been an inability to identify a 'pain centre' in the brain. This is probably because pain is of multiple dimensions which include sensory-discriminative, affective-motivational, and cognitive-evaluative components (Melzack & Casey, 1968). The specific role of cerebral cortex in pain perception has been a matter of debate for many decades. The notion that pain is perceived in the thalamus can be traced back to the report by Head and Holmes, which was based on careful clinical observations in patients (Head & Holmes, 1911). This belief was further supported by the observations of Penfield and Boldrey, where electrical stimulation of S1 cortex rarely, if ever, evoked pain sensation in conscious patients (Penfield & Boldrey, 1937). These observations had questioned the participation of the cerebral cortex in human pain perception for many years. However, other authors have also shown evidence that cortical wounds impaired pain sensation and neurosurgical experience has emphasized the long-term unpredictability of the results obtained following most ablative procedures of cerebral structures (Sweet, 1982; White & Sweet, 1969). This failure to identify a "pain centre" in the brain is in accord with the results of current electrophysiological and functional imaging studies of pain (for review see Peyron et al. (2000); Casey and Tran (2006); Apkarian et al. (2005) or Kakigi et al. (2004)) which demonstrate the involvement of widely distributed cortical areas in pain perception.

Central processing of the sensory-discriminative component of pain has been ascribed to the lateral nociceptive system, whereas the medial nociceptive system processes the affective-emotional component of pain. In the lateral system, the spinothalamic tract originating in the nociceptive areas of the spinal dorsal horn projects to nuclei in the lateral thalamus, whereas the spinothalamic tract of the medial system projects to nuclei in the medial thalamus. From the thalamus, the thalamocortical pathways in turn project to the cortical areas, with S1 and S2 belonging to the lateral system, and anterior cingulate cortex to the medial system. The insular cortex forms a communication channel between the sensory-discriminative function of the somatosensory cortex and limbic cortical structures mediating the affective component of pain.

Given the present state of the science, we now know there are many cortical areas involved in the sensory-discriminative, affective-emotional and cognitive-motivational aspects of pain perception, and these cortical structures may have partially overlapping functions. Therefore, the S1, S2, anterior insula (AI), posterior insula (PI), premotor cortex (PreMot) and inferior parietal cortex (InfPar) all play a role in the sensory aspect of pain; and again AI, PS, PreMot and InfPar contribute to the affective aspect of pain along with anterior cingulate cortex (ACC), posterior cingulate cortex (PCC), orbitofrontal cortex (OFC), medial prefrontal cortex (MedPFC), hippocampus and entorhinal cortex (Hip/Ento). In turn, the OFC, MedPFC and Hip/Ento, along with the dorsal lateral prefrontal cortex (DLPFC), are also involved in cognitive-motivational aspect of pain.

Electrophysiological and functional imaging studies of pain reveal that the most commonly reported areas in MEG studies are S1, S2 and ACC; and in functional imaging studies the most commonly reported areas (PET and fMRI) are S1, S2, ACC, insular cortex, and the thalamus (Apkarian et al., 2005). In this section, we will present what specific functions these cortical areas subserve in pain perception based on the different aspects of pain experience. Yet, many lines of evidence suggest that sensory, affective and other dimensions of pain are likely to be processed in parallel by different parts of the nociceptive system.

Sensory-Discriminative Aspect of Pain

The sensory-discriminative component of pain refers to the capacity to discriminate the spatial, temporal, intensity and quality domains of a painful stimulus. In other words, this component accounts for our capacity to know "where does it hurt?", "how long does it last?", and "how intense is it?".

Primary somatosensory cortex (S1). Electrophysiological studies in humans with noxious laser or brief mechanical stimulation revealed that the earliest nociceptive information, the pain-related MEG and EEG evoked signals, arrives nearly simultaneously in the S1 and S2 (Arendt-Nielsen et al., 1999; Kakigi et al., 1995; Kanda et al., 2000; Schnitzler & Ploner, 2000). A recent MEG study with laser-evoked selective stimulation of C-fibers also found nearly simultaneously responses within approximately 750 ms in both S1 and S2 cortices (Tran et al., 2002). In the S1, electrophysiological studies show that the primary activities following painful electrical and ascorbic acid stimulation of finger and leg are in hand and foot areas, respectively (Kitamura et al., 1995; Kitamura et al., 1997; Porro et al., 1998). Moreover, using painful CO_2 stimulation of the nasal membrane, Huttunen and colleagues revealed a cortical response near the lateral end of the central sulcus, which is close to the face area in the S1 (Huttunen et al., 1986).

Early functional imaging studies inconsistently showed S1 activation following painful stimuli. In a meta-analysis, Peyron and colleagues suggested that the discrepancy was probably due to the stimulated size, and that the spatial summation was more critical than temporal summation to elicit S1 activity (Peyron et al., 2000). In fact, S1 is one of the most common areas which shows activity following pain stimuli in many functional imaging studies (Apkarian et al., 2005). In accord with electrophysiological studies, a PET study using intracutaneous injection of capsaicin also revealed different locations along the central sulcus for hand pain and foot pain (Andersson et al., 1997). These findings support the role of S1 in spatial discrimination in pain perception. To investigate the involvement of human cortical areas encoding temporal and intensive aspects of pain, Porro and colleagues using subcutaneous ascorbic acid induced pain have demonstrated that S1 responses were specifically related to pain intensity and duration in an fMRI study (Porro et al., 1998). This result is also consistent with more recent studies that used the stimulus-response function to define the brain regions responsible for intensity encoding (Alkire, White, Hsieh, & Haier, 2004; Bornhövd et al., 2002; Büchel et al., 2002; Kong et al., 2006). Evidence from other functional imaging studies also supports the concept that the S1 cortex participates in the sensory-discriminative aspect of pain (Bushnell et al., 1999; Chen et al., 2002; Coghill et al., 1999; Duncan & Albanese, 2003; Peyron et al., 1999), although cognitive variables may further modify the intensity of the response significantly (see below).

The weight of evidence from a variety of sources favors the view that S1 cortex is specialized to engage in the earliest processes mediating the discriminative aspects of pain sensation. Clinical observations also suggest that this cortical area is essential for nociceptive discriminative functions, but is less essential for mediating or modulating the affective or cognitive aspects of chronically painful conditions (Casey & Tran, 2006; Ploner et al., 1999).

Secondary somatosensory cortex (S2). The MEG is considered a highly sensitive technique to detect S2 activity due to its tangential and superficial current dipole. Consequently, almost all MEG studies report S2 activity following pain stimuli. The simultaneous activation of S1 and S2 indicates parallel thalamocortical processing of pain signals (Ploner et al., 1999; Tran et al., 2002). Furthermore, it is found that the duration of neuronal activity in S2 is significantly longer than in the S1 cortex (Inui et al., 2002; Kanda et al., 2000; Ploner et al., 2002).

The S2 cortex is also one of the most consistently activated structures in PET and fMRI studies (Burton et al., 1993; Casey, 1999; Davis, 2000; Derbyshire, 2003; Peyron et al., 2000). For review see also Apkarian et al. (2005). An fMRI study that applied electrical stimulation on different fingers demonstrated that there was a coarse somatotopic organization within the S2 cortex (Ruben et al., 2001). Another fMRI study also provided evidence that both S1 and S2 encode spatial information of nociceptive stimuli without additional information from the tactile system (Bingel et al., 2004). In contrast, other functional imaging studies provided evidence against the role of the S2 in spatial-discriminative aspects of pain perception (Ferretti et al., 2004; Timmermann et al., 2001; Xu et al., 1997). However, S2 activation is well correlated with pain intensity as shown in a fMRI study (Coghill et al., 1999).

In brief, many lines of evidence support the view that S2 is probably not critical for spatial discrimination. Instead, the early S2 activation appears to be intensity-dependent, and therefore, involved in the early identification of noxious nature and attention toward more painful stimuli.

Functional imaging studies also reveal many other cortical areas, whose activities are related to some domains of the sensory-discriminative component of pain, e.g. intensity and duration (Coghill et al., 1999; Craig et al., 2000; Peyron et al., 1999; Porro et al., 1998). Those cortical areas include anterior insula and ACC, which are essential to the cortical network mediating some early aspects of pain perception including anticipation and attention rather than the sensory-discriminative aspect of pain (Davis et al., 1997; Ploghaus et al., 1999); and the premotor and medial prefrontal cortices, which are more likely to be involved in developing a motor response to stimulus and the emotional impact and evaluative aspects of pain perception (Wager et al., 2003).

Affective-Motivational Aspect of Pain

The affective-motivational component is an essential part of pain sensation, because pain always has some hedonic aspects. The affective-motivational aspect imparts aversive qualities and emotional reactions to noxious stimuli ("I don't like it"), and the cognitive-motivational aspect represent the evaluation of pain in terms of past experience, enviromental context, expectation and its significance for daily life (e.g. "What will this do to me?") (Melzack & Casey, 1968).

Anterior cingulate cortex (ACC). Electrophysiological studies in humans revealed that the earliest nociceptive information, the pain-related MEG and EEG evoked signals, arrives nearly simultaneously not only in the S1 and S2, but also in the AI and ACC (Arendt-Nielsen et al., 1999; Kakigi et al., 1995; Kanda et al., 2000; Ploner et al., 1999; Schnitzler & Ploner 2000), indicating that spatiotemporal and intensity analysis begins in parallel with the processing of affective-related information (Ploner et al., 2002; Schnitzler & Ploner 2000).

Functional imaging studies show that either the rostral or mid-anterior or both sectors of ACC are activated consistently during pain (Bushnell et al., 1999; Casey 1999; Derbyshire, 2000; Derbyshire 2003). In a beautiful experiment designed to differentiate cortical areas involved in pain affect, Rainville and colleagues used hypnotic suggestions to alter selectively the unpleasantness of noxious stimuli, without changing the perceived intensity. This PET study revealed significant changes in pain-evoked activity within ACC, consistent with the encoding of perceived unpleasantness, whereas S1 cortex activation was unchanged. These findings provide direct experimental evidence in humans linking the ACC activity with pain affect and a less likely role of the S1 in mediating the affective components of pain (Rainville et al., 1997). There is evidence in pain imaging studies that the ACC is also involved in attention-demanding cognitive tasks (Davis et al., 1997; Peyron et al., 1999). Another PET study showed that the most rostral sector of the ACC is active only during the early phase of repetitive heat stimulation and the activation of the more caudal part of the ACC appears during the later phase (Casey et al., 2001). This result is in accord with the observation that the most rostral sector of the ACC is associated with the anticipation of pain (Ploghaus et al., 1999). Sawamoto and colleagues further showed that the uncertain expectation of painful stimulus enhanced ACC responses to non-painful stimulus (Sawamoto et al., 2000). Interestingly, a recent fMRI study reported anterior insula and ACC activation when female subjects experienced pain and when they witnessed a loved one experiencing pain (Singer et al., 2004). Furthermore, the areas activated by empathy with another's pain closely matched areas activated by cognitive evaluation (Kong et al., 2006).

Taken together, the results suggest that the ACC is activated very early in the course of nociceptive processing. The early parallel processing of affective and sensory information is consistent with the concept that noxious stimuli have an intrinsic, primary unpleasantness (Fields, 1999; Melzack & Casey 1968; Price, 2000). In brief, the ACC participates in the affective and cognitive aspects of pain perception.

Insular cortex. The insular cortex, which gives rise to a radial current dipole, is not sensitive to MEG recording, but is more sensitive to other functional imaging techniques that measure haemodynamic changes.

Many functional imaging studies show pain-related activity in the anterior insula (AI) (Casey et al., 1996; Coghill et al., 1994; Davis et al., 1998; Hsieh et al., 1994; Svensson et al., 1997). Moreover, a PET imaging study shows that the AI is active during the early phase of a series of repetitive noxious heat stimuli, but not after the stimulation continues for 45 s (Casey et al., 2001). This is consistent with the findings that the AI was activated specifically during the anticipation of experimentally induced pain rather than during the experience of pain itself (Ploghaus et al., 1999). There is also evidence that activity in AI cortex is increased not only during anticipation of pain but also correlated with perceived pain intensity (Peyron et al., 1999; Porro et al., 2002). A recent fMRI study showed that AI specifically responded to stimulus novelty (Downar et al., 2002). The AI is activated when female subjects experienced pain and when they witnessed a loved one experiencing pain (Singer et al., 2004), and it is also activated by cognitive evaluation (Kong et al., 2006). These results suggest that the AI is an essential component of the cortical network mediating some early aspects of pain perception including the anticipation and cognitive evaluation of pain.

The mid-posterior insula is among the most regularly responsive regions found among a variety of functional imaging studies (Casey 1999; Craig et al., 2000; Peyron et al., 2002, 2000). Derbyshire (2003) has reviewed evidence showing that visceral distention activates both the AI and PI cortices. However, the most posterior insular activation is observed during esophageal stimulation and the most anterior activation during rectal stimulation. These findings may imply a functional anatomical distinction between the two areas of insular cortex.

There is very little evidence which indicates that the insular activity related to attention (Peyron et al., 2000). Although no pain studies have directly investigated the correlation of insular activity and the affective and emotional component of pain, there is evidence of insular involvement with emotional tasks with negative affective component such as stimulation with fearful faces, emotional voices or aversive conditions (Buchel et al., 1999; Morris et al., 1998; Phillips et al., 1997).

The anatomical connectivity, functional imaging results and clinical observations (see below) note that the insular cortex forms a communication channel between the discriminative functions of the somatosensory cortex and limbic cortical structures mediating the affective components of pain. Activity in the mid-and posterior insula follows that in the S1, S2, and AI cortices and is associated with a clear recognition of the intensity of the noxious stimulus, its affective quality, and its biological significance (Casey & Tran 2006).

In summary, many lines of evidence in pain studies demonstrate the involvement of widely distributed cortical structures in pain perception. These cortical areas may have partially overlapping functions. There are cortical areas mediating early identification of the spatial localization, intensity, and affective quality of noxious stimuli. These cortical activities may occur at preconscious levels or at the earliest stages of conscious experience. As the nociceptive identification process is sustained, even for a brief period, there are cortical areas that participate in the conscious awareness of the noxious event, leading to the subsequent allocation of attentional resources and the recognition of stimulus identity for further analysis and immediate response. Following this recognition and immediate reaction, other cortical structures mediate a more prolonged and detailed analysis of the physical nature of the stimulus for the evaluation and sustained behavior (for detail see Casey and Tran (2006)).

Pain Modulation

The transmission of nociceptive signals is continuously modulated by networks in the central nervous system (CNS). Modulation depends on a host of variables; other somatic stimuli, social, environmental and psychological factors such as arousal, attention and expectation (Fields et al., 2005; Osborne et al., 2007). These variables may contribute to development and maintenance of chronic pain states. Development of low back pain disability, for example, depends on psychosocial factors (Gatchel et al., 1995) and pain catastrophizing (responses to pain that characterize it as being awful, horrible and unbearable) is increasingly recognized as an extremely important contributor to the experience of pain in fibromyalgia patients (Gracely et al., 2004). Cognitive evaluation of pain states depends on prior experience and involves memory (Gedney et al., 2003; Petrovic et al., 2005; Ploghaus et al., 2003).

A challenge when studying brain regions involved in pain modulation is that little is known about which regions are involved in which components of the pain experience (Wager, 2005). Many of these same gross anatomical regions are activated by nonpainful cognitive and emotional demands, making it unclear whether activations represent pain-specific processes or the attentional and behavioral responses elicited by pain. The areas involving cognitive evaluation of pain does not even require somatic input to be activated, as empathy with another's pain, and expectation of pain, closely match areas activated by cognitive evaluation of pain (Koyama et al., 2005; Singer et al., 2004).

Below we will provide some examples of how functional imaging has contributed to understanding how psychological factors such as attention, expectation and emotion modulate pain.

Impact of Attention and Distraction

For pain of weak to moderate intensity distraction is probably one of the more frequently used self-treatments. When a child cries after a minor injury, parents use distraction as the most natural treatment. Distraction is a cognitive coping strategy and distraction from a painful event is usually reported to decrease the level of reported pain intensity and unpleasantness, compared with attention to the stimulus (Bushnell et al., 1999; Dowman, 2001; Eccleston, 1995). Distraction-studies are, however, not always easy to interpret given a paradox inherent in studies of divided attention: one cannot simultaneously attend to pain in order to give a rating while being distracted (Roelofs et al., 2003).

Neural correlates of reported pain reduction during distraction have been found in several structures in the pain matrix that encode both sensory and affective information. Regions showing reduced activity during distraction correspond to the pain matrix and include S1, S2, thalamus, insular cortex and anterior cingulate cortex (area 24) (Bantick et al., 2002; Petrovic et al., 2000; Peyron et al., 2000; Valet et al., 2004). Figure 2 is taken from Valet et al (2004) and shows the cerebral processing of a 40-s heat pain stimulus without (A) and with (B) distraction by the colour Stroop task. Without distraction noxious stimulation evokes activation of the sensory-discriminative pain system (e.g.: S1, S2, lateral thalamus, posterior insular cortex) and the affective-motivational system (medial thalamus, ACC, anterior insular cortex). During distraction the same noxious stimulation is no longer able to activate the former pain network. There are MEG studies which attempt to identify brain regions involved in attentional modulation of pain as well. A MEG study demonstrated cognitive modulation on early pain processing in S2 cortex; S2 activity was enhanced by attention (Nakamura et al., 2002).

In contrast to Valet et al (2004), who found elimination of almost all pain-related activity during distraction, Seminowicz and Davis recently showed that although activity in several pain-related regions was attenuated, all pain-related areas (S1/M1, S2, paracentral lobule, SMA, caudal ACC, AI, and cerebellum) were nonetheless significantly activated by painful stimuli during distraction (Seminowicz & Davis, 2007). The authors explain their results by pointing to the extremely important biological role of nociceptive pain, rendering it likely that pain, and pain-related activity may not be entirely diminished by cognitive disruption. A variance in experimental design may also contribute to explaining the differences between the contrasting findings of Valet et al (2004) and

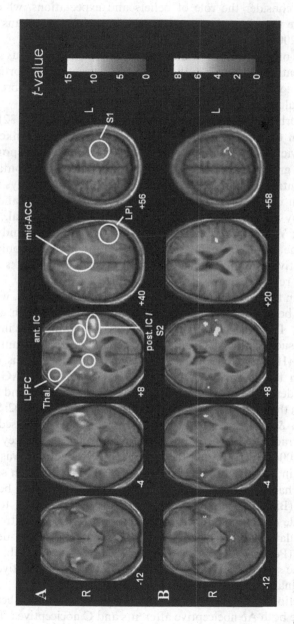

Fig. 2 Effects of distraction on cerebral pain processing. (A) Without distraction heat stimulation activates the sensory-discriminative pain coding system (e.g.: S1, S2, lateral thalamus, posterior insular cortex) and affective-motivational system (medial thalamus, ACC, anterior insular cortex). (B) With distraction, induced by the Stroop-task, the same noxious stimulation is no longer able to activate the former pain network. Image right is brain left. (From Valet et al., 2004; reprinted with permission. Pain 109, 399–408)

Seminowicz and Davis (2007), namely that in the latter study the subjects were not instructed to rate the pain intensity while in the scanner. Studies where subjects know they will be required to provide ratings, such as that of Valet and co-authors, should consider the role of beliefs and expectations, which are known to contribute to pain and pain-related brain activity (Ploghaus et al., 2003; Wager et al., 2004).

There are reports of a shift in the insular region activated by noxious stimuli (from anterior to central insula) when the subject is distracted, supporting the view that the insula consists of discrete functional/anatomic units whose activity depends on stimulus attention (Brooks et al., 2002).

The prefrontal, orbitofrontal and anterior cingulate cortex (area 32) show increased activation during distraction (Bantick et al., 2002; Frankenstein et al., 2001; Petrovic et al., 2000; Valet et al., 2004). This corresponds to findings by several groups suggesting that the dorsoloateral prefrontal cortex exerts active control on pain perception by modulating pathways within the cortex, between cortex and subcortical structures (thalamus and midbrain), as shown by functional connectivity analyses (Lorenz et al., 2002; Lorenz et al., 2003; Valet et al., 2004). According to Seminowicz and Davis (2007), however, the bilateral dorsolateral prefrontal cortex was only activated at high cognitive demand, indicating that lower difficulty tasks can be performed without reliance on this prefrontal area.

A key structure in the midbrain is the periaqueductal gray (PAG), which is also considered to be a site for modulation of higher cortical pain activity (Tracey et al., 2002). PAG has connections to several key brain areas involved in pain processing, such as the ACC, amygdala, thalamus, hypothalamus and prefrontal cortices (Hadjipavlou et al., 2006). Caudally the PAG is closely interconnected with the rostroventral medulla (RVM) and the PAG/RVM system is thus considered the final common pathway of facilitatory and inhibitory influences from the brain on spinal excitability (Porreca et al., 2002; Suzuki et al., 2004; Urban & Gebhart, 1999). Some studies report increased PAG activity during distraction when compared to a control task (Tracey et al., 2002; Valet et al., 2004). In one study the increase in PAG activity was correlated with changes in perceived intensity (Tracey et al., 2002), which seem to correspond with what happens during anticipation of pain relief before a placebo treatment (Bingel et al., 2006; Wager et al., 2004). Taken together these studies provide evidence supporting the notion that PAG controls descending pain modulation. PAG activity has also been reported to decrease during distraction (Petrovic et al., 2000), which could reflect inhibition of noxious input at the spinal level since the structure receives nociceptive input directly through spinal pathways (Blomqvist & Craig, 1991).

Most of the functional imaging studies described above used tonic heat pain stimuli that activate both $A\delta$ nociceptive afferents and C nociceptive afferents. Using MEG, Qiu and colleagues have shown that distraction reduce the amplitude of C-fiber evoked MEG responses in S1, S2 and the cingulate gyrus (Qiu et al., 2004). This implies that distraction is able to affect processing of nociceptive information rather early in the signal pathway. Also, C fibers are considered particularly important in several chronic pain conditions including musculoskeletal pain and neuropathic pain (Djouhri et al., 2006). Although distraction seems to influence experimental pain at a statistically significant level, the clinical significance of distraction in inhibiting pain is not evident. The general clinical consensus is that pain must be reduced by at least 30% for it to be meaningful to patients (Farrar et al., 2003; Farrar et al., 2001; Salaffi et al., 2004). The majority of experimental studies report reductions in the order of 5% (Todd, 1996; Turk, 2000). One clinical example of distraction is the use of virtual reality during burn wound dressing changes. Compared to a control situation, virtual reality produced a decline in subjective pain ratings, accompanied by large decreases in pain-related brain activity in ACC, S1, S2, insula and thalamus (Hoffman et al., 2006).

The tendency to "catastrophize" during painful stimulation contributes to more intense pain experience and increased emotional distress (Sullivan et al., 2001). Several theoretical models have tried to explain pain catastrophizing, one being the attention model that describes a difficulty in disengaging from pain (Van Damme et al., 2004). The attention model is supported by neuroimaging data in subjects with chronic fibromyalgia pain, showed a correlation between catastrophizing scores and activity in the dorsolateral prefrontal cortex, rostral anterior cingulate cortex, and medial prefrontal cortex (Gracely et al., 2004). Also in healthy individuals, catastrophizing affects brain activity involved in pain perception. Individuals with higher catastrophizing scores seemed to engage more a cortical network implicated in affective, attention, and motor responses (Seminowicz & Davis, 2006). During intense pain, however, these individuals showed little engagement in cortical areas implicated in top-down modulation of pain, indicating a lack of pain control in people considered to be catastrophizers (Seminowicz & Davis 2006). Catastrophizing can be treated through manipulations designed to change the threat value of the stimulus, or attention to the stimulus. The findings also suggest that behavioral interventions designed to alter attention to or the perceived threat of clinical pain may be beneficial among persons with pain who catastrophize about their condition (Gracely et al., 2004).

Taken together, functional imaging studies of distraction from pain seem to modulate activity in areas involved in both sensory-discriminative and affective-motivational pain processing. The degree of modulation seems to originate in prefrontal areas, and possibly activate PAG, which in turn controls descending inhibition of nociceptive signals. As such, the effect of distraction depends on cognitive complexity, timing of subjective pain rating, as well as, on emotional components such as catastrophic thinking.

Impact of Expectation and Emotion

Expectation plays a significant role in modulation of pain and predicts recovery after painful episodes. In placebo analgesia, expectation is considered a key element along with conditioning (Amanzio & Benedetti, 1999; Benedetti, F, Pollo A. this volume). In situations of fear or anxiety expectation interacts with emotion to influence the pain experience (Gedney & Logan, 2007; Rhudy & Meagher, 2000). Fear and anxiety has been conceptualized into 'certain expectations' and 'uncertain expectations', respectively, which seem to be mediated by different neural pathways (Ploghaus et al., 2003).

The present section gives an overview of neural networks of pain modulation in the cognitive and emotional context by presenting selected studies of how pain and neural correlates of pain is modulated by expectation, emotion and hypnosis.

Expectation. Expectation is defined as "a strong belief that something will happen or be the case" (Expectation, 2006). That expectation of reduced pain leads to lower subjective pain ratings has been shown in numerous reports (e.g. Benedetti et al. (1999); Dannecker et al. (2003); Hirsch and Liebert (1998)).Yet, some researchers question the existence of expectation-induced analgesia, such as placebo-analgesia. The arguments presented are that the placebo response results from effects such as spontaneous recovery or a social contract between therapist and patient (Hrobjartsson & Gotzsche, 2001). Several epidemiological studies, however, show quite clearly that expectation has health effects, e.g. by predicting work-disability after episodes of back pain (Heymans et al., 2006; Turner et al., 2006), supporting the view that expectation may contribute significantly in the clinical setting.

The placebo-model has in recent years been used extensively to study expectation. Functional imaging studies have found correlations between brain regions activated during anticipation and brain regions encoding pain intensity, suggesting that expectation-induced pain-reduction is much more than reporting bias (Koyama et al., 2005; Petrovic et al., 2002; Wager et al., 2004). During expectation-induced analgesia the subject is led to anticipate reduced pain given a certain context. The context can be a pain-killer (such as a pill) administered by a health care provider, as is usually the case in placebo studies. Alternatively a Pavlovian conditioning task can be used, where a conditioning stimulus (such as a symbol) precedes an unconditioned stimulus (such as a painful stimulus). By repeated pairings of different symbols and different stimulus intensities, learning is induced. Conditioning in this regard is mediated through expectancy (Benedetti et al., 2003; Montgomery & Kirsch, 1997) and the subject learns to expect a certain stimulus intensity when he/she sees a certain symbol.

If some of the somatic stimuli are falsely signaled, e.g. a painful stimulus follows a symbol signaling a non-painful stimulus; it is possible to study the effect of expectancy on the experience of pain. This paradigm was recently used by Koyama and colleagues (Koyama et al., 2005). Their objective was to identify whether brain regions activated during expectation interacted with brain regions encoding pain intensity, thus identifying brain regions encoding the subjective experience of reduced pain intensity. They found significant overlap between regions activated during a 50°C heat stimulus and during expectation of the same stimulus in insula, ACC and supplementary motor

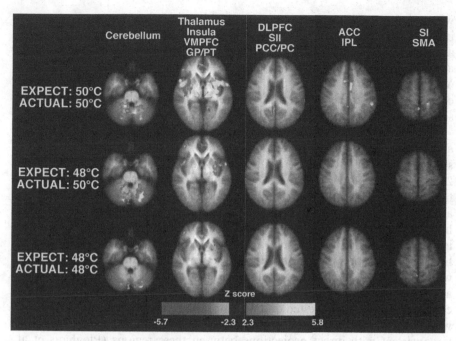

Fig. 3 Expectations for decreased pain significantly reduce pain-related brain activation during 50°C stimulation. Image right is brain left. (From Koyama et al., 2005; Copyright (2005) National Academy of Sciences, U.S.A)

area. Rostral ACC portions tended to have greater expectation-related activation, and caudal portions tended to have greater pain-intensity-related activation. When subjects expected a 48°C stimulus, but received a 50°C stimulus, no detectable activation was found in ACC and S1 (Fig. 3, middle row), when compared to a correctly signaled 50°C stimulus (Fig. 3, upper row). The degree of activation in the insula, dorsolateral prefrontal cortex, S2 and other areas were also significantly reduced. In fact, after decreased expectations of pain the pain-intensity-related activation closely resembled that evoked by correctly signaled 48°C stimuli (Fig. 3, bottom row).

Taken together, ACC, S1 and S2 likely represent critical pathways for the integration of expectation-related information with afferent sensory information (Koyama et al., 2005). Connections exist between ACC/insula and S1/S2, thus, all of these cortical areas receiving afferent nociceptive information can be modulated by expectation-induced information. There is emerging, although still incomplete evidence that at least part of the expectancy effect is mediated by descending pain modulatory circuits (Matre et al., 2006; Wager et al., 2006).

Emotion. Emotion may be defined as a physiological state in which an intense affective experience is accompanied by physiological reactions to the inciting event (eg: laughter, crying, preparations to attack or flee, etc.). Emotions such as fear and anxiety have divergent effects on human pain thresholds;

whereas fear leads to reduced pain sensitivity, anxiety has been shown to increase pain sensitivity (Rhudy & Meagher 2000). In the clinical setting, anxiety levels have been reported to predict pain severity and behavior in acute and chronic pain patients (Kain et al., 2000; van den Hout et al., 2001). Yet the relationship between pain and anxiety is not always positive or unidirectional. For instance, anxiety that is irrelevant to the source of pain does not seem to increase pain (al Absi & Rokke, 1991).

In a conditioning study, similar to Koyama et al (2005) (see above), Ploghaus and colleagues induced expectations of high and low anxiety in a group of subjects receiving high and low intensity thermal stimulation (Ploghaus et al., 2001). High anxiety was induced by giving the subjects intermittent stimuli of high intensity when they received a signal for low-intensity stimulation. Low anxiety was induced by correctly signaling a low-intensity stimulus. During high anxiety, the low-intensity stimulus was perceived as significantly more intense than during low anxiety. Event-related fMRI analysis comparing the high and low anxiety conditions revealed activation in the left entorhinal cortex, which is consistent with observations of left-lateralized processing of explicit aversive conditioning in the medial temporal lobes (Ploghaus et al., 2001). A correlation analysis suggested that the entorhinal cortex correlated significantly with time courses in the perigenual cingulate cortex and in the mid-insula, which is consistent with direct projections between these regions (Ploghaus et al., 2001). The perigenual cingulate cortex, involved in affective processing (Bush et al., 2000), is activated by aversive conditioned stimuli (Buchel et al., 1999) and during symptom provocation in patients with anxiety disorders (Rauch et al., 1995). Ploghaus and co-workers (2001) further suggest that the entorhinal cortex mediated anxiety-induced hyperalgesia by influencing intensity coding in the mid-insula, an area which mediates thermosensitivity (Craig et al., 2000).

The data presented above provides a neural mechanism which can, in part, explain the positive impact of optimism in chronic disease states (Drossman et al., 1988). That multiple brain regions are affected by expectation is likely, given the highly distributed and parallel nature of pain processing. For instance, during anxiety, the entorhinal cortex seems to play a vital role. A better understanding of the neural processes underlying different forms of expectation is of great interest from a basic science perspective, as it can potentially assist in the development of novel therapeutic strategies (Ploghaus et al., 2003), as well as, potentially modulate the clinical context where care is provided (Benedetti et al., 2007; Colloca & Benedetti, 2006).

Hypnosis. Hypnosis has three main components: absorption, dissociation and suggestibility (Spiegel, 1991). Absorption is the tendency to become fully involved in an experience. Dissociation is the mental separation of components of behavior that would ordinarily be processed together. Suggestibility leads to an enhanced tendency to comply with hypnotic instructions.

Studies using hypnotic analgesia have contributed to improved understanding of cerebral processing of the sensory and affective components of pain. By giving hypnotic suggestions to reduce pain unpleasantness (affective component of pain) there is a correlation in ACC activity (area 24) accompanied by reduced pain unpleasantness ratings while pain intensity ratings is unchanged (Rainville et al., 1997). This study was the first to provide direct evidence of a specific encoding for pain unpleasantness in the ACC. In another study by the same group, suggestions were given to reduce pain intensity (Hofbauer et al., 2001). This time pain intensity ratings were accompanied by changes in S1 activity without changing ACC activity.

Faymonville and colleagues, using hypnosis and PET, confirmed the role of ACC (area 24) in encoding pain affect and showed that it also plays a role in encoding pain intensity (Faymonville et al., 2000). This has later been confirmed (Büchel et al., 2002). A subsequent study, by the same authors, used a functional connectivity approach to demonstrate that area 24 modulates a large cortical and subcortical network. Compared to normal alertness (rest and mental imagery), the hypnotic state enhanced the functional modulation between midcingulate cortex (area 24) and bilateral insula, pregenual anterior cingulate cortex, pre-supplementary motor area, right prefrontal cortex and striatum, thalamus and brainstem (Faymonville et al., 2003), see Fig. 4. Two recent connectivity analyses also confirms that the rostral ACC is capable of activating caudal regions involved in nociceptive modulation, such as PAG and nucleus cuneiformis (Bingel et al., 2006; Wager, Scott, & Zubieta, 2007).

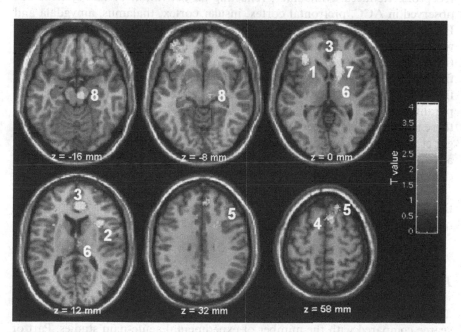

Fig. 4 Regions that showed an increased functional connectivity with midcingulate cortex in hypnosis relative to normal alertness rest and mental imagery. 1,2: Insula, 3: pregenual cortex, 4: Pre-supplementary motor area, 5: superior frontal gyrus, 6: Thalamus, 7: Caudate nucleus, 8: Midbrain/brainstem. (From Faymonville et al., 2003; reprinted with permission)

Taken together, the anterior cingulate cortex is confirmed as a region that orchestrates caudal cortical and subcortical networks crucial for learning and descending inhibition.

Effects of opiates. The opioid system is a vital antinociceptive system and is activated endogenously during painful stimulation (Sprenger et al., 2006; Zubieta et al., 2001), during placebo analgesia (Petrovic et al., 2002; Zubieta et al., 2005), and during the exogenous administration of opioid compounds (Casey et al., 2000; Wagner et al., 2007). An example of the latter is the study by Casey and colleagues where they report reduced rCBF in most brain regions responsive to pain during a cold stimulation with and without fentanyl (a mu-opioid agonist) (Casey et al., 2000). This confirms an inhibitory effect of fentanyl on pain-induced neuronal activity. Casey et al. (2000) also showed that fentanyl activates the rostral ACC, known for its involvement in pain inhibition. A similar approach was used by Petrovic and colleagues using heat pain, remifentanil and placebo (Petrovic et al., 2002). They revealed overlaps in terms of rCBF increases in dorsal ACC during active the drug and placebo, suggesting that this brain region may be involved in placebo effects.

With ligand PET techniques, it is possible to investigate the opioid system in vivo. Using sustained muscle pain combined with the mu-opioid radiotracer ^{11}C-carfentanil, Zubieta et al (2001) determined the availability of mu-opioid receptors. Reduced availability, reflecting an activation of this system, was observed in ACC, prefrontal cortex, insular cortex, thalamus, amygdala and PAG. Subjectively assessed pain affect is associated with activity in an area within ACC, an area that has previously been associated with pain affect (Rainville et al., 1997). Supporting the role of ACC in pain modulation are findings by Sprenger and colleagues. Using heat pain and the radiotracer ^{18}F-fluorodiprenorphine they demonstrated reduced receptor binding in limbic and paralimbic brain areas including the rostral ACC and insula, indicating that these regions are activate in pain modulation during a painful stimulus (Sprenger et al., 2006). Considering the complex functions of the insula, opioids may alter pain perception directly at the insular level, or by insular influences on the descending inhibitory system (i.e. PAG/RVM) (Sprenger et al., 2006).

An understanding of the opioid receptor system is likely to be improved by the use of receptor binding studies in the coming years, by probing into the neurochemical changes in response to acute and chronic pain conditions.

Pain Imaging in Patients

The number of functional imaging studies in patients with long-lasting pain is scarce compared with the number of experimental acute-pain studies. Part of the explanation may be that patient populations vary largely in terms of pain history, pain distribution, cause of pain and psychological factors; posing a challenge when designing studies. The present section provides a few examples on how functional imaging has proved useful in understanding clinical pain states. For a more extensive review of brain imaging of clinical states, the reader is referred to a recently published a review by Kupers and Kehlet (2006).

One area in clinical pain research that has been studied is neuropathic pain. Neuropathic pain is when trauma or disease affecting peripheral nerves result in development of chronic pain (Devor, 2005). Spontaneous pain and hypersensitivity are usually present and there is a general consensus today that both peripheral and central nervous system processes play a role (Devor 2005). Functional brain imaging has been used in a number of studies to reveal abnormal nociceptive brain processing in patients with neuropathic pain (Casey et al., 2003; Petrovic et al., 1999; Peyron et al., 1998; Peyron et al., 2004; Schweinhardt et al., 2006).

Insights into the pathophysiology of painful sensory disorders was provided by Lorenz and colleagues using fMRI (Lorenz et al., 2002, 2003). In an experimental model of heat allodynia (hypersensitivity to heat), topical capsaicin (the pungent ingredient in chili pepper) was used to increase the sensitivity to contact heat such that a normally warm stimulus (approx. 43°C) became as intense as noxious heat (approx. 47°C). Comparing rCBF during equally perceived intensity, the authors revealed that the forebrain activity during heat allodynia is different from that during normal heat pain. This show that heat allodynia, and possibly inflammatory pain, cannot be regarded as simply an enhanced normal pain response. These data, and other data from studies on patients with mononeuropathy, suggests that the brain employs different central mechanisms for chronic neuropathic pain and experimentally induced acute pain, respectively (Casey et al., 2003; Hsieh et al., 1995; Petrovic et al., 1999). During experimental heat allodynia, for instance, the dorsolateral prefrontal cortex seems to attenuate the affective component of the pain experience by reducing the functional connectivity of subcortical pathways (Lorenz et al., 2003).

A stroke involving the lower brainstem or thalamus is sometimes accompanied by a neuropathic pain called 'central poststroke pain' (CPSP) (Leijon et al., 1989). Treatment of CPSP is challenging, because the exact role of the lesion within the pain processing systems is not fully understood (Seghier et al., 2005b). In a case study of a CPSP-patient, Seghier and collegues combined diffusion tensor imaging (DTI; imaging anatomical connections in the brain) and fMRI and were able to show a residual hemorrhagic cavity within the right VPL nucleus and the posterior arm of the internal capsule, as well as a selective loss of the lateral thalamoparietal fibers (Seghier et al., 2005a). This indicates how functional neuroimaging is not only valuable in understanding basic neuroscientific mechanisms, but can also become a useful diagnostic aid for individual patients (Peyron et al., 1998; Willoch et al., 2004).

MEG studies have advanced our understanding of phantom-limb pain, another neuropathic pain syndrome (Flor et al., 2006). Studies demonstrated that the magnitude of phantom-limb pain is strongly correlated to the amount of S1 cortical reorganization (Flor et al., 1995), and that the extent of cortical reorganization contralateral to the amputation is an indicator of a more widespread plastic change in the brain involving bilateral pathways (Knecht et al., 1995). In addition, the cortical reorganization is not a stationary change but rather an extensive, inaccurate and highly fluctuating reorganized network (Knecht et al., 1998).

The approach of inducing experimental pain in patients is also used in non-pain patients, such as those diagnosed with psychiatric disorders, in order to provide evidence for altered pain processing. Using fMRI, Stoeter and colleagues showed that patients with somatoform pain disorders showed increased activations, in response to pinprick pain, in the known pain-processing areas (Stoeter et al., 2007). The authors interpreted this as support for exaggerated memory and/or anticipation of pain exposure. A functional imaging study of patients with borderline personality disorder (BPD), who have reduced pain sensitivity, show that the dorsolateral prefrontal cortex modulate pain circuits by deactivation of the anterior cingulate and amygdala (Schmahl et al., 2006). People with Alzheimer's disease are administered fewer analgesics than cognitively intact controls, which has prompted speculation about whether the neurodegeneration of Altzheimer's impact central pain processing (Cole et al., 2006). Results from this study by Cole and colleagues do suggest that pain perception and pain processing are not diminished in Alzheimer's disease, thereby raising concerns about the current inadequate treatment of pain in this patient group population.

In brief, few functional imaging studies have been devoted to the mechanisms associated with chronic pain. More effort to develop good clinical pain models is necessary. In the future we will probably see studies using a multidisciplinary approach, that combine blood flow-based methods with genetic analysis, receptor-binding techniques and techniques with high temporal resolution (such as MEG) (Kupers & Kehlet, 2006).

Future Perspectives

Functional imaging studies of pain have changed substantially over the last decade. Early imaging studies were used to identify those brain areas that are involved in pain perception (brain activation studies). These studies revealed that there is no "pain centre" but rather the involvement of widely distributed cortical areas in pain perception. Many recent sophisticated and intelligent studies have been designed to explore how different brain regions participate in pain processing. We now know that there are specific brain networks, which may overlap, that participate in the sensory-discriminative, affective-emotional and cognitive-motivational aspects of pain perception. The distributed cortical areas responding to pain stimuli, however, remain a challenge. It appeals to our curiosity to discover the functional connectivity of the involved cortical areas in pain sensation. For example, in a recent study, Lorenz and colleagues used principle component analysis to explore the specific role of subregions of the frontal cortex in pain perception (Lorenz et al., 2003). Furthermore, Wager and colleagues, in a receptor-binding PET study, revealed that placebo treatment increased functional connectivity among a number of limbic and prefrontal regions, suggesting increased functional integration of opioid responses (Wager et al., 2007).

The combination of electrophysiological methods and hemodynamic based methods provides an opportunity to understand the sequential activation of the widely distributed cortical areas responding to pain. Recent simultaneous recordings of laser-evoked EEG signals and fMRI responses is a move in this direction (Christmann et al., 2007; Iannetti et al., 2005). The technical combination provides unique spatial and temporal information, a combination that is going to blossom in the coming years.

Most pain imaging studies use acute experimental pain to understand normal pain processing, that is influenced by psychological variables such as attention and distraction, anticipation and anxiety. To explore how the brain is involved in pathological pain states, there are attempts to use experimental pain that mimic a clinical situation, such as the capsaicin model or burn injury model to mimic cutaneous hyperalgesia. These approaches in healthy subjects pose limitations. Few imaging studies have been devoted to investigations of clinical pain in patients, and those few have yielded inconclusive results. This discrepancy can be explained in part by the small sample sizes, the different pain pathologies of recruited patients, and a lack of controls. In a recent review, Kupers and Kehlet argue that post-operative pain is a highly appealing model since it opens perspectives for prospective longitudinal studies with repeated assessments and it enables control for many confounding factors, which hamper the interpretation of most current studies (Kupers & Kehlet 2006). More efforts to develop good clinical pain models are also necessary. Another approach to clinical pain is the use of PET receptor-binding studies, which probe neurochemical changes in response to an acute, or a chronic pain condition. Recently, the opioidergic and dopaminergic neurotransmitter systems have also been investigated (Scott, Heitzeg, Koeppe, Stohler, & Zubieta, 2006; Sprenger et al., 2006; Zubieta et al., 2005).

In summary, the challenge today in understanding pain goes far beyond the mapping of activation. Hypothesis-driven studies and intelligently designed models are necessary to discover how different regions participate in normal and clinical pain processing. Other advanced non-invasive methods may also be fully utilized in pain studies in the future. These include proton magnetic resonance spectroscopy (H-MRS) to measure the concentrations or synthesis rates of neurotransmitters such as glutamate, glycine, and GABA; diffusion tensor imaging (DTI) that allows in-vivo study of anatomical connectivity in the human brain; voxel-based morphometry (VBM) that measures differences in local concentrations of brain tissue through a voxel-wise comparison of multiple brain images; pharmacological fMRI that measure the direct modulation of regional brain activity by drugs that act within the central nervous system or the indirect modulation of regional brain activity through pharmacologically modified afferent input; and non-pharmacological imaging that measure the modulation effect of psychological factors, such as placebo effect, on pain-related brain activity (Kupers & Kehlet 2006). All will advance our understanding of the brain's perception of pain and contribute to the care of pain patients.

Acknowledgment We thank Kenneth L. Casey for critically reading a previous version of this manuscript.

References

al Absi, M., Rokke, P. D. (1991) Can anxiety help us tolerate pain? *Pain* 46: 43–51

Alkire, M. T., White, N. S., Hsieh, R., Haier, R. J. (2004) Dissociable brain activation responses to 5-Hz electrical pain stimulation: a high-field functional magnetic resonance imaging study. *Anesthesiology* 100: 939–946

Amanzio, M., Benedetti, F. (1999) Neuropharmacological dissection of placebo analgesia: expectation – activated opioid systems versus conditioning-activated specific subsystems. *Journal of Neuroscience* 19: 484–494

Andersson, J. L., Lilja, A., Hartvig, P., Langstrom, B., Gordh, T., Handwerker, H., Torebjork, E. (1997) Somatotopic organization along the central sulcus, for pain localization in humans, as revealed by positron emission tomography. *Experimental Brain Research* 117: 192–199

Apkarian, A. V., Bushnell, M. C., Treede, R. D., Zubieta, J. K. (2005) Human brain mechanisms of pain perception and regulation in health and disease. *European Journal of Pain* 9: 463–484

Arendt-Nielsen, L., Graven-Nielsen, T., Svarrer, H., Svensson, P. (1996) The influence of low back pain on muscle activity and coordination during gait – A clinical and experimental study. *Pain* 64: 231–240

Arendt-Nielsen, L., Yamasaki, H., Nielsen, J., Naka, D., Kakigi, R. (1999) Magnetoencephalographic responses to painful impact stimulation. *Brain Research* 839: 203–208

Bailey, D. L. (1992) 3D acquisition and reconstruction in positron emission tomography. *Annals of Nuclear Medicine* 6: 123–130

Bandettini PA (2001) Selection of the optimal pulse sequence for functional MRI. In: Jezzard P, Matthews PB, Smith SM (eds) Functional MRI. An introduction to methods. Oxford University Press, New York, pp. 123–143

Bantick, S. J., Wise, R. G., Ploghaus, A., Clare, S., Smith, S. M., Tracey, I. (2002) Imaging how attention modulates pain in humans using functional MRI. *Brain* 125: 310–319

Baumgartner, U., Buchholz, H. G., Bellosevich, A., Magerl, W., Siessmeier, T., Rolke, R., Hohnemann, S., Piel, M., Rosch, F., Wester, H. J., Henriksen, G., Stoeter, P., Bartenstein, P., Treede, R. D., Schreckenberger, M. (2006) High opiate receptor binding potential in the human lateral pain system. *Neuroimage* 30: 692–699

Beckmann, C. F., DeLuca, M., Devlin, J. T., Smith, S. M. (2005) Investigations into resting-state connectivity using independent component analysis. *Philosophical transactions of the Royal Society of London. Series B, Biological sciences* 360: 1001–1013

Benedetti, F., Arduino, C., Amanzio, M. (1999) Somatotopic activation of opioid systems by target-directed expectations of analgesia. *Journal of Neuroscience* 19: 3639–3648

Benedetti, F., Lanotte, M., Lopiano, L., Colloca, L. (2007) When words are painful: Unraveling the mechanisms of the nocebo effect. *Neuroscience* 147: 260–271

Benedetti, F., Pollo, A., Lopiano, L., Lanotte, M., Vighetti, S., Rainero, I. (2003) Conscious expectation and unconscious conditioning in analgesic, motor, and hormonal placebo/nocebo responses. *Journal of Neuroscience* 23: 4315–4323

Bingel, U., Lorenz, J., Glauche, V., Knab, R., Glascher, J., Weiller, C., Büchel, C. (2004) Somatotopic organization of human somatosensory cortices for pain: a single trial fMRI study. *Neuroimage* 23: 224–232

Bingel, U., Lorenz, J., Schoell, E., Weiller, C., Buchel, C. (2006) Mechanisms of placebo analgesia: rACC recruitment of a subcortical antinociceptive network. *Pain* 120: 8–15

Blomqvist A, Craig AD (1991) Organization of spinal and trigeminal input to the PAG. In: Depaulis A, Bandler R (eds) The midbrain periaqueductal gray matter:

functional, anatomical and neurochemical organization. Plenum Press, New York, pp. 345–363

Bornhövd, K., Quante, M., Glauche, V., Bromm, B., Weiller, C., Büchel, C. (2002) Painful stimuli evoke different stimulus-response functions in the amygdala, prefrontal, insula and somatosensory cortex: a single-trial fMRI study. *Brain* 125: 1326–1336

Brooks, J. C., Nurmikko, T. J., Bimson, W. E., Singh, K. D., Roberts, N. (2002) fMRI of thermal pain: effects of stimulus laterality and attention. *Neuroimage* 15: 293–301

Bruckbauer, T., Christian, B., Mantil, J., Valk, P. (2000) 9:–9:15. 3D Data Acquisition for Whole Body Images on the ECAT HR +. *Clin.Positron.Imaging* 3: 145

Büchel, C., Bornhövd, K., Quante, M., Glauche, V., Bromm, B., Weiller, C. (2002) Dissociable neural responses related to pain intensity, stimulus intensity, and stimulus awareness within the anterior cingulate cortex: a parametric single-trial laser functional magnetic resonance imaging study. *Journal Of Neuroscience* 22: 970–976

Buchel, C., Dolan, R. J., Armony, J. L., Friston, K. J. (1999) Amygdala-hippocampal involvement in human aversive trace conditioning revealed through event-related functional magnetic resonance imaging. *Journal of Neuroscience* 19: 10869–10876

Bullmore, E., Fadili, J., Breakspear, M., Salvador, R., Suckling, J., Brammer, M. (2003) Wavelets and statistical analysis of functional magnetic resonance images of the human brain. *Statistical Methods in Medical Research.* 12: 375–399

Burton, H., Videen, T. O., Raichle, M. E. (1993) Tactile-vibration-activated foci in insular and parietal-opercular cortex studied with positron emission tomography: mapping the second somatosensory area in humans. *Somatosensory Motor Research* 10: 297–308

Bush, G., Luu, P., Posner, M. I. (2000) Cognitive and emotional influences in anterior cingulate cortex. *Trends in Cognitive Sciences* 4: 215–222

Bushnell, M. C., Duncan, G. H., Hofbauer, R. K., Ha, B., Chen, J. I., Carrier, B. (1999) Pain perception: is there a role for primary somatosensory cortex? *Proceedings of The National Academy of Science of the USA* 96: 7705–7709

Buxton, R. B., Uludag, K., Dubowitz, D. J., Liu, T. T. (2004) Modeling the hemodynamic response to brain activation. *Neuroimage* 23(Suppl 1): S220–S233

Casey, K. L. (1999) Forebrain mechanisms of nociception and pain: analysis through imaging. *Proceedings of The National Academy of Science of the USA* 96: 7668–7674

Casey, K. L., Lorenz, J., Minoshima, S. (2003) Insights into the pathophysiology of neuropathic pain through functional brain imaging. *Experimental Neurology* 184 Suppl 1: S80–S88

Casey, K. L., Minoshima, S., Morrow, T. J., Koeppe, R. A. (1996) Comparison of human cerebral activation pattern during cutaneous warmth, heat pain, and deep cold pain. *Journal of Neurophysiology* 76: 571–581

Casey, K. L., Morrow, T. J., Lorenz, J., Minoshima, S. (2001) Temporal and spatial dynamics of human forebrain activity during heat pain: analysis by positron emission tomography. *Journal of Neurophysiology* 85: 951–959

Casey, K. L., Svensson, P., Morrow, T. J., Raz, J., Jone, C., Minoshima, S. (2000) Selective opiate modulation of nociceptive processing in the human brain. *Journal of Neurophysiology* 84: 525–533

Casey KL, Tran DT (2006) Cortical mechanisms and chronic pain in humans. In: Cervero F, Jensen TS (eds) Handbook of Clinical Neurology. Elsevier, pp. 159–177

Chen, J. I., Ha, B., Bushnell, M. C., Pike, B., Duncan, G. H. (2002) Differentiating noxious- and innocuous-related activation of human somatosensory cortices using temporal analysis of fMRI. *Journal of Neurophysiology* 88: 464–474

Christmann, C., Koeppe, C., Braus, D. F., Ruf, M., Flor, H. (2007) A simultaneous EEG-fMRI study of painful electric stimulation. *Neuroimage* 34: 1428–1437

Coghill, R. C., Sang, C. N., Maisog, J. M., Iadarola, M. J. (1999) Pain intensity processing within the human brain: a bilateral, distributed mechanism. *Journal of Neurophysiology* 82: 1934–1943

Coghill, R. C., Talbot, J. D., Evans, A. C., Meyer, E., Gjedde, A., Bushnell, M. C., Duncan, G. H. (1994) Distributed processing of pain and vibration by the human brain. *Journal of Neuroscience* 14: 4095–4108

Cohen, D. (1972) Magnetoencephalography: detection of the brain's electrical activity with a superconducting magnetometer. *Science* 175: 664–666

Cole, L. J., Farrell, M. J., Duff, E. P., Barber, J. B., Egan, G. F., Gibson, S. J. (2006) Pain sensitivity and fMRI pain-related brain activity in Alzheimer's disease. *Brain* 129: 2957–2965

Colloca, L., Benedetti, F. (2006) How prior experience shapes placebo analgesia. *Pain* 124: 126–133

Craig, A. D., Chen, K., Bandy, D., Reiman, E. M. (2000) Thermosensory activation of insular cortex. *Nature Neuroscience* 3: 184–190

Dannecker, E. A., Price, D. D., Robinson, M. E. (2003) An examination of the relationships among recalled, expected, and actual intensity and unpleasantness of delayed onset muscle pain. *Journal of Pain* 4: 74–81

Davis, K. D. (2003) Neurophysiological and anatomical considerations in functional imaging of pain. *Pain* 105: 1–3

Davis KD (2000) Studies of pain using functional magnetic resonance imaging. In: Casey KL, Bushnell MC (eds) Pain Imaging. Progress in pain research and management. IASP Press, Seattle, pp. 195–210

Davis, K. D., Kwan, C. L., Crawley, A. P., Mikulis, D. J. (1998) Functional MRI study of thalamic and cortical activations evoked by cutaneous heat, cold, and tactile stimuli. *Journal of Neurophysiology* 80: 1533–1546

Davis, K. D., Taylor, S. J., Crawley, A. P., Wood, M. L., Mikulis, D. J. (1997) Functional MRI of pain- and attention-related activations in the human cingulate cortex. *Journal of Neurophysiology* 77: 3370–3380

Derbyshire, S. W. (2000) Exploring the pain "neuromatrix". *Current Review of Pain* 4: 467–477

Derbyshire, S. W. (2003) A systematic review of neuroimaging data during visceral stimulation. *American Journal of Gastroenterology* 98: 12–20

Devor M (2005) Response of nerves to injury in relation to neuropathic pain. In: McMahon S, Koltzenburg M (eds) Wall and Melzack's Textbook of Pain. Elsevier, pp. 905–928

Djouhri, L., Koutsikou, S., Fang, X., McMullan, S., Lawson, S. N. (2006) Spontaneous pain, both neuropathic and inflammatory, is related to frequency of spontaneous firing in intact C-fiber nociceptors. *Journal of Neuroscience* 26: 1281–1292

Dowman, R. (2001) Attentional set effects on spinal and supraspinal responses to pain. *Psychophysiology* 38: 451–464

Downar, J., Crawley, A. P., Mikulis, D. J., Davis, K. D. (2002) A cortical network sensitive to stimulus salience in a neutral behavioral context across multiple sensory modalities. *Journal of Neurophysiology* 87: 615–620

Drossman, D. A., McKee, D. C., Sandler, R. S., Mitchell, C. M., Cramer, E. M., Lowman, B. C., Burger, A. L. (1988) Psychosocial factors in the irritable bowel syndrome. A multivariate study of patients and nonpatients with irritable bowel syndrome. *Gastroenterology* 95: 701–708

Druschky, K., Lang, E., Hummel, C., Kaltenhauser, M., Kohlloffel, L. U., Neundorfer, B., Stefan, H. (2000) Pain-related somatosensory evoked magnetic fields induced by controlled ballistic mechanical impacts. *Journal of Clinical Neurophysiology* 17: 613–622

Duncan, G. H., Albanese, M. C. (2003) Is there a role for the parietal lobes in the perception of pain? *Advances in Neurology* 93: 69–86

Eccleston, C. (1995) The attentional control of pain: methodological and theoretical concerns. *Pain* 63: 3–10

Eccleston, C., Crombez, G. (1999) Pain demands attention: A cognitive-affective model of the interuptive function of pain. *Psychological Bulletin* 125: 356–366

Ernst, T., Hennig, J. (1994) Observation of a fast response in functional MR. *Magnetic Resonance Medicine* 32: 146–149

Expectation. "expectation n." The Concise Oxford English Dictionary, Eleventh edition revised .Ed. Catherine Soanes and Angus Stevenson. Oxford University Press 2006. *Oxford Reference Online.Oxford University Press.STAMI.25 June 2007* www.oxfordreference.com/views/ENTRY.html?subview=Main&entry=t23.e19371. 2006.

Fair, D. A., Brown, T. T., Petersen, S. E., Schlaggar, B. L. (2006) A comparison of analysis of variance and correlation methods for investigating cognitive development with functional magnetic resonance imaging. *Developmental Neuropsychology* 30: 531–546

Farrar, J. T., Berlin, J. A., Strom, B. L. (2003) Clinically important changes in acute pain outcome measures: a validation study. *Journal of Pain and Symptom Management* 25: 406–411

Farrar, J. T., Young, J. P., Jr., LaMoreaux, L., Werth, J. L., Poole, R. M. (2001) Clinical importance of changes in chronic pain intensity measured on an 11-point numerical pain rating scale. *Pain* 94: 149–158

Faymonville, M. E., Laureys, S., Degueldre, C., DelFiore, G., Luxen, A., Franck, G., Lamy, M., Maquet, P. (2000) Neural mechanisms of antinociceptive effects of hypnosis. *Anesthesiology* 92: 1257–1267

Faymonville, M. E., Roediger, L., Del, F. G., Delgueldre, C., Phillips, C., Lamy, M., Luxen, A., Maquet, P., Laureys, S. (2003) Increased cerebral functional connectivity underlying the antinociceptive effects of hypnosis. *Brain Research. Cognitive Brain Research* 17: 255–262; Copyright Elsevier.

Ferretti, A., Del, G. C., Babiloni, C., Caulo, M., Arienzo, D., Tartaro, A., Rossini, P. M., Romani, G. L. (2004) Functional topography of the secondary somatosensory cortex for nonpainful and painful stimulation of median and tibial nerve: an fMRI study. *Neuroimage* 23: 1217–1225

Fields, H. L. (1999) Pain: an unpleasant topic. *Pain* 83(Suppl 6): S61–S69

Fields HL, Basbaum AI, Heinricher MM (2005) Central nervous system mechanisms of pain modulation. In: McMahon S, Koltzenburg M (eds) Wall and Melzack's Textbook of Pain. Elsevier.

Flandin, G., Penny, W. D. (2007) Bayesian fMRI data analysis with sparse spatial basis function priors. *Neuroimage* 34: 1108–1125

Flor, H., Elbert, T., Knecht, S., Wienbruch, C., Pantev, C., Birbaumer, N., Larbig, W., Taub, E. (1995) Phantom-limb pain as a perceptual correlate of cortical reorganization following arm amputation. *Nature* 375: 482–484

Flor, H., Nikolajsen, L., Staehelin, J. T. (2006) Phantom limb pain: a case of maladaptive CNS plasticity? *Nature Reviews Neuroscience* 7: 873–881

Frankenstein, U. N., Richter, W., McIntyre, M. C., Remy, F. (2001) Distraction modulates anterior cingulate gyrus activations during the cold pressor test. *Neuroimage* 14: 827–836

Friston, K. (1994) Functional and effective connectivity in neuroimaging: A synthesis. *Human Brain Mapping* 2: 56–78

Friston, K. J. (2005) Models of brain function in neuroimaging. *Annual Review of Psychology* 56: 57–87

Gatchel, R. J., Polatin, P. B., Mayer, T. G. (1995) The dominant role of psychosocial risk factors in the development of chronic low back pain disability. *Spine* 20: 2702–2709

Gedney, J. J., Logan, H. (2007) Perceived control and negative affect predict expected and experienced acute clinical pain: a structural modeling analysis. *Clinical Journal of Pain* 23: 35–44

Gedney, J. J., Logan, H., Baron, R. S. (2003) Predictors of short-term and long-term memory of sensory and affective dimensions of pain. *J Pain* 4: 47–55

Gracely RH (2005) Studies of pain in human subjects. In: McMahon S, Koltzenburg M (eds) Wall and Melzack's Textbook of Pain. Elsevier.

Gracely, R. H., Geisser, M. E., Giesecke, T., Grant, M. A., Petzke, F., Williams, D. A., Clauw, D. J. (2004) Pain catastrophizing and neural responses to pain among persons with fibromyalgia. *Brain* 127: 835–843

Hadjipavlou, G., Dunckley, P., Behrens, T. E., Tracey, I. (2006) Determining anatomical connectivities between cortical and brainstem pain processing regions in humans: a diffusion tensor imaging study in healthy controls. *Pain* 123: 169–178

Hamalainen, M., Hari, R., Ilmoniemi, R. J., Knuutila, J., Lounasmaa, O. V. (1993) Magnetoencephalography—theory, instrumentation, and applications to noninvasive studies of the working human brain. *Reviews of Modern Physics* 65: 413–97

Hari, R., Hamalainen, M., Kaukoranta, E., Reinikainen, K., Teszner, D. (1983) Neuromagnetic responses from the second somatosensory cortex in man. *Acta Neurologica Scandinavica* 68: 207–212

Hari, R., Joutsiniemi, S. L., Sarvas, J. (1988) Spatial resolution of neuromagnetic records: theoretical calculations in a spherical model. *Electroencephalography and Clinical Neurophysiology* 71: 64–72

Head, H., Holmes, G. (1911) Sensory disturbances from cerebral lesions. *Brain* 34:

Heymans, M. W., de Vet, H. C., Knol, D. L., Bongers, P. M., Koes, B. W., van, M. W. (2006) Workers' beliefs and expectations affect return to work over 12 months. *Journal of Occupational Rehabilitation* 16: 685–695

Hirsch, M. S., Liebert, R. M. (1998) The physical and psychological experience of pain: the effect of labelling and cold pressor temperature on three pain measures in college women. *Pain* 77: 41–48

Hofbauer, R. K., Rainville, P., Duncan, G. H., Bushnell, M. C. (2001) Cortical representation of the sensory dimension of pain. *Journal of Neurophysiology* 86: 402–411

Hoffman, H. G., Richards, T. L., Bills, A. R., Van, O. T., Magula, J., Seibel, E. J., Sharar, S. R. (2006) Using FMRI to study the neural correlates of virtual reality analgesia. *CNS Spectrums* 11: 45–51

Hrobjartsson, A., Gotzsche, P. C. (2001) Is the placebo powerless? An analysis of clinical trials comparing placebo with no treatment. *The New England Journal of Medicine* 344: 1594–1602

Hsieh, J. C., Belfrage, M., Stone-Elander, S., Hansson, P., Ingvar, M. (1995) Central representation of chronic ongoing neuropathic pain studied by positron emission tomography. *Pain* 63: 225–236

Hsieh, J. C., Hagermark, O., Stahle-Backdahl, M., Ericson, K., Eriksson, L., Stone-Elander, S., Ingvar, M. (1994) Urge to scratch represented in the human cerebral cortex during itch. *Journal of Neurophysiology.* 72: 3004–3008

Hu, D., Yan, L., Liu, Y., Zhou, Z., Friston, K. J., Tan, C., Wu, D. (2005) Unified SPM-ICA for fMRI analysis. *Neuroimage* 25: 746–755

Huttunen, J., Kobal, G., Kaukoranta, E., Hari, R. (1986) Cortical responses to painful $CO2$ stimulation of nasal mucosa; a magnetoencephalographic study in man. *Electroencephalography And Clinical Neurophysiology* 64: 347–349

Iannetti, G. D., Niazy, R. K., Wise, R. G., Jezzard, P., Brooks, J. C., Zambreanu, L., Vennart, W., Matthews, P. M., Tracey, I. (2005) Simultaneous recording of laser-evoked brain potentials and continuous, high-field functional magnetic resonance imaging in humans. *Neuroimage* 28: 708–719

Inui, K., Tran, T. D., Qiu, Y., Wang, X., Hoshiyama, M., Kakigi, R. (2002) Pain-related magnetic fields evoked by intra-epidermal electrical stimulation in humans. *Clinical Neurophysiology* 113: 298–304

Jones, A. K., Cunningham, V. J., Ha-Kawa, S., Fujiwara, T., Luthra, S. K., Silva, S., Derbyshire, S., Jones, T. (1994) Changes in central opioid receptor binding in relation to inflammation and pain in patients with rheumatoid arthritis. *British Journal of Rheumatology* 33: 909–916

Kain, Z. N., Sevarino, F., Alexander, G. M., Pincus, S., Mayes, L. C. (2000) Preoperative anxiety and postoperative pain in women undergoing hysterectomy. A repeated-measures design. *Journal of Psychosomatic Research* 49: 417–422

Kakigi, R., Inui, K., Tran, D. T., Qiu, Y., Wang, X., Watanabe, S., Hoshiyama, M. (2004) Human brain processing and central mechanisms of pain as observed by electro- and magneto-encephalography. *Journal of Chinese Medical Association* 67: 377–386

Kakigi, R., Koyama, S., Hoshiyama, M., Kitamura, Y., Shimojo, M., Watanabe, S. (1995) Pain-related magnetic fields following painful CO_2 laser stimulation in man. *Neuroscience Letters* 192: 45–48

Kanda, M., Nagamine, T., Ikeda, A., Ohara, S., Kunieda, T., Fujiwara, N., Yazawa, S., Sawamoto, N., Matsumoto, R., Taki, W., Shibasaki, H. (2000) Primary somatosensory cortex is actively involved in pain processing in human. *Brain Research* 853: 282–289

Kiebel, S. J., Friston, K. J. (2004) Statistical parametric mapping for event-related potentials: I. Generic considerations. *Neuroimage* 22: 492–502

Kitamura, Y., Kakigi, R., Hoshiyama, M., Koyama, S., Shimojo, M., Watanabe, S. (1995) Pain-related somatosensory evoked magnetic fields. *Electroencephalography and Clinical Neurophysiology* 95: 463–474

Kitamura, Y., Kakigi, R., Hoshiyama, M., Koyama, S., Watanabe, S., Shimojo, M. (1997) Pain-related somatosensory evoked magnetic fields following lower limb stimulation. *Journal of Neurology and Science* 145: 187–194

Knecht, S., Henningsen, H., Elbert, T., Flor, H., Hohling, C., Pantev, C., Birbaumer, N., Taub, E. (1995) Cortical reorganization in human amputees and mislocalization of painful stimuli to the phantom limb. *Neuroscience Letters* 201: 262–264

Knecht, S., Soros, P., Gurtler, S., Imai, T., Ringelstein, E. B., Henningsen, H. (1998) Phantom sensations following acute pain. *Pain* 77: 209–213

Kong, J., White, N. S., Kwong, K. K., Vangel, M. G., Rosman, I. S., Gracely, R. H., Gollub, R. L. (2006) Using fMRI to dissociate sensory encoding from cognitive evaluation of heat pain intensity. *Human Brain Mapping* 27: 715–721

Koyama, T., McHaffie, J. G., Laurienti, P. J., Coghill, R. C. (2005) The subjective experience of pain: where expectations become reality. *Proceedings of the National Academy of Science of the USA* 102: 12950–12955

Kupers, R., Kehlet, H. (2006) Brain imaging of clinical pain states: a critical review and strategies for future studies. *Lancet Neurology* 5: 1033–1044

Leijon, G., Boivie, J., Johansson, I. (1989) Central post-stroke pain – neurological symptoms and pain characteristics. *Pain* 36: 13–25

Logothetis, N. K., Pauls, J., Augath, M., Trinath, T., Oeltermann, A. (2001) Neurophysiological investigation of the basis of the fMRI signal. *Nature* 412: 150–157

Lorenz, J., Cross, D., Minoshima, S., Morrow, T., Paulson, P., Casey, K. (2002) A unique representation of heat allodynia in the human brain. *Neuron* 35: 383

Lorenz, J., Minoshima, S., Casey, K. L. (2003) Keeping pain out of mind: the role of the dorsolateral prefrontal cortex in pain modulation. *Brain* 126: 1079–1091

Maihofner, C., Kaltenhauser, M., Neundorfer, B., Lang, E. (2002) Temporo-spatial analysis of cortical activation by phasic innocuous and noxious cold stimuli – a magnetoencephalographic study. *Pain* 100: 281–290

Matre, D., Casey, K. L., Knardahl, S. (2006) Placebo-induced changes in spinal cord pain processing. *Journal of Neuroscience* 26: 559–563

Melzack R, Casey KL (1968) Sensory, motivational, and central control determinants of pain: a new conceptual model. In: Kenshalo D, Thomas CC (eds) The skin senses. Springfield, IL, pp. 423–439

Minoshima S, Cross DJ, Koeppe RA, Casey KL (2000) Brain activation studies using PET and SPECT: Execution and analysis. In: Casey KL, Bushnell MC (eds) Pain Imaging. IASP Press, Seattle, pp. 95–121

Mitiche, A., Sekkati, H. (2006) Optical flow 3D segmentation and interpretation: a variational method with active curve evolution and level sets. *IEEE Transactions On Pattern Analysis and Machine Intelligence* 28: 1818–1829

Montgomery, G. H., Kirsch, I. (1997) Classical conditioning and the placebo effect. *Pain* 72: 107–113

Morris, J. S., Ohman, A., Dolan, R. J. (1998) Conscious and unconscious emotional learning in the human amygdala. *Nature* 393: 467–470

Nakamura, Y., Paur, R., Zimmermann, R., Bromm, B. (2002) Attentional modulation of human pain processing in the secondary somatosensory cortex: a magnetoencephalographic study. *Neuroscience Letters* 328: 29–32

Ninomiya, Y., Kitamura, Y., Yamamoto, S., Okamoto, M., Oka, H., Yamada, N., Kuroda, S. (2001) Analysis of pain-related somatosensory evoked magnetic fields using the MUSIC (multiple signal classification) algorithm for magnetoencephalography. *Neuroreport*. 12: 1657–1661

Ogawa, S., Menon, R. S., Tank, D. W., Kim, S. G., Merkle, H., Ellermann, J. M., Ugurbil, K. (1993) Functional brain mapping by blood oxygenation level-dependent contrast magnetic resonance imaging. A comparison of signal characteristics with a biophysical model. *Biophysical Journal* 64: 803–812

Osborne, T. L., Jensen, M. P., Ehde, D. M., Hanley, M. A., Kraft, G. (2007) Psychosocial factors associated with pain intensity, pain-related interference, and psychological functioning in persons with multiple sclerosis and pain. *Pain* 127: 52–62

Parker, G. J., Roberts, C., Macdonald, A., Buonaccorsi, G. A., Cheung, S., Buckley, D. L., Jackson, A., Watson, Y., Davies, K., Jayson, G. C. (2006) Experimentally-derived functional form for a population-averaged high-temporal-resolution arterial input function for dynamic contrast-enhanced MRI. *Magnetic Resonance on Medicine* 56: 993–1000

Penfield, W., Boldrey, E. (1937) Somatic motor and sensory representation in the cerebral cortex of man as studied by electrical stimulation. *Brain* 60: 389–443

Petersen, E. T., Zimine, I., Ho, Y. C., Golay, X. (2006) Non-invasive measurement of perfusion: a critical review of arterial spin labelling techniques. *British Journal of Radiology* 79: 688–701

Petrovic, P., Dietrich, T., Fransson, P., Andersson, J., Carlsson, K., Ingvar, M. (2005) Placebo in emotional processing – induced expectations of anxiety relief activate a generalized modulatory network. *Neuron* 46: 957–969

Petrovic, P., Ingvar, M., Stone-Elander, S., Petersson, K. M., Hansson, P. (1999) A PET activation study of dynamic mechanical allodynia in patients with mononeuropathy. *Pain* 83: 459–470

Petrovic, P., Kalso, E., Petersson, K. M., Ingvar, M. (2002) Placebo and opioid analgesia – imaging a shared neuronal network. *Science* 295: 1737–1740

Petrovic, P., Petersson, K. M., Ghatan, P. H., Stone-Elander, S., Ingvar, M. (2000) Pain-related cerebral activation is altered by a distracting cognitive task. *Pain* 85: 19–30

Peyron, R., Frot, M., Schneider, F., Garcia-Larrea, L., Mertens, P., Barral, F. G., Sindou, M., Laurent, B., Mauguiere, F. (2002) Role of operculoinsular cortices in human pain processing: converging evidence from PET, fMRI, dipole modeling, and intracerebral recordings of evoked potentials. *Neuroimage* 17: 1336–1346

Peyron, R., Garcia-Larrea, L., Gregoire, M. C., Convers, P., Lavenne, F., Veyre, L., Froment, J. C., Mauguiere, F., Michel, D., Laurent, B. (1998) Allodynia after lateral-medullary (Wallenberg) infarct. A PET study. *Brain* 121 (Pt 2): 345–356

Peyron, R., Garcia-Larrea, L., Gregoire, M. C., Costes, N., Convers, P., Lavenne, F., Mauguiere, F., Michel, D., Laurent, B. (1999) Haemodynamic brain responses to acute pain in humans: sensory and attentional networks. *Brain* 122 (Pt 9): 1765–1780

Peyron, R., Laurent, B., Garcia-Larrea, L. (2000) Functional imaging of brain responses to pain. A review and meta-analysis (2000). *Neurophysiologie Clinique*. 30: 263–288

Peyron, R., Schneider, F., Faillenot, I., Convers, P., Barral, F. G., Garcia-Larrea, L., Laurent, B. (2004) An fMRI study of cortical representation of mechanical allodynia in patients with neuropathic pain. *Neurology* 63: 1838–1846

Phelps, M. E., Kuhl, D. E., Mazziota, J. C. (1981) Metabolic mapping of the brain's response to visual stimulation: studies in humans. *Science* 211: 1445–1448

Phillips, M. L., Young, A. W., Senior, C., Brammer, M., Andrew, C., Calder, A. J., Bullmore, E. T., Perrett, D. I., Rowland, D., Williams, S. C., Gray, J. A., David, A. S. (1997) A specific neural substrate for perceiving facial expressions of disgust. *Nature* 389: 495–498

Ploghaus, A., Becerra, L., Borras, C., Borsook, D. (2003) Neural circuitry underlying pain modulation: expectation, hypnosis, placebo. *Trends in Cognitive Sciences* 7: 197–200

Ploghaus, A., Narain, C., Beckmann, C. F., Clare, S., Bantick, S., Wise, R., Matthews, P. M., Rawlins, J. N., Tracey, I. (2001) Exacerbation of pain by anxiety is associated with activity in a hippocampal network. *Journal of Neurosciences* 21: 9896–9903

Ploghaus, A., Tracey, I., Gati, J. S., Clare, S., Menon, R. S., Matthews, P. M., Rawlins, J. N. (1999) Dissociating pain from its anticipation in the human brain. *Science* 284: 1979–1981

Ploner, M., Gross, J., Timmermann, L., Schnitzler, A. (2002) Cortical representation of first and second pain sensation in humans. *Proceedings of the National Academy of Science of the USA* 99: 12444–12448

Ploner, M., Schmitz, F., Freund, H. J., Schnitzler, A. (1999) Parallel activation of primary and secondary somatosensory cortices in human pain processing. *Journal of Neurophysiology* 81: 3100–3104

Porreca, F., Ossipov, M. H., Gebhart, G. F. (2002) Chronic pain and medullary descending facilitation. *TINS* 25: 319–325

Porro, C. A., Baraldi, P., Pagnoni, G., Serafini, M., Facchin, P., Maieron, M., Nichelli, P. (2002) Does anticipation of pain affect cortical nociceptive systems? *Journal of Neuroscience* 22: 3206–3214

Porro, C. A., Cettolo, V., Francescato, M. P., Baraldi, P. (1998) Temporal and intensity coding of pain in human cortex. *Journal of Neurophysiology* 80: 3312–3320

Price, D. D. (2000) Psychological and neural mechanisms of the affective dimension of pain. *Science* 288: 1769–1772

Price DD, Bushnell MC (2004) Overview of pain dimensions and their psychological modulation. In: Price DD, Bushnell MC (eds) IASP Press, Seattle, pp. 3–17

Qiu, Y., Inui, K., Wang, X., Nguyen, B. T., Tran, T. D., Kakigi, R. (2004) Effects of distraction on magnetoencephalographic responses ascending through C-fibers in humans. *Clinical Neurophysiology* 115: 636–646

Raichle, M. E., MacLeod, A. M., Snyder, A. Z., Powers, W. J., Gusnard, D. A., Shulman, G. L. (2001) A default mode of brain function. *Proceedings of the National Academy of Science of the USA* 98: 676–682

Rainville, P., Duncan, G. H., Price, D. D., Carrier, B., Bushnell, M. C. (1997) Pain affect encoded in human anterior cingulate but not somatosensory cortex. *Science* 277: 968–971

Rauch, S. L., Savage, C. R., Alpert, N. M., Miguel, E. C., Baer, L., Breiter, H. C., Fischman, A. J., Manzo, P. A., Moretti, C., Jenike, M. A. (1995) A positron emission tomographic study of simple phobic symptom provocation. *Archives of General Psychiatry* 52: 20–28

Rhudy, J. L., Meagher, M. W. (2000) Fear and anxiety: divergent effects on human pain thresholds. *Pain* 84: 65–75

Roelofs, J., Peters, M. L., McCracken, L., Vlaeyen, J. W. (2003) The pain vigilance and awareness questionnaire (PVAQ): further psychometric evaluation in fibromyalgia and other chronic pain syndromes. *Pain* 101: 299–306

Ruben, J., Schwiemann, J., Deuchert, M., Meyer, R., Krause, T., Curio, G., Villringer, K., Kurth, R., Villringer, A. (2001) Somatotopic organization of human secondary somatosensory cortex. *Cerebral Cortex* 11: 463–473

Salaffi, F., Stancati, A., Silvestri, C. A., Ciapetti, A., Grassi, W. (2004) Minimal clinically important changes in chronic musculoskeletal pain intensity measured on a numerical rating scale. *European Journal of Pain* 8: 283–291

Sawamoto, N., Honda, M., Okada, T., Hanakawa, T., Kanda, M., Fukuyama, H., Konishi, J., Shibasaki, H. (2000) Expectation of pain enhances responses to nonpainful somatosensory stimulation in the anterior cingulate cortex and parietal operculum/posterior insula: an event-related functional magnetic resonance imaging study. *Journal of Neuroscience* 20: 7438–7445

Schmahl, C., Bohus, M., Esposito, F., Treede, R. D., Di, S. F., Greffrath, W., Ludaescher, P., Jochims, A., Lieb, K., Scheffler, K., Hennig, J., Seifritz, E. (2006) Neural correlates of antinociception in borderline personality disorder. *Archives of General Psychiatry* 63: 659–667

Schnitzler, A., Ploner, M. (2000) Neurophysiology and functional neuroanatomy of pain perception. *Journal of Clinical Neurophysiology* 17: 592–603

Schweinhardt, P., Glynn, C., Brooks, J., McQuay, H., Jack, T., Chessell, I., Bountra, C., Tracey, I. (2006) An fMRI study of cerebral processing of brush-evoked allodynia in neuropathic pain patients. *Neuroimage* 32: 256–265

Scott, D. J., Heitzeg, M. M., Koeppe, R. A., Stohler, C. S., Zubieta, J. K. (2006) Variations in the human pain stress experience mediated by ventral and dorsal basal ganglia dopamine activity. *Journal of Neuroscience* 26: 10789–10795

Seghier, M. L., Lazeyras, F., Vuilleumier, P., Schnider, A., Carota, A. (2005b) Functional magnetic resonance imaging and diffusion tensor imaging in a case of central poststroke pain. *Journal of Pain* 6: 208–212

Seghier, M. L., Lazeyras, F., Vuilleumier, P., Schnider, A., Carota, A. (2005a) Functional magnetic resonance imaging and diffusion tensor imaging in a case of central poststroke pain. *Journal of Pain* 6: 208–212

Seminowicz, D. A., Davis, K. D. (2007) Interactions of pain intensity and cognitive load: the brain stays on task. *Cerebral Cortex* 17: 1412–1422

Seminowicz, D. A., Davis, K. D. (2006) Cortical responses to pain in healthy individuals depends on pain catastrophizing. *Pain* 120: 297–306

Shepp, L. A., Logan, B. F. (1974) The Fourier reconstruction of a head section. *IEEE Transactions on Nuclear Science* NS-21: 21–43

Sheth, S. A., Nemoto, M., Guiou, M., Walker, M., Pouratian, N., Toga, A. W. (2004) Linear and nonlinear relationships between neuronal activity, oxygen metabolism, and hemodynamic responses. *Neuron* 42: 347–355

Singer, T., Seymour, B., O'Doherty, J., Kaube, H., Dolan, R. J., Frith, C. D. (2004) Empathy for pain involves the affective but not sensory components of pain. *Science* 303: 1157–1162

Smith SM (2001) Overview of fMRI analysis. In: Jezzard P, Matthews PB, Smith SM (eds) Functional MRI. An introduction to methods. Oxford University Press, New York, pp. 215–227

Spiegel, D. (1991) Neurophysiological correlates of hypnosis and dissociation. *Journal of Neuropsychiatry Clinical Neuroscience* 3: 440–445

Sprenger, T., Valet, M., Boecker, H., Henriksen, G., Spilker, M. E., Willoch, F., Wagner, K. J., Wester, H. J., Tolle, T. R. (2006) Opioidergic activation in the medial pain system after heat pain. *Pain* 122: 63–67

Stoeter, P., Bauermann, T., Nickel, R., Corluka, L., Gawehn, J., Vucurevic, G., Vossel, G., Egle, U. T. (2007) Cerebral activation in patients with somatoform pain disorder exposed to pain and stress: An fMRI study. *Neuroimage* 36: 418–430

Sullivan, M. J., Thorn, B., Haythornthwaite, J. A., Keefe, F., Martin, M., Bradley, L. A., Lefebvre, J. C. (2001) Theoretical perspectives on the relation between catastrophizing and pain. *Clinical Journal of Pain* 17: 52–64

Suzuki, R., Rygh, L. J., Dickenson, A. H. (2004) Bad news from the brain: descending 5-HT pathways that control spinal pain processing. *Trends in Pharmacological Science* 25: 613–617

Svensson, P. (2007) What can human experimental pain models teach us about clinical TMD? *Archives of Oral Biology* 52: 391–394

Svensson, P., Minoshima, S., Beydoun, A., Morrow, T. J., Casey, K. L. (1997) Cerebral processing of acute skin and muscle pain in humans. *Journal of Neurophysiology* 78: 450–460

Sweet WH (1982) Cerebral localization of pain. In: Thompson RA, Green JR (eds) New Perspectives in Cerebral Localization. Raven Press, New York, pp. 205–242

Timmermann, L., Ploner, M., Haucke, K., Schmitz, F., Baltissen, R., Schnitzler, A. (2001) Differential coding of pain intensity in the human primary and secondary somatosensory cortex. *Journal of Neurophysiology.* 86: 1499–1503

Todd, K. H. (1996) Clinical versus statistical significance in the assessment of pain relief. *Annals of Emerging Medicine.* 27: 439–441

Tracey, I. (2005) Functional connectivity and pain: how effectively connected is your brain? *Pain* 116: 173–174

Tracey, I., Ploghaus, A., Gati, J. S., Clare, S., Smith, S., Menon, R. S., Matthews, P. M. (2002) Imaging attentional modulation of pain in the periaqueductal gray in humans. *Journals of Neuroscience* 22: 2748–2752

Tran, T. D., Inui, K., Hoshiyama, M., Lam, K., Qiu, Y., Kakigi, R. (2002) Cerebral activation by the signals ascending through unmyelinated C-fibers in humans: a magnetoencephalographic study. *Neuroscience* 113: 375–386

Turk, D. C. (2000) Statistical significance and clinical significance are not synonyms!. *Clinical Journal of Pain* 16: 185–187

Turner, J. A., Franklin, G., Fulton-Kehoe, D., Sheppard, L., Wickizer, T. M., Wu, R., Gluck, J. V., Egan, K. (2006) Worker recovery expectations and fear-avoidance predict work disability in a population-based workers' compensation back pain sample. *Spine* 31: 682–689

Urban, M. O., Gebhart, G. F. (1999) Supraspinal contributions to hyperalgesia. *Proceeding of the National Academy of Science of the USA* 96: 7687–7692

Valet, M., Sprenger, T., Boecker, H., Willoch, F., Rummeny, E., Conrad, B., Erhard, P., Tolle, T. R. (2004) Distraction modulates connectivity of the cingulo-frontal cortex and the midbrain during pain – an fMRI analysis. *Pain* 109: 399–408

Van Damme, S., Crombez, G., Eccleston, C. (2004) Disengagement from pain: the role of catastrophic thinking about pain. *Pain* 107: 70–76

van den Hout, J. H., Vlaeyen, J. W., Houben, R. M., Soeters, A. P., Peters, M. L. (2001) The effects of failure feedback and pain-related fear on pain report, pain tolerance, and pain avoidance in chronic low back pain patients. *Pain* 92: 247–257

Wager, T. D. (2005) The neural bases of placebo effects in anticipation and pain. *Seminars in Pain Medicine* 3: 22–30

Wager, T. D., Matre, D., Casey, K. L. (2006) Placebo effects in laser-evoked pain potentials. *Brain, Behavior, and Immunity* 20: 219–230

Wager, T. D., Phan, K. L., Liberzon, I., Taylor, S. F. (2003) Valence, gender, and lateralization of functional brain anatomy in emotion: a meta-analysis of findings from neuroimaging. *Neuroimage* 19: 513–531

Wager, T. D., Rilling, J. K., Smith, E. E., Sokolik, A., Casey, K. L., Davidson, R. J., Kosslyn, S. M., Rose, R. M., Cohen, J. D. (2004) Placebo-induced changes in FMRI in the anticipation and experience of pain. *Science* 303: 1162–1167

Wager, T. D., Scott, D. J., Zubieta, J. K. (2007) Placebo effects on human {micro}-opioid activity during pain. *Proceedings of the National Academy of Science of the USA*

Wagner, K. J., Sprenger, T., Kochs, E. F., Tolle, T. R., Valet, M., Willoch, F. (2007) Imaging human cerebral pain modulation by dose-dependent opioid analgesia: a positron emission tomography activation study using remifentanil. *Anesthesiology* 106: 548–556

White JC, Sweet WH (1969) Pain and the Neurosurgeon. A Forty-Year Experience. C.C. Thomas, Springfield Illinois

Willoch, F. PET studies on pain and analgesia: brain activity changes & opioidergic mechanisms. 2001. Dept of Pharmacology, University of Oslo, Norway. Ref Type: Thesis/Dissertation

Willoch, F., Schindler, F., Wester, H. J., Empl, M., Straube, A., Schwaiger, M., Conrad, B., Tolle, T. R. (2004) Central poststroke pain and reduced opioid receptor binding within pain processing circuitries: a [11C]diprenorphine PET study. *Pain* 108: 213–220

Wise, R. G., Tracey, I. (2006) The role of fMRI in drug discovery. *Journal of Magnetic Resonance Imaging* 23: 862–876

Woolrich, M. W., Behrens, T. E. (2006) Variational Bayes inference of spatial mixture models for segmentation. *IEEE Transactions on Medical Imaging* 25: 1380–1391

Worsley K (2001) Statistical activation of activation images. In: Jezzard P, Matthews PB, Smith SM (eds) Functional MRI. An introduction to methods. Oxford University Press, New York, pp. 251–270

Xu, X., Fukuyama, H., Yazawa, S., Mima, T., Hanakawa, T., Magata, Y., Kanda, M., Fujiwara, N., Shindo, K., Nagamine, T., Shibasaki, H. (1997) Functional localization of pain perception in the human brain studied by PET. *Neuroreport* 8: 555–559

Zimmerman, J. E., Thiene, P., Harding, J. T. (1970) Design and operation of stable rf-biased superconductiong point-contact quantum devices and a note on the properties of perfectly clean metal contacts. *Journal of Applied Physiology* 41: 1572–1580

Zubieta, J. K., Bueller, J. A., Jackson, L. R., Scott, D. J., Xu, Y., Koeppe, R. A., Nichols, T. E., Stohler, C. S. (2005) Placebo effects mediated by endogenous opioid activity on mu-opioid receptors. *Journal of Neuroscience* 25: 7754–7762

Zubieta, J. K., Smith, Y. R., Bueller, J. A., Xu, Y., Kilbourn, M. R., Jewett, D. M., Meyer, C. R., Koeppe, R. A., Stohler, C. S. (2001) Regional mu opioid receptor regulation of sensory and affective dimensions of pain. *Science* 293: 311–315

Pain, Transportation Issues and Whiplash

Michele Sterling

The development of pain following a motor vehicle crash (MVC) is a common occurrence. The most frequently reported and investigated pain condition following such trauma is neck pain or whiplash associated disorders (WAD), which are usually associated with rear-end collision. However, WAD can also be caused by any event that results in the hyperextension and flexion of the cervical spine (Malanga & Peter, 2005; Sizer, Poorbaugh, & Phelps, 2004). Following such injuries the development of chronic musculoskeletal pain affects many and this condition is also burdensome both in terms of the financial costs associated with those who develop chronic symptoms and personal costs to these individuals (Ferrari, Russell, Carroll, & Cassidy, 2005).

Some studies suggest that the development of more widespread musculoskeletal pain (that is pain throughout numerous body areas) is also associated with MVC trauma. Buskila, Neumann, Vaisberg, Alkalay, and Wolfe (1997) reported a 10-fold increased risk of developing fibromylagia ,a chronic pain disorder characterized by widespread muscle tenderness and associated with disordered central pain processing, in individuals with a MVC induced neck injury. McLean, Williams, and Clauw (2005) argued that there is substantial evidence to support a causal relationship between MVC trauma and the development of fibromyalgia. However this relationship is the site of vigorous controversy given the obvious medico-legal ramifications if such an association was accepted (Shir, Pereira, & Fitzcharles, 2006).

A more recent large longitudinal study (Tishler, Levy, Maslakov, Bar-Chaim, & Amit-Vazina, 2006) showed no association between whiplash injury, road trauma and increased risk of fibromyalgia. Similarly Wynne-Jones, Macfarlane, Silman, and Jones (2006) found that the rate of onset of widespread pain following a MVC is not statistically significant. Most recently, Holm, Carroll, Cassidy, Skillgate, and Ahlbom (2007) reported that whilst the incidence of

M. Sterling (✉)
Associate Director, Centre for National Research on Disability and Rehabilitation Medicine (CONROD) and Director of the Rehabilitation (Medical and Allied Health) Research Program (CONRD). The University of Queensland, Brisbane, Australia
e-mail: m.sterling@uq.edu.au

R.J. Moore (ed.), *Biobehavioral Approaches to Pain*,
DOI 10.1007/978-0-387-78323-9_18, © Springer Science+Business Media, LLC 2009

widespread pain following whiplash injury may be low, people who report early depressive symptoms and more severe neck symptoms are at increased risk of developing widespread pain especially if there was early onset and widespread pain after injury.

From these findings it would appear that the associations between the onset of more widespread pain conditions, including fibromyalgia, following MVC requires further investigation before firm conclusions can be made. For this reason, this chapter will focus on whiplash associated disorders (WAD), a condition that is more readily accepted to arise as a consequence of motor vehicle trauma. The symptoms, possible injury mechanisms and manifestations, both physical and psychological of the condition will be outlined. There are overlapping features between WAD and conditions with more widespread pain and these will be described. Finally evidence based best practices for the assessment and management of whiplash will be discussed, and future therapeutic strategies explored.

The Whiplash Injury

The rather simplistic model of a flexion, hyperextension action of the head and neck during a rear-end impact has been recently replaced by a more sophisticated injury model as new evidence has emerged. Bioengineering studies where cadavers were subjected to simulated rear end crashes have demonstrated perturbations in segmental movement including intersegmental hyperextension in the lower cervical spine, S-curve formation and differential acceleration of the upper cervical spine (Cusick, Pintar, & Yoganandan, 2001; Stemper, Yoganandan, Rao, & Pintar, 2005). The cervical spine has been shown to assume a S-shape shortly after impact where the lower segments extend as the upper segments are still undergoing flexion (Sizer et al., 2004). Secondary thoracic spine movement also occurs including superiorly directed acceleration and extension/ rotation of the upper thoracic spine which has been referred to as thoracic ramping (Stemper et al., 2005). Axial and shear forces also occur which cause intervertebral rotation and translation movements (Ivancic & Panjabi, 2006).

The determination of specific injured neck structures remains difficult and most likely due to the insensitivity of current imaging technologies (Ronnen, de Korte, & Brink, 1996; Steinberg, Ovadia, Nissan, Menahem, & Dekel, 2005). This is not to say that such injuries do not occur. When evidence is taken together from bioengineering studies identifying the potential for lesions to occur (Yoganandan, Pintar, & Cusick, 2002); and cadaveric studies where clear lesions are demonstrated in non-survivors of a MVC (Taylor & Taylor, 1996), there is reasonable justification for the presence of pathoanatomical lesions in at least some of the injured people (Bogduk, 2002). Damaged structures may include zygapophyseal joints, intervertebral discs, synovial folds, vertebral bodies and nerve tissue (including dorsal root ganglia, spinal cord or brainstem) (Uhrenholt,

Grunnet-Nilsson, & Hartvigsen, 2002). Unfortunately for the injured person, this (circumstantial) evidence in the majority of whiplash cases but without a clear pathoanatomical diagnosis via an imaging modality, has been extrapolated to assume that there is no objective measurable tissue injury in this condition leading to speculation of the injured person's motives (Shir et al., 2006).

Clinical studies provide additional support for the findings of potential structural lesions from both bioengineering and cadaveric studies. Lord, Barnsley, Wallis, and Bogduk (1996) linked zygapophyseal arthropathy with chronic WAD by achieving substantial pain relief in some patients with persistent pain following a whiplash injury using placebo-controlled zygapophyseal joint blocks. The zygapophyseal joint may be vulnerable due to the orientation of the articular surfaces that allow movement coupling and compressive forces during the trauma (Sizer et al., 2004). In addition, gender differences have also been observed where females may be more at risk of zygapophyseal joint damage due to decreased cartilage thickness on the articular surfaces (Yoganandan, Knowles, Maiman, & Pintar, 2003). This may be one possible explanation for the higher number of females who present with persistent whiplash symptoms.

Findings from clinical studies also implicate injury to peripheral nerve tissue. Clinical tests designed to provoke upper quadrant peripheral nerve structures have demonstrated the presence of apparently mechanosensitive nerve tissue (Ide, Ide, Yamaga, & Takagi, 2001; Sterling, Treleaven, & Jull, 2002) and mechanically hyperalgesic nerve trunks have been shown to be a feature of chronic whiplash (Greening, Dilley, & Lynn, 2005; Sterling et al., 2002). Studies utilising quantitative electromyography have also demonstrated abnormalities suggestive of neural injury; particularly involving the lower cervical segments (Chu, Eun, & Schwartz, 2005; Steinberg et al., 2005). Magnetic resonance imaging (MRI) and functional MRI (fMRI) have also shown lesions of the cranio-cervical regions in participants with chronic whiplash (Johansson, 2006; Kaale, Krakenes, Albrektsen, & Webster, 2005; Krakenes et al., 2002, 2003). A drawback of this MRI work is that all of the studies have involved patients with chronic WAD, a substantial time after the initial injury (approximately 2–9 years post-injury). Moreover, this selected study group of chronic whiplash injured people also fails to take the acutely injured patient into account and thus may considerably overestimate the actual incidence of these changes. Nevertheless, these studies demonstrate that at least in some individuals with chronic whiplash, the possibility of cranio-vertebral injures should also be considered.

Symptoms

Symptoms following whiplash injury can be quite diverse in nature. The predominant symptom is neck pain that typically occurs in the posterior region of the neck but can also radiate to the head, shoulder and arm, thoracic, interscapular and lumbar regions (Barnsley, Lord, & Bogduk, 1998). Additional common symptoms include headache, dizziness/loss of balance, visual disturbances, para-esthesia, anaesthesia, weakness and cognitive disturbances such as concentration and memory difficulties (Barnsley et al., 1998; Radanov & Sturzenegger, 1996; Treleaven, Jull, & Sterling, 2003). The onset of symptoms may occur immediately or, in many patients the expression of symptoms may be delayed for up to 12 to 15 hours (Provinciali & Baroni, 1999).

It could be argued that the identification of the pathoanatomical source of symptoms provides little basis for appropriate assessment and management of WAD and that the emphasis should instead be placed on treatment approaches directed toward mechanisms and processes underlying the development of this painful condition. Some authors have argued for this approach to the manage-ment and investigation of neuropathic pain syndromes (Jensen & Baron, 2003; Woolf & Mannion, 1999) but a similar approach to the treatment of musculoske-letal conditions should also be considered. In the case of whiplash associated disorders (WAD), there is additional clinical evidence that a variety of motor, sensory and psychological disturbances also characterize the condition. Therefore, understanding and clinical recognition of these factors will likely underpin the development of improved treatment strategies. This is important since treatment strategies evaluated to date in the acute stages of the whiplash injury have failed to demonstrate efficacy in terms of decreasing the incidence of those who develop persistent symptoms (Borchgrevink et al., 1998; Provinciali, Baroni, Illuminati, & Ceravolo, 1996; Rosenfeld, Gunnarsson, & Borenstein, 2000; Rosenfeld, Seferiadis, Carllson, & Gunnarsson, 2003).

Physical Characteristics of the Whiplash Condition

Motor and Sensori-Motor Dysfunction

Motor and sensori-motor dysfunction, including loss of neck movement, altered cervical and shoulder girdle muscle recruitment patterns and kinaesthetic deficits have been identified in both the acute and chronic stages of the condition (Dall'Alba, Sterling, Trealeven, Edwards, & Jull, 2001; Nederhand, Hermens, Ijzerman, Turk, & Zilvold, 2002; Sterling, Jull, Vizenzino, Kenardy, & Darnell, 2003; Treleaven et al., 2003). Individuals with chronic whiplash also demonstrate balance loss with less demanding tasks (for example, comfortable standing with eyes open) and higher levels tasks (for instance, standing on a soft surface with eyes closed) (Treleaven, Jull, & Low choy, 2005). Disturbances in eye movement control whilst the neck is rotated or torsioned have also been described in individuals with chronic whiplash (Tjell, Tenenbaum, & Sandstrom, 2002; Tre-leaven, Jull, & LowChoy, 2005). Interestingly greater deficits in postural control (loss of balance, disturbed eye movement control, increased joint repositioning error in the neck) are seen in whiplash injured people who also report associated dizziness as a symptom of their condition (Treleaven, Jull, & LowChoy, 2005;

Treleaven, Jull, & LowChoy, 2005). The mechanisms underlying these features are not fully understood but are proposed to reflect alteration in cervical afferentation as a consequence of injury to neck structures or related functional deficits (Heikkila & Astrom, 1996; Treleaven et al., 2003).

Recent investigations, using MRI, has shown marked structural changes to cervical spine muscles in people with chronic whiplash. Elliott et al (2006) showed that the presence of fatty infiltrate in both deep and superficial cervical extensor muscles compared to a asymptomatic control group. Although the fatty infiltrate was generally higher in all muscles investigated in the patient group, it was highest in the deeper muscles; the rectus capitis minor / major and multifidi. The causes of these fatty muscle changes are not known, but these authors suggest several possibilities including general muscle disuse, inflammation, or muscle denervation (Elliott et al., 2006). That said, the relevance of the muscle changes in terms of pain, disability or functional recovery is still unclear.

Many motor deficits (movement loss, altered muscle recruitment patterns) seem to be present to various degrees in whiplash injured individuals irrespective of reported pain and disability levels and rate or level of recovery (Sterling, Jull, Vizenzino et al., 2003). Additionally, these features may not be unique to whiplash and have also been identified in chronic neck pain of an idiopathic (non-traumatic) nature (Jull, Kristjansson, & Dall'Alba, 2004; Sterling, Jull, & Wright, 2001). Furthermore treatment directed at rehabilitating motor dysfunction and improving general movement shows only modest effects on reported pain and disability levels (Jull, Sterling, Kenardy, & Beller, 2007; Stewart et al., 2007). Together these findings suggest that motor deficits, although present, may not play a key role in the development of chronic or persistent symptoms following whiplash injury.

Evidence for Augmented Central Pain Processes in WAD

In contrast to the apparently uniform presence of motor dysfunction, sensory hypersensitivity (central hyperexcitability) may be a feature that could differentiate whiplash from less severe neck pain conditions and whiplash sub-groupings into higher or lower levels of reported pain and disability. Whilst other chronic painful musculoskeletal conditions also demonstrate hypersensitivity to nociceptive input (Shir et al., 2006) there appears to be a relationship between the extent of reported symptoms and sensory hypersensitivity (Carli, Suman, Biasi, & Marcolongo, 2002). Scott, Jull, & Sterling (2005) recently showed that people with chronic WAD had a more complex presentation involving lowered pain thresholds to pressure, heat and cold stimuli in areas remote to the cervical spine that were not present in those with chronic idiopathic (non-traumatic) neck pain. The latter group also reported much lower levels of pain and disability (Scott et al., 2005). In contrast, widespread sensory hypersensitivity is a feature of cervical radiculopathy and individuals with this condition reported similar pain and disability levels to those with chronic whiplash (Chien, Eliav, & Sterling, 2008a). This suggests that chronic whiplash and chronic cervical radiculopathy share similar underlying mechanisms, but differ from idiopathic neck pain illustrating the diversity of processes involved in these various neck pain conditions.

There is now consistent evidence from numerous cohorts that demonstrate the presence of sensory hypersensitivity (or decreased pain thresholds) to a variety of stimuli in WAD (Table 1). For example, Koelbaek-Johansen, Graven-Nielsen, Schou-Olesen, and Arendt-Nielsen (1999) reported larger referred pain areas (proximal and even in the contralateral limb) in whiplash subjects following intramuscular saline injection into Tibialis Anterior and Infraspinatus. Moog, Quintner, Hall, and Zusman (2002) reported the presence of allodynia with innocuous vibration stimuli and Sterling et al. (2002) demonstrated a generalized lowering of pressure pain thresholds in areas both local (neck) and remote (upper and lower limbs) to the site of injury. These findings indicate the involvement of augmented central pain processing mechanisms or central hyperexcitability as contributing to chronic whiplash pain.

Most, if not all of these studies relied on the patient to provide a cognitive response following the stimulus application and as such it could be argued that

Table 1 Studies supporting the presence of central hyperexcitability in whiplash. WAD: whiplash associated disorders

Study	Findings	Study cohort
Sheather Reid and Cohen (1998)	Lowered pain threshold and pain tolerance to electrical stimulation – neck	Chronic neck pain including WAD
Koelbaek-Johansen et al (1999)	Widespread pain responses following injection of intramuscular hypertonic saline	Chronic WAD
Curatolo et al (2001)	Lowered pain thresholds for electrical stimulation – neck and lower limbs	Chronic WAD
Sterner et al (2001)	Sensory disturbance in trigeminal distribution	Chronic WAD
Ide et al (2001)	Mechanosensitivity to brachial plexus provocation manoeuvres	Chronic WAD
Sterling et al. (2002)	Lowered pressure pain thresholds throughout body areas both local and remote to injury site	Chronic WAD
Sterling et al (2002)	Hypersensitive responses to brachial plexus provocation test	Chronic WAD
Moog et al (2002)	Pain on non noxious stimulation (vibration) Hyperalgesia to heat and cold stimuli	Chronic WAD
Sterling et al (2003, 2005)	Cold hyperalgesia, sympathetic disturbances predictive of poor outcome.	Acute to chronic WAD
Banic et al (2004) Sterling et al (2008)	Decreased threshold for activation of flexor withdrawal reflex	Chronic WAD
Scott et al (2005)	Mechanical and thermal hyperalgesia – present in chronic WAD but not idiopathic neck pain	Chronic WAD and idiopathic neck pain
Kasch et al (2005)	Reduced cold pressor pain tolerance associated with poor recovery	Acute to chronic WAD

the response may be feigned or at least cognitively influenced in some way. In an attempt to account for bias, Banic et al (2004) demonstrated facilitated flexor withdrawal reflexes (using electromyography of biceps femoris muscle) in the lower limbs of chronic WAD subjects following electrical stimulation of the sural nerve. In this test (termed the Nociceptive Flexion Reflex), less electrical current was required to elicit a reflex in the whiplash group compared to controls thus providing evidence of spinal cord hypersensitivity (central sensitisation) without relying on the subject's self reported response. More recent evidence shows that the heightened reflex responses are not associated with psychological factors such as catastrophisation and distress (Sterling, Pettiford, Hodkinson, & Curatolo, 2008).

Mechanical hyperalgesia locally over the cervical spine appears to be common to both chronic whiplash and idiopathic neck pain and may indicate an ongoing peripheral nociceptive source of pain (Chien, Eliav, & Sterling, 2005; Scott et al., 2005). In addition to its presence in the chronic stages of neck pain conditions, local mechanical hyperalgesia has also been shown to occur following acute whiplash injury irrespective of symptom intensity and disability levels reported by the patient (Kasch, Stengaard-Pedersen, Arendt-Nielsen, & Staehelin Jensen, 2001; Sterling, Jull, Vicenzino, & Kenardy, 2004). However this local mechanical hyperalgesia usually resolves within several weeks in those patients who recover or report continuing milder symptoms but persist in whiplash patients with chronic symptoms at six months post injury (Sterling, Jull, Vicenzino, & Kenardy, 2003).

In contrast, the phenomena of widespread (throughout the body and away from the cervical spine) sensory hypersensitivity has been shown to be an early and persistent characteristic of those whiplash injured patients with poor functional recovery (Sterling, Jull, Vicenzino et al., 2003). Mechanical hyperalgesia has been shown to occur in both the upper and lower limbs from within a few weeks of injury in those with poor recovery and persisted virtually unchanged at long-term follow up (6 months and 2 years) (Sterling, Jull, & Kenardy, 2006; Sterling, Jull, Vicenzino et al., 2003). In contrast these changes were never a feature for those participants who recovered well or reported only milder levels of ongoing pain. Furthermore the picture of those individuals with poor functional recovery becomes more complex, where the presence of both thermal (cold and heat) hyperalgesia and diminished sympathetic vasoconstriction are also early and persistent features of this group (Sterling, Jull, Vicenzino et al., 2003). In fact, cold hyperalgesia, decreased cold tolerance and diminished sympathetic vasoconstriction have been shown to be predictive of poor functional recovery at 6 months, one and two years post MVC (Kasch, Qerama, Bach, & Jensen, 2005; Sterling, Jull, Vicenzino, Kenardy, & Darnell, 2005). The mechanisms underlying these sensory disturbances are not well understood, but these factors are also features of peripheral neuropathic pain conditions (Bennett, 2006). Although preliminary at this stage, recent findings of hypoaesthetic responses (increased detection threshold) to vibration, electrical and heat stimuli in the hands of people with chronic WAD does indicate potential dysfunction of peripheral nerve fibres (Chien, Eliav, & Sterling, 2008b).

While it is clear that the phenomena of widespread sensory hypersensitivity is associated with poorer functional recovery; it is also apparent that the sensory presentation of whiplash is still markedly heterogeneous. Some whiplash injured individuals present with only local cervical mechanical hyperalgesia with no evidence of more widespread disturbance, cold hyperalgesia, or sympathetic nervous system dysfunction (Sterling, 2004). In contrast there appears to be greater sensory disturbance (both hypersensitivity and hypoaesthesia) in those with poor recovery and who reported higher levels of pain and disability. The sensory hypersensitivity in this whiplash sub-group occurs not only locally within the cervical spine but additionally at more peripheral or remote body sites away from the injured area including both the upper and lower limbs (Sterling, 2004). As previously stated, the sensory presentation of this whiplash group seems quite different from neck pain of an idiopathic nature but quite similar to cervical radiculopathy. Such varied sensory manifestations would suggest that different mechanisms underlie sub-groups that exist within the whiplash condition. Those with persistent moderate to severe levels of pain and disability display a complex presentation that indicates the involvement of augmented central pain processing mechanisms. The reason why this group of whiplash injured develops a hypersensitive state is not clear. As outlined earlier in this chapter, numerous cervical spine structures are implicated as possible sources of nociception following whiplash injury. It is also possible that injuries to deep cervical structures do not rapidly heal and thus become a nociceptive 'driver' of central nervous system hyperexcitability. Moreover there is evidence from cadaver studies that certain lesions can persist unresolved in MVC survivors who die of unrelated causes some years later (Taylor & Finch, 1993).

Whilst this argument may meet opposition from those who believe injured soft tissues are healed within several weeks, it is gaining an increasing amount of support from researchers as a possible contributor to the development of chronic musculoskeletal pain including whiplash (Curatolo, Arendt-Nielsen, & Petersen-Felix, 2006; Vierck, 2006).

Psychological Features of the Whiplash Condition

Psychological factors have been shown to be consistently associated with both acute and chronic musculoskeletal conditions as well as involved in the transitions between these two states (Linton, 2000). This has perhaps inadvertently led to two misconceptions. Firstly, that similar (if not the same) psychological factors are involved in all painful musculoskeletal conditions and secondly that a Cartesian or dichotomous separation of the mind from the physical manifestations (body) of such conditions can be made.

If we take the first example, it is apparent that unique psychological factors may be involved in the etiology and development of chronic whiplash pain when compared with other conditions such as low back pain (Sterling, Kenardy, Jull, & Vicenzino, 2003). There is no doubt that persistent neck pain from whiplash injury (similarly to low back pain) is also associated with psychological distress and may include affective disturbances, anxiety, depression, as well as, behavioural abnormalities such as fear of movement (Nederhand, Ijzerman, Hermens, Turk, & Zilvold, 2004; Peebles, McWilliams, & MacLennan, 2001; Sterling, Kenardy, et al., 2003; Wenzel, Haug, Mykletun, & Dahl, 2002).

Psychological distress is also a feature of whiplash in the acute stages of the condition, with most people reporting some distress, even in those patients who report low levels of pain (Sterling, Kenardy et al., 2003). Data from several studies indicates that persistent levels of psychological distress are associated with ongoing or non-resolved pain and disability. Sterling et al (2003) showed that initial levels of psychological distress (measured with GHQ-28) decreased by two to three months post injury in those patients who recovered and in those with lesser symptoms, seemingly paralleling decreasing levels of pain and disability. In contrast, the whiplash group who continued to report moderate to severe levels of pain and disability at this time point and later at six months and two years post injury also showed above threshold scores on the GHQ-28 throughout this entire period (Sterling, Kenardy et al., 2003). A recent large cross-sectional study showed an association between anxiety and depression with pain and disability in whiplash patients whose accidents occurred over two years previously, but not in those with acute injury, suggesting that symptom persistence is the trigger for psychological distress (Wenzel et al., 2002). This view is supported by other prospective studies where delayed recovery following whiplash injury could not be predicted from psychological factors alone such as personality traits or self rated well being. Instead delayed recovery after whiplash injury was related to initial symptom severity (Borchgrevink, Stiles, Borchgrevink, & Lereim, 1997; Radanov, Sturzenegger, & Di Stefano, 1995).

The role of fear of movement or fear avoidance beliefs and behaviors in whiplash pain is not clear. Nederhand et al (2004) found that scores on the Tampa Scale of Kinesiphobia (TSK) were predictive of poor recovery following whiplash injury. These findings would appear to be consistent with investigations of chronic low back pain where it has been proposed that fear of movement plays a role in the transition from acute to chronic pain (Vlaeyen & Linton, 2000). However other studies have provided conflicting evidence. Sterling et al (2003) noted that in the acute stage of whiplash, patients who eventually recovered quite well showed high initial scores on the TSK that were no different from this who developed chronic pain. In this longitudinal study, where several psychological substrates were measured, fear avoidance beliefs did not emerge as a predictor of poor recovery at any stage (Sterling et al., 2006, 2005). These findings suggest that fear of movement may be justified in the acute stage of injury as a protective mechanism against further injury and to allow healing to occur, as has been proposed by other investigators (Vlaeyen, Kole-Snijders, & Boeren, 1995), but is often overlooked when considering acute spinal pain.

Maladaptive coping strategies such as catastrophising have also been shown to be associated with persistent low back pain (Pincus, Burton, Vogel, & Field, 2002) but have not been well investigated in neck pain cohorts. Buitenhuis, Spanjer, & Fidler (2003) evaluated the association between the coping styles used by participants and the duration of neck complaints following whiplash injury. A palliative reaction or one where the patient seeks palliative relief of their symptoms such as distraction, smoking or drinking was significantly associated with a longer duration of neck symptoms at 12 months post injury. Those participants who sought social support and shared their concerns with others showed a better outcome with less symptom duration (Buitenhuis et al., 2003). Carroll, Cassidy, & Cote (2006) also showed that passive coping strategies were associated with slower recovery following whiplash injury. They suggest that attention to the types of coping styles adopted by the whiplash patient in the early stages of their condition and behavioral interventions to promote active coping may decrease the length of time that symptoms are reported. In contrast Kivioja, Jensen, & Lindgren (2005) found no evidence that different coping styles in the early stage of injury influenced the outcome at one year post accident. These studies involved different inception times and were conducted in different cultural contexts which may explain the variation in study findings. The participants of Carroll et al's study were recruited within six weeks of injury, with the inception time of the latter study being within hours of the injury. Thus coping strategies may vary depending on the stage of the condition or injury and this requires further investigation. Nevertheless whilst coping styles may not be independently associated with poor recovery, improvement of the individual patient's coping mechanisms via education and assurance is recommended and in keeping with current evidence-based treatment guidelines for whiplash (MAA, 2007; Scholten-Peeters et al., 2002).

Posttraumatic Stress Symptoms – An Important Factor in Whiplash?

Post-traumatic stress disorder (PTSD) is a psychiatric disorder that results from the experience or witnessing of traumatic or life-threatening events. PTSD has profound psychobiological correlates, which can impair the person's daily life and be life threatening (Iribarren, Prolo, Neagos, & Chiappelli, 2005).Whiplash injury differs from most other musculoskeletal pain syndromes, including low back pain, in that it is generally precipitated by a significant traumatic event, namely a MVC. The effect of the psychological stress surrounding the crash itself as opposed to distress about neck pain complaints may have an influence on outcome. The stress that results from this traumatic event precipitates a spectrum of psycho-emotional and physiopathological outcomes. Posttramatic stress disorder is a common sequalae of severe injuries following a MVC (Kuch, Cox, Evans, & Shulman, 1994). Yet, it is only recently that evidence has emerged to show that that it may also play a role in less severe road accident injuries including whiplash.

Posttraumatic stress disorder has been diagnosed in some patients with chronic whiplash associated disorders (WAD) (Freidenberg, Hickling, Blanchard, & Malta, 2006). In addition an acute posttraumatic stress reaction appears to be present in some whiplash injured individuals soon after injury with moderate to high levels of distress (measured with the Impact of Events Scale), being demonstrated both within days of injury and within three to four weeks of injury (Drottning, Staff, Levin, & Malt, 1995; Sterling, Jull, Vicenzino et al., 2003). The presence of posttraumatic stress symptoms has been shown to be associated with greater levels of pain and disability, more severe whiplash complaints and poor functional recovery after injury (Buitenhuis, DeJong, Jaspers, & Groothoff, 2006; Sterling, Kenardy et al., 2003). Furthermore following a motor vehicle crash, those with a diagnosis of whiplash (neck pain) are significantly more likely to express posttraumatic stress disorder symptoms at 12 months post-accident compared to those who never reported neck pain post accident (Freidenberg et al., 2006). A moderate posttraumatic stress reaction, present within a month of injury, is also a strong predictor of poor outcome at both six months and 2 years post injury being stronger than both general psychological distress (GHQ-28) and fear of movement and reinjury (TSK) (Sterling et al., 2006, 2005).

Symptoms of posttraumatic stress may include intrusive thoughts and/or images of the event (in this case the motor vehicle crash); avoidance behaviour associated with the event such as driving avoidance or avoidance behavior via substance abuse; hyperarousal such as panic attacks, hypervigilance and sleep disturbance. Yet it is not clear if any of these symptoms play a specific or greater role than the others in the development of whiplash pain, disability or related adverse health outcomes. Sterling, Kenardy et al (2003) showed that avoidance behaviour may have a stronger influence on recovery and more recently Buitenhuis et al (2006) showed that a greater number of hyperarousal symptoms (panic attacks, hypervigilance, sleep disturbance, easily startled) in the acute stage of injury was a stronger predictor of symptom persistence. Further investigation is required to determine the relative importance of the substrates of posttraumatic stress as this may provide fruitful direction in terms of approaches for the the psychological management and treatment of the whiplash patient.

In summary the available data to date indicate that posttraumatic stress symptoms play an important role in functional recovery from a whiplash injury, at least in some individuals. The treatment of PTSD is complex, both in terms of available treatments and the myriad of traumatic possibilities that cause it. Properly diagnosing PTSD according to DSM-IV criteria should be the first step, including assessments for co-morbidity. This should be followed by treatments with various degrees of demonstrated efficacy (Iribarren et al., 2005). This suggests that specific treatments directed toward understanding and treating these factors which may be more efficacious than a broadly applied cognitive behavioural approach in the management of pain after whiplash.

Relationships Between Physical and Psychological Factors

The biopsychsocial model considers pain and disability as the result of multiple factors, including both biomedical (physical) and psychological factors. However it is not clear, nor is it usually investigated, what the relative role of each factor may be or how they potentially interact.

Widespread mechanical and thermal hyperalgesia seem to be a feature of whiplash injury which is not apparent in neck pain of insidious origin (Scott et al., 2005). The sensory changes observed in whiplash are not only a feature of the chronic stage of thise condition but are present from soon after the initial injury in those who develop persistent pain and disability, remaining virtually unchanged from the acute to chronic stages of the condition (Sterling, Jull, Vicenzino et al., 2003). Whilst it is not a universal phenomenon, psychological factors including general distress, posttraumatic stress reaction and fears of movement and reinjury generally occur concomitantly with the sensory hypersensitivity seen in whiplash (Sterling et al., 2005). It is also generally recognized that psychological factors such as depression and anxiety can also modulate pain threshold responses (Chiu et al., 2005). Posttraumatic stress reaction may also be associated with heightened reactivity to stimuli as well being manifested by sympathetic nervous system changes in some individuals (Harvey & Bryant, 2002). It is likely that the co-occurrence of sensory hypersensitivity, increased muscle activity and psychological distress observed in some whiplash injured individuals is not merely coincidental. Potentially, these domains are related and knowledge of these relationships is important in order to improve our clinical understandings of the processes underlying the condition.

There does appear to be some relationship between psychological factors and sensory disturbance. Sterling et al (2008) recently demonstrated moderate associations between pain thresholds (pressure and cold) at some sites, particularly at more remote sites such as in the lower limb, and both psychological distress (General Health Questionnaire [GHQ-28]) and catastrophisation (Pain Catastrophising Scale -PCS). Notably there was no relationship between catastrophisation and the intensity of electrical stimulation required to elicit a flexor withdrawal response in biceps femoris in the same patient group (Sterling et al., 2007). The latter test is a measure of spinal cord hyperexcitability requiring no cognitive response from the participant (Banic et al., 2004). These findings indicate that psychological factors play a role in central hypersensitivity. However, they do not support the assumption that psychological factors are the only or main factors responsible for central hypersensitivity in whiplash patients. In particular, spinal cord hyperexcitability appears not to be affected, at least significantly, by the psychological factors that were assessed.

The relationships between sensory and sympathetic changes and posttraumatic stress reaction have also been explored. Sterling and Kenardy (2006) (Sterling & Kenardy, 2006) showed that the early presence of mechanical and cold hyperalgesia was associated with posttraumatic stress symptoms at six months post MVC, but this relationship was also mediated by initial pain and disability levels (in this case, Neck Disability Index scores). In contrast, early sympathetic disturbance (impaired peripheral vasoconstriction) was associated with persistent posttraumatic stress symptoms and showed no relationship with initial pain and disability levels (Fig. 1). Although speculative, the impaired vasoconstrictive response may be an indication of a biological vulnerability in some patients with acute whiplash injury which could be a trigger for PTSR seen in the chronic stages of the condition. Certainly it would appear that there are common pathways and associations between pain levels, sensory changes, posttraumatic stress reactions and outcome following MVC.

When taken together, these findings suggest that psychological factors such as distress, catastrophisation and posttraumatic stress symptoms show some association with the development of sensory hypersensitivity in chronic whiplash. However this relationship is not consistent for all modalities, measures or at all body sites tested and may be mediated by levels of pain and disability. As such, psychological factors are not the only or main issues responsible for central hypersensitivity in whiplash patients. Central hyperexcitability after whiplash is therefore a complex phenomenon that probably involves both neurobiological changes as well as psychological factors.

It is clear that central hyperexcitability plays a significant role in the development of chronic whiplash pain. More importantly, the sensory changes reflective of central hyperexcitability occur very soon after injury. More widespread pain

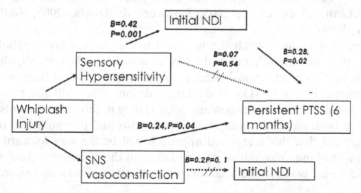

Fig. 1 Relationships between sensory and sympathetic disturbances and persistent posttraumatic stress symptoms following whiplash injury. The relationship between sensory hypersensitivity and PTSS is moderated by pain and disability (NDI) levels. SNS vasoconstriction independently predicts persistent PTSS (Sterling & Kenardy, 2006). NDI: Neck Disability Index; PTSS: posttraumatic stress symptoms; SNS: sympathetic nervous system

conditions such as fibromyalgia demonstrate a remarkably similar sensory pre-sentation with both conditions featuring hyperalgesic responses to numerous stimuli including pressure, light touch, heat, cold and electric current (Sterling, 2007; Vierck, 2006). Thus it would seem feasible that the early central hyperexcit-ability of whiplash could further develop and lead to extended peripheral pain in areas away from the neck, head and upper limbs. However current data would suggest that this more widespread pain occurs in a small subsample of patients with whiplash (Holm et al., 2007; Tishler et al., 2006). Moreover it is also clear that not all whiplash injured individuals develop sensory hypersensitivity as it seems to occur to a greater degree in those reporting higher levels of pain and disability. The reasons underlying the apparently greater central changes in some and not others are perplexing. Numerous hypotheses could be put forward including a more severe initial injury; involvement of injured peripheral nerve tissue; contribution of psychological factors and even a genetic predisposition to such changes.

Recently several authors have proposed the potential role of stress related factors and subsequent influence on nociceptive pathways on the development of WAD. Of particular interest is the hypothalamic-pituitary-adrenal (HPA) axis, since alterations of the HPA axis, the sympathetic-adrenal-medullary (system) and the immune system may mediate or facilitate somatic conditions such as chronic pain, fatigue and traumatic stress (Gaab et al., 2005; McLean, Clauw, Abelson, & Liberzon, 2005). Dysregulations of the HPA axis in terms of reduced reactivity and enhanced negative feedback suppression has also been shown to exist in chronic WAD and the observed endocrine abnormalities could serve as a systemic mechanism of symptoms experienced by chronic WAD patients (Gaab et al., 2005). Other research indicates that sympathetic activation (as a consequence of stress or arousal) in the early stages following injury interacts with neurobiological pain processing mechanisms. This inter-action may be a critical step in the development of persistent or chronic pain.(McLean, Clauw et al., 2005; Passatore & Roatta, 2006; Sterling & Kenardy, 2006).

Models such as these which aim to integrate the physical and psychological manifestations of whiplash and neck pain are overdue in the conceptualization and investigation of musculoskeletal pain and will provide a framework for future investigation of WAD and similar conditions. They will also provide an improved basis for the integration and appropriate timing of treatments direc-ted toward both physical (biological) impairments and psychological factors. It is suggested that this integrated approach will be the way forward in the management of musculoskeletal pain rather than the dichotomous separation of physical and psychological factors that so often occurs in research and practice.

There has also been some preliminary exploration of the relationship between the motor dysfunction seen in whiplash injured persons and fears of movement/reinjury. Psychological factors such as fear of movement and dis-tress have been associated with altered lumbar paraspinal muscle activity in chronic low back pain (Verbunt et al., 2005; Watson, Booker, & Main, 1997). Sterling et al. (2003) have shown that motor dysfunction including cervical range of movement loss, kinaesthetic deficits and altered cervical flexor muscle recruitment patterns occurred independently (statistically) of TSK scores with this relationship being consistent at both the acute and chronic stages of whiplash injury. These findings have been interpreted as an indication of physiological disturbances in motor function, as opposed to fears of movement. In contrast to these findings, Nederhand et al. (2006) showed that fear of movement (TSK scores) were independently associated with decreased activity in the upper trapezius in a prospective whiplash cohort. These two studies appear to provide conflicting results. However different muscles were measured in each study with the cervical flexors in Sterling et al.'s study showing increased activity and the upper trapezius in Nederhand et al's study decreased activity. It is therefore feasible that the psychological factors such as fear of movement influence the motor system in different ways, or that both physiological and psychological factors are inter-relating in their effects on the motor system.

There is still much to be learned about the nexus between physical (sensory and motor) manifestations and psychological aspects of WAD. For practitioners it is also important to realise the potential influence of psychological factors on the patient's physical presentation and vice versa. The challenge is to disentangle these relationships in both the research environment, and in the clinical setting.

The Prediction of Outcome Following Whiplash Injury

The capacity to predict outcome following whiplash injury is important because of the need to institute appropriate early intervention for those deemed at risk of a poorer outcome and the possible curtailment of costs. Many studies have investigated the prognostic capability of various factors such as sociodemographic status; crash related variables; compensation/litigation, psychosocial and physical factors (Cassidy et al., 2000; Kasch, Flemming, & Jensen, 2001; Radanov et al., 1995). However two recent systematic reviews of prospective cohort studies on whiplash could agree on only high initial pain intensity as showing strong evidence for delayed functional recovery (Cote, Cassidy, Carroll, Frank, & Bombardier, 2001; Scholten-Peeters et al., 2003). Knowledge of this factor may offer some assistance in identifying that sub-group of patients who may go on to develop persistent symptoms. However, it has also been shown that pain and disability levels alone whilst having high specificity had relatively low sensitivity to predict those with ongoing moderate to severe symptoms at six months post accident (Sterling et al., 2005). In addition, the sole measurement of pain and disability levels is unlikely to alter the direction of secondary and tertiary management stages of this condition.

Since the time of these systematic reviews (Cote et al., 2001; Scholten-Peeters et al., 2003) other factors have emerged as potentially useful prognostic indicators of outcome. These include physical factors of decreased range of neck movement, cold hyperalgesia or intolerance and impaired sympathetic vasoconstriction (Kasch et al., 2005; Sterling et al., 2006, 2005) as well as the psychological substrates of posttraumatic stress symptoms (Sterling et al., 2006, 2005). These factors are in addition to high levels of pain and disability which consistently emerges as an important predictor of adverse outcomes (Hendricks et al., 2005; Rebbeck, Sindhausen, & Cameron, 2006). When included together, the sensitivity of the combined factors increased to 69%, compared to 37%, when pain and disability levels are the sole measures (Sterling et al., 2005).

Two studies have demonstrated that symptoms of posttraumatic stress are also predictive of poor functional recovery (Buitenhuis et al., 2006; Sterling et al., 2006), with the latter study demonstrating superior predictive capacity of this variable, when compared to other psychological domains (Sterling et al., 2006). Additional psychological factors such as high levels of catastrophising, low self efficacy and palliative coping strategies have also been identified, in some studies, as potentially influencing the course of recovery in WAD patients (Buitenhuis et al., 2003; Hendricks et al., 2005). At this stage, the strongest psychosocial predictor appears to be low-educational attainment (Ottoson, Nyren, Johansson, & Ponzer, 2005; Sterner, Toolanen, Gerdle, & Hildingson, 2003). The role of the controversial issue of compensation related factors is still inconclusive with some studies showing it has predictive capacity (Dufton et al., 2006) and others reporting no predictive capacity for this particular factor (Sterling et al., 2006).

It is apparent that understanding of factors associated with poor functional recovery following whiplash injury has progressed substantially in recent years. Whilst initially high levels of pain and disability are the most consistent predictors, studies including a more broad range of factors have provided important additional information. What has also emerged is that the transition from the acute to chronic stage of whiplash is multifactorial, involving physical factors indicative of central hyperexcitability, as well as, psychological and psychosocial factors. No doubt complex inter-relationships between these factors exist and have yet to be illuminated. The implications for the management of whiplash are that a full and comprehensive assessment of these factors will likely be necessary, particularly in the important acute stages of injury.

Implications for Assessment and Management of Whiplash

Currently available evidence –based guidelines for the management of acute WAD promote reassurance to the patient, the maintenance of activity levels, range of movement exercises, simple analgesics and the adoption of active coping strategies (MAA, 2007; Scholten-Peeters et al., 2002). However, the emerging multifactorial nature of WAD suggests that whilst the current guidelines may benefit some whiplash patients with a less complex presentation, they are unlikely to be adequate for the management of those with a complex phenotype, which includes both marked physical dysfunction (including sensory hypersensitivity) and psychological distress.

There is some support for this argument where randomized controlled trials of interventions for acute whiplash have shown that whilst the maintenance of activity levels and exercise is more efficacious than rest and the use of a neck collar or advice only, a substantial proportion of patients still develop chronic symptoms (Rosenfeld et al., 2003; Rosenfeld, Seferiadis, & Gunnarsson, 2006). One reason for these findings may be that those patients with a more complex presentation require a more specific or concerted approach to their management.

Surprisingly few randomized controlled intervention studies have been conducted for chronic WAD. The only therapy to demonstrate clear evidence of efficacy is radiofrequency neurotomy for zygapophyseal joint pain (Lord, Barnsley, Wallis, McDonald, & Bogduk, 1996), but this difficult procedure is only performed in a highly selected sub-group with pain arising from lower cervical zygapophyseal joints identified using placebo, controlled blocks. Conservative treatment approaches such as a submaximal graded exercise program and a more specific physical therapy approach utilizing manual therapy and specific neck exercise have demonstrated only modest effects with approximately 25% of patients not responding to the intervention (Jull et al., 2007; Stewart et al., 2007). However interesting findings emerged from the latter clinical trial when sub-group analysis was performed. They found that the presence of cold and mechanical hyperalgesia moderated the effects of the physical therapy program (Jull et al., 2007). Fibromyalgia is a condition with a similar sensory presentation as the moderate/severe whiplash group. In this condition, there is some evidence that exercise may actually increase pain and sensory hypersensitivity (Vierck et al., 2001). If a similar scenario exists for whiplash, then stratifying sub-group classifications within treatment trials would be a prudent approach in the investigation of the most efficacious physical interventions.

The complex presentation of some of the whiplash injured, including central hyperexcitability and the presence of psychological factors including posttraumatic stress suggests that interventions directed toward these characteristics may be required. However, it is not yet clear whether or not modulation of sensory hypersensitivity is possible and if this would be reflected in reduced levels of pain and disability. Curatolo et al (2006) outlined three theoretical approaches to the treatment of central hypersensitivity. These include pharmacological interventions such as NSAIDS or opioids, directed at blocking or decreasing peripheral nociceptive input; pharmacological interventions (eg NSAIDS, NMDA antagonists) directed at modulating spinal cord hyperexcitability or pharmacological or psychological interventions acting at a supraspinal level and influencing descending inhibitory pathways. Trials of pharmacological interventions for whiplash are scarce but this also may be an area for future research. Theoretically, physical interventions such as Transcutaneous Electrical Nerve Stimulation (TENS) and acupuncture may also be useful in modulating sensory hypersensitivity. Yet these interventions have not been specifically investigated in WAD.

Few studies have investigated the effects of psychologically based interventions on this condition. Oliveira, Gevirtz, & Hubbard (2006) found that a short psycho-educational video (including education of the whiplash condition, exercises to reduce muscle tension and relaxation breathing exercises) shown in the emergency department soon after injury resulted in substantially less pain and disability at one, three and six months post injury when compared to usual care. However a similar approach using video as an educational tool for early whiplash patients found no significant difference between this approach and usual medical care (Brison et al., 2005). The differential results of these studies indicate that further research is required to determine the role and nature of education delivered to individuals following whiplash injury. Only one study has investigated specific psychological intervention directed toward PTSD in chronic whiplash. Blanchard et al., (2003) showed that this form of intervention, whilst improving posttraumatic stress symptoms, had no effect on pain levels in this group. The obvious question arising from this study is whether a combined approach to management of WAD that addresses both the psychological and physical manifestations of the condition may be of greater benefit than psychological or physical treatments alone.

It may be the case that an integrated multidisciplinary and multi-professional approach is required to adequately address the complexities of the physical and psychological presentations of whiplash injured people. Whilst this statement may appear hackneyed in terms of the arguments for treatment approaches for this and other musculoskeletal conditions, it should be noted that many patients do not receive adequate management and treatment until their condition has become chronic. Thus it is time to re-evaluate this situation and provide *early* and targeted interventions to those individuals at risk for developing chronic pain. This is not to say that such treatment should occur in the already overstretched multidisciplinary pain clinic environment. To the contrary, a well integrated and co-operative approach amongst community primary care practitioners may be the most appropriate and cost effective approach.

Summary

The available literature consistently shows that whiplash is a condition involving both physical and psychological manifestations. The sub-group of whiplash injured who do not recover well and who contribute substantially to the costs of this condition, manifest a more complex presentation. Those who recover well are characterised by milder initial levels of pain and disability, some motor dysfunction and local cervical hyperalgesia. In contrast the former group with poor functional recovery are characterised by the presence of widespread sensory hypersensitivity and posttraumatic stress symptoms in addition to higher initial pain and disability. It is generally acknowledged that sensory hypersensitivity represents augmented central pain processing mechanisms. Moreover, while there is some relationship between the sensory responses and psychological factors but these relationships are not consistent across modalities, measures or body sites tested. This suggests that psychological factors alone cannot fully explain the sensory disturbances seen in whiplash. A likely scenario is a complex interplay between these factors.

Currently utilised therapeutic approaches consider whiplash to be a homogenous condition and fail to account for the complex multifaceted presentation that occurs in some of the whiplash injured. This may be one reason for the generally modest effects of treatments for both acute and chronic WAD. Future management strategies may need to be directed toward physical (motor and sensory) dysfunctions and psychological factors identified in individual whiplash patients. Whilst those with a more straight forward presentation will likely respond to minimalist intervention approaches, the whiplash sub-group with central hypersensitivity and psychological distress, particularly posttraumatic stress may need a more concerted multidisciplinary treatment approach. In view of findings that many of these changes occur within a few weeks of injury, the management of patients in this sub-group may need to be aggressively instituted in the early acute stage of the condition. This may help to lessen the transition to chronicity that commonly occurs in this condition.

References

Banic, B., Petersen-Felix, S., Andersen, O., Radanov, B., Villiger, P., Arendt-Nielsen, L., et al. (2004). Evidence for spinal cord hypersensitivity in chronic pain after whiplash injury and in fibromyalgia. *Pain, 107*(1–2), 7–15.

Barnsley, L., Lord, S., & Bogduk, N. (1998). The pathophysiology of whiplash. *Spine; State of the Art Reviews, 12*(2), 209–242.

Bennett, G. (2006). Can we distinguish between inflammatory and neuropathic pain? *Pain Research and Managment, 11*(Supp A), 11–15.

Blanchard, E., Hickling, E., Devineni, T., Veazey, C., Galovski, T., Mundy, E., et al. (2003). A controlled evaluation of cognitive behaviour therapy for posttraumatic stress in motor vehicle accident survivors. *Behavior Research and Therapy, 41*, 7996.

Bogduk, N. (2002). Point of view. *Spine, 27*(17), 1940–1941.

Borchgrevink, G., Kaasa, A., McDonagh, D., Stiles, T., Haraldseth, O., & Lereim, I. (1998). Acute treatment of whiplash neck sprain injuries. A randomized trial of treatment during the first 14 days after a car accident. *Spine, 23*(1), 25–31 *LHM: Herston Medical, Biological Sciences *LHC: RD768.S767.

Borchgrevink, G., Stiles, T., Borchgrevink, P., & Lereim, I. (1997). Personality profile among symptomatic and recovered patients with neck sprain injury, measured by mcmvi acutely and 6 months after car accidents. *Journal of Psychosomatic Research, 42*(4), 357–367.

Brison, R., Hartling, L., Dostaler, S., Leger, A., Rowe, B., Stiell, I., et al. (2005). A randomised controlled trial of an educational intervention to prevent the chronic pain of whiplash associated disorders following rear-end motor vehicle collisions. *Spine, 30*(16), 1799–1807.

Buitenhuis, J., DeJong, J., Jaspers, J., & Groothoff, J. (2006). Relationship between post-traumatic stress disorder symptoms and the course of whiplash complaints. *Journal of Psychosomatic Research, 61*(3), 681–689.

Buitenhuis, J., Spanjer, J., & Fidler, V. (2003). Recovery from acute whiplash – the role of coping styles. *Spine, 28*(9), 896–901.

Buskila, D., Neumann, L., Vaisberg, G., Alkalay, D., & Wolfe, F. (1997). Increased rates of fibromyalgia following cervical spine injury. A controlled study of 161 cases of traumatic injury. *Arthritis and Rheumatism, 40*(3), 446–452 *LHM: Herston Medical, PA Hospital, Mater Hospital *LHC: RC927.A447.

Carli, G., Suman, A., Biasi, G., & Marcolongo, R. (2002). Reactivity to superficial and deep stimuli in patients with chronic musculoskeletal pain. *Pain, 100*, 259–269.

Carroll, L., Cassidy, D., & Cote, P. (2006). The role of pain coping strategies in prognosis after whiplash injury: Passive coping predicts slowed recovery. *Pain, 124*(1–2), 18–26.

Cassidy, J. D., Carroll, L. J., Cote, P., Lemstra, M., Berglund, A., & Nygren, A. (2000). Effect of eliminating compensation for pain and suffering on the outcome of insurance claims for whiplash injury. *The New England Journal of Medicine, 20*, 1179–1213.

Chien, A., Eliav, E., & Sterling, M. (2005). *Sensory function in chronic whiplash associated disorders.* Paper presented at the 11th World Congress on Pain, Sydney.

Chien, A., Eliav, E., & Sterling, M. (2008a). Whiplash (Grade II) and Cervical Radiculopathy Share a similar sensory presentation: An investigation using quantitative sensory testing. *Clinical Journal of Pain* (in press).

Chien, A., Eliav, E., & Sterling, M. (2008b). Hypoaesthesia occurs with sensory hypersensitivity in chronic whiplash-further evidence of a neuropathic condition. *Manual Therapy* (in press) doi:10.1016/j.math.2007.12.004/.

Chiu, Y., Sillman, A., Macfarlane, G., Ray, D., Gupta, A., Dickens, C., et al. (2005). poor sleep and depression are independently associated with a reduced pain threshold. results of a population based study. *Pain, 115*(3), 316–321.

Chu, J., Eun, S., & Schwartz, J. (2005). Quantitative motor unit action potentials (QUAMP) in whiplash patients with neck and upper limb pain. *Electromyography and clinical neurophysiology, 45*(6), 323–328.

Cote, P., Cassidy, D., Carroll, L., Frank, J., & Bombardier, C. (2001). A systematic review of the prognosis of acute whiplash and a new conceptual framework to synthesize the literature. *Spine, 26*(19), E445–E458.

Curatolo, M., Arendt-Nielsen, L., & Petersen-Felix, S. (2006). Central hypersensitivity in chronic pain: Mechanisms and clinical implications. *Physical Medicine Rehabilitation Clinics of North America, 17*, 287–302.

Curatolo, M., Petersen-Felix, S., Arendt-Nielsen, L., Giani, C., Zbinden, A., & Radanov, B. (2001). Central hypersensitivity in chronic pain after whiplash injury. *Clinical Journal of Pain, 17*(4), 306–315.

Cusick, J., Pintar, F., & Yoganandan, N. (2001). Whiplash syndrome: Kinematic factors influencing pain patterns. *Spine, 26*(11), 1252–1258.

Dall'Alba, P., Sterling, M., Trealeven, J., Edwards, S., & Jull, G. (2001). Cervical range of motion discriminates between asymptomatic and whiplash subjects. *Spine, 26*(19), 2090–2094.

Drottning, M., Staff, P., Levin, L., & Malt, U. (1995). Acute emotional response to common whiplash predicts subsequent pain complaints: A prospective study of 107 subjects sustaining whiplash injury. *Nordic Journal of Psychiatry, 49*(4), 293–299.

Dufton, J., Kopec, J., Wong, H., Cassidy, J., Quon, J., McIntosh, G., et al. (2006). Prognostic factors associated with minimal improvement following acute whiplash associated disorders. *Spine, 31*(20), E759–765.

Elliott, J., Jull, G., Noteboom, T., Darnell, R., Galloway, G., & Gibbon, W. (2006). Fatty infiltration in the cervical extensor muscles in persistent whiplash associated disorders: An MRI analysis. *Spine, 31*(22).

Ferrari, R., Russell, A., Carroll, L., & Cassidy, D. (2005). A re-examination of the whiplash associated disorders (WAD) as a systemic illness. *Annals of Rheumatic Disease, 64*(9), 1337–1142.

Freidenberg, B., Hickling, E., Blanchard, E., & Malta, L. (2006). Posttraumatic stress disorder and whiplash after motor vehicle accidents. In G. Young, A. Kane & K. Nicholson (Eds.), *Psychological knowledge in court* (pp. 215–224). New York: Springer.

Gaab, J., Baumann, S., Budnoik, A., Gmunder, H., Hottinger, N., & Ehlert, U. (2005). Reduced reactivity and ehnanced negative feedback sensitivity of the hypothalamus-pituitary-adrenal axis in chronic whiplash associated disorders. *Pain, 119*, 219–224.

Greening, J., Dilley, A., & Lynn, B. (2005). In vivo study of nerve movement and mechanosensitivity of the median nerve in whiplash and non-specific arm pain patients. *Pain, 115*(3), 248–253.

Harvey, A., & Bryant, R. (2002). Acute stress disorder: A synthesis and critique. *Psychological Bulletin, 128*(6), 886–902.

Heikkila, H., & Astrom, P. (1996). Cervicocephalic kinesthetic sensibility in patients with whiplash injury. *Scandinavian Journal of Rehabilitation, 28*, 133–138.

Hendricks, E., Scholten-Peeters, G., van der Windt, D., Neeleman-van der Steen, C., Oostendorp, R., & Verhagen, A. (2005). Prognostic factors for poor recovery in acute whiplash patients. *Pain, 114*, 408–416.

Holm, L., Carroll, L., Cassidy, D., Skillgate, E., & Ahlbom, A. (2007). Widespread pain following whiplash associated disorders: Incidence, course and risk factors. *Journal of Rheumatology, 34*, 193–200.

Ide, M., Ide, J., Yamaga, M., & Takagi, K. (2001). Symptoms and signs of irritation of the brachial plexus in whiplash injuries. *The Journal of Bone and Joint Surgery (British), 83*, 226–229.

Iribarren, J., Prolo, P., Neagos, N., & Chiappelli, F. (2005). Post-traumatic stress disorder: Evidence based research for the third millennium. *Evidence Based Complementary and Alternative Medicine, 2*(4), 503–512.

Ivancic, P., & Panjabi, M. (2006). Cervical spine loads and intervertebral motions during whiplash. *Traffic Injury Prevention, 7*, 389–399.

Jensen, T., & Baron, R. (2003). Translation of symptoms and signs into mechanisms in neuropathic pain. *Pain, 102*(2), 1–8.

Johansson, B. (2006). Whiplash injuries can be visible by functional magnetic resonance imaging. *Pain Research and Managment, 11*(3), 197–199.

Jull, G., Kristjansson, E., & Dall'Alba, P. (2004). Impairment in the cervical flexors: A comparison of whiplash and insidious onset neck pain patients. *Manual Therapy, 9*(2), 89–94.

Jull, G., Sterling, M., Kenardy, J., & Beller, E. (2007). Does the presence of sensory hypersensitivity influence outcomes of physical rehabilitation for chronic whiplash? – A preliminary RCT. *Pain, 129*, 28–34.

Kaale, B., Krakenes, J., Albrektsen, G., & Webster, K. (2005). WAD impairment rating: Neck Disability Index score according to severity of MRI findings of ligaments and membranes in the upper cervical spine. *Journal of Neurotrauma, 4*, 466–475.

Kasch, H., Flemming, W., & Jensen, T. (2001). Handicap after acute whiplash injury. *Neurology, 56*, 1637–1643.

Kasch, H., Qerama, E., Bach, F., & Jensen, T. (2005). Reduced cold pressor pain tolerance in non-recovered whiplash patients: A 1 year prospective study. *European Journal of Pain, 9*(5), 561–569.

Kasch, H., Stengaard-Pedersen, K., Arendt-Nielsen, L., & Staehelin Jensen, T. (2001). Pain thresholds and tenderness in neck and head following acute whiplash injury: A prospective study. *Cephalalgia, 21*, 189–197.

Kivioja, J., Jensen, I., & Lindgren, U. (2005). Early coping strategies do not influence the prognosis after whiplash injuries. *Injury, 36*, 935–940.

Koelbaek-Johansen, M., Graven-Nielsen, T., Schou-Olesen, A., & Arendt-Nielsen, L. (1999). Muscular hyperalgesia and referred pain in chronic whiplash syndrome. *Pain*, *83*, 229–234.

Krakenes, J., Kaale, B., Moen, G., Nordli, H., Gilhus, N., & Rorvik, J. (2002). MRI assessment of the alar ligaments in the late stage of whiplash injury – a study of structural abnormalities and observer agreement. *Neuroradiology*, *44*(7), 617–624.

Krakenes, J., Kaale, B., Moen, G., Nordli, H., Gilhus, N., & Rorvik, J. (2003). MRI of the tectorial and posterior atlanto-occipital membranes in the late stage of whiplash injury. *Neuroradiology*, *44*(6), 637–644.

Kuch, K., Cox, B., Evans, R., & Shulman, I. (1994). Phobias, panic and pain in 55 survivors of road vehicle accidents. *Journal of Anxiety Disorders*, *8*(2), 181–187.

Linton, S. (2000). A review of psychological risk factors in back and neck pain. *Spine*, *25*(9), 1148–1156.

Lord, S., Barnsley, L., Wallis, B., & Bogduk, N. (1996). Chronic cervical zygapophysial joint pain after whiplash: A placebo-controlled prevalence study... including commentary by Derby R Jr. *Spine*, *21*(15), 1737–1745.

Lord, S., Barnsley, L., Wallis, B., McDonald, G., & Bogduk, N. (1996). Percutaneous radiofrequency neurotomy for chronic cervical zygapophyseal joint pain. *New England Journal of Medicine*, *335*(23), 1721–1726.

MAA. (2007). *Guidelines for the management of whiplash associated disorders*. Sydney: Motor accidents authority.

Malanga, G., & Peter, J. (2005). Whiplash Injuries. *Current Pain and Headache Reports*, *9*(5), 322–325.

McLean, S., Clauw, D., Abelson, J., & Liberzon, I. (2005). The development of persistent pain and psychological morbidity after motor vehicle collision: Intergrating the potential rle of stress response systems into a biopsychosocial model. *Psychosomatic Medicine*, *67*, 783–790.

McLean, S., Williams, D., & Clauw, D. (2005). Fibromyalgia after motor vehicle collision: Evidence and implications. *Traffic Injury Prevention*, *6*(2), 97–104.

Moog, M., Quintner, J., Hall, T., & Zusman, M. (2002). The late whiplash syndrome: A psychophysical study. *European Journal of Pain*, *6*(4), 283–294.

Nederhand, M., Hermens, H., Ijzerman, M., Groothuis, K., & Turk, D. (2006). The effect of fear of movement on mucle activation in posttraumatic neck pain disability. *Clinical Journal of Pain*, *22*(6), 519–525.

Nederhand, M., Hermens, H., Ijzerman, M., Turk, D., & Zilvold, G. (2002). Cervical muscle dysfunction in chronic whiplash associated disorder grade 2. The relevance of trauma. *Spine*, *27*(10), 1056–1061.

Nederhand, M., Ijzerman, M., Hermens, H., Turk, D., & Zilvold, G. (2004). Predictive value of fear avoidance in developing chronic neck pain disability: Consequences for clinical decision making. *Archives of Physical Medicine and Rehabilitation*, *85*, 496–501.

Oliveira, A., Gevirtz, R., & Hubbard, R. (2006). A psycho-educational video used in the emergency department provides effective treatment for whiplash injuries. *Spine*, *31*(15), 1652–1657.

Ottoson, C., Nyren, O., Johansson, S., & Ponzer, S. (2005). Outcome after minor taffic accidents: A follow-up study of orthopedic patients in an inner city area emergency room. *Journal of Trauma*, *58*, 553–560.

Passatore, M., & Roatta, S. (2006). Influence of sympathetic nervous system on sensorimotor function: Whiplash associated disorders (WAD) as a model. *European Journal of Applied Physiology*, *98*(5), 423–449.

Peebles, J., McWilliams, L., & MacLennan, R. (2001). A comparison of symptom checklist 90-revised profiles from patients with chronic pain from whiplash and patients with other musculoskeletal injuries. *Spine*, *26*(7), 766–770.

Pincus, T., Burton, A., Vogel, S., & Field, A. (2002). A systematic review of psychological factors as predictors of chronicity/disability in prospective cohorts of low bcak pain. *Spine*, *27*(5), E109–E120.

Provinciali, L., & Baroni, M. (1999). Clinical approaches to whiplash injuries: A review. *Critical Reviews in Physical and Rehabilitation Medicine, 11,* 339–368.

Provinciali, L., Baroni, M., Illuminati, L., & Ceravolo, M. (1996). Multimodal treatment to prevent the late whiplash syndrome. *Scandinavian Journal of Rehabilitation Medicine, 28*(2), 105–111.

Radanov, B., & Sturzenegger, M. (1996). Predicting recovery from common whiplash. *European Neurology, 36,* 48–51.

Radanov, B., Sturzenegger, M., & Di Stefano, G. (1995). Long-term outcome after whiplash injury. A 2-year follow-up considering features of injury mechanism and somatic, radiologic, and psychological findings. *Medicine, 74*(5), 281–297.

Rebbeck, T., Sindhausen, D., & Cameron, I. (2006). A prospective cohort study of health outcomes following whiplash associated disorders in an Australian population. *Injury Prevention, 12,* 86–93.

Ronnen, J., de Korte, P., & Brink, P. (1996). Acute whiplash injury: Is there a role for MR imaging. *Radiology, 201,* 93–96.

Rosenfeld, M., Gunnarsson, R., & Borenstein, P. (2000). Early intervention in whiplash-associated disorders. A comparison of two protocols. *Spine, 25,* 1782–1787.

Rosenfeld, M., Seferiadis, A., Carllson, J., & Gunnarsson, R. (2003). Active intervention in patients with whiplash associated disorders improves long-term prognosis: A randomised controlled clinical trial. *Spine, 28*(22), 2491–2498.

Rosenfeld, M., Seferiadis, A., & Gunnarsson, R. (2006). Active involvement and intervention in patients exposed to whiplash trauma in automobile crashes reduces costs. *Spine, 31*(16), 1799–1804.

Scholten-Peeters, G., Bekkering, G., Verhagen, A., van der Windt, D., Lanser, K., Hendriks, E., et al. (2002). Clinical practice guideline for the physiotherapy of patients with whiplash associated disorders. *Spine, 27*(4), 412–422.

Scholten-Peeters, G., Verhagen, A., Bekkering, G., van der Windt, D., Barnsley, L., Oostendorp, R., et al. (2003). Prognostic factors of Whiplash Associated Disorders: A systematic review of prospective cohort studies. *Pain, 104*(1–2), 303–322.

Scott, D., Jull, G., & Sterling, M. (2005). Sensory hypersensitivity is a feature of chronic whiplash associated disorders but not chronic idiopathic neck pain. *Clinical Journal of Pain, 21*(2), 175–181.

Sheather-Reid, R., & Cohen, M. (1998). Psychophysical evidence for a neuropathic component of chronic neck pain. *Pain, 75,* 341–347.

Shir, Y., Pereira, J., & Fitzcharles, M.-A. (2006). Whiplash and fibromyalgia: An ever widening gap. *The Journal of Rheumatology, 33,* 1045–1047.

Sizer, P., Poorbaugh, K., & Phelps, V. (2004). Whiplash associated disorders: Pathomechanics, diagnosis and management. *Pain Practice, 4*(3), 249–266.

Steinberg, E., Ovadia, D., Nissan, M., Menahem, A., & Dekel, S. (2005). Whiplash injury: Is there a role for electromyographic studies. *Archives of Orthopaedic Trauma Surgery, 125*(1), 46–50.

Stemper, B., Yoganandan, N., Rao, R., & Pintar, F. (2005). Influence of thoracic ramping on whiplash kinematics. *Clinical Biomechanics, 20,* 1019–1028.

Sterling, M. (2004). A proposed new classification system for whiplash associate disorders – implications for assessment and management. *Manual Therapy, 9*(2), 60–70.

Sterling, M. (2007). Whiplash injury pain: Basic science and current/future therapeutics. *Reviews in Analgesia, 9,* 105–116.

Sterling, M., Jull, G., & Kenardy, J. (2006). Physical and psychological predictors of outcome following whiplash injury maintain predictive capacity at long term follow-up. *Pain, 122,* 102–108.

Sterling, M., Jull, G., Vicenzino, B., & Kenardy, J. (2003). Sensory hypersensitivity occurs soon after whiplash injury and is associated with poor recovery. *Pain, 104,* 509–517.

Sterling, M., Jull, G., Vicenzino, B., & Kenardy, J. (2004). Characterisation of acute whiplash associated disorders. *Spine, 29*(2), 182–188.

Sterling, M., Jull, G., Vicenzino, B., Kenardy, J., & Darnell, R. (2005). Physical and psychological factors predict outcome following whiplash injury. *Pain, 114*, 141–148.

Sterling, M., Jull, G., Vizenzino, B., Kenardy, J., & Darnell, R. (2003). Development of motor system dysfunction following whiplash injury. *Pain, 103*, 65–73.

Sterling, M., Jull, G., & Wright, A. (2001). Cervical mobilisation: Concurrent effects on pain, sympathetic nervous system activity and motor activity. *Manual Therapy, 6*(2), 72–81.

Sterling, M., & Kenardy, J. (2006). The relationship between sensory and sympathetic nervous system changes and acute posttraumatic stress following whiplash injury – a prospective study. *Journal of Psychosomatic Research, 60*, 387–393.

Sterling, M., Kenardy, J., Jull, G., & Vicenzino, B. (2003). The development of psychological changes following whiplash injury. *Pain, 106*(3), 481–489.

Sterling, M., Pettiford, C., Hodkinson, E., & Curatolo, M. (2008). Psychological factors are related to some sensory pain thresholds but not nociceptive flexion reflex threshold in chronic whiplash. *24*, 124–130.

Sterling, M., Treleaven, J., Edwards, S., & Jull, G. (2002). Pressure pain thresholds in chronic whiplash associated disorder: Further evidence of altered central pain processing. *Journal of Musculoskeletal Pain, 10*(3), 69–81.

Sterling, M., Treleaven, J., & Jull, G. (2002). Responses to a clinical test of mechanical provocation of nerve tissue in whiplash associated disorders. *Manual Therapy, 7*(2), 89–94.

Sterner, Y., Toolanen, G., Gerdle, B., & Hildingson, C. (2003). The incidence of whiplash trauma and the effects of different factors on recovery. *Journal of Spinal Disorders, 16*, 195–199.

Sterner, Y., Toolanen, G., Knibestol, M., Gerdle, B., & Hildingsson, C. (2001). Prospective study of trigeminal sensibility after whiplash trauma. *Journal of Spinal Disorders, 14*(6), 479–486.

Stewart, M., Maher, C., Refshauge, K., Herbert, R., Bogduk, N., & Nicholas, M. (2007). Randomised controlled trial of exercise for chronic whiplash associated disorders. *Pain, 128*(1–2), 59–68.

Taylor, J., & Finch, P. (1993). Acute injury of the neck: Anatomical and pathological basis of pain. *Annals of the Academy of Medicine Singapore, 22*(2), 187–192.

Taylor, J., & Taylor, M. (1996). Cervical spinal injuries: An autopsy study of 109 blunt injuries. *Journal of Musculoskeletal Pain, 4*(4), 61–79.

Tishler, M., Levy, O., Maslakov, I., Bar-Chaim, S., & Amit-Vazina, M. (2006). Neck injury and fibromyalgia – are they really associated? *Journal of Rheumatology, 33*, 1183–1185.

Tjell, C., Tenenbaum, A., & Sandstrom, S. (2002). Smooth pursuit neck torsion test – a specific test for whiplash associated disorders. *Journal of Whiplash and Related Disorders, 1*(2), 9–24.

Treleaven, J., Jull, G., & LowChoy, N. (2005). Standing balance in persistent whiplash: A comparison between subjects with and without dizziness. *Journal of Rehabilitation Medicine, 37*, 224–229.

Treleaven, J., Jull, G., & LowChoy, N. (2005). Smooth pursuit neck torsion test in whiplash associated disorders: Relationship to self-eports of neck pain and disability, dizziness and anxiety. *Journal of Rehabilitation Medicine, 37*, 219–223.

Treleaven, J., Jull, G., & Sterling, M. (2003). Dizziness and unsteadiness following whiplash injury – characteristic features and relationship with cervical joint position error. *Journal of Rehabilitation, 34*, 18.

Uhrenholt, L., Grunnet-Nilsson, N., & Hartvigsen, J. (2002). Cervical spine lesions after road traffic accidents. A systematic review. *Spine, 27*(17), 1934–1941.

Verbunt, J., Seelen, H., Vlaeyen, J., Bousema, E., van der Heijden, G., Heuts, P., et al. (2005). Pain related factors contributing to muscle inhibition in patients with chronic low back pain. *Clinical Journal of Pain, 21*(3), 232–240.

Vierck, C. (2006). Mechanisms underlying development of spatially distributed chronic pain (fibromyalgia). *Pain, 124*, 242–263.

Vierck, C., Staud, R., Price, D., Cannon, R., Mauderli, A., & Martin, A. (2001). The effect of maximal exercise on temporal summation of second pain (windup) in patients with fibromyalgia syndrome. *The Journal of Pain, 2*(6), 334–344.

Vlaeyen, J., Kole-Snijders, A., & Boeren, R. (1995). Fear of movement/reinjury in chronic low back pain patients and its relation to behavioural performance. *Pain, 1995*(62), 363–372.

Vlaeyen, J., & Linton, S. (2000). Fear-avoidance and its consequences in chronic musculoskeletal pain: A state of the art. *Pain, 85,* 317–332.

Watson, P., Booker, C., & Main, C. (1997). Evidence for the role of psychological factors in abnormal paraspinal activity in patients with chronic low back pain. *Journal of Musculoskeletal Pain, 5*(4), 41–56.

Wenzel, H., Haug, T., Mykletun, A., & Dahl, A. (2002). A population study of anxiety and depression among persons who report whiplash traumas. *Journal of Psychosomatic Research, 53*(3), 831.

Woolf, C., & Mannion, R. (1999). Neuropathic pain: Aetiology, symptoms, mechanisms and management. *Lancet, 353,* 1959–1964.

Wynne-Jones, G., Macfarlane, G., Silman, A., & Jones, G. (2006). Does physical trauma lead to an increase in the risk of new onset widespread pain? *Annals of Rheumatic Disease, 65,* 391–393.

Yoganandan, N., Knowles, S., Maiman, D., & Pintar, F. (2003). Anatomic study of the morphology of the human cervical facet joint. *Spine, 28,* 2317–2323.

Yoganandan, N., Pintar, F., & Cusick, J. (2002). Biomechanical analyses of whiplash injuries using an experimental model. *Accident Analysis and Prevention, 34,* 663–671.

Gene Therapy for Chronic Pain

William R. Lariviere and Doris K. Cope

Abstract Gene therapy shows great potential to assist numerous patients with inadequate relief of inflammatory or neuropathic pain, or intractable pain associated with advanced cancer. A brief overview is provided of the methods of gene therapy and of preclinical findings in animal models of prolonged inflammatory, neuropathic and cancer pain. Preclinical findings demonstrate no efficacy of gene therapy on basal thermal nociception and mechanical sensitivity, and almost universal effects on pathological nociception and hypersensitivity models. The status of human trials is provided with recommendations for future directions and precautions. This early stage of development of gene therapy for chronic pain will likely be followed by an increased number of human clinical trials aimed specifically at the relief of chronic, unrelenting pain.

Introduction

Remarkable advances in the understanding of chronic pain have occurred over the past few decades since the beginning of the field of pain research and the recognition of chronic pain as a disease entity. However, many patients continue to suffer due to unresponsiveness to analgesic therapies and our still incomplete understanding of the basic underlying mechanisms of many chronic pain conditions including pain in advanced cancer and in chronic diseases such as autoimmune and neuropathic pain syndromes (Dworkin et al. 2003; Dray 2004). The inability to adequately relieve pain in these conditions often calls for higher doses of analgesics, leading to intolerable side effects for the patient. Thus, there is a continuing need for novel therapies with greater specificity for individual molecular targets and for specific pain-related tissues.

W.R. Lariviere (✉)
Assistant Professor, Department of Anesthesiology, University of Pittsburgh School of Medicine, A-1305 Scaife Hall, 3550 Terrace Street, Pittsburgh, PA 15261, USA
e-mail: lariwr@upmc.edu

R.J. Moore (ed.), *Biobehavioral Approaches to Pain*,
DOI 10.1007/978-0-387-78323-9_19, © Springer Science+Business Media, LLC 2009

Gene therapy, in which genetic material is introduced into the individual for therapeutic purposes, is a promising approach to provide a highly target- and tissue- specific treatment for chronic pain patients (Pohl and Braz 2001; Pohl et al. 2003; Glorioso et al. 2003; Meunier et al. 2004). This chapter will briefly review the various methods of introducing genetic material to highlight the strengths and weaknesses of the methods. Next, the universally successful preclinical studies of gene therapy in animal models of pain are reviewed with emphasis on the desirable specificity of effects that leave normal sensitivity intact, and the unexpected lack of specificity across pain models. Finally, the current status of clinical trials will be described demonstrating that, despite the profound need of severe pain sufferers, few trials of gene therapy for pain relief are actually in progress.

Methods of Gene Therapy

Gene therapy (or molecular therapy) for pain relief is the introduction of genetic material with the goal of decreasing signaling of noxious input to the central nervous system. This can be accomplished by introduction of genetic material to overexpress endogenous analgesic (or antinociceptive) or anti-inflammatory compounds, or to inhibit the transcription of nociceptive compounds released from nociceptive primary afferent neurons or glial cells that contribute to increased excitability of neighboring neurons. The desired result is decreased activity or excitability of spinal cord dorsal horn neurons that signal nociceptive input to higher central nervous system structures. (Pohl et al. 2003; Beutler et al. 2005; Hao et al. 2007; Mata and Fink 2007)

A number of methods of introduction of transgenic material are available (Weichselbaum and Kufe 1997; Smith 1999; Pohl and Braz 2001), each with differing levels of transgene insert capability, target cell selectivity and efficiency of gene transduction. These properties, in addition to the immunogenicity and toxicity of each method, render each method more or less suitable for the treatment of chronic pain.

Liposomes and Naked Plasmid DNA

Liposomes are positively charged lipid membranes that complex with DNA. The liposome-DNA complex fuses with negatively charged cell membranes and results in transfer of the DNA with therapeutic potential into the cells. Advantages of the method are that there is no immune response induced by liposomes and that there are a variety of liposomes available for gene transfer to a wide range of cell targets (but with relatively low target cell specificity) (Weichselbaum and Kufe 1997; Smith 1999; Pohl and Braz 2001). This method has shown to be useful for gene therapy targeting cancer cells, and improvements of the method continue to be made to increase target cell specificity (Shiota et al. 2007). However, due in part to the low gene transduction efficiency of the method often requiring microgram to milligram quantities (Goss 2007), there has been little interest in this method of gene transfer for pain relief.

Naked plasmid double stranded (ds) DNA (without viral vector components) can also be introduced without evoking an immunological response rendering *in vivo* use safe. However, *in vitro* transgene expression is variable in efficiency and duration (Weichselbaum and Kufe 1997). That said, even though the method can be limited by short term expression of transgenes and lower efficiency, gene gun injection of naked plasmid DNA has been shown to be effective in animal models of pain (Chuang et al. 2003, 2005).

Viral Vectors

Viral vectors including adenovirus, adeno-associated virus (AAV), retrovirus, and HSV vectors are much more commonly used for in vivo testing in animal models of pain. Systemic injection of recombinant viral vectors results in transduction seen mostly in hepatocytes (Wirtz and Neurath 2003). This requires vector delivery directly to the targeted or innervated tissue to achieve an efficient level of transduction.

Adenoviral Vectors

The adenovirus genome is a dsDNA, core-protein complex surrounded by a protein capsid. High-affinity binding of the adenovirus vector to the coxsackie/adenovirus receptor on the cell membrane is followed by endocytosis-mediated internalization and results in release of the viral vector into the nucleus where transcription and replication occur. For all viral vectors, genes necessary for normal viral replication must be removed (Glorioso et al. 2003). For adenovirus vectors, deletion of adenovirus E1 genes and replacement by non-viral genes renders the virus replication deficient while maintaining the ability to transduce an inserted transgene (Hao et al. 2007).

Adenovirus exhibits high efficiency for the infection of both dividing and non-dividing cells, unlike a ssRNA retrovirus vector that requires dividing cells. Adenoviral infection normally targets intestinal epithelial cells and the elderly and children may also develop respiratory infections (Wirtz and Neurath 2003). Adenoviral vectors show little cell specificity of infection and transduction, although some cell-type specificity can be induced with changes in viral coat proteins. Lumbosacral intrathecal (i.th.) injection of adenoviral vectors results in infection of predominantly meningeal cells surrounding the lower spinal cord

CSF space (Mannes et al. 1998). Accordingly, i.th. injection of adenoviral vectors has proven to be effective in reducing pain behaviors in animals (see Tables 2–3).

Adenoviral vectors induce antiviral cellular and humoral immune responses, representing the major limitation of the method. Infected cells can be detected and eliminated, and the high turnover of target cells (gut epithelium) leads to transient expression of only days to weeks (Gudmundsson et al. 1998). In addition, adenovirus induces proinflammatory factors (e.g., proinflammatory cytokines) that may increase nociceptive signaling and limit the therapeutic potential (Tsai et al. 2000, Castro et al. 2001). Removal of most, or all adenovirus protein coding genes to produce gutless adenovirus vectors can extend the transgene expression period, decrease proinflammatory responses and allow for larger packets of DNA to be inserted.

Adeno-Associated Virus and Lentivirus Vectors

Adeno-associated virus (AAV) vectors, harmless by themselves, do not stimulate inflammation or antibody production and can produce persistent transgene expression. With AAV infection of the sciatic nerve, for instance, small, medium and large afferent fiber types of the dorsal root ganglion have been shown to be effectively targeted (Gu et al. 2005). Retrovirus lentivirus vectors can also be used to transfect motor neurons of the spinal cord via retrograde axonal transport from muscle, but transfection of sensory neurons remains to be demonstrated. Despite persistent transgene expression with AAV vectors, the possible risks associated with integration of AAV and lentiviruses into the host genome will likely remain a drawback for clinical applications (Pohl et al. 2003; Yanez-Munoz et al. 2006).

Herpes Simplex Virus (HSV)-1

Of greatest potential for somatic chronic pain therapy is HSV vector-mediated gene therapy due to its target cell specificity, lack of integration in the host genome, large transgene insert capability, efficient transgene expression, and limited immunogenic and toxic effects (Mata et al. 2003; Berto et al. 2005; Goss 2007). Primary afferent neurons are the natural targets of HSV, allowing this method to target cells that may be affected by a peripheral source of nociception, or by nerve injury in addition to targeting their central terminals in the spinal cord dorsal horn. Following a simple subcutaneous injection, the dsDNA HSV vector infects epithelial cells (or neurons directly), goes through several cycles of replication and penetrates the peripheral afferent nerve terminals. The HSV vector is retrogradely transported to afferent nerve cell bodies in sensory dorsal root ganglia, and remains as chromatin structure without integration into the host genome. In one study, one to two hundred neurons per animal were labeled as HSV vector-infected for at least two weeks, with 10–20% remaining at four to six weeks (Wilson and Yeomans 2002). The LAT promoter, particularly active in neurons, can produce efficient transgene expression of neuroactive peptides that become incorporated into large dense-core vesicles and released into the synapse. Over 30 kb of foreign DNA, or three to four times that which can be inserted in the adenovirus vector, can be inserted in recombinant HSV vectors. The target cell specificity, the possibility of introducing several synergistic transgenes, the simple mode of administration and limited side effects make the HSV vector particularly suited to the gene therapy of chronic pain.

Preclinical Studies of Gene Therapy

Transgenes have been delivered by naked plasmid DNA, naked RNA, adenovirus, AAV, and HSV vector systems to reduce nociception in animals (see Tables 1–3). Both the over-expression of genes whose products are analgesic, including enkephalins, and the inhibition of genes whose products are nociceptive, including calcitonin gene-related peptide (CGRP), have been studied (Glorioso et al. 2003; Pohl et al. 2003; Kurreck 2004). Effective gene therapy has also targeted non-neuronal cells such as astrocytes and microglia, which are now known to modulate spinal cord neuron activity, including by the introduction of interleukin-10 (IL-10) genes whose products act on glial cell receptors not found on spinal cord neurons (see Tables 1–3) (Milligan et al. 2005a,b).

Basal Nociceptive and Mechanical Sensitivity

An ideal pain therapy should reduce spontaneous pain, or evoked hypersensitivity of a pathological origin, but leave normal, nonpathological sensitivity to stimuli intact. Almost all studies have shown that gene therapy, while universally exhibiting antinociceptive, anti-hyperalgesic, or anti-allodynic effects, does not affect basal mechanical sensitivity to von Frey monofilaments, or thermal nociception from radiant heat focused on the hind paw of the rat (see Table 1) (Finegold et al. 1999; Wilson et al. 1999; Lu et al. 2002; Yao et al. 2003; Gu et al. 2005; Milligan et al. 2005a,b; Tan et al. 2005). Only one exception without any clear explanation has been reported: i.th. adenovirus vector delivery of interleukin-2 (IL-2) produced significant thermal antinociception for up to three weeks (Yao et al. 2003). It is most likely that the particular transgene is responsible for the effect since i.th. delivery of transgenes for β-endorphin and IL-10 via adenovirus vector does not affect

Table 1 Effect of gene therapy on basal thermal nociception and mechanical sensitivity in rodents

Study	Vector	Administration site	Transgene	Pain model	Result
Finegold et al. 1999	Adenovirus	Intrathecal	β-endorphin	Radiant heat to hind paw	No effect
Gu et al. 2005	AAV	Sciatic nerve	μ-opioid receptor	Radiant heat to hind paw	No effect
Lu et al. 2002	Plasmid DNA	Plantar hind paw	Proopio-melanocortin	Radiant heat to hind paw	No effect
Milligan et al. 2005a,b	Adenovirus	Intrathecal	Interleukin-10	Radiant heat, Von Frey monofilaments to hind paw	No effect
Tan et al. 2005	Naked RNA	Intrathecal	NMDA receptor NR2B subunit siRNA	Radiant heat to hind paw	No effect
Wilson et al. 1999	HSV	Hind paw	Proenkephalin A	Radiant heat to hind paw	No effect
Yao et al. 2003	Adenovirus	Intrathecal	Interleukin-2	Radiant heat to hind paw	Antinociception

Table 2 Effect of gene therapy on inflammatory nociception and hypersensitivity in rodents

Study	Vector	Administration site	Transgene	Pain model	Result
Braz et al. 2001	HSV	Plantar hind paw	Proenkephalin A	Adjuvant-induced polyarthritis, thermal hyperalgesia	Decreased hyperalgesia
Chuang et al. 2005	Plasmid DNA	Bladder wall	Preproenkephalin	Capsaicin-induced bladder irritation, intercontraction interval	Reduction of capsaicin-induced decrease of interval
Finegold et al. 1999	Adenovirus	Intrathecal	β-endorphin	Subcutaneous carrageenan to hind paw, thermal hyperalgesia	Decreased hyperalgesia
Garry et al. 2000	Naked DNA	Intrathecal	NMDA-R1 artisense oligonucleotides	Subcutaneous formalin to hind paw	Antinociception
Goss et al. 2001	HSV	Hind paw	Proenkephalin	Subcutaneous formalin to hind paw	Antinociception
Gu et al. 2005	AAV	Sciatic nerve	μ-opioid receptor	Adjuvant-induced monoarthritis, thermal hyperalgesia	No effect
Kang et al. 1998	HSV	Bilateral amygdalae	Proenkephalin	Subcutaneous formalin to hind paw	Antinociception
Lu et al. 2002	Plasmid DNA	Plantar hind paw	Proopio-melanocortin	Subcutaneous formalin to hind paw	Antinociception

Table 2 (continued)

Study	Vector	Administration site	Transgene	Pain model	Result
Milligan et al. 2005a,b	Adenovirus	Intrathecal	Interleukin-10	Peri-sciatic zymosan; Intrathecal HIV-1 gp120, mechanical allodynia	Decreased allodynia
Tan et al. 2005	Naked RNA	Intrathecal	NMDA receptor NR2B subunit siRNA	Subcutaneous formalin to hind paw	Antinociception
Wilson et al. 1999	HSV	Hind paw	Proenkephalin A	DMSO; capsaicin, thermal hyperalgesia	Decreased hyperalgesia
Wilson and Yeomans 2002	HSV	Hind paw	CGRP antisense	Capsaicin to hind paw skin, thermal hyperalgesia	Decreased hyperalgesia
Yao et al. 2002b	Plasmid DNA	Intrathecal; hind paw	Interleukin-2	Subcutaneous carrageenan to hind paw, thermal hyperalgesia	Decreased hyperalgesia

Table 3 Effect of gene therapy on neuropathic pain hypersensitivity models in rodents

Study	Vector	Administration site	Transgene	Pain model	Result
Eaton et al. 2002	AAV	Spinal cord dorsal horn	Brain-derived neurotrophic factor	Chronic constriction of sciatic nerve, thermal and mechanical hyperalgesia, mechanical allodynia	Decreased hyperalgesia and allodynia
Hao et al. 2003b	HSV	Plantar hind paw	Glial cell-derived neurotrophic factor	L5 spinal nerve ligation, mechanical allodynia	Decreased allodynia
Hao et al. 2003a	HSV	Plantar hind paw	Proenkephalin	L5 spinal nerve ligation, mechanical allodynia	Decreased allodynia
Hao et al. 2005	HSV	Plantar hind paw	Glutamic acid decarboxylase	L5 sciatic nerve ligation, thermal hyperalgesia, mechanical allodynia	Decreased hyperalgesia and allodynia
Lin et al. 2002	Naked DNA	Intrathecal	Proopio-melanocortin	Chronic constriction of common sciatic, thermal hyperalgesia	Decreased hyperalgesia
Liu et al. 2004	HSV	Plantar hind paw	Glutamic acid decarboxylase	T13 spinal cord hemisection; mechanical allodynia	Decreased allodynia
Meunier et al. 2005	HSV	Vibrissal pad territory	Preproenkephalin A	Chronic constriction of left infraorbital nerve, mechanical responsiveness	Decreased mechanical hyper-responsiveness
Milligan et al. 2005a, b	Adenovirus	Intrathecal	Interleukin-10	Chronic constriction of sciatic nerve, thermal hyperalgesia, mechanical allodynia	Decreased hyperalgesia and allodynia

Table 3 (continued)

Study	Vector	Administration site	Transgene	Pain model	Result
Pradat et al. 2001b	Adenovirus	Skeletal muscle	Neurotrophin-3	Streptozotocin diabetic peripheral neuropathy, acrylamide intoxication	Decreased hyperalgesia
Yao et al. 2002a	Plasmid DNA	Intrathecal	Interleukin-2	Chronic constriction of sciatic nerve; thermal hyperalgesia	Decreased hyperalgesia
Yao et al. 2003	Adenovirus	Intrathecal	Interleukin-2	Chronic constriction of sciatic nerve; thermal hyperalgesia	Decreased hyperalgesia
Yeomans et al. 2004	HSV	Dorsal hind paw	Preproenkephalin	Intrathecal pertussis toxin; thermal hyperalgesia	Decreased hyperalgesia

thermal nociception assessed similarly. At this time, however, it is still not known why IL-2 would have this effect.

Inflammatory Nociception and Hypersensitivity

Several studies have shown significant effects of gene therapy on inflammatory nociception and hypersensitivity in the rat or mouse (see Table 2). Inflammatory nociception models are most commonly characterized by subcutaneous injection of an inflammatory irritant such as formalin in the plantar hind paw, evoking spontaneous nociceptive behaviors of paw licking, shaking and elevation. HSV vector delivery of pEnkA to the hind paw or amygdala of the rat and gene gun administration of plasmid POMC gene DNA to the hind paw all produce significant antinociceptive effects in the intraplantar formalin test. Reinoculation with the vector-mediated transgene can reinstate effectiveness after transgene expression and significant antinociceptive effects have diminished (Goss et al. 2001).

In models of inflammatory hypersensitivity, an inflammatory irritant is most commonly injected subcutaneously in the hind paw evoking hypersensitivity to mechanical and noxious thermal stimuli. When the hypersensitivity causes a previously non-noxious stimulus to become nociceptive, it is referred to as allodynia; when the hypersensitivity causes greater sensitivity to a previously noxious stimulus, it is referred to as hyperalgesia. In inflammatory hypersensitivity models, including those shown to be genetically distinct from the formalin test (Lariviere et al. 2002), peripheral subcutaneous delivery of HSV vector encoding pEnkA produces significant inhibition of thermal hyperalgesia in the hind paw induced by injection of capsaicin, DMSO, and complete-Freund's adjuvant (Wilson et al. 1999; Braz et al. 2001). Similarly, gene gun delivery of plasmid DNA of pEnkA to the bladder wall is effective in the visceral pain model of capsaicin-induced bladder hyperactivity (Chuang et al. 2005). For instance, HSV vector delivery of CGRP antisense oligonucleotides that block transcription of CGRP decreases swelling in the complete Freund's adjuvant-induced rheumatoid arthritis model (Pohl and Braz 2001) and decreases capsaicin-induced thermal hyperalgesia with direct application to lumbar primary sensory neurons (Wilson and Yeomans 2002). For example, cytokine directed gene therapy has also been shown to be effective. Plasmid delivery of IL-2 or adenovirus vector containing β-endorphin reduces subcutaneous carrageenan-induced thermal hyperalgesia, and spinal cord intrathecal injection of adenovirus vector containing IL-10 is effective against prolonged inflammatory hypersensitivity models, despite the pro-inflammatory effect of adenovirus administration (Yao et al. 2002b; Milligan et al. 2005a,b).

Neuropathic Pain Models of Allodynia and Hyperalgesia

Gene therapy is also effective in animal models of neuropathic pain (see Table 3) (Hao et al. 2006; Goss 2007). Vector mediated introduction of trans-genes for proenkephalins, POMC, IL-10, and IL-2 has been shown to be effective against the mechanical allodynia and thermal hyperalgesia induced in several rodent neuropathic pain models including chronic constriction injury (CCI) of the sciatic nerve or infraorbital nerve, tight ligation of the fifth lumbar nerve distal to the dorsal root ganglion, and intrathecal pertussis toxin injection (see Table 3) (Lin et al. 2002; Yao et al. 2002a, 2003; Hao et al. 2003a; Yeomans et al. 2004; Meunier et al. 2005; Milligan et al. 2005a,b). Gene therapy to increase the expression of neurotrophic factors with known roles in neuropathic pain models is also effective. Vector mediated increases in expression of neuro-trophin-3, glial cell-derived and brain-derived neurotrophic factors (GDNF and BDNF) has been shown to effectively decrease hypersensitivity evoked by spinal nerve ligation, CCI, and the acrylamide intoxication diabetic neuropathy model for up to eight weeks (Pradat et al. 2001a,b, 2002; Eaton et al. 2002; Hao et al. 2003a). Studies which target the role of GABA in neuropathic pain models, HSV vector mediated gene therapy to overexpress glutamic acid dec-arboxylase has also proven effective, whereas attempts to increase GABA expression have fallen short of successful (Glorioso and Fink 2004; Liu et al. 2004; Hao et al. 2005). As for the inflammatory nociception models, the dura-tion of effect ranges widely from less than a week to eight weeks, with reinstate-ment of effects after reinoculation (Hao et al. 2003a,b; Liu et al. 2004).

Cancer Pain Models

One study has shown that inoculation with the pEnkA-encoding HSV vector produces significant antinociception mediated by opioid receptors in the spinal cord in a rodent femoral bone cancer pain model (Goss et al. 2002).

Specificity of Effects of Preclinical Studies

Gene therapies which target pronociceptive and antinociceptive compounds are unequivocally effective, and in animal models, generally without effect on normal sensation assessed with mechanical and thermal stimuli. Further speci-ficity of effect has been observed in the formalin inflammatory nociception model. In the formalin test, a dilute solution of formaldehyde is injected sub-cutaneously in the hind paw evoking a biphasic response of spontaneous nociceptive behaviors of paw licking, lifting and shaking (Dubuisson and Dennis 1977). HSV vector delivery of pEnkA to the hind paw or amygdala of the rat, gene gun administration of plasmid POMC gene DNA, and knockdown of NMDA receptors with intrathecal administration of antisense NMDA-R1 oligonucleotides or siRNA to the NR2B subunit all have significant antinociceptive effects only in the second phase of the biphasic formalin pain response. (Kang et al. 1998; Garry et al. 2000; Goss et al. 2001; Lu et al. 2002; Tan et al. 2005). The second phase of the formalin response is considered the 'inflammatory' phase and has been associated with hyperalgesia. This is in contrast to the first phase that is considered due to the direct action of formalin on peripheral afferent fibers and shows pharmacological sensitivity more like that of brief thermal nociception assays than the second phase of the formalin response. Gene therapy results are consistent with other pharmacological findings in this respect.

However, the lack of specificity of effect across types of pain model is unexpected. Models of inflammatory and neuropathic mechanical allodynia and thermal hyperalgesia, for instance, are genetically distinct from the formalin test of inflammatory nociception and from each other (Lariviere et al. 2002). Neuropathic pain differs in clinical presentation, mechanisms and treatments from somatic and visceral pain. As a consequence, it is unexpected that vector-mediated introduction of the same transgenes of proenkephalins, POMC, IL-10, and IL-2 are effective against the nociception and hypersensitivity induced in all of the inflammatory, neuropathic, and cancer pain models examined. It is also unlikely that this single treatment modality with a single transgene will be effective against all types of human chronic pain, since no other existing treatment has this ability. Indeed, additional data on the specificity of effects is needed for the judicious application of this treatment method to specific chronic pain conditions.

Human Clinical Trials

Specificity of effects notwithstanding, the ever-increasing literature reporting almost universal success of gene therapy in rodent pain models indicates that more clinical trials are warranted. In favor of proceeding, significant effects have been shown to be due to increased transgene expression in the appropriate tissue space, and to be blocked by antagonists of the receptors at which the transgene product acts (e.g. Goss et al. 2001). The duration of transgene expression and effect ranges from seven days up to fourteen weeks, even several months, and can be reinstated by reinoculation (Goss 2007). Furthermore, studies in animal models have also demonstrated a lack of adverse effects, and issues regarding replication of viral DNA and oncogenic transformation are not of primary concern, although large-scale clinical trials in human patients have not yet been performed to assess and evaluate the long-term risk.

According to the *Journal of Gene Medicine*, there were 1,309 active clinical gene therapy trials with 2.4% in Phase III (n = 32) as of July 2007 (http://www.abedia.com/wiley/indications.php). The vast majority were trials of cancer therapies (n = 861; 66.5%).A combination of monogenetic, vascular, and infectious diseases, (n = 313) comprised 24% of all clinical trials. The majority of these studies are being conducted in North America (67%) and Europe (27%). The most common vectors currently being used in these clinical trials are adenovirus and adeno-associated virus vectors (28.6%) followed by lipofection (7.8%) and herpes simplex virus vectors (3.3%).Other vectors being trialed in human studies comprise approximately 2% of current studies, including the following vectors: adenovirus + retrovirus; flavivirus; gene gun; lentivirus; listeria monocytogenes; and measles virus. (http://www.abedia.com/wiley/indications.php)

Gene therapies are also moving from the laboratory to Phase I/II clinical trials primarily in the area of localized cancer pain. Clinical trials with isolated vertebral metastases are in the planning stage. In contrast to the specific cell targets of herpes simplex viral vectors, intrathecal delivery of adeno-associated virus vectors can potentially deliver the transgene to multiple sites in the spinal canal (Touitou et al. 2004). In an early study in humans, intraprostatically-injected adenovirus that delivered suicide genes to sensitize malignant cells to radiation and chemotherapy in sixteen patients with local recurrent prostate cancer (Freytag et al. 2002). There was a response or partial response in over half of the patients and there were no treatment-related serious adverse effects. This early success was followed by further successful Phase I and Phase I/II clinical trials and led to the conclusion that this treatment modality may become part of prostate cancer management (Freytag et al. 2007).

Despite success of the method, caution is still required in considering the widespread use of gene therapy. For example, one increasingly common application of gene therapy uses naked plasma DNA encoding for vascular endothelial growth factor-2 (VEGF-2) to increase myocardial blood flow reducing myocardial ischemia and angina. Unfortunately, in one patient, VEGF-2 DNA injected via a thoracotomy into ischemic myocardium resulted in immediate death. A later study from the same group (Reilly et al. 2005) noted significant reduction in pain and angina class for two years post treatment with further outcome data pending completion of a large, proposed phase III trial. Other rare cases of unexpected serious and fatal adverse effects of gene therapy indicate that the benefits and risks of the therapy need to be weighed carefully, screening trial participants for those who may benefit the most and for co-morbid immunological events that may contribute to adverse reactions (Hughes 2007). Non-replicating HSV vectors have been shown to produce high titers of missing gene products in rodent models of brain tumors, Parkinsonism, and spinal root and spinal cord injuries (Glorioso and Fink 2004). These vectors can be produced in pure preparations to high titers with low immunogenicity and toxicity and thus may be more appropriate for clinical trials in human patients.

One interesting approach would be to identify combinations of specific genetic mutations in a disease state such as autoinflammatory disorders and to tailor therapy appropriately. An example is classifying autoimmune disorders such as Crohn's disease and hereditary periodic fevers by constellations of causation genes rather than prescribing treatment based on physiological symptoms, which frequently overlap. Pain is also a common response to many different syndromes and types of pain as well as underlying disorders can vary widely. Genetic screening may not only help diagnose a disorder but also direct gene therapy to rationally treat the specific mutations. In this same manner patients with various pain syndromes may be genotyped in the future for greater specificity in both diagnosis and treatment.

Conclusions

The potential of emerging gene therapies as an effective treatment for human chronic pain is supported by the numerous preclinical studies. The available results from rodent studies of gene therapy for prolonged pain show that gene therapy is unequivocally effective with little dependence on the test used to assess effects, regardless of the etiological mechanisms, and regardless of whether trigeminal or lower spinal somatic or visceral systems are targeted. This pattern may be due to an early bias to publish positive results as is commonly seen for emerging methods. Based on the current review of the preclinical studies, it is recommended that future studies simultaneously examine the effect of a particular transgene and vector system on several pain model types (e.g. inflammatory versus neuropathic pain). This can be achieved by determining the effective dose ranges for the particular treatment across several pain models in the same study. With such data, indications and contraindications that still remain to be determined will be better understood prior to moving toward widespread clinical application.

Since the vast majority of human clinical trials have been used to treat recognizable disease states, trials for the treatment of chronic pain have been sparse, in part due to the inaccurate consideration of pain as secondary to the underlying disease. Pain should be also considered as a primary disease with mechanisms that can become independent of an underlying disease due to sensitization of central and peripheral nervous system mechanisms (Woolf and Salter 2000). In other words, the effects of gene therapy on pain outcomes can occur independently of effects on the injury or pathology of the affected tissue. Thus, targeting both the pathology and pain mechanisms may represent a critical approach. For this reason, the use of HSV vectors, in which several transgenes can be inserted to act synergistically, is an especially promising future direction of research and human clinical trials.

Improvement of vector systems is continuously under investigation, including enhancement of target cell selectivity, reduction of inflammatory and toxic responses, and increasing the efficiency and duration of transgene expression (Smith 1999; Noureddini et al. 2006). For instance, transduction promoters are being varied to increase expression while minimizing toxicity. Moreover, although severe adverse reactions to gene therapy in clinical trials have been rare, careful screening of trial participants for immunological conditions that may provoke adverse reactions is essential. In addition, careful selection of patients with the greatest need of treatment of specific types of refractory pain will ensure the safety and success of what promises to be a highly effective treatment modality for future generations.

References

Berto, E., Bozac, A. and Marconi, P. (2005) Development and application of replication-incompetent HSV-1-based vectors. *Gene Ther* 12, S98–S102

Beutler, A.S., Banck, M.S., Walsh, C.E. and Milligan, E.D. (2005) Intrathecal gene transfer by adeno-associated virus for pain. *Curr Opin Mol Ther* 7, 431–439

Braz, J., Beaufour, C., Coutaux, A., Epstein, A.L., Cesselin, F., Hamon, M. and Pohl, M. (2001) Therapeutic efficacy in experimental polyarthritis of viral-driven enkephalin over-production in sensory neurons. *J Neurosci* 21, 7881–7888

Castro, M., Hurtado-Lorenzo, A., Umana, P., Smith-Arica, J.R., Zermansky, A., Abordo-Adesida, E. and Lowenstein, P.R. (2001) Regulatable and cell-type specific transgene expression in glial cells: prospects for gene therapy for neurological disorders. *Prog Brain Res* 132, 655–681

Chuang, Y.C., Chou, A.K., Wu, P.C., Chiang, P.H., Yu, T.J., Yang, L.C., Yoshimura, N. and Chancellor, M.B. (2003) Gene therapy for bladder pain with gene gun particle encoding pro-opiomelanocortin cDNA. *J Urol* 170, 2044–2048

Chuang, Y.C., Yang, L.C., Chiang, P.H., Kang, H.Y., Ma, W.L., Wu, P.C., DeMiguel, F., Chancellor, M.B. and Yoshimura, N. (2005) Gene gun particle encoding preproenkephalin cDNA produces analgesia against capsaicin-induced bladder pain in rats. *Urology* 65, 804–810

Dray, A. (2004) Future pharmacologic management of neuropathic pain. *J Orofac Pain* 18, 381–385

Dubuisson, D. and Dennis, S.G. (1977) The formalin test: a quantitative study of the analgesic effects of morphine, meperidine, and brain stem stimulation in rats and cats. *Pain* 4, 161–174

Dworkin, R.H., Backonja, M., Rowbotham, M.C., Allen, R.R., Argoff, C.R., Bennett, G.J., Bushnell, M.C., Farrar, J.T., Galer, B.S., Haythornthwaite, J.A., Hewitt, D.J., Loeser, J.D., Max, M.B., Saltarelli, M., Schmader, K.E., Stein, C., Thompson, D., Turk, D.C., Wallace, M.S., Watkins, L.R. and Weinstein, S.M. (2003) Advances in neuropathic pain: diagnosis, mechanisms, and treatment recommendations. *Arch Neurol* 60, 1524–1534

Eaton, M.J., Blits, B., Ruitenberg, M.J., Verhaagen, J. and Oudega, M. (2002) Amelioration of chronic neuropathic pain after partial nerve injury by adeno-associated viral (AAV) vector-mediated over-expression of BDNF in the rat spinal cord. *Gene Ther* 9, 1387–1395

Finegold, A.A., Mannes, A.J. and Iadarola, M.J. (1999) A paracrine paradigm for in vivo gene therapy in the central nervous system: treatment of chronic pain. *Hum Gene Ther* 10, 1251–1257

Freytag, S.O., Khil, M. Stricker, H., Peabody, J., Menon, M., DePeralta-Venturina, M., Nafziger, D., Pegg, J., Paielli, D., Brown, S., Barton, K., Lu, M., Aguilar-Cordova, E. and Kim, J.H. (2002) Phase I study of replication-competent adenovirus-mediated double suicide gene therapy for the treatment of locally recurrent prostate cancer. *Cancer Res* 62, 4968–4976

Freytag, S.O., Stricker, H., Movsas, B. and Kim, J.H. (2007) Prostate cancer gene therapy clinical trials. *Mol Ther* 15, 1042–1052

Garry, M.G., Malik, S., Yu, J., Davis, M.A. and Yang, J. (2000) Knock down of spinal NMDA receptors reduces NMDA and formalin evoked behaviors in rat. *Neuroreport* 11, 49–55

Glorioso, J.C. and Fink, D.J. (2004) Herpes vector-mediated gene transfer in treatment of diseases of the nervous system. *Annu Rev Microbiol* 58, 253–271.

Glorioso, J.C., Mata, M. and Fink, D.J. (2003) Gene therapy for chronic pain. *Curr Opin Mol Ther* 5, 483–488

Goss, J.R. (2007) The therapeutic potential of gene transfer for the treatment of peripheral neuropathies. *Expert Rev Mol Med* 9, 1–20

Goss, J.R., Harley, C.F., Mata, M., O'Malley, M.E., Goins, W.F., Hu, X., Glorioso, J.C. and Fink, D.J. (2002) Herpes vector-mediated expression of proenkephalin reduces bone cancer pain. *Ann Neurol* 52, 662–665

Goss, J.R., Mata, M., Goins, W.F., Wu, H.H., Glorioso, J.C. and Fink, D.J. (2001) Antinociceptive effect of a genomic herpes simplex virus-based vector expressing human proenkephalin in rat dorsal root ganglion. *Gene Ther* 8, 551–556

Gu, Y., Xu, Y., Li, G.W. and Huang, L.Y. (2005) Remote nerve injection of mu opioid receptor adeno-associated viral vector increases antinociception of intrathecal morphine. *J Pain* 6, 447–454

Gudmundsson, G., Bosch, A., Davidson, B.L., Berg, D.J. and Hunninghake, G.W. (1998) Interleukin-10 modulates the severity of hypersensitivity pneumonitis in mice. *Am J Respir Cell Mol Biol* 19, 812–818

Hao, S., Mata, M., Fink, D.J. (2007) Viral vector-based gene transfer for treatment of chronic pain. *Int Anesthesiol Clin* 45, 59–71

Hao, S., Mata, M., Glorioso, J.C. and Fink, D.J. (2006) HSV-mediated expression of interleukin-4 in dorsal root ganglion neurons reduces neuropathic pain. *Mol Pain* 2, 6

Hao, S., Mata, M., Goins, W., Glorioso, J.C. and Fink, D.J. (2003a) Transgene-mediated enkephalin release enhances the effect of morphine and evades tolerance to produce a sustained antiallodynic effect in neuropathic pain. *Pain* 102, 135–142

Hao, S., Mata, M., Wolfe, D., Huang, S., Glorioso, J.C. and Fink, D.J. (2003b) HSV-mediated gene transfer of the glial cell-derived neurotrophic factor provides an antiallodynic effect on neuropathic pain. *Mol Ther* 8, 367–375

Hao, S., Mata, M., Wolfe, D., Huang, S., Glorioso, J.C. and Fink, D.J. (2005) Gene transfer of glutamic acid decarboxylase reduces neuropathic pain. *Ann Neurol* 57, 914–918

Hughes, V. (2007) Therapy on trial. *Nature Med* 13, 1008–1009

Kang, W., Wilson, M.A., Bender, M.A., Glorioso, J.C. and Wilson, S.P. (1998) Herpes virus-mediated preproenkephalin gene transfer to the amygdala is antinociceptive. *Brain Res* 792, 133–135

Kurreck, J. (2004) Antisense and RNA interference approaches to target validation in pain research. *Curr Opin Drug Discov Devel* 7, 179–187

Lariviere, W.R., Wilson, S.G., Laughlin, T.M., Kokayeff, A., West, E.E., Adhikari, S.M., Wan, Y. and Mogil, J.S. (2002) Heritability of nociception. III. Genetic relationships among commonly used assays of nociception and hypersensitivity. *Pain* 97, 75–86

Lin, C.R., Yang, L.C., Lee, T.H., Lee, C.T., Huang, H.T., Sun, W.Z. and Cheng, J.T. (2002) Electroporation-mediated pain-killer gene therapy for mononeuropathic rats. *Gene Ther* 9, 1247–1253

Liu, J., Wolfe, D., Hao, S., Huang, S., Glorioso, J.C., Mata, M. and Fink, D.J. (2004) Peripherally delivered glutamic acid decarboxylase gene therapy for spinal cord injury pain. *Mol Ther* 10, 57–66

Lu, C.Y., Chou, A.K., Wu, C.L., Yang, C.H., Chen, J.T., Wu, P.C., Lin, S.H., Muhammad, R. and Yang, L.C. (2002) Gene-gun particle with pro-opiomelanocortin cDNA produces analgesia against formalin-induced pain in rats. *Gene Ther* 9, 1008–1014

Mata, M. and Fink, D.J. (2007) Gene therapy for pain. *Anesthesiology* 106, 1079–1080

Mata, M., Glorioso, J. and Fink, D.J. (2003) Development of HSV-mediated gene transfer for the treatment of chronic pain. *Exp Neurol* 184 Suppl 1, S25–29

Mannes, A.J., Caudle, R.M., O'Connell, B.C. and Iadarola, M.J. (1998) Adenoviral gene transfer to spinal-cord neurons: intrathecal vs. intraparenchymal administration. *Brain Res* 793, 1–6

Meunier, A., Braz, J., Cesselin, F., Hamon, M. and Pohl, M. (2004) [From inflammation to pain: experimental gene therapy]. *Med Sci (Paris)* 20, 325–330

Meunier, A., Latremoliere, A., Mauborgne, A., Bourgoin, S., Kayser, V., Cesselin, F., Hamon, M. and Pohl, M. (2005) Attenuation of pain-related behavior in a rat model of trigeminal neuropathic pain by viral-driven enkephalin overproduction in trigeminal ganglion neurons. *Mol Ther* 11, 608–616

Milligan, E.D., Langer, S.J., Sloane, E.M., He, L., Wieseler-Frank, J., O'Connor, K., Martin, D., Forsayeth, J.R., Maier, S.F., Johnson, K., Chavez, R.A., Leinwand, L.A. and Watkins, L.R. (2005a) Controlling pathological pain by adenovirally driven spinal production of the anti-inflammatory cytokine, interleukin-10. *Eur J Neurosci* 21, 2136–2148

Milligan, E.D., Sloane, E.M., Langer, S.J., Cruz, P.E., Chacur, M., Spataro, L., Wieseler-Frank, J., Hammack, S.E., Maier, S.F., Flotte, T.R., Forsayeth, J.R., Leinwand, L.A., Chavez, R. and Watkins, L.R. (2005b) Controlling neuropathic pain by adeno-associated virus driven production of the anti-inflammatory cytokine, interleukin-10. *Mol Pain* 1, 9

Noureddini, S.C., Krendelshchikov, A., Simonenko, V., Hedley, S.J., Douglas, J.T., Curiel, D.T. and Korokhov, N. (2006) Generation and selection of targeted adenoviruses embodying optimized vector properties. *Virus Res* 116, 185–195

Pohl, M. and Braz, J. (2001) Gene therapy of pain: emerging strategies and future directions. *Eur J Pharmacol* 429, 39–48

Pohl, M., Meunier, A., Hamon, M. and Braz, J. (2003) Gene therapy of chronic pain. *Curr Gene Ther* 3, 223–238

Pradat, P.F., Finiels, F., Kennel, P., Naimi, S., Orsini, C., Delaere, P., Revah, F. and Mallet, J. (2001a) Partial prevention of cisplatin-induced neuropathy by electroporation-mediated nonviral gene transfer. *Hum Gene Ther* 12, 367–375

Pradat, P.F., Kennel, P., Naimi-Sadaoui, S., Finiels, F., Orsini, C., Revah, F., Delaere, P. and Mallet, J. (2001b) Continuous delivery of neurotrophin 3 by gene therapy has a neuro-protective effect in experimental models of diabetic and acrylamide neuropathies. *Hum Gene Ther* 12, 2237–2249

Pradat, P.F., Kennel, P., Naimi-Sadaoui, S., Finiels, F., Scherman, D., Orsini, C., Delaere, P., Mallet, J. and Revah, F. (2002) Viral and non-viral gene therapy partially prevents experimental cisplatin-induced neuropathy. *Gene Ther* 9, 1333–1337

Reilly, J.P., Grise, M.A., Fortuin, F.D., Vale, P.R., Schaer, G.L., Lopez, J., Van Camp, J.R., Henry, T., Richenbacher, W.E., Losordo, D.W., Schatz, R.A. and Isner, J.M. (2005) Long-term (2-year) clinical events following transthoracic intramyocardial gene transfer of VEGF-2 in no-option patients. *J Interven Cardiol* 18, 27–31

Shiota, M., Ikeda, Y., Kaul, Z., Itadani, J., Kaul, S.C. and Wadhwa, R. (2007) Internalizing antibody-based targeted gene delivery for human cancer cells. *Hum Gene Ther* 18, 1153–1160

Smith, A.E. (1999) Gene therapy – where are we? *Lancet* 354 Suppl 1, SI1–4

Tan, P.H., Yang, L.C., Shih, H.C., Lan, K.C. and Cheng, J.T. (2005) Gene knockdown with intrathecal siRNA of NMDA receptor NR2B subunit reduces formalin-induced nociception in the rat. *Gene Ther* 12, 59–66

Tsai, S.Y., Schillinger, K. and Ye, X. (2000) Adenovirus-mediated transfer of regulable gene expression. *Curr Opin Mol Ther* 2, 515–523

Touitou, I., Notarnicola, C., and Grandemange, S. (2004) Identifying mutations in autoin-flammatory diseases: towards novel genetic tests and therapies? *Am J Pharmacogenomics* 4, 109–118

Weichselbaum, R.R. and Kufe, D. (1997) Gene therapy of cancer. *Lancet* 349 Suppl 2, SII10–12

Wilson, S.P. and Yeomans, D.C. (2002) Virally mediated delivery of enkephalin and other neuropeptide transgenes in experimental pain models. *Ann NY Acad Sci* 971, 515–521

Wilson, S.P., Yeomans, D.C., Bender, M.A., Lu, Y., Goins, W.F. and Glorioso, J.C. (1999) Antihyperalgesic effects of infection with a preproenkephalin-encoding herpes virus. *Proc Natl Acad Sci USA* 96, 3211–3216

Wirtz, S. and Neurath, M.F. (2003) Inflammatory bowel disorders: gene therapy solutions. *Curr Opin Mol Ther* 5, 495–502

Woolf, C.J. and Salter, M.W. (2000) Neuronal plasticity: increasing the gain in pain. *Science* 288, 1765–1769.

Yanez-Munoz, R.J., Balaggan, K.S., Macneil, A., Howe, S.J., Schmidt, M., Smith, A.J., Buch, P., Maclaren, R.E., Anderson, P.N., Barker, S.E., Duran, Y., Bartholomae, C., von Kalle, C., Heckenlively, J.R., Kinnon, C., Ali, R.R. and Thrasher, A.J. (2006) Effective gene therapy with nonintegrating lentiviral vectors. *Nat Med* 12, 348–353

Yao, M.Z., Gu, J.F., Wang, J.H., Sun, L.Y., Lang, M.F., Liu, J., Zhao, Z.Q. and Liu, X.Y. (2002b) Interleukin-2 gene therapy of chronic neuropathic pain. *Neuroscience* 112, 409–416

Yao, M.Z., Gu, J.F., Wang, J.H., Sun, L.Y., Liu, H. and Liu, X.Y. (2003) Adenovirus-mediated interleukin-2 gene therapy of nociception. *Gene Ther* 10, 1392–1399

Yao, M.Z., Wang, J.H., Gu, J.F., Sun, L.Y., Liu, H., Zhao, Z.Q. and Liu, X.Y. (2002b) Interleukin-2 gene has superior antinociceptive effects when delivered intrathecally. *Neuroreport* 13, 791–794

Yeomans, D.C., Jones, T., Laurito, C.E., Lu, Y. and Wilson, S.P. (2004) Reversal of ongoing thermal hyperalgesia in mice by a recombinant herpesvirus that encodes human preproenkephalin. *Mol Ther* 9, 24–29

Palliative Care and Pain Management in the United States

James Hallenbeck and Shana McDaniel

Introduction

In approaching the topic of pain and palliative care, we will first discuss the cultural evolution of the modern palliative care movement. This should help establish a foundation for a more detailed discussion of the relationship between palliative care and pain management in the United States and in the United Kingdom. We believe some understanding of this history is important in fleshing out this relationship. Then, we will contrast the clinical worlds of "palliative care" and "pain management" as specifically practiced in the United States. We will then review and discuss the impact the palliative care field has had on evidence based practice. Finally, we discuss future directions for this field.

The Cultural Evolution of the Modern Palliative Care Movement: A Brief History

Palliative care is a relatively modern term for a most ancient practice – the relief of suffering associated with illness. The root word, *palliare*, in Latin means to cloak or to shield. The term, palliative care, was first coined by Dr. Balfour Mount in 1974. Mount first studied with the founder of the modern hospice movement, Dr. Cicely Saunders, in England in 1973 and went on to establish the Royal Victoria Palliative Care Service in Montreal, Canada in 1975 [1, 2]. From medieval times "hospice" had referred to shelters or sanctuaries often run by religious orders for the needy, the poor, and for travelers [3]. In English the word, hospice, had largely fallen out of use [4]. In French speaking Quebec, however, the older meaning was better retained. Thus, as the story goes, Mount believed it was necessary to find an alternate term for hospice care [5]. From early on, Mount also envisioned the application of skills associated with hospice

J. Hallenbeck (✉)
Stanford University School of Medicine, VA Palo Alto Health Care System, Stanford, CA, USA
e-mail: james.hallenbeck@va.gov

R.J. Moore (ed.), *Biobehavioral Approaches to Pain*,
DOI 10.1007/978-0-387-78323-9_20, © Springer Science+Business Media, LLC 2009

in venues such as acute care hospitals beyond hospice communities. He borrowed "palliative" from the related terms, palliative chemotherapy and radiation therapy, and added "care."

Since that point in time, the meaning of palliative care has continued to diverge from that of hospice. Hospice care in the United States has come to be understood as care for overtly terminal and dying patients, delivered primarily in patients' homes, which is directed toward enhancing quality of life and relief of suffering. Palliative care, as currently conceived, similarly has as a goal the improvement in quality of life, but now differs from hospice in that the provision of care is not exclusively for the dying. As the recently published American Clinical Practice Guidelines for Quality Palliative Care state, "The goal of palliative care is to prevent and relieve suffering and to support the best quality of life for patients and their families, *regardless of the stage of the disease* [italics ours] or the need for other therapies."[6]. Such care is not restricted to any particular care venue. Indeed, while the majority of formal palliative care services are still provided for patients with advanced chronic, life-limiting, or frankly terminal illnesses, this distinction is important. It is not just the imminently dying who wish not to suffer in their illness. While such a definition of palliative care is important conceptually, it risks being so broad as to lose all sense of meaning; by this definition, every time people use over-the-counter pain relievers they are practicing "palliative care." Palliative care is also a social movement, advancing the position that attention to quality of life and relief of suffering are fundamental to the practice of medicine. Access to palliative care can be considered a basic human right and as such should be available in all venues at all stages of illness [7]. This movement is becoming incorporated into discrete social and organizational structures [8]. Many hospitals now have palliative care consultation teams and palliative care clinics are beginning to appear [9, 10]. In 2006 the Accreditation Council on Graduate Medical Education (ACGME) and the American Board of Medical Specialties (ABMS), the oversight bodies governing physician accreditation and credentialing respectively, deemed Hospice and Palliative Medicine a new subspecialty of medicine [11]. This subspecialty now enjoys the same status as specialties, such as Cardiology or Oncology.

We offer the above discussion because misunderstandings regarding palliative care abound. While modern palliative care is historically the child of the hospice movement, it is not synonymous with hospice. Still, if we are to better grasp what palliative care has to offer to the consideration of pain we must first reflect on the relationship between pain management and hospice in a historical context.

The Clinical Worlds of "Palliative Care" and "Pain Management"

Pain Management and Hospice

A primary motivation for Saunders in establishing the first modern hospice in 1967 was to develop and disseminate better methods of pain control for patients with advanced and terminal illness. As a nurse in the 1940's Dr. Saunders experienced first hand how many patients suffered terrible pain toward the end of their lives. Chronic back pain brought an end to her nursing career and she became an almoner (similar to a modern social worker) in the mid-1940s [12]. In 1948 she sought a position at St. Luke's, a "home for the dying and the poor." It was there that she first observed the regular giving of morphine around the clock – a local practice that by report dated back to at least to 1935 [12]. This approach stood in sharp contrast to the (still) far too common practice whereby patients were (and are) required to "earn" their medication, as Saunders often put it, by crying out and displaying other pain behaviors. Saunders noted not only better patient pain relief but also greater lucidity and general sense of well-being with this approach. Encouraged by this, but still frustrated by how little was understood about pain management and other aspects of care for patients with advanced illness, she became determined to do something about it. She was urged to become a physician. She was told, "[S]he would only get frustrated as a nurse, because people wouldn't listen to her; in any case there was so much to be learnt about pain control and she really ought to do it properly. 'Go and read Medicine …It's the doctors who desert the dying.'" [12].

Following medical training Saunders began her career as a pain research fellow. At the time she was one of 20 research fellows working in pain at her institution, but the first one to specialize in care of patients with advanced illness. In this capacity she began working at St. Joseph's Hospice in Hackney in 1958 [12]. There, she introduced the regular administration of opioids, which was soon adopted as a standard of care in hospice for patients with chronic pain. Building on this experience she began planning a new venture, which was to become St. Christopher's, the first modern hospice.

In keeping with the older notion of hospice, well known to Saunders, St Christopher's was envisioned as sanctuary or community for patients suffering from advanced, chronic, and terminal illness. While hospice care in the United States has become exclusively associated with care of the terminally ill, Saunders emphatically rejected this tight association. She argued that:

> "St Christopher's is unique in that it offers care, research and teaching into the problems of patients with *chronic* [italics ours] and terminal pain, and the needs of their families both at home and in the Hospice." [1]. "It will concentrate upon the understanding and management of chronic and terminal pain both in the 54 beds of the first stage of building and in an out-patient pain clinic." ([13], copied in Saunders, Selected Writings 1958–2004, Clark (ed) 2006, Oxford U. Press).

In the quoted sentences, we see the great importance attached to pain management in hospice care. St Christopher's was (and is) an academic center, stressing research and education in addition to clinical care.

Total Pain

Arguably, Saunders' greatest contribution to the larger world of pain management was her elucidation of the concept of "total pain": pain with physical, emotional (psychological), social, and spiritual dimensions [14, 15]. She often cited a conversation with a patient (1963) in making the point that pain must be approached comprehensively.

> I asked her to describe her pain. She said, without further prompting, 'Well, doctor, it began in my back but now it seems that all of me is wrong.' She spoke of several other symptoms and went on- "I could have cried for the pills and the injections but I knew that I mustn't. Nobody seemed to understand how I felt and it was as if the world was against me. My husband and son were marvelous, but they were having to stay off work and lose their money. But it's wonderful to begin to feel safe again.' Physical, emotional and social pain and the spiritual need for security, meaning and self-worth, all in one answer. [16]

While certainly not unique in drawing attention to the multi-faceted nature of the pain experience, Saunders incorporated this concept into the very fabric of hospice care. Appropriate staffing, including mental health workers and spiritual care providers, was not optional on the care team; it was an expectation. Such an interdisciplinary emphasis has been maintained in palliative care programs, evolving years later. As the recent National Consensus Project for Quality Palliative Care stated: "Palliative care services must organize and maintain an interdisciplinary team that can provide sufficient services including support for the family, continuity of care, optimal use of institutional and community resources, and close collaboration with other professionals involved with the care of the patient." [6].

In the same article referenced above [16] Saunders begins a section on total pain with a discussion of the confrontation of two "myths" – that use of "narcotics" replaced the misery of pain with the misery of addiction and that their use quickly resulted in tolerance, thereby making them ineffectual (See also Heit/ Lipman, Chapter 15, This Volume). The inclusion of this discussion in this section is curious as the issues of addiction and tolerance do not appear to be directly related to the far broader concept of total pain. We suspect she did so to highlight the very practical problem patients in pain, particularly those with cancer, often face – grossly inadequate analgesia, in part because of serious misunderstandings about the principle class of medications used to treat pain, the opioids [17].

Attention to such nitty-gritty details of pain management in a discussion of total pain seem an appropriate counter-balance to her broader philosophical discussion of suffering. This indicates that for Saunders, effective pain management must attend as much to the therapeutic details as to broader issues of experience, context, and meaning. The inclusion also suggests that while attention to the individual's "total pain" is important, research, education, and advocacy are also obligations for the field. Saunders' writing and the writing of later champions in the field repeatedly stress that the proper response to total pain requires both a multi-dimensional approach to the individual and a systematic approach to the underlying conditions that give rise to so many people suffering so unnecessarily.

Saunders' Total Pain, Engels' Biopsychosocial Model, and Bonica's Multidisciplinary Pain Centers

While Saunders' model of total pain had a major impact on pain management in palliative care, available evidence suggests that Saunders' conceptualization of total pain had minimal direct influence on the evolution of the modern pain management movement. To the extent there is recognition of the importance of non-medical aspects of pain in traditional pain management, this appears to represent a relatively independent, parallel evolution. Records from the first international symposium on pain, organized by Dr. John Bonica in 1973 make no reference to Saunders or total pain, although presentations were made on psychological and psychiatric aspects of pain. Later textbooks and articles in this lineage commonly discuss *biopsychosocial* aspects of pain management, referencing the work of George Engel and his followers, but generally do not reference Saunders, or the total pain concept [18, 19].

As implied in the term, the biopsychosocial model stresses that illness is more than physical disease. Psychological and social aspects of the experience of illness must also be considered by the clinician in tailoring an appropriate therapeutic response. Engel first put forth this model in 1977, well after Saunders elucidation of the concept of "total pain" in the early 1960's. Of note, he makes no reference Saunders or her work [20, 21]. Similar to Saunders, Engel, a physician, also developed his model in response to what was perceived to be an reductionist conceptualization of illness that overly stressed biology and neglected more human aspects of the experience of illness. Their models differed, however, in ways that may have influenced the divergent evolution of palliative care and pain management. Moreover, we note the inclusion of the spiritual domain in the total pain model. While Engel recognized the importance of *meaning* in his model, the issue of spirituality as Saunders understood it, his and subsequent work along his line tended not to invoke spirituality directly. Saunders originally used the term, *emotional*, to describe psychological aspects of pain, thereby stressing affective aspects of the experience, although later writers in the total pain tradition seemed to have interpreted this more broadly as the psychological aspects of pain [22, 68, 67, 69]. In contrast, the biopsychosocial line tends to be more "clinical" in its analysis, seeing affect as but one psychological dimension among many others, including cognitive and behavioral aspects. From early on Saunders' model seemed to demand an interdisciplinary approach to understand the problem of suffering. Interestingly, in Engel's original *Science* article, the initial discussion was also more narrowly focused on the role of psychiatry as a physician specialty. The emphasis was on the multidimensional aspects of illness in the *patient* and how *physicians* should approach patients using the biopsychosocial model, with less of an emphasis on an interdisciplinary professional response.

Of note, Saunders' model was developed explicitly in response to *pain* (and was later more broadly applied to other aspects of suffering). As Arber put it,

"It is significant that the concept of total pain emerged from the patient experience that Saunders captured by listening to patients talking about their experience of pain." [23] In contrast Engel's original paper does not discuss pain directly. His more general model of illness was later adapted by pain management specialists and expanded to fit Bonica's multidisciplinary approach to pain management [26].

Well prior to Engel's 1977 *Science* article, Bonica, the founder of modern pain management, had stressed the importance of interdisciplinary care, in his advocacy for multi-disciplinary pain centers [24]. Bonica and Saunders were well aware of each others work, having corresponded as early as 1966 [1]. Saunders was clearly influenced by Bonica's work. Indeed, the first reference in her first publication in 1958 is to Bonica's 1953 classic text, *The Management of Pain* [25]. It seems probable that Bonica was similarly influenced by Saunders, as the following quote suggests:

> "Cancer pain is of particular importance because of its special attributes and significance to the patient and his family. Usually the physiologic and psychologic impact of cancer pain on the patient is greater than that of nonmalignant chronic pain. The physical deterioration is much more severe because the patients have greater problems through lack of sleep, lack of appetite, nausea and vomiting. Equally important is the mental depression caused not only by the persistent pain but its prognostic significance. In the usual setting, the physical appearance and suffering stresses the family emotionally, and this in turn enhances the patients pain and suffering." [26].

In 1977 Bonica invited Saunders to lecture at the first International Congress on Cancer Pain, again suggesting his awareness of and respect for her work [1]. Thus, Saunders may have had some indirect influence on Bonica and the field of pain management, although direct references to her work are strikingly absent in the pain literature reviewed.

Hospice Care Comes to the United States

The first three hospice/palliative care programs in North America (in New Haven Connecticut, New York, and Montreal) were started from 1974–1975. In 1982 Medicare established the Medicare Hospice Benefit, the first public reimbursement system to provide dedicated funding for hospice care in the United States [2, 3]. While the establishment of this benefit was a great boon for many, associated eligibility criteria and reimbursement policies significantly shaped the way hospice and palliative care evolved in the United States for better and for worse.

Under the Benefit eligibility for hospice is limited to Medicare recipients with prognoses of six months or less "if the illness runs its normal course." [27]. In restricting eligibility based on estimated life-expectancy, hospice care became exclusively associated with care for the terminally ill – in contrast to Saunders' original vision. The Hospice Benefit also requires that patients and/or proxies accept a "palliative approach to care." While not unreasonable on the face of it, in practice this policy is often interpreted as to mean that patients and families must make a difficult choice; either they could pursue aggressive care oriented to prolongation of life, but too often with inadequate attention to comfort, or they could choose a comfort-oriented approach, which made little if any effort to prolong life. Such a stark and dichotomous choice was and is resisted by many patients, families, and clinicians, who rightly consider efforts at life-prolongation to exist along a continuum with efforts directed toward comfort. The benefit also strongly biased hospice care toward care in the home. While funding mechanisms exist under the benefit for hospice care in acute care or nursing homes, by policy most care must be delivered in the home. No independent option existed under the benefit for outpatient care [27].[1]

Reimbursement under the Medicare Hospice Benefit is on a per-diem basis. That is, virtually all services delivered, including medications, are "packaged" within this daily rate. While such bundling enabled a more comprehensive approach to care, it also discouraged the use of more expensive therapies (such as certain medications and therapies for pain) even where they might be most appropriate [28, 29].

The Medicare Hospice Benefit stressed the provision of care by an inter-disciplinary team, lead most commonly by nurses and social workers. While such an interdisciplinary approach was quite consistent with original hospice values the same cannot be said for the role of the physician in hospice, whose contribution to the provision of care was systematically devalued under the Benefit [2].[2] While all Medicare-certified hospices require a physician hospice medical director, no requirements yet exist for physician training or competency [31].[3] The medical director is to provide oversight of medical care, but in most cases does not serve as attending of record. The attending role is most commonly filled by physicians not affiliated with the hospice, many of whom lack basic palliative care competencies, including pain management skills. Many patients admitted to hospice under Medicare will never see a physician prior to death, as home visits are rare (and poorly reimbursed). Finally, the Medicare

---

[1] Bonica had stressed the importance of multidisciplinary outpatient clinics in pain management. This emphasis stands in sharp contrast with the neglect of outpatient care under the Medicare Hospice Benefit. This difference in emphasis may have contributed to the divergent evolution of pain management from that of hospice and palliative care.

[2] Saunders was concerned about these developments in the United States. In a letter to the editors of the Journal of Chronic Diseases in 1984, just after the institution of the Medicare benefit she commented, "Experience of work in two older and one modern (1967) Hospice has convinced me that this work should not be seen as encouraging doctors to leave care for the end of life to other professionals, still less the inadequately informed or supported family. The careful analysis and control of physical symptoms and the answering of the patient's and the family's questions concerning the progress of the disease and the nature of its likely end may be shared with other staff but still remain the prime responsibility of the clinician." [30].

[3] The Joint Commission, which accredits American healthcare organizations, has general standards for all clinicians regarding assessment of competency, but no specific requirements regarding competency standards for medical directors.

Hospice Benefit is exclusively a clinical program. There are no provisions supporting education or research. In contrast, significant monies are provided for physician training in acute care hospitals associated with Medicare reimbursement [32].

As originally implemented in England at St. Christopher's, hospice care was actively involved in efforts to improve pain management through both research and education. The same, unfortunately, cannot be said for hospice as it evolved under the Medicare Hospice Benefit. America's hospices certainly value relief of suffering from pain and other debilitating symptoms. However, the sharp delineation of terminal from non-terminal patients, the general restriction to home care, the fiscal bias toward inexpensive therapies under a per-diem system, the relative neglect of the role of the physician and the lack of any emphasis on research and education all create serious barriers to the use of certain pain management approaches. While the Medicare Hospice Benefit did much to legitimize hospice care and provided a funding stream for care, an unintended consequence of the benefit was to put hospice in the United States on a very different evolutionary path from that of more traditional pain management.

The Growth of Palliative Care Services in the United States

Following early euphoria associated with the establishment of a funding mechanism for hospice through the Medicare Hospice Benefit, certain problems became apparent. Growth in the number of patients receiving hospice care was relatively stagnant in the late 1980's and early 1990's.[4] Contrary to hopes, most Americans continued to die in institutional settings, primarily acute care hospitals [34]. Hospice providers often pleaded with physicians and hospitals to 'hand-over' their dying patients to their care and then became frustrated when there was some reluctance to do so. Physicians not affiliated with hospices tended to resent the implication that they were providing "bad" care for dying patients and that hospice could do better. Patients, families, and clinicians commonly balked at being forced to make stark choices between hospice and traditional medical care. Studies demonstrated that hospice care tended to be used primarily by well educated, well-to-do Americans of

---

[4] In 1985 158,000 Americans received hospice care. By 1992 this number had grown only to 246,000. The rate of growth in hospice utilization did pick up substantially from 1992 onward. By 2005 1.2 million Americans had received some hospice care. Even today, the majority of Americans die in institutional settings without the benefit of hospice care. It is interesting to note that the rapid growth in hospice enrollment is temporally correlated with emergence of palliative care in the United States. While some in the American hospice movement expressed concern that palliative care might threaten hospice by re-medicalizing dying and caring for dying patients in hospitals, this correlation suggests that palliative care has had a beneficial effect in terms of hospice utilization [33]. This represents approximately one third of the deaths in America.

European descent [35, 36]. Hospice care, while institutionalized under the Medicare Hospice Benefit, remained in many ways an alternative form of care for the privileged, outside the mainstream of Medicine.

On a positive note, and informed by a growing literature largely from outside the United States, clinicians started to gain a better understanding of the scope of what was possible in the provision of symptom management and related care. The Oxford Textbook of Palliative Medicine (out of England), the first major palliative care textbook, was first published in 1993 [37]. This was a revelation for many hospice physicians in the United States. Practitioners began to understand that pain management and other skills being learned in the care of the dying could often be extrapolated to patient populations not so imminently dying. By the early 1990's it also became clear that the majority of Americans would continue to die in institutional settings, either acute care or nursing homes, and equally clear that most of these patients were not benefiting from the advances reflected in this textbook and in the emerging hospice and palliative care literature.

But why was this the case? From the 1960's within mainstream Medicine in the United States the dominant approach to problems arising at the end-of-life was ethical. 'If only the clinician knew what the patient had wanted when lucid (presumably most would not want to die in an intensive care unit for example), then everything would be alright'. The focus was on getting patients to complete advance directives and for healthcare systems to recognize these advance directives. Medical education to the extent it addressed end-of-life issues, similarly focused on matters of ethics [38]. These efforts culminated in the Patient Self-Determination Act of 1991, wherein healthcare organizations are mandated to inquire about patient's advance directives on admission to a healthcare facility [39].

In 1995 a major study was published, the SUPPORT study, which was a watershed in the evolution of palliative care in the United States [40]. Growing out of the continuing belief that the key to good end-of-life care was "knowing what the patient wanted," this was a large interventional study in which half the population was supported by a nurse, whose job it was to elicit patient preferences. The other half of the population was a control group. The premise was that if a nurse took the time to ask patients about their preferences (regarding their resuscitation status, for example) and their condition (how much pain they were in, most notably) and communicated this information to the physician, there would be improvement in care delivery – except it did not work. There was no difference between the two groups on a host of measures, including their reports of pain. In this study 50% of dying hospitalized patients were reported as being in moderate to severe pain at least 50 percent of the time in the last 3 days of life by their relatives. This study was a major wake-up call. The study painted a bleak picture of end-of-life care in the dominant venue where Americans die: the acute care hospital. It suggested (as supported by later studies) that whatever the problem was, it was not as simple as just finding out what patients wanted [41–43]. A different approach was clearly needed.

Palliative Care Post – SUPPORT

Leaders in the hospice and emerging palliative care movement regrouped in light of the SUPPORT study and related literature, which demonstrated that most Americans continued to die outside of hospice and that physicians and other clinicians were poorly taught even the basics of pain and other symptom management. Supported largely by two philanthropic organizations, the Robert Wood Johnson Foundation and the SOROS Foundation, clinical and political efforts shifted toward a more systems-based approach. The goal was to improve care for patients with advanced and terminal illness. Major initiatives were launched to improve clinician education, to explore new models of palliative care delivery outside of hospice, and in support of research. Physician subspecialty status for hospice and palliative medicine was sought and gained in 2006 [44]. As a result of these efforts new requirements for education and accreditation in symptom assessment and management have been promulgated [45]. Palliative care has thus evolved into a formal system of care, now within the world of traditional medicine, with all the rights, honors, privileges, and bureaucratic headaches that come with such status.

Palliative Care and Pain Management

We are now, finally, able to address the key question for this chapter: What contribution has palliative care made to the management of pain in the United States? As the previously described history reflects, palliative care has evolved beyond its early American roots of a home-based hospice program for dying patients. Yet, philosophically, much has been retained.[5] Perhaps most importantly, palliative care highlights the fact that patients with advanced and terminal illnesses have special needs and that therapeutic approaches must be adjusted accordingly. While Bonica, like Saunders had made very strong statements as early as 1955 regarding the importance of pain management for patients with terminal illness, especially cancer, historically this population has largely been neglected by most clinicians and researchers, including many pain specialists [46]. Pain management as a field tended to focus more on isolated, difficult pain syndromes in patients with far greater life-expectancies.

For the majority of patients seen in the practice of palliative care, little doubt exists as to whether they are in pain, or why. No one (patient or clinician) would question, for example, why a patient with diffuse bony metastases might hurt. In contrast, the cause (and "veracity") of pain in many overtly "healthy" patients seen by pain specialists is often less clear. These differences in patient populations

---

[5] The Clinical Practice Guidelines for Quality Palliative Care, the major consensus document on standards for palliative care in the United States, were developed by hospice and palliative care leaders and modeled to a large degree on older hospice guidelines. The importance of an interdisciplinary approach, addressing physical, psychological, social, and spiritual aspects of care is stressed, consistent with Saunder's total pain philosophy [6].

have given rise, in our opinion, to very different philosophies of care and significant differences in practice. In palliative care there is a strong bias towards giving patients the benefit of the doubt, for example, if opioids are being considered, as to whether there is a physical cause for the pain. A phrase often heard in hospice and palliative care is, "Pain is what the patient says hurts." [22, 23]. This bias is often quite reasonable in the presence of physical disease which is overwhelmingly likely to cause pain. A limited life-expectancy, almost by definition, removes the potential for long-term "abuse" of opioids and tolerance. Malingering and secondary gain are also rarely major issues. Complications of long-term opioid use and other medications such as steroids are also reduced by limited life-expectancies. By contrast the pain management literature more often addresses questions of addiction, malingering, and secondary gain, and raises questions of the veracity of pain complaints. Such suspicion makes some sense in light of etiologic uncertainty and often very different motivations for seeking care in more overtly healthy populations (see also Heit and Lipman, This Volume).

Palliative care also continues to emphasize the importance of a broad, "total pain" approach to pain management and to emphasize an interdisciplinary approach to care. This is both a philosophical and a most practical bias. While most patients with advanced and terminal illness have an easily understood cause for their physical pain, the complexity of their illness requires a comprehensive approach. Well-trained pain specialists certainly recognize the interplay between physical and psychosocial/spiritual dimensions of pain and suffering in patients. However, advanced illness presents special challenges. Even if restricting the discussion to physical symptomatology, most patients with advanced illness and pain also suffer from a number of other common symptoms and ailments – most commonly dyspnea, constipation, nausea, cachexia, and asthenia. The interplay among these symptoms physiologically and experientially is complex. Pain medications are often adjusted both to avoid certain side-effects common in advanced illness (such as choosing certain opioids over others in patients with renal or hepatic insufficiency) and in hopes of improving more than one symptom at a time. By way of example, opioids are commonly used for both pain and dyspnea management. Steroids are often useful both for compression neuropathies and for anorexia. Expert palliative care pain management requires an intimate understanding of these related physiologies and options for treatment. Further, while most pain specialists have valuable added knowledge and expertise in specific pain procedures, such as the use of nerve blocks, it is also safe to say that palliative care experts usually have greater understanding and expertise in managing complex and overlapping symptoms [47, 48].

Evidence Based Pain Management and Palliative Care

The most important contribution to evidence based pain management by palliative care has been to broaden the scope of questions where evidence is thought to be important. Some of the larger questions include:

- How does pain fit into the larger constellation of symptoms and suffering as experienced by patients?
- How do social and cultural forces influence the experience of pain and clinicians' responses to pain?
- What system barriers exist to effective pain management?
- In assessing efforts to improve the quality of pain management, what outcomes are most important to measure?

At a more basic level, palliative care research has significantly influenced pain management by calling into question certain common practices with poor evidence bases. Perhaps the best historical example was Twycross' early work, validated by others, demonstrating that morphine was equally efficacious in the provision of pain relief as Brompton's cocktail, a popular mixture of ingredients, which contained opioids and cocaine and which caused greater side-effects [49, 50, 51]. Some other evidence-based practices in which palliative care played a major role are listed in Table 1 [52, 53, 54, 55, 56].

Beyond any specific contributions to evidence-based pain management, palliative care has contributed to a much broader discussion of the role of evidence-based medicine in medical practice and research. While recognizing the importance and value of evidence in guiding practice, significant criticism has arisen within the palliative care movement regarding what is perceived to be at times a narrow and rigidly constructed conceptualization of what constitutes "good evidence." [57].

Three concerns tend to dominate such criticism. First, is a recognition that for certain types of research questions, especially those germane to palliative care (and by extension pain management), randomized-controlled trials, generally considered the highest-level of evidence, are not feasible or frankly are not

Table 1 Contributions of palliative care to evidence-based pain management

Issue	Evidence Based Practice
Chronic pain is best treated with regular, not as-needed, medication "by the clock"	• Use of long-acting oral opioids are generally favored over short-acting parenteral doses for chronic pain [52]
Management of opioid-related side-effects	• Use of antiemetics with dopamine-blocking activity are favored agents for centrally mediated opioid-related nausea [53] • Use of prokinetics for opioid-related dysmotility and constipation [54]
Pain Assessment	• Use of alternative methods of pain assessment are needed in special populations, such as non verbal patients and patients with dementia [55]
Opioids and hastening of death	• Use of opioids in dying patients: Evidence suggests that the use of opioids within standard practice guidelines at the end-of-life does not significantly increase the chance of a hastened death [56]

the best available research methodology [58, 59 60]. Greater consideration and respect should be given to alternate approaches such as systematic reviews, qualitative, and narrative analysis [61]. Second, biases, both fiscal and cultural, tend to encourage greater attention to certain types of research and evidence at the expense of others. In pain management a great deal of money has been spent exploring expensive procedural and pharmacologic approaches to pain management. Yet, to date there is not one good randomized controlled trial comparing prochlorperazine and promethazine in the treatment of opioid-related nausea. Finally, a more general worry has been expressed by researchers in this field, regarding inherent dangers in the objectification of suffering [57]. If only objective evidence is considered legitimate, more subjective aspects of human experience, particularly pain and suffering proportionately are de-legitimized. Indeed, the most popular "evidence-based medicine" texts tend to discuss pain and other major symptoms, such as nausea and dyspnea rather superficially in the context of specific disorders, if at all [62, 63]. Pain, and related suffering also often fail to appear in and of themselves to be considered legitimate topics for inquiry. We suspect this is not intentional, but rather reflects difficulties arising from the objectification of what is inherently a subjective phenomenon.

System Change and Advocacy

While palliative care experts possess rather different but quite complementary skills to those of pain specialists, we would argue that the greatest contribution palliative care has made to the broader field of pain management is in terms of advocacy and system change. Following the SUPPORT study, research conducted in nursing homes and pediatric populations by palliative care researchers similarly demonstrated grossly inadequate pain management [64, 65]. No one would or could defend such practices. As a society it would seem we could at least keep dying elders and children comfortable. Despite major advances in the understanding and treatment of pain the palliative care literature revealed that the vast majority of patients suffering from pain were not benefiting from these clinical advances.[6] No simple solution exists to this problem. However, palliative care has worked systematically to improve access to appropriate pain management. Here, we will highlight some major achievements.

(Note: these achievements were not uniquely dependent on palliative care leadership. Varying degrees of collaboration with pain management leaders

---

[6] Bonica is his preface to the report on the first international symposium on pain makes just this point. "It is a distressing fact that in this age of marvelous scientific and technologic advances which permit us to send people to the moon, there are still hundreds of thousands, and indeed millions, of suffering patients who are not getting the relief they deserve." However, system aspects of pain management are otherwise largely ignored in this historically important symposium and much subsequent literature of the mainstream pain management movement [66].

existed. However, palliative care leadership was critical to the success of these ventures):

- **Education:** Formal requirements regarding palliative care education (including pain management) have been promulgated for major clinical disciplines at both undergraduate and graduate levels for physicians. To date the greatest impact appears to have been on the disciplines of Internal Medicine, Geriatrics, and Neurology [67]. Faculty Development and continuing education courses on palliative and pain management have been created [68 69 70]. In some states continuing education credits in pain management and end-of-life care are required. Fellowships in palliative medicine have been developed and hospice & palliative medicine was acknowledged as a medical subspecialty by the American Board of Medical Specialties in 2006 [71]. [7]
- **Regulatory Bodies:** The Joint Commission, the major accrediting body for healthcare in the United States, has incorporated formal standards for pain assessment and expectations regarding pain management into their accreditation process in part in response to advocacy from palliative care leaders [45]. Regulatory bodies at all levels (national, state, county, healthcare facility) have been encouraged to liberalize policies that restrict access to the appropriate use of controlled substances and to issue statements supporting proper use of these medications.
- **System factors contributing to inadequate pain management:** While education can help address misguided attitudes regarding pain management and improve skills, research in palliative care has demonstrated that these are not enough. Systems of care can either promote or hinder patients' access to proper pain management. A superb example of such can be found in Morrison's study, which demonstrated that opioids simply were not available in many pharmacies in inner-city New York. People living in those areas could not get their prescriptions filled [75]. Various projects have demonstrated much improved pain scores and patient satisfaction followed the implementation of quality improvement projects addressing such system problems [76, 77].
- **A re-examination of the use of opioids in relation to the risk of addiction and tolerance:** Pain management as a field in its early years was and is much concerned with the use of opioids in terms of their potential for abuse and the risk of tolerance [78, 79]. It is our impression that work in hospice and palliative care has had some influence on softening what was a relatively

---

[7] Palliative medicine became a medical specialty in 1987 in the UK, almost 20 years earlier than in the United States. American standards require one year of clinical training for board eligible status. A second year is sometimes included in fellowship programs for those interested in academic careers. In the UK four years of specialty training are required for recognition as a sub-specialist in palliative medicine. While differences exist in specialty training requirements for physicians and other clinicians working in palliative care between the US and the UK, both countries appear to face a similar educational challenge: balancing specialty training in palliative care with the need to incorporate palliative care content into curricula for non-specialists [72, 73, 74].

hard-line stance on these issues in the traditional world of pain management in the United States and abroad. Historically both hospice and pain management camps were overtly characterized by what now appear to be rather extreme positions. Pain management tended to view the risk of addiction and tolerance in the use of opioids as a very serious problem, especially when used for "non-malignant" pain [80]. In a paper entitled, "The use and misuse of narcotics in the treatment of chronic pain," presented at the first International Symposium on Pain (one of only 2 papers on the use of opioids in the symposium), Houde, arguably the preeminent leader representing the dominant pain management perspective on this topic at the time stated, "...

[T]he narcotics are felt to excel in their capabilities of producing psychological dependence or craving and it is this property that sets the narcotics apart from the other classes of drugs" and "...tolerance and physical dependence will undoubtedly develop on the repeated administration of even moderate doses of potent narcotics within a period as short as 2 to 3 weeks..." [81]

At the other extreme Twycross, who was based at St. Christophers' Hospice, represented the hospice point of view, championing the position that addiction and tolerance were not major issues. "Tolerance to morphine is not a practical problem. Psychological dependence (addiction) does not occur if morphine is used correctly."[22]. In truth, as Meldrum observed in her excellent article detailing the history of the development of the WHO pain ladder, these two towering figures were not as far apart as these statements might imply. "Houde and Twycross could not agree on the inevitability of tolerance, but they concurred that it was manageable."[79]. Meldrum goes on to suggest that neuro-oncologist Kathleen Foley, who had trained with Houde at Memorial Sloan-Kettering, was pivotal in negotiating an agreement that enabled the codification of the WHO pain ladder in Milan, Italy in 1982. Fishbain and colleagues in their 1992 systematic review of drug abuse, dependence, and addiction in chronic pain identify Drs. Foley and Portenoy, a neurologist, as two investigators whose work challenged commonly held assumptions about the risk of these problems [82, 83 84]. This review found, "There is little evidence in these studies that addictive behaviors are common within the chronic pain population." Foley and Portenoy emerged as interesting and important figures in this regard. Both rose to prominence in the culture of traditional pain management. Yet, they are also recognized as pioneers in American palliative care and thus have served as a bridge between the worlds of pain management and palliative care. Today, a more centrist view, recognizing that tolerance and addiction can be significant problems (but often are not) seems to dominate both the pain and palliative care literature.

Palliative Care and Pain Management – Still Worlds Apart

In the above section, we contrasted palliative care with traditional pain management. Palliative care has clearly benefited from research done by pain specialists. We would like to think that in turn pain management has been aided by the palliative care movement, which has strongly advocated that pain can only be understood within in a broader context of suffering. Increasingly, pain management texts explicitly reference palliative care. For example, a core curriculum for pain management fellows begins its section on cancer pain with the following:

1. "Recognize that pain management is part of a broader therapeutic endeavor known as palliative care.
2. Know that palliative care is defined as the active, total care of the patient with active, progressive, life threatening disease.
3. Recognize that palliative care involves a variety of health care professionals.
4. Know that palliative care provides a model for continuing management including control of pain and symptoms, maintenance of function, psychosocial and spiritual support for the patient and family, and comprehensive care at the end of life." [85].

Unquestionably, leaders such as Portenoy, Foley, and Twycross have reached across their special fields to find commonalities of interest and purpose, which have benefited both pain and palliative care specialists. However we are left with an uncomfortable truth : in practice palliative care and pain management specialists more often than not work in separate clinical worlds. Given the primacy of pain to both fields, how could this be? As discussed above, differences in populations served are responsible to some extent. We have also suggested that the structure of hospice as it evolved under the Medicare Hospice Benefit was not conducive to collaborative efforts between the two fields. On the pain management side we also note a greater and growing emphasis on interventional pain management. In part this has resulted from major improvements in technique and associated efficacy in pain relief [86].

In addition, we must also note that fee-for-service reimbursement systems, including Medicare, are strongly biased toward technologic interventions and against time and knowledge-based practice. To put it bluntly, under the dominant reimbursement schemes in the United States, high tech procedures, such as nerve blocks and pump insertions, are considerably more profitable than relatively low-tech, interdisciplinary care. Thus, almost overwhelming fiscal incentives encourage pain management specialists to treat principally through procedures. This strong fiscal bias sadly tends to segregate pain and palliative care specialists into high and low-tech medical worlds of "haves" and "have-nots." Interventional pain specialists are among the most highly reimbursed physicians in America. In contrast many palliative medicine physicians and palliative care programs are still struggling for fiscal viability.

An Eye to the Future

Summarizing the above :historically, there was a close connection and mutual respect between leaders in pain management and hospice/palliative care in the early 1960's. However, a variety of factors resulted in a divergent evolution.

Must this divergence continue or could a new synergy come into being? Here, we are somewhat optimistic. Palliative care has benefited immensely from advances in understanding and techniques developed in traditional pain management. However, we believe that even in very good hospice and palliative care programs too many patients do not have access to procedures such as nerve blocks, epidural, and intrathecal infusions, which might be of benefit. In part this is because of reimbursement system barriers and practical limitations regarding what can be done in certain venues, such as the home. We must also admit that at times access to such procedures appears to be limited by ignorance of their potential benefits on the part of palliative care clinicians and lack of collaboration with pain specialists.

As palliative medicine clinicians do become more sophisticated in their understanding of pain and the use of pain management techniques, we are beginning to see a confluence of interest with pain specialists. A better understanding of psychosocial as well as physiologic mechanisms for pain relief and mechanisms of complications of pain management, such as opioid tolerance and hyperalgesia, is moving the field to consider the therapeutic implications of such discoveries. We hope that pain specialists will similarly come to better appreciate the contributions palliative care can make to pain management. Palliative care specialists can help pain specialists better understand and treat pain patients with complex medical comorbidities. Beyond this, we believe pain specialists could learn much from palliative care experts about effective education strategies and methods for creating systematic change.

Acknowledgments We would like to acknowledge David Clark and Russell Portenoy for kindly reviewing the manuscript for this chapter and for their contributions to the field, without which this work would not have been possible.

References

1. Clark D. *Cicely Saunders – founder of the hospice movement selected letters 1959–1999*. Oxford: Oxford University Press; 2005.
2. Lewis M. *Medicine and the Care of the Dying*. Oxford: Oxford University Press; 2007.
3. Stoddard S. *The Hospice Movement*. NY: Vintage; 1992.
4. Saunders C. The modern hospice. In: Wald F, ed. *Quest of the Spiritual Component of Care for the Terminally Ill: Proceedings of a Colloquium*. New Haven: Yale Unveristy School of Nursing; 1986:41–48.
5. Mount B. The Royal Victoria Hospital Palliative Care Service: a Canadian experience. In: Saunders C, Kastenbaum R, eds. *Hospice Care on the International Scene*. New York: Saunders; 1997:73–85.
6. Clinical Practice Guidelines for Quality Palliative Care. *National Concensus Project for Quality Palliative Care*. 2003;http://www.nationalconsensusproject.org/, last accessed 4/23/07.
7. Brennan F. Palliative care as an international human right. *J Pain Symptom Manage*. 2007;33(5):494–499.
8. Clark D, Seymour J. *Reflections on Palliative Care*. Philadelphia: Open University Press; 1999.

9. Morrison RS, Maroney-Galin C, Kralovec PD, Meier DE. The growth of palliative care programs in United States hospitals. *J Palliat Med.* Dec 2005;8(6):1127–1134.
10. von Gunten CF. Secondary and tertiary palliative care in US hospitals. *JAMA.* Feb 20 2002;287(7):875–881.
11. American Academy of Hospice and Palliative Medicine Website.http://www.aahpm.org/about/recognition(Last accessed 4/23/07).
12. Du Boulay S. *Ciceley Saunders.* 2 ed. London: Hodder & Stoughton; 1994.
13. Saunders C. St. Christopher's Hospice. *Br Hosp J Soc Serv Rev.* 1967;77(10):2127–2130.
14. Clark D. 'Total pain', disciplinary power and the body in the work of Cicely Saunders, 1958–1967. *Soc Sci Med.* 1999;49(6):727–736.
15. Saunders C, Baines M. *Living with Dying – The management of terminal disease.* Oxford: Oxford University Press; 1983.
16. Saunders C. The evolution of palliative care. *Patient Education and Counseling.* 2000;41:7–13, cited in Saunders, C. Selected Writings 1958–2004.
17. Cleeland CS, Gonin R, Hatfield AK, et al. Pain and its treatment in outpatients with metastatic cancer. *N Engl J Med.* 1994;330(9):592–596.
18. Gallagher R. Treatment planning in pain management – integrating medical, phyhsical, and behavioral therapies. *Med Clin North America.* 1999;83(3):823–847.
19. Warfield C, Bajwa Z, eds. *Principles and Practice of Pain Medicine.* 2nd ed. NY: Mcgraw-Hill; 2004.
20. Engel g. The need for a new medical model: a challenge for biomedicine. *Science.* 1977;196:129–136.
21. Borrell-Carrio F, Suchman AL, Epstein RM. The biopsychosocial model 25 years later: principles, practice, and scientific inquiry. *Ann Fam Med.* 2004;2(6):576–582.
22. Twycross R. *Introducing Palliative Care.* NY: Radcliffe Medical Press; 1995.
23. Arber A. Is pain what the patient says it is? Interpreting an account of pain. *Int J Palliat Nurs.* 2004;10(10):491–496.
24. Bonica JJ. Evolution and current status of pain programs. *J Pain Symptom Manage.* 1990;5(6):368–374.
25. Saunders C. Dying of Cancer. *St. Thomas's Hospital Gazette.* 1958;56(2):37–47, cited in Clark 2006, Cicely Saunders -selected writings 1958–2004,pp2001–2011.
26. Bonica JJ. Cancer pain: a major national health problem. *Cancer Nurs.* 1978;1(4):313–316.
27. Medicare Benefit Policy Manual. www.cms.hhs.gov/manuals/Downloads/bp102c09.pdf. Last accessed 4/17/07.
28. Joranson DE. Are health-care reimbursement policies a barrier to acute and cancer pain management? *J Pain Symptom Manage.* 1994;9(4):244–253.
29. Ferrell BR, Griffith H. Cost issues related to pain management: report from the Cancer Pain Panel of the Agency for Health Care Policy and Research. *J Pain Symptom Manage.* 1994;9(4):221–234.
30. Saunders C. Evaluation of hospice activities. *J. Chronic Disease.* 1984;37(11):871, cited by Clark, 2006.
31. *Standards for Hospice 2004–5:* Joint Commission; 2005.
32. Billings JA. A primer on training slots for graduate medical education. *J Palliat Med.* 2007;10(1):12–16.
33. *National Hospice and Palliative Care Organization.*Available at: www.nhpco.org/files/public/Patients_served_1985–2005.pdf (Last accessed 6/27/07).
34. Field MJ, Cassel CK, Institute of Medicine (U.S.). Committee on Care at the End of Life. *Approaching death: improving care at the end of life.* Washington, D.C.: National Academy Press; 1997.
35. Greiner KA, Perera S, Ahluwalia JS. Hospice usage by minorities in the last year of life: results from the National Mortality Followback Survey. *J Am Geriatr Soc.* 2003;51(7):970–978.

36. Kapo J, MacMoran H, Casarett D. "Lost to follow-up": ethnic disparities in continuity of hospice care at the end of life. *J Palliat Med.* 2005;8(3):603–608.
37. Doyle D, Hanks GWC, MacDonald N. *Oxford Textbook of Palliative Medicine.* Oxford; New York: Oxford University Press; 1993.
38. Billings JA, Block S. Palliative care in undergraduate medical education. Status report and future directions. *JAMA.* 1997;278(9):733–738.
39. Greco PJ, Schulman KA, Lavizzo-Mourey R, Hansen-Flaschen J. The Patient Self-Determination Act and the future of advance directives. *Ann Intern Med.* Oct 15 1991;115(8):639–643.
40. SUPPORT. A controlled trial to improve care for seriously ill hospitalized patients. The study to understand prognoses and preferences for outcomes and risks of treatments (SUPPORT). *JAMA.* 1995;274(20):1591–1598.
41. Lynn J, Arkes HR, Stevens M, et al. Rethinking fundamental assumptions: SUPPORT's implications for future reform. Study to Understand Prognoses and Preferences and Risks of Treatment. *J Am Geriatr Soc.* 2000;48(5 Suppl):S214–221.
42. Teno J, Lynn J, Wenger N, et al. Advance directives for seriously ill hospitalized patients: effectiveness with the patient self-determination act and the SUPPORT intervention. SUPPORT Investigators. Study to Understand Prognoses and Preferences for Outcomes and Risks of Treatment. *J Am Geriatr Soc.* Apr 1997;45(4):500–507.
43. Pritchard RS, Fisher ES, Teno JM, et al. Influence of patient preferences and local health system characteristics on the place of death. SUPPORT Investigators. Study to Understand Prognoses and Preferences for Risks and Outcomes of Treatment. *J Am Geriatr Soc.* 1998;46(10):1242–1250.
44. Portenoy RK, Lupu DE, Arnold RM, Cordes A, Storey P. Formal ABMS and ACGME recognition of hospice and palliative medicine expected in 2006. *J Palliat Med.* Feb 2006;9(1):21–23.
45. JCAHO. Pain Standards. *at* www.jcaho.org/standard/stds2001_mpfrm.html. 2001.
46. Bonica JJ, Backup PH. Control of cancer pain. *Northwest Med.* 1955;54(1):22–28.
47. Berger A, Shuster J, von Roenn J, eds. *Principles and Practice of Palliative Care and Supportive Oncology.* 3rd ed. Philidelphia: Lippincott Williams & Wilkins; 2007.
48. Doyle D, Hanks GW, Cherny N, Calman K, eds. *Oxford Textbook of Palliative Medicine.* 3rd ed. Oxford: Oxford University Press; 2005.
49. Cark D. The rise and demise of the Brompton Cocktail. In: Meldrum M, ed. *Opioids and Pain Relief: A Historical Perspective. Progress in Pain Research and Management.* Vol 25. Seattle: IASP press; 2003:85–98.
50. Twycross RG, Gilhooley RA. Letter: Euphoriant elixirs. *Br Med J.* 1973;4(5891):552.
51. Kaiko RF, Kanner R, Foley KM, et al. Cocaine and morphine interaction in acute and chronic cancer pain. *Pain.* 1987;31(1):35–45.
52. Twycross RG. *Introducing palliative care.* 2nd ed. Oxford; New York: Radcliffe Medical Press; 1997
53. Dalal S, Palat G, Bruera E. Chronic nausea and vomiting. In: Berger A, Shuster J, von Roenn J, eds. *Principles and Practice of Palliative Care and Supportive Oncology.* 3rd ed. Philadelphia: Lippincott Williams &Wilkins; 2007:151–162.
54. Herndon CM, Jackson KC, 2nd, Hallin PA. Management of opioid-induced gastrointestinal effects in patients receiving palliative care. *Pharmacotherapy.* 2002;22(2):240–250.
55. Zwakhalen SM, Hamers JP, Abu-Saad HH, Berger MP. Pain in elderly people with severe dementia: a systematic review of behavioural pain assessment tools. *BMC Geriatr.* 2006;6:3.
56. Portenoy RK, Sibirceva U, Smout R, et al. Opioid use and survival at the end of life: a survey of a hospice population. *J Pain Symptom Manage.* 2006;32(6):532–540.
57. Hallenbeck J. Evidence-based medicine and palliative care. *J Palliat Med.* 2008;11(1):2–4.
58. Higginson IJ. Evidence based palliative care. There is some evidence-and there needs to be more. *Bmj.* 1999;319(7208):462–463.

59. Aoun SM, Kristjanson LJ. Evidence in palliative care research: How should it be gathered? *Med J Aust*. 2005;183(5):264–266.
60. Aoun SM, Kristjanson LJ. Challenging the framework for evidence in palliative care research. *Palliat Med*. 2005;19(6):461–465.
61. Devery K. The framework for evidence in palliative care: narrative-based evidence. *Palliat Med*. 2006;20(1):51.
62. Sackett DL, Strause S, Richardson WS, Rosenberg WM, Haynes RB. *Evidence-based medicine*. 2nd ed. Edinburgh: Chruchill Livingstone; 2000.
63. *Clinical Evidence Handbook*. London: BMJ Publishing Group; 2007.
64. Bernabei R, Gambassi G, Lapane K, et al. Management of pain in elderly patients with cancer. SAGE Study Group. Systematic Assessment of Geriatric Drug Use via Epidemiology. *Jama*. 1998;279(23):1877–1882.
65. Wolfe J, Grier HE, Klar N, et al. Symptoms and suffering at the end of life in children with cancer. *N Engl J Med*. 2000;342(5):326–333.
66. Bonica J, ed. *International Symposium on Pain*. NY: Raven Press; 1974. Advances in Neurology; No. 4.
67. Weissman DE, Block SD. ACGME requirements for end-of-life training in selected residency and fellowship programs: a status report. *Acad Med*. 2002;77(4):299–304.
68. VanGeest JB. Process evaluation of an educational intervention to improve end-of-life care: the Education for Physicians on End-of-Life Care (EPEC) program. *Am J Hosp Palliat Care*. Jul-Aug 2001;18(4):233–238.
69. Stratos GA, Katz S, Bergen MR, Hallenbeck J. Faculty development in end-of-life care: evaluation of a national train-the-trainer program. *Acad Med*. Nov 2006;81(11):1000–1007.
70. Sullivan AM, Lakoma MD, Billings JA, Peters AS, Block SD. Creating enduring change: demonstrating the long-term impact of a faculty development program in palliative care. *J Gen Intern Med*. Sep 2006;21(9):907–914.
71. von Gunten CF. Fellowship training in palliative medicine. *J Palliat Med*. Apr 2006;9(2):234–235.
72. Miller M, Wee B. Medical Education. In: Wee B, Hughes N, eds. *Education in Palliative Care*. Oxford: Oxford University Press; 2006:14–22.
73. Wee B, Hughes N. *Education in Palliative Care – Building a culture of learning*. Oxford: Oxford University Press; 2007.
74. Hallenbeck J. Palliative care training for the generalist a luxury or a necessity? *J Gen Intern Med*. 2006;21(9):1005–1006.
75. Morrison RS, Wallenstein S, Natale DK, Senzel RS, Huang LL. "We don't carry that" – failure of pharmacies in predominantly nonwhite neighborhoods to stock opioid analgesics. *N Engl J Med*. 2000;342(14):1023–1026.
76. Byock I, Twohig JS, Merriman M, Collins K. Promoting excellence in end-of-life care: a report on innovative models of palliative care. *J Palliat Med*. Feb 2006;9(1):137–151.
77. Lynn J, Chaudry E, Noyes Simon L, Wilkinson A. *The Common Sense Guide to Improving Palliative Care*. NY: Oxford University Press; 2007.
78. Seymour J, Clark D, Winslow M. Pain and palliative care: the emergence of new specialties. *J Pain Symptom Manage*. Jan 2005;29(1):2–13.
79. Meldrum M. The ladder and the clock: cancer pain and public policy at the end of the twentieth century. *J Pain Symptom Manage*. 2005;29(1):41–54.
80. Schofferman J. Long-term use of opioid analgesics for the treatment of chronic pain of nonmalignant origin. *J Pain Symptom Manage*. 1993;8(5):279–288.
81. Houde R. The use and misuse or narcotics in the treatment of chronic pain. In: Bonica J, ed. *International Symposium on Pain*. New York: Raven Press; 1974:527–536.
82. Fishbain DA, Rosomoff HL, Rosomoff RS. Drug abuse, dependence, and addiction in chronic pain patients. *Clin J Pain*. 1992;8(2):77–85.
83. Portenoy RK. Chronic opioid therapy in nonmalignant pain. *J Pain Symptom Manage*. 1990;5(1 Suppl):S46–62.

84. Portenoy RK, Foley KM. Chronic use of opioid analgesics in non-malignant pain: report of 38 cases. *Pain*. 1986;25(2):171–186.

85. Charlton J, ed. *Core curriculum for professional education in pain*. Seattle: IASP Press; 2005.

86. Manchikanti L, Boswell MV, Raj PP, Racz GB. Evolution of interventional pain management. *Pain Physician*. 2003;6(4):485–494.

Pain in Society: Ethical Issues and Public Policy Concerns

Ben A. Rich

Introduction

This volume appears in the second half of the congressionally declared "Decade of Pain Control and Research" (H.R. 3244, 2000). Such a declaration by the Congress of the United States generates a perception that we are in the midst of a major national public policy initiative promoting the importance of pain relief to the health and well-being of all citizens who are currently or at some time in the future may become the victims of pain. Such a perception would not, however, necessarily comport with reality. Indeed, the very context in which H.R. 3244 arose was the persistent efforts of the opponents of physician-assisted suicide in general, and the Oregon Death With Dignity Act in parti-cular, to enact federal legislation (under the guise of promoting pain relief) that would make it a federal offence for a physician to provide a competent, terminally ill patient who requested it with a lethal prescription, even if state law and public policy supported it. Such a tension is emblematic of tensions and conflicts inherent in how western culture thinks about and responds to the phenomenon of pain.

Until recently (the last fifteen years), there was virtually no discussion, even in the literature of the health professions, of the role of ethics, law, or public policy on the subject of pain and its relief. The objective of this chapter is to provide an overview of the ambivalence that western society has demonstrated toward those who suffer pain and how those who are in a position to provide relief should respond to it. Despite an incredible amount and diversity of activity in recent years, particularly in the United States, the ambivalence persists and manifests itself in law and public policy that prompts many health care professionals to decry that they are truly between the proverbial "rock and hard place" when it comes to caring for patients who report and seek prompt and effective relief from pain.

B.A. Rich (✉)
University of California, Davis School of Medicine, Sacramento, CA, USA
e-mail: barich@ucdavis.edu

R.J. Moore (ed.), *Biobehavioral Approaches to Pain*,
DOI 10.1007/978-0-387-78323-9_21, © Springer Science+Business Media, LLC 2009

Ethical Dimensions of Pain and Its Relief

As the physician Eric Cassell observed 25 years ago, acknowledgement of the physician's duty to relieve human suffering stretches back into antiquity. Nevertheless, he continues, little attention is given to it in medical education, research, or practice (Cassell, 1982). We should note at the outset that pain and suffering are not synonymous, inasmuch as pain can exist without suffering (a paradigm case is childbirth) and suffering can exist without pain (there are many examples of "existential suffering" completely unassociated with physical pain). Nevertheless, our focus in this chapter will be the experience of pain which, when it persists without adequate treatment, can be a significant source of human suffering.

In ancient, and even early modern medicine, the relief of pain held a prominent position in the priorities of patient care. To some extent this may have been because there was so little else that physicians could do for their patients. Even when the state of their art (and rudimentary medical science) enabled them to diagnose a patient's disease, more often then not cure, or even significant remediation, eluded them. But particularly with the discovery of the analgesic properties of opium, and its derivative morphine, the relief of pain was within their power. Great figures in the history of medicine proclaimed the marvelous powers of these substances, from Thomas Sydenham's paen declaring that "among the remedies which it has pleased Almighty God to give to man to relieve his sufferings, none is so universal and so efficacious as opium" to Sir William Osler's reference to opium as "God's own medicine."

During the Twentieth Century, two phenomena converged to produce the crisis that we currently face – an epidemic of undertreated pain (Rich, 2000). The first was the remarkable advance in medical science and technology, particularly in the last half of the century. A longstanding balance between curative and palliative medicine, based in significant part on medicine's earlier limitations, gave way to the reign of the curative (disease-directed) model of patient care in which the primary focus was on making the diagnosis and designing and implementing therapeutic measures (Fox, 1997). The second was the imposition of a rigid and often punitive regime of federal control over opioid analgesics, in which the DEA and federal prosecutors argued that physicians whose prescribing of controlled substances fell outside certain parameters were guilty of drug diversion (Musto, 1999). Mounting evidence, particularly in the later decades of the Century, suggested that all types of pain, acute, chronic nonmalignant, and even cancer pain, were routinely undertreated (Cleeland, et al., 1994). In extreme cases, health care professionals appeared to be in the grip of a phenomenon that came to be characterized as "opiophobia," believing that the risks and side-effects of opioid analgesia almost always outweighed the benefits of pain relief (Morgan, 1985). Patients with pain began with increasing frequency to manifest a newly diagnosed condition, pseudo-addiction, which consisted of behaviors consistent with addiction but which were in fact the product of severe, chronic undertreated pain. Pseudo-addiction is an iatrogenic condition (Weissman and Haddox, 1989).

The next section of this chapter will identify and briefly analyze the most commonly identified barriers to effective pain management, link them to the phenomena noted in the previous paragraph, and offer an ethical analysis of their consequences. Section 3 will provide a concise review of the regulatory environment for opioid analgesics. Section 4 will consider a few legal cases that have driven home the point, seemingly lost heretofore, that the failure to provide necessary and appropriate pain relief constitutes both unethical and substandard medical practice (Pellegrino, 1998). Section 5 will review some of the most important public policy responses to the growing recognition that undertreated pain was pervasive, pernicious in that it constituted a major public health problem, and constituted a significant and unacceptable departure from a traditional core value of the health professions – the relief of pain and suffering.

Barriers to Effective Pain Relief

There has been remarkable consistency in discussions of the barriers to good pain management, at least with regard to what arguably constitute "the usual suspects." The first, and perhaps most surprising and disconcerting to lay persons, is ignorance. The clinical literature readily acknowledges that health care professionals, physicians and nurses, quite simply, are not trained adequately in the assessment and management of pain (Von Roenn, et al., 1993). The training that clinicians generally do receive, often serendipitous and anecdotal, serves only to perpetuate myths and misinformation about the risks of opioids and the penchant for patients who complain of pain to be routinely characterized as "drug seeking" rather than genuine victims of a condition that warrants palliation (Hill, 1995).

The failure of health professional schools, particularly medical and nursing, to bring their curricula in line with current national standards for the assessment and management of pain, and to consistently impart the requisite knowledge, skills, and attitudes in their graduates, in and of itself constitutes a major pedagogical deficiency. But while these curricular deficits do constitute one of the reasons why health care professionals undertreat pain, it does not constitute an excuse upon which those professionals can escape responsibility for causing or allowing their patients to suffer unnecessarily. The reason is that medicine and nursing are true professions, an essential aspect of which is a moral obligation to engage in lifelong learning so as to possess and consistently provide competent care and treatment to patients. The fact that an important aspect of patient care was not included in a professional's primary training in no way absolves them from a responsibility for acquiring the requisite knowledge and skills subsequently.

The most obvious way for health professionals to remediate such deficits is through continuing professional education. A few states have actually mandated, and some others have recommended, that physicians obtain continuing medical education in pain management and the treatment of terminally ill patients (Pain & Policy Studies Group, 2005). In a subsequent section of this chapter, we will consider legal cases in which health care professionals were held liable in civil actions for failure to provide appropriate pain relief to their patients.

It is not only health care professionals, but patients and, indeed, many lay persons who have major knowledge deficits concerning the proper role of pain relief in patient care, and more particularly, the relative risks and benefits of opioid analgesia for the relief of moderate to severe pain. One of the pervasive myths is that anyone who receives opioids for more than a few days is at a high risk of becoming addicted. The primary basis for this myth is a failure to distinguish between the development of physical dependence and true addiction. While all patients who receive opioids for an extended period of time will become physically dependent, this simply means that such patients must be gradually tapered off such medications rather than having them precipitously discontinued. By contrast, addiction is a craving for (compulsive use of) a drug, and the continued use of it despite obvious harmful consequences (See Chapter 15 of this volume). The primary responsibility for educating patients and their families about the importance of pain relief in patient care and the actual risks and benefits of opioids must lie with the health care professional. For that reason, ignorance and misinformation on the part of the lay public is not really a separate barrier, but directly related to ignorance and misinformation in the health professions.

A second barrier to effective pain relief is the failure of health care institutions to make pain relief a priority in patient care. Given that the relief of suffering was historically a core value of medicine, the identification, and to a remarkable degree, acceptance of this barrier boggles the mind. How, one might reasonably ask, could modern medicine have strayed so far from one of its core values that the relief of pain could cease to be a priority in patient care? There may be no definitive answer to this question, but here is one theoretical possibility. As modern medicine demonstrated the capacity to cure or significantly address many heretofore life-threatening conditions, the focus of the medical gaze shifted from caring for the patients who could not be cured to making an accurate diagnosis and formulating and implementing appropriate (and often effective) therapeutic measures for the increasing percentage of patients who could be. This was the hallmark of the curative model of medicine, which has reigned supreme since at least the last half of the Twentieth Century.

The major problem with the curative model of medicine is its failure to accommodate the unique personal identity of the patient. It is in this regard that the curative model appears to be the diametric opposite of the palliative model, as astutely noted by one commentator (Fox, 1997). While the curative model is essentially objective, scientific, rational, impersonal, and reductionistic, the palliative model is subjective, humanistic, empathetic, personal, and holistic. This is why Eric Cassell charges that if "the test of a system of medicine is its adequacy in the face of suffering," then "modern medicine fails that test." Indeed, Cassell contends that "the central assumptions on which twentieth-century medicine is founded provide no basis for an understanding of suffering" (Cassell, 1991). Given the essential features of the reigning curative model, we can readily discern why this is so. Bodies do not suffer, as Cassell so pithily puts it, persons suffer. If the clinician cannot engage the patient as person, the clinician will never be able to acknowledge and effectively address pain and suffering, for pain and suffering are inherently subjective and personal, and a humane response to them must be holistic and empathic.

Finally, and perhaps most importantly when it comes to pain associated with grave or terminal illness, in the curative model death equals failure, whereas in the palliative model it is not death, but unnecessary pain and suffering that constitutes medical failure. Yet herein lies another conundrum about how the practitioners of modern medicine think about palliation, when they think about it at all. Palliative care is commonly conceived of as the appropriate therapeutic response when "medicine has nothing more to offer," meaning that curative (disease-directed) therapies have demonstrably failed and the patient's prognosis has been acknowledged as grim. But the advocates for comprehensive pain care dispute this narrow and rigid scope for the application of the palliative model. They assert that the proper definition of palliative care is the relief of pain and suffering, whenever and wherever it occurs in the experience of illness or, stated in curative model terminology, at anywhere along the trajectory of the disease. One of the reasons for the monumental failure of the health professions to provide good care of the dying patient is that significant palliative measures are rarely initiated so long as disease-directed therapies are still under way. This failure of the curative model to acknowledge the important role of pain and symptom management in good patient care also goes a long way toward explaining why patients are referred to hospice, if at all, so very late (Taylor, 2004).

The third and final barrier that is most frequently identified is fear of regulatory scrutiny or legal liability. The sources of that scrutiny – real or imagined – that has come to be so profoundly feared is that of state medical licensing boards and/or the federal Drug Enforcement Administration. The focus of that scrutiny is the physician's prescribing of controlled substances, particularly the heavy-duty Schedule II drugs such as oxycodone, fentanyl, and hydromorphone. One might naturally think that the genesis of such fear would be that patently inappropriate prescribing would raise red flags and place professionals at risk. But instead, the exquisite irony of the situation is that many professionals believe that they are likely to be investigated and sanctioned for the appropriate provision of controlled substances to relieve pain. The reason such fears cannot be dismissed as groundless is that studies of the knowledge, skills, and attitudes of state medical board members revealed that many of them believed that opioid analgesia was so fraught with risks and side-effects that physicians who provided such medications to any patients who were not actively dying must be violating professional standards, and probably the law (Gilson and Joranson, 2001). In section 4 we will consider a policy initiative designed to move state medical boards away from being part of the problem of undertreated pain and toward being part of the solution to it.

These concerns were exacerbated by the existence in a number of states of triplicate form requirements for Schedule II drugs. The very purpose of the triplicate form, at least in theory, was to provide a paper trail for regulators to monitor a professional's prescribing practices. The root of the problem, however, was not so much the fact that such monitoring took place, but the standards or criteria that were applied by those doing the monitoring. For far too long these were woefully outdated or based upon myths and misinformation about the risks and side-effects of opioid analgesia that went on for more than a few days (Fohr,1998). More recently, there has been a trend away from triplicate forms toward prescription monitoring programs designed and intended to balance the sometimes competing goals of insuring appropriate pain management and prevention of drug abuse and diversion (Joranson, et al., 2002).

Regulation of Opioid Analgesics

Opioids have been regulated in the United States for purposes of prevention or punishment of diversion and misuse since the passage of the Harrison Act in 1914, prior to which, as surprising as it now may seem, there was essentially no regulation. In 1970, the current regime of the federal Controlled Substances Act (CSA) began. Despite the more than half century that separated the two enactments, they both emphasize some of the same key terms and phrases. The primary thrust of both was to make it a federal offence to prescribe certain types of drugs except "in the course of professional practice" and "for legitimate medical purposes." The CSA divided federally controlled substances into 5 schedules based upon abuse potential and whether or not it was deemed to have any recognized medical use. Schedule I drugs have high abuse potential and no currently accepted medical use. Schedule II drugs are also considered to have a high abuse potential, but are also deemed to have a currently accepted medical use. Schedule III-V drugs have a progressively diminishing abuse potential and recognized medical uses. The Schedule II drugs, such as morphine, have tended to receive the most attention, since they are viewed by pain management specialists as often essential to provide effective relief of moderate to severe pain. Prosecutions of prescribers under the CSA raised significant concerns as to whether the federal Drug Enforcement Administration and law enforcement agencies were purporting to set the criteria for what constituted a legitimate medical purpose and when a particular physician had stepped outside the bounds of acceptable medical practice, matters which were not considered within the purview of nonphysicians. Two recent federal court cases highlight the tensions in this area.

In 2005, a federal jury in Virginia convicted William Hurwitz, M.D., of 58 counts of drug trafficking, and the trial judge subsequently sentenced him to 25 years in prison. Hurwitz conducted a pain management practice that drew patients complaining of chronic nonmalignant pain whom other physicians had refused to treat. He was, by any measure, out of the mainstream of pain practitioners with regard to his liberal philosophy of prescribing opioids and giving his patients the benefit of the doubt about their stories and their prior experience with controlled substances. In the period between 1998 and 2002, Hurwitz acknowledged that the median daily dosage for his patients was roughly 2000 miligrams (2 grams) of morphine or its equivalent. The federal government took the position that Hurwitz was little more than a drug dealer who operated out of a medical office, an argument which the conviction suggests the jury accepted.

There are several significant aspects of the trial and the subsequent reversal of the conviction on appeal. First, the testimony of the prosecution's chief medical expert, Dr. Michael Ashburn, was so controversial that it prompted six past presidents of the American Pain Society to write a letter expressing their profound concerns about his contentions that:

- "high dose" opioid therapy is an indication of drug abuse in chronic non-malignant pain patients
- a dosage of 195 mg/day of morphine is high
- opioid therapy for a patient with a known addiction disorder is wrong
- high dose opioids produce hyperanalgesia
- high dose opioids may compromise the immune system

Each of the above contentions the signatories to the letter asserted to be either patently false or highly speculative and without foundation in the medical literature, at least when made as sweeping generalizations.

Second, when the defense indicated its intention to introduce into evidence a document then posted on the DEA website entitled Prescription Pain Medications: Frequently Asked Questions for Health Care Professionals and Law Enforcement Personnel (FAQ), the DEA precipitously pulled the document from the site and posted the following statement: "The document contained misstatements and has therefore been removed ... [it] was not approved as an official statement of the agency and does not have the force and effect of law." The FAQ document was, in fact, the product of an extended collaborative effort among experts in pain management, pain policy, and representatives of the DEA. The revocation by the DEA, initially without any indication of the nature of the misstatements it allegedly contained, provoked statements of frustration and concern not only by the other collaborators, but also the National Association of Attorneys General, the organization representing the chief law enforcement officers of the states.

The third, and perhaps most significant aspect of the Hurwitz case was the reversal of the conviction, and the ordering of a new trial by the Fourth Circuit Court of Appeals. The critical issue on appeal was whether or not Dr. Hurwitz was entitled to an instruction to the jury that it could take into consideration when evaluating his practice the question of whether his prescribing of controlled substances was done in a good faith effort to provide them with medical care. The government argued that the evidence presented at trial so overwhelmingly demonstrated that he was acting "beyond the bounds of accepted medical practice" that the jury could not reasonably have found that he acted in good faith even if it had been provided with such an instruction. The Court of Appeals was unwilling to accept that argument. However, neither was it willing to accept Dr. Hurwitz's contention that the relevant "good faith" criterion should be based upon a subjective, rather than an objective standard. In the language of the court: "A physician is not allowed to apply his own idiosyncratic view of what constitutes acceptable prescribing. Thus good faith in this context can only be demonstrated by evidence of [the physician's] sincerity in attempting to conduct himself in accordance with a standard of medical practice generally recognized and accepted in the country" (USA v. Hurwitz, 2006).

In the mid- Twentieth Century, a number of states sought to increase their regulatory oversight of Schedule II drugs by enacting triplicate prescription laws, which imposed, at least in theory, a heightened level of scrutiny on professionals who prescribed them (Joranson et al., 2002). While the public policy argument in support of such laws was to deter inappropriate prescribing and drug diversion, studies of the impact of these laws strongly suggested that they constituted a significant barrier to prescribing these drugs to patients who had a legitimate need for them. Some physicians simply declined to acquire and utilize the special triplicate forms, thereby relegating all of their patients to the weaker drugs in the lower schedules. Others began to significantly curtail the number of prescriptions they wrote for Schedule II drugs in states that required triplicate forms (Weintraub, et al., 1991).

More recently, states have begun to utilize electronic prescription monitoring programs (PMP), which are said to be more effective yet at the same time less overt and presumably less intimidating to prescribing professionals than triplicate forms (Fishman et al., 2004). By 2006, 26 states had implemented some form of electronic prescription monitoring system (Pain and Policy Studies Group, 2006). While all such programs have as their primary goal the reduction of prescription drug diversion and abuse, they vary in such aspects as which drugs are covered, how prescriptions for those drugs are monitored and collected, and which agency is given the responsibility for the administering the program (GAO Report, 2002). State and federal agencies that promote and administer PMPs emphasize that their concern is strictly illegitimate prescribing, drug diversion, and abuse, and disclaim any intent to curtail or otherwise restrict prescribing of these drugs for legitimate medical purposes. Nevertheless, studies in the clinical literature continue to report that such monitoring of prescribing practices has created a fear on the part of both physicians and patients (Fishman, et al., 2004).

Litigating the Right to Pain Relief

A curious situation existed as the decade of the 1990's began. The reports of widespread undertreated pain had continued to multiply, and the fledgling initiatives to change professional perceptions and practices continued to be ignored by many health care institutions and professionals outside of the small community of pain advocates. Nevertheless, no health care professional, or institution, had ever been held liable for substandard pain management that led to unnecessary pain and suffering on the part of a patient. This inattentiveness, verging on indifference, to the ethical, legal, and professional implications of the failure to treat pain prompted scholar David Morris to predict: "The ethics of pain management, unfortunately, may not receive proper attention until the first doctor is successfully sued for failing to provide adequate relief. At that point, the need for a full and reflective dialogue on ethical questions about pain will be preempted – as so often happens in American life – in favor of the slowly grinding mills of the law" (Morris, 1991).

Why, one might reasonably ask, in the midst of a medical malpractice crisis that had prompted major tort reform legislation, was undertreated pain never the basis of a claim for medical malpractice? Could it be that there is no standard of care for the management of pain? Is pain relief not a part of the physician's responsibility to the patient? One possible explanation is that lay persons simply presumed that physicians were able and willing to treat pain effectively to the fullest extent that medical science would allow. Hence the significant pain that patients nevertheless experienced must be that which is truly intractable, i.e., beyond the capacity of available therapies to relieve.

The very year that Morris wrote the passage quoted above, a completely unprecedented case was tried to a jury in rural, northeastern North Carolina. It involved an elderly patient, Henry James, with metastatic prostate cancer who was admitted to a skilled nursing facility (SNF) owned and operated by the Hillhaven Corporation (Estate of James v. Hillhaven, 1989). Just prior to his arrival, he had been placed on a pain management regimen at the local hospital that included opioid analgesics to manage the pain commonly associated with the terminal stage of that disease. Presumably there was an expectation that this regimen would be continued at the Hillhaven facility as his disease progressed, with possible increases in dosage should his pain become unmanaged. In fact, quite the opposite happened.

A nursing supervisor at the SNF decided that Mr. James was either addicted to opioids or in serious risk of becoming so, and that the pain regimen he was on was excessive. She promptly began to wean him off of the opioids. A subsequent investigation of the SNF found that on many days during his 3-week stay at the facility, Mr. James received little, if any, of the analgesics he had been prescribed prior to admission. When the Hillhaven facility was sanctioned by the State of North Carolina, the family retained legal counsel and filed a civil action seeking damages for the unnecessary pain and suffering that he had experienced prior to his death. Estate of Henry James v. Hillhaven Corporation was what is known as a "case of first impression," since previously no case had ever examined the critical issues of whether there is a standard of care for the management of pain and if so, what would be the basis for and extent of damages for the unnecessary pain and suffering that would be caused by such negligent acts or omissions. The jury decided there was such a standard that could be established by competent, credible expert medical testimony, and that the several weeks of unnecessary pain Mr. James endured justified an award of $7.5 million in compensatory damages. Furthermore, the jury was so outraged that an elderly, dying patient would be allowed to suffer that they assessed another $7.5 million in punitive damages. Despite its novelty, the defendant's liability insurance carrier chose to settle the case rather than appeal it.

Ten years following, the Morris prophecy was fully realized in the case of Bergman v. Chin, when a northern California physician was found guilty of elder abuse for failure to provide adequate pain relief for an 85-year old patient in an acute care hospital who died of advanced lung cancer within a week following discharge (Bergman v. Chin, 2001). This was a civil, not a criminal proceeding, but the claim of elder abuse required that the plaintiffs (the deceased patient's family) prove not just a departure from the standard of care but gross negligence. This case, like that of Henry James, was settled in lieu of an appeal.

A third case, this one, like *Bergman*, in northern California, involved an elderly patient with terminal cancer whose pain management at both an acute care hospital and a nursing home were alleged to be substandard (Tomlinson v. Bayberry Care Center, 2003). All defendants elected to settle with the plaintiff prior to trial. Furthermore, the defendant physician responsible for the patient's medical care at the SNF was disciplined by the Medical Board of California because of his inadequate knowledge of the analgesics he prescribed (Accusation of Whitney, 2004). This was only the second instance in which a state medical board had taken disciplinary action against a physician for conduct associated with undertreatment of pain. The first was by the Oregon Board of Medical Examiners (In re Bilder, 1999).

Public Policy Responses to the Phenomenon of Undertreated Pain

Beginning in the 1990's, a series of public policy initiatives began to address the barriers to pain relief and the epidemic of undertreated pain that their persistence had spawned. Some states adopted what have come to be called intractable pain treatment laws (Joranson, 1995). Their primary purpose was to send a legislative message to the state's medical licensing board that it was no longer deemed appropriate, as a matter of public policy, for such boards to initiate a disciplinary action against a physician solely because she prescribed opioid analgesics to patients with chronic nonmalignant pain, as some boards had been doing in the past. By 2003, twelve states had adopted such statutes (AACPI, 2003). According to this type of legislation, the board must present evidence that such prescribing constituted unprofessional or substandard practice because of circumstances pertinent to the patient for whom opioids had been prescribed. Although well-intentioned, common terms and provisions of these statutes proved to be problematic. For example, many contained language strongly suggesting that opioids could only be provided to such patients after all other treatment options had been exhausted, or unless and until it could be established that there was no disease-directed therapy available for the underlying condition with which the pain was likely to be associated (Joranson, 1995).

Also in the early 1990's, the Agency for Health Care Policy and Research (AHCPR – now the Agency for Health Care Research and Quality) brought together interdisciplinary panels of experts and issued clinical practice guidelines on acute and cancer pain (AHCPR, 1992, 1994). These guidelines were the first comprehensive national guidelines on the assessment and management of these types of pain. Subsequently, other national organizations, e.g., the American Academy of Pain Medicine and the American Pain Society, have issued similar guidelines for the management of various types of pain. In 1998, the Federation of State Medical Boards (FSMB) issued model guidelines for the use of opioids in the management of pain, and urged all state boards to adopt those or comparable policies so as to encourage physicians to make pain relief a priority in patient care (FSMB, 1998). In 2003, the FSMB expanded and reissued these as a model policy, and for the first time urged that both over and underprescribing of opioids be considered grounds for disciplinary action (FSMB 2004).

The policy initiative that appeared to offer the greatest promise for addressing the epidemic of undertreated pain was undertaken in 1999 by the Joint Commission for the Accreditation of Healthcare Organizations (JCAHO). In July of that year JCAHO adopted pain management standards that would be incorporated into the formal accreditation survey process in 2001. Developed through a collaboration with the University of Wisconsin Medical School funded by the Robert Wood Johnson Foundation, the objective was "to integrate pain assessment and management into standards to accredit the nation's healthcare organizations to make pain management a priority in the healthcare system" (Dahl and Gordon, 2002). One of the pain standards quite literally states: "patients have the right to appropriate assessment and management of pain" (JCAHO, 2007). In addition to assuring that an accredited health care institution implements policies and procedures to insure that pain is assessed and treated promptly and effectively, the standards charge institutions with the responsibility to assure the competency of its clinical staff to provide pain management.

Conclusion

For over thirty-five years the United States, largely through its law enforcement agencies, spearheaded by the federal Drug Enforcement Administration, has been waging a declared "War on Drugs," the war having been initially declared in June of 1971 by President Nixon at a press conference in which he asserted that drug abuse was "public enemy number one in the United States" (PBS, 2001). The focus of this war, of course, is ostensibly illicit drug use, the abuse and diversion of drugs regulated by the Controlled Substances Act. Nevertheless, in the absence of a commensurate "War on Pain," legitimate pain patients have become the noncombatant casualties of the War on Drugs. Health care professionals with prescribing privileges are regularly admonished that they must balance the needs of their patients for controlled substances with a commensurate societal responsibility to prevent drug abuse and diversion. Moreover, a failure on the part of any professional to act in this dual capacity, by, for example, erring on the side of pain relief in ambiguous situations, will create a real risk of legal sanctions. Because physicians are risk averse by nature, many have erred on the side of pain rather than pain relief; hence, the epidemic of undertreated pain has persisted despite the many reform measures discussed in the previous section (Hill, 1996).

Quite recently the DEA has issued policy statements on dispensing controlled substances for the treatment of pain that are intended to blunt charges that the agency targets physicians who prescribe controlled substances for pain. The DEA disclaims either the authority or the inclination to regulate the practice of medicine or to interfere with the legitimate prescribing of controlled substances for pain relief. In an effort to reassure physicians, the policy statement declares: "the overwhelming majority of physicians who prescribe controlled substances do so for legitimate medical purposes . . . in a manner that will never warrant scrutiny by Federal or State law enforcement officials" (DEA Final Policy, 2006). Such statements to the contrary notwithstanding, physician fears of legal sanctions (civil and criminal) continue to be one of the major barriers to effective pain management in patient care.

It is a perplexing and disturbing sign of our times that physicians who pursue the relief of their patients' pain by following nationally recognized clinical practice guidelines nevertheless fear that they are at risk in doing so. There is a pervasive perception among clinicians that caring for more than a few patients with major chronic pain syndromes requiring opioid analgesia demands that one regularly engage in acts of moral courage. While doing the right thing may sometimes demand personal sacrifice, an enduring state of affairs in which that is often the case should be a cause of profound concern for all of us.

References

Accusation against Eugene B. Whitney, M.D. Medical Board of California Case # 12 2002 133376, Decision December 15, 2004.
American Alliance of Cancer Pain Initiatives (2003). Statement on Intractable Pain Treatment Acts.
Agency for Healthcare Policy and Research (1992). Acute Pain Management. Rockville, MD.
Agency for Healthcare Policy and Research (1994). Management of Cancer Pain. Rockville, MD.

Bergman v. Chin., 2001 No. H205732-1 (Cal App Dept Super Ct 1999).
Cassell, E.J. (1982). The nature of suffering and the goals of medicine. *New Eng J Med,* 306: 639–645.
Cassell, E.J. (1991). *The Nature of Suffering and the Goals of Medicine.* New York: Oxford University Press.
Cleeland, C.S., Gonin, R., Hatfield. A.K., Pandya, K.J. (1994). Pain and its treatment in outpatients with metastatic cancer. *New Eng J Med,* 330: 592–596.
Dahl, J.L, Gordon, D.B. (2002). Joint commission pain standards: a progress report. *American Pain Society Bulletin,* 12: 1,11, 12.
Drug Enforcement Administration. Final Policy on Dispensing Controlled Substances for the Treatment of Pain. (2006) Vol. 71 *Fed. Reg.* available at wais.access.gps.gov (DOCID: fr06se06-137).
Estate of Henry James v. Hillhaven Corp., No. 89 CVS 64 (N.C. Super. Ct. Jan. 15, 1991).
Federation of State Medical Boards (1998). Model Guidelines for the Use of Controlled Substances for the Treatment of Pain.
Federation of State Medical Boards (2004). Model Policy for the Use of Controlled Substances for the Treatment of Pain Available at http://www.fsmb.org/pdf/2004_grpol_controlled_ substances.pdf.
Fishman, S.M., Papazian, J.S., Gonzalez, B.S., Riches, P.S., Gilson, A. (2004). Regulating opioid prescribing through prescription monitoring programs: balancing drug diversion and treatment of pain. *Pain Medicine,* 5: 309–324.
Fohr, S.A. (1998). The double effect of pain medication: separating myth from reality. *J Palliative Med,* 1: 315–328.
Fox, E. (1997). Predominance of the curative model of medical care – a residual problem. *JAMA,* 278: 761–763.
General Accounting Office. (2002). Prescription Drugs – State Monitoring Programs Provide Useful Tool to Reduce Diversion.
Gilson, A.M, Joranson, D.E. (2001). Controlled substances and pain management: changes in knowledge and attitudes of state medical regulators. *Journal Pain Symp Mgmt,* 21: 227–237.
Hill, C.S., Jr., (1995), When will adequate pain treatment be the norm? JAMA, 274: 1870–73
Hill, C.S., Jr. (1996). Government regulatory influences on opioid prescribing and their impact on the treatment of pain of nonmalignant origin. *Journal Pain Symp Mgmt,* 11: 287–298.
House Resolution 3244 (2000). Title VI, Sec. 1603. Decade of Pain Control and Research.
In re Paul Bilder, M.D. Oregon Board of Medical Examiners, 1999.
Joint Commission for the Accreditation of Health care Institutions (2007). Comprehensive Accreditation Manual for Hospitals.
Joranson, D.E. (1995). Intractable pain treatment laws and regulations. *American Pain Society Bulletin,* 5: 1–3, 15–17.
Joranson, D.E. et al. (2002). Pain management and prescription monitoring. *Journal Pain Symp Mgmt,* 23: 231–238.
Morgan, J.P. (1985). American opiophobia: customary underutilization of opioid analgesics. *Adv Alcohol Subst Abuse,* 5: 163–173.
Morris, D.B. (1991). *The Culture of Pain.* Berkeley: University of California Press.
Musto, D.F. (1999). *The American Disease: Origins of Narcotic Control.* New York: Oxford University Press.
Pain & Policy Studies Group. University of Wisconsin Comprehensive Cancer Center (2005). State Continuing Medical Education Policies for Pain and Palliative Care.
Pain & Policy Studies Group. University of Wisconsin Comprehensive Cancer Center (2006). States with Prescription Monitoring Programs.
Pellegrino, E.D. (1998). Emerging ethical issues in palliative care. *JAMA,* 279: 1521–1522.
Public Broadcasting System (2001). Thirty Years of America's Drug War – A Chronology. available at www.pbs.org/wgbh/pages/frontline/shows/drugs/cron.

Rich, B.A. (2000). A prescription for the pain: the emerging standard of care for pain management. *William Mitchell L Rev*, 26: 1–91.

Rosa Tomlinson, et al. v. Bayberry Care Center, et. al., 2003 Contra Costa County Superior Court, No. C-02-00120.

Taylor, C.L. (2004). Improving referral of patients to hospice through community physician outreach. *Journal Pain Symp Mgmt*, 28: 294–295.

United States v. Hurwitz, United States Court of Appeals for the Fourth Circuit, No. 05-4474 (2006).

Von Roenn, J.H, Cleeland, C.S., Gonin, R., Hatfield, A.K., Pandya, K.J. (1993). Physician attitudes and practice in cancer pain management: a survey from the eastern cooperative oncology group. *Ann Int Med*, 119: 121–126.

Weintraub, M., Satesh, S., Byrne, L., Maharaj, K., Guttmacher, L. (1991). Consequences of the 1989 New York state triplicate benzodiazepine prescription regulations. *JAMA*, 266: 2392–2397.

Weissman, D.E., Haddox, J.D. (1989). Opioid pseudoaddiction. *Journal Pain Symp Mgmt*, 36: 363–366.

Index